T0281054

Safe Liposuction and Fat Transfer

BASIC AND CLINICAL DERMATOLOGY

Series Editors

ALAN R. SHALITA, M.D.

Distinguished Teaching Professor and Chairman
Department of Dermatology
State University of New York
Health Science Center at Brooklyn
Brooklyn, New York

DAVID A. NORRIS, M.D.

Director of Research
Professor of Dermatology
The University of Colorado
Health Sciences Center
Denver, Colorado

1. Cutaneous Investigation in Health and Disease: Noninvasive Methods and Instrumentation, *edited by Jean-Luc Lévêque*
2. Irritant Contact Dermatitis, *edited by Edward M. Jackson and Ronald Goldner*
3. Fundamentals of Dermatology: A Study Guide, *Franklin S. Glickman and Alan R. Shalita*
4. Aging Skin: Properties and Functional Changes, *edited by Jean-Luc Lévêque and Pierre G. Agache*
5. Retinoids: Progress in Research and Clinical Applications, *edited by Maria A. Livrea and Lester Packer*
6. Clinical Photomedicine, *edited by Henry W. Lim and Nicholas A. Soter*
7. Cutaneous Antifungal Agents: Selected Compounds in Clinical Practice and Development, *edited by John W. Rippon and Robert A. Fromtling*
8. Oxidative Stress in Dermatology, *edited by Jürgen Fuchs and Lester Packer*
9. Connective Tissue Diseases of the Skin, *edited by Charles M. Lapière and Thomas Krieg*
10. Epidermal Growth Factors and Cytokines, *edited by Thomas A. Luger and Thomas Schwarz*
11. Skin Changes and Diseases in Pregnancy, *edited by Marwali Harahap and Robert C. Wallach*
12. Fungal Disease: Biology, Immunology, and Diagnosis, *edited by Paul H. Jacobs and Lexie Nall*
13. Immunomodulatory and Cytotoxic Agents in Dermatology, *edited by Charles J. McDonald*

14. Cutaneous Infection and Therapy, *edited by Raza Aly, Karl R. Beutner, and Howard I. Maibach*
15. Tissue Augmentation in Clinical Practice: Procedures and Techniques, *edited by Arnold William Klein*
16. Psoriasis: Third Edition, Revised and Expanded, *edited by Henry H. Roenigk, Jr., and Howard I. Maibach*
17. Surgical Techniques for Cutaneous Scar Revision, *edited by Marwali Harahap*
18. Drug Therapy in Dermatology, *edited by Larry E. Millikan*
19. Scarless Wound Healing, *edited by Hari G. Garg and Michael T. Longaker*
20. Cosmetic Surgery: An Interdisciplinary Approach, *edited by Rhoda S. Narins*
21. Topical Absorption of Dermatological Products, *edited by Robert L. Bronaugh and Howard I. Maibach*
22. Glycolic Acid Peels, *edited by Ronald Moy, Debra Luftman, and Lenore S. Kakita*
23. Innovative Techniques in Skin Surgery, *edited by Marwali Harahap*
24. Safe Liposuction and Fat Transfer, edited by Rhoda S. Narins

ADDITIONAL VOLUMES IN PREPARATION

Safe Liposuction and Fat Transfer

edited by

Rhoda S. Narins

Dermatology Surgery and Laser Center
New York and White Plains
and New York University Medical Center
New York, New York, U.S.A.

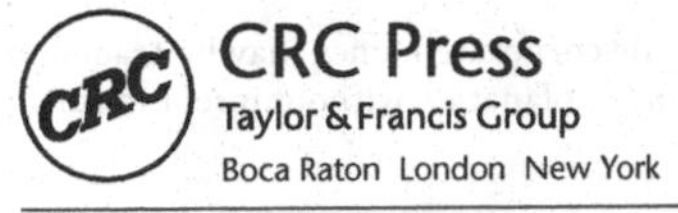

CRC Press is an imprint of the
Taylor & Francis Group, an **informa** business

CRC Press
Taylor & Francis Group
6000 Broken Sound Parkway NW, Suite 300
Boca Raton, FL 33487-2742

First issued in paperback 2019

ISBN-13: 978-0-8247-0852-8 (hbk)
ISBN-13: 978-0-367-39548-3 (pbk)

Visit the Informa Web site at
www.informa.com

and the Informa Healthcare Web site at
www.informahealthcare.com

To my husband, David, who has always supported my every endeavor

Series Introduction

Over the past decade, there has been a vast explosion in new information relating to the art and science of dermatology as well as fundamental cutaneous biology. Furthermore, this information is no longer of interest only to the small but growing specialty of dermatology. Scientists from a wide variety of disciplines have come to recognize both the importance of skin in fundamental biological processes and the broad implications of understanding the pathogenesis of skin disease. As a result, there is now a multidisciplinary and worldwide interest in the progress of dermatology.

With these factors in mind, we have undertaken to develop this series of books specifically oriented to dermatology. The scope of the series is purposely broad, with books ranging from pure basic science to practical, applied clinical dermatology. Thus, while there is something for everyone, all volumes in the series will ultimately prove to be valuable additions to the dermatologist's library.

The latest addition to the series by Rhoda S. Narins is both timely and pertinent. *Safe Liposuction and Fat Transfer* focuses on the common goal of all liposuction surgeons and I believe this book will be a valuable resource for those involved in the pursuit of that goal.

Alan R. Shalita
SUNY Health Science Center
Brooklyn, New York

Foreword

Safe liposuction and fat transfer is the focus of this book and an ardent concern of the editor, Dr. Rhoda Narins. Safety is a relative term. No surgical procedure is completely safe; one can only say that one procedure is safer than another. This book will help liposuction surgeons reduce the risks of complications and improve the safety of their liposuction procedures.

It is axiomatic that the occurrence of complications in liposuction surgery is a matter of probability. Our goal as surgeons is to prevent and reduce the probability of complications by every possible means. Only by reading the literature and attending lectures can the surgeon hope to attain the ability to effectively prevent, diagnose, and treat liposuction complications.

Prevention of complication is obviously the most important aspect of safe liposuction surgery. Safe liposuction requires that surgeons avoid unnecessary risks. The vast majority of liposuction-related deaths have been associated with either doing too much liposuction on a single day or combining liposuction with unrelated surgical procedures. For example, liposuction together with gynecological surgical procedures is particularly dangerous. Excessively obese patients are associated with significantly higher risks of liposuction-related complications and malpractice litigation.

A controversial aspect of liposuction safety is the choice of anesthesia. Liposuction is unusual in that it is commonly performed either entirely by local anesthesia or by general anesthesia. Although general anesthesia is inherently more dangerous, liposuction can be done safely under general anesthesia. The use of general anesthesia for liposuction has a permissive effect in facilitating unnecessarily large liposuction cases and encouraging patients and surgeons to include unrelated surgical procedures with liposuction. Excessive surgical trauma together with prolonged exposure to general anesthesia and subsequent excessive immobility seem to explain why pulmonary thromboembolism is a leading cause of death associated with liposuction. The permissive aspect of inhalational and intravenous (IV) anesthetics accounts for the observation that virtually all liposuction-related deaths have been associated with the use of general anesthesia or heavy IV sedation.

In contrast, surgeons who do liposuction entirely by local anesthesia must always consider the limitations imposed by not exceeding the safe dosages of lidocaine. The surgeon can treat multiple areas and remove large volumes of fat, but this can be accomplished only by splitting the case into smaller sequential procedures performed separately, preferably several weeks apart. The fact that there has never been a death associated with liposuction performed entirely by local anesthesia attests to its superior safety compared with liposuction under general anesthesia.

Lidocaine toxicity with tumescent liposuction is rare. The already low risk of lidocaine toxicity can be further reduced by limiting the dosage of tumescent lidocaine to less than 50 mg/kg and by avoiding drug interactions that interfere with lidocaine metabolism. If a patient cannot discontinue a drug that inhibits the hepatic isoenzyme cytochrome P450 3A4 responsible for lidocaine metabolism, then the total dosage of lidocaine must be reduced to 35 mg/kg or less. Another means of reducing the risk of lidocaine toxicity is facilitating the postoperative drainage of residual subcutaneous tumescent anesthetic solution, which in turn reduces the total amount of systemic lidocaine absorption. This postoperative drainage can be encouraged by allowing incision sites to remain open and not closing them with sutures.

Early diagnosis of a complication can prevent significant morbidity. For example, the surgeon should suspect necrotizing fasciitis whenever a patient complains of intense pain exceeding the patient's clinical appearance. Necrotizing fasciitis is a surgical emergency that requires immediate consultation with a general surgeon.

Admission to hospital for observation should be considered whenever there is a likelihood of a liposuction complication. If there is concern about possible lidocaine toxicity, the patient should be admitted to an intensive care unit for observation and sequential measurement of plasma lidocaine concentrations.

Safe liposuction requires the surgeon to have extensive knowledge of reported liposuction complications. If a surgeon has never read or heard about a specific complication, then the diagnosis will likely be delayed. This book will help surgeons to improve the safety of liposuction surgery.

Jeffrey A. Klein, M.D.
Associate Professor of Dermatology
University of California, Irvine
Irvine, California

Preface

This book provides the reader with information on how and when to perform safe liposuction and fat transfer. The tumescent technique of local anesthesia, introduced by Dr. Jeffrey Klein, a dermatological surgeon, is the safest way to perform liposuction.

Safe Liposuction and Fat Transfer is meant for the neophyte as well as the experienced liposuction surgeon. The book discusses study and training, design of a surgical suite, techniques of liposuction surgery and tumescent anesthesia, and safety and risk management. Complications and repair of defects are also presented, as are dietary guidelines and nonsurgical fat-removal procedures. The related topic of fat transfer is discussed in detail along with the various techniques used today worldwide.

Tumescent liposuction is the standard of care for safe liposuction and fat transfer. This technique allows liposuction to be performed in an ambulatory setting using only local anesthesia. The tumescent technique is the infiltration into the fatty tissue of a large volume of fluid with a dilute anesthetic, lidocaine. There are many reasons why tumescent liposuction is the best and safest way to perform liposuction. These include: minimal blood loss, making transfusions unnecessary; no need for general anesthesia and its accompanying risks; minimal postoperative pain, as the anesthesia is long-lasting; and a limit to the amount of liposuction and the number of ancillary procedures that can be done at one time based on the safe amount of tumescent solution (lidocaine) that can be used at one time. In addition, the ability of the awake patient to move during surgery makes it easier for the surgeon to get to the fat pockets more exactly; lessens the occurrence of thrombophlebitis, which can lead to a pulmonary embolus; and reduces the risk of perforation of the abdominal or thoracic cavities. There is decreased chance of infection because of the antibacterial nature of the tumescent solution; it is possible to use smaller cannulas with concomitant smaller incisions; and the tumescent solution provides fluid replacement. The patient recovers from surgery much more quickly and can return to work in 1–3 days and to nonjarring, noncontact activities and exercise immediately.

Safe liposuction and fat transfer is our goal as liposuction surgeons and this book discusses how to achieve that goal.

Rhoda S. Narins

Contents

Surgical Tips and Pearls

Liposuction Beyond Tumescent Technique

Postoperative Care, Complications, and Touch-Ups

Safety and Risk Management

Advanced Repair of Liposuction Defects

Fat Transfer Techniques

Nonsurgical Fat Reduction Techniques

Contributors

Michael Bermant, M.D. Bermant Plastic and Cosmetic Surgery, Richmond, Virginia, U.S.A.

Kimberly J. Butterwick, M.D. Dermatology Associates, La Jolla, California, U.S.A.

Sydney R. Coleman, M.D. Centre for Aesthetic Rejuvenation and Enhancement, New York, New York, U.S.A.

W. Patrick Coleman IV, M.D. Tulane University School of Medicine, New Orleans, Louisana, U.S.A.

William P. Coleman III, M.D. Department of Dermatology, Tulane University Health Sciences Center, New Orleans, Louisana, U.S.A.

Kim K. Cook, M.D. Coronado Skin Medical Center, Inc., Coronado, California, U.S.A.

William R. Cook, Jr., M.D. Coronado Skin Medical Center, Inc., Coronado, California, U.S.A.

Susan Ellen Cox, M.D. Cosmetic Surgery Center of North Carolina, Durham, North Carolina, U.S.A.

Lisa M. Donofrio, M.D. Department of Dermatology, Yale University School of Medicine, New Haven, Connecticut, U.S.A.

Zoe Diana Draelos, M.D. Department of Dermatology, Wake Forest University School of Medicine, Winston-Salem, North Carolina, U.S.A.

Timothy Corcoran Flynn, M.D. University of North Carolina, Chapel Hill, North Carolina, U.S.A.

Pierre F. Fournier, M.D. Private Practice, Paris, France

Paul Jarrod Frank, M.D. Department of Dermatology, New York University Medical Center, New York, New York, U.S.A.

Roy C. Grekin, M.D. University of California, San Francisco, San Francisco, California, U.S.A.

C. William Hanke, M.D. Laser and Skin Surgery Center of Indiana, Carmel, and Indiana University School of Medicine, Indianapolis, Indiana, U.S.A.

Carolyn I. Jacob, M.D. Northwestern University, Chicago, Illinois, U.S.A.

Michael S. Kaminer, M.D. Dartmouth Medical School, Chestnut Hill, Massachusetts, and Yale University School of Medicine, New Haven, Connecticut, U.S.A.

Bruce E. Katz, M.D. Department of Dermatology, College of Physicians and Surgeons, Columbia University, and Juva Skin and Laser Center, New York, New York, U.S.A.

Edward B. Lack, M.D. The Center for Liposculpture and Cosmetic Laser Surgery, Chicago, Illinois, U.S.A.

Naomi Lawrence, M.D. Department of Dermatologic Surgery, Cooper Health System, Marlton, New Jersey, U.S.A.

Min-Wei Christine Lee, M.D. University of California, San Francisco, San Francisco, and The East Bay Laser and Skin Care Center, Inc., Walnut Creek, California, U.S.A.

Patrick J. Lillis, M.D. New York University Medical Center, New York, New York, U.S.A.

Gary D. Monheit, M.D., F.A.A.D. University of Alabama at Birmingham, Birmingham, Alabama, U.S.A.

Ronald L. Moy, M.D. Division of Dermatology, David Geffen School of Medicine at UCLA, Los Angeles, and West Los Angeles Veterans Administration Hospital, Los Angeles, California, U.S.A.

David J. Narins, M.D., F.A.C.S. New York University School of Medicine, New York, New York, U.S.A.

Rhoda S. Narins, M.D. Dermatology Surgery and Laser Center, New York and White Plains, and Department of Dermatology, New York University Medical Center, New York, New York, U.S.A.

Neil S. Sadick, M.D., F.A.C.P. Department of Dermatology, Weill Medical College of Cornell University, New York, New York, U.S.A.

Ziya Saylan, M.D. Saylan Cosmetic Surgery Center, Düsseldorf, Germany

Brian Shafa, M.D. Los Angeles, California, U.S.A.

Abel Torres, M.D. Division of Dermatology, Department of Internal Medicine, Loma Linda University School of Medicine, Loma Linda, California, U.S.A.

Jean-Francois Tremblay, M.D. Department of Dermatology, University of Montreal Hospital Centre, Montreal, Quebec, Canada

David A. Wrone, M.D. Department of Dermatology, Northwestern University, Chicago, Illinois, U.S.A.

Safe Liposuction and Fat Transfer

1

History and Development of Tumescent Liposuction

Rhoda S. Narins
Dermatology Surgery and Laser Center
New York and White Plains, and
New York University Medical Center
New York, New York, U.S.A.

The history of practical modern liposuction in the United States began in 1982, when several physicians, including the author, visited Paris to take courses given by Yves Illouz and Pierre Fournier of France and Georgio Fischer of Italy. The experience of these physicians plus the innovations by Illouz made liposuction a technique destined to become the most popular cosmetic surgery within only a few years [1]. Illouz pioneered three innovative changes. These included the use of blunt cannulas to push vital tissues such as blood vessels and nerves out of the way, the injection of small amounts of a hypotonic saline solution into the tissue prior to surgery, and the popularization of the technique worldwide. The use of blunt cannulas and a wet technique markedly decreased bleeding and left vertical septae, which kept the blood and nerve supply to the overlying tissue [2]. The honeycombed tunnels produced in the fat allowed the skin to collapse rather than form large cavities in which fluid or blood could accumulate as hematomas or seromas. Illouz calls this "adipoaspiration by tunnelization." He started using these improvements in 1977 to suck out a lipoma on the back of a French movie actress who wanted only a small scar on her décolleté.

After experience with many patients he presented the findings at a meeting of the American Society for Plastic and Reconstructive Surgery in Hawaii in October 1982 [2,3]. The procedure had already been presented in France in the late 1970s and in Japan in 1980. The following year, 1983, these findings were published [2,3].

Prior to these improvements, the history of liposuction was marked by complications. In 1921, Charles Dujarrier performed the first known lipectomy on a ballerina's knees and calves using a sharp curette with resulting blood vessel injury necessitating amputation. In the 1960s Schrudde used sharp curettage to remove fat through small incisions. This technique produced bleeding, seromas, and other complications [4,5]. Other physicians also attempted sharp curettage and *en bloc* resection without success until the Fischers in the mid 1970s [4,6,7]. The Fishers invented a blunt hollow electric cannula attached to a suction machine but unfortunately had problems with bleeding and hematomas from the sharp blade within the cannula that cut off fat. The incidence of seroma reported by Fischer was 30% [5].

Many surgeons such as Pierre Fournier preferred the dry technique with no fluid injection. They felt that the fluid distorted the tissue and the results were harder for the surgeon to judge. This technique required drains and a hospital stay because of bleeding and was soon totally replaced by the wet technique [3,7]. Experienced surgeons do not find the fluid distortion a problem. In fact, Dr. Fournier, using a wet technique, has tirelessly taught tumescent liposuction around the world and we are all grateful to him. He has kindly authored several chapters in this text.

In 1977, Larry Field, a dermatologic surgeon attended a cosmetic surgery meeting in Paris, where he observed the Fischers and Pierre Fournier perform liposuction using the Fischer's machine [8]. Other physicians in several specialties visited Illouz and Fournier to study liposuction in the early 1980s, including Claude Caver and Arthur Sumrall, two dermatologists who learned the technique in mid-1982 [4,6–8].

In the fall of 1982, during the course in liposuction given by Illouz, Fournier, and Fischer that I took, members of a task force from the American Society of Plastic and Reconstructive Surgery came to observe. I brought a suction aspiration machine and Illouz cannulas home from Paris and started doing small procedures. I used a wet technique, injecting a few cubic centimeters of the hypotonic saline solution every 2 cm as described by Illouz. Subsequently, I went back to Paris several times over the next year to study with him [2].

Larry Field and I taught one of the first dermatologic courses on liposuction at the International Society for Dermatologic Surgery in the early 1980s and Tromovitch, Stegman, and Glogau discussed liposuction in December 1983 at the American Academy of Dermatology. Liposuction was also presented at the American Society for Dermatologic Surgery. Other cosmetic surgeons such as Jules Newman and Richard Dolsky gave courses and live workshops in the United States under the auspices of the American Academy of Cosmetic Surgery and started The American Society of Liposuction Surgery in 1984. It was Newman who first coined the term "*Lipo Suction*" [4,6]. Training was available in liposuction in some dermatology resident programs in 1984. Liposuction became part of the core surgical curriculum in dermatology in 1987 [4,6].

The next and certainly one of the most important innovations in liposuction was the development of the tumescent technique of local anesthesia by Jeffrey Klein, a dermatologic surgeon from California [4,6–8]. This technique radically changed the future of liposuction. The tumescent fluid was a dilute saline solution of lidocaine and epinephrine. Jeff Klein called me in the mid 1980s to ask if I would try the new technique he had developed for liposuction using only local anesthesia. As I had a patient just at that time on whom I did not want to use general anesthesia, I agreed to try it and he sent me the equipment and gave me the formula for the tumescent solution. The procedure was simple and required injecting the solution into the tissue using a large cannula and a 60-cc syringe attached to a three-way stopcock. I liked the procedure so much and there was such an improvement in what the patient felt post-op and in the diminished amount of blood in the canister that I was amazed. I never went back to using general anesthesia. Klein presented the technique at the Second World Congress of Lipo-Suction Surgery in June 1986 and published it in 1987 [9,10].

The tumescent technique has many benefits, which are summarized in Table 1. The most important improvement is the marked decrease in bleeding, making transfusions unnecessary [7,9,11]. Other advantages include minimal pain, as the anesthesia is long lasting; decreased infection, as the tumescent fluid is antibacterial; the ability of the awake patient to move (1) makes it easier for the surgeon to take out the fat, (2) markedly decreases the possibility of thrombophlebitis and therefore pulmonary emboli as well as (3) reduces the risk of perforation into the abdominal or chest cavity. In addition, with no need of general anesthesia and the risks that go along with it, the procedure is safer and patients feel better postoperatively. The amount of lidocaine that can safely be used limits both the liposuction and any ancillary procedures, making for a safer procedure with rapid recovery.

During the next few years Patrick Lillis, this author, Saul Asken, William Coleman, William Hanke, Gerald Bernstein, Bruce Chrisman, Ronald Moy, and many other dermatologic surgeons wrote articles and made many advances in the use and safety of tumescent anesthesia for liposuction [11–18]. Hands-on training courses were given by Patrick Lillis, Jeffrey Klein, and the author. The first Guidelines of Care for Liposuction by any specialty

Table 1 Benefits of Tumescent "Safe" Liposuction

Benefit	Result
Minimal blood loss	No transfusions necessary
Anesthesia long lasting	Minimal pain
General anesthesia not needed (patient awake)	Quicker recovery
	Patient move into position needed
	Less thrombophlebitis/pulmonary embolism
	None of general anesthesia's risks
	Less risk of perforation of body cavities
	Patients feel better post-op
Surgery limited by safe amount of lidocaine	Fewer ancillary procedures (e.g., facelifts)
	Quicker recovery
	Shorter procedures
Tumescent solution antibacterial	Fewer infections
High volume solution	Provides fluid replacement
Infiltration of fluid into fat	Smaller cannulas and smaller incisions
Maximizes tissue	

was by the American Academy of Dermatology in 1989, which was published in 1991 [19].

Other improvements made over the years include the development of smaller and different types of cannulas that allow us to make smaller incisions; criss-crossing the cannula tunnels for a smoother result; quieter and more efficient aspiration units; the replacement of hand-held syringes for infiltration by electric infiltration pumps; Occupational Safety and Health Administration-acceptable disposable tubing, canisters, and viral filters; a different way of visualizing the body so that circumferential liposuction could be done in various areas such as the abdomen and thighs; and better ways of approaching gynecomastia, buffalo humps, microliposuction of the face, and liposuction for axillary hyperhidrosis. Also, undermining of grafts was explored [20–22].

Ultrasonic liposuction was introduced by Zocchi in 1992 and has proven a useful adjunct to regular liposuction for some surgeons as has powered liposuction [23–25]. These newer types of liposuction make it easier to get through fibrous tissue and make it easier for the surgeon and patient. Ultrasonic liposuction breaks up the fat cells using ultrasound prior to suctioning. This technique requires the use of tumescent fluid in order to work. Plastic surgeons were at first amazed at the benefits of ultrasonic liposuction despite problems with burns and seromas, incorrectly attributing the marked decrease in bleeding and pain to the ultrasonic technique instead of realizing they were from the use of tumescent fluid. The other benefits of the tumescent technique were not realized because, despite the use of the tumescent solution, general anesthesia was still used. Ultrasonic liposuction is still useful for areas where there is a lot of fibrous tissue. It is only used for a short time as an adjunct to regular or powered liposuction.

Tumescent liposuction is an extremely safe procedure. The use of general anesthesia and iv fluid with the tumescent anesthetic solution used locally is not the true tumescent technique of local anesthesia. When iv fluids and general anesthesia are used, the patient is more prone to fluid overload with the possibility of pulmonary edema [26]. In addition, all the problems with the unconscious patient, including thrombophlebitis and pulmonary embolus, longer recovery, and problems with ancillary procedures are also seen. The tumescent technique should not be blamed for these complications [27]. When the true tumescent technique is used, no deaths or serious complications have been reported [15]. In fact, the number of lawsuits is dramatically decreased when liposuction is performed in an office facility rather than a hospital [28].

Many dermatologic surgeons such as Naomi Lawrence, Tim Flynn, and Kimberly Butterwick have continued to push ahead with new studies on liposuction [4,10,29]. In addition, liposuction has been reported to be useful in diabetes, lymphedema, and breast reduction [30,31].

Although liposuction is a multispecialty procedure there have unfortunately through the years been some turf wars. Some specialties have tried to prevent other specialties from performing this surgery by limiting where the procedure can be done. I was able to get OR privileges in my local hospital many years ago although like most liposuction surgeons, I do most procedures in my office operating rooms, which are AAAHC accredited.

I believe, as stated by William Coleman, that the safest liposuction is done using the tumescent technique and is performed by a board-certified dermatologic surgeon in an outpatient setting [6].

REFERENCES

1. Lewis CM. Early history of lipoplasty in the United States. Aesth Plast Surg 1990; 14:123–126.
2. Illouz YG. Body contouring by lipolysis: a 5-year experience with over 3,000 cases. Plast Reconstr Surg 1993; 72:511.
3. Illouz YG. History and current concepts of lipoplasty. Clin Plastic Surg 1996; 23(4):721–730.

4. Flynn TC, Coleman WP III, Field L, Klein JA, Hanke CW. History of liposuction. Dermatol Surg 2000; 26:515–520.
5. Dolsky RL, Newman J, Fetzek JR, Anderson RW. Liposuction history, techniques, and complications. Dermatol Clin 1987; 5(2):313–333.
6. Coleman WP III. The History of Liposuction and Fat Transplantation in America. Dermatol Clin 1999; 17(4):723–727.
7. Field L, Narins RS. Liposuction surgery. In: Epstein E, ed. Skin Surgery. 6th ed. Philadelphia: WB Saunders, 1987.
8. Field L. The dermatologist and liposuction—a history. J Dermatol Surg Oncol 1987; 13:1040–1041.
9. Klein JA. The tumescent technique for liposuction surgery. Am J Cosmet Surg 1987; 4:263–267.
10. Coleman WP III, Lawrence N, Lillis PJ, Narins RS. The tumescent technique. Plast Reconstr Surg 1998; 101(6):1751–1753.
11. Lillis PJ. The tumescent technique for liposuction surgery. Dermatol Clin 1990; 8:439.
12. Lillis PJ. Liposuction surgery under local anesthesia: limited blood loss and minimal lidocaine absorption J Dermatol Surg Oncol 1998;14:1145–1148.
13. Narins RS. Liposuction and anesthesia. Dermatol Clin 1990; 8(3):421–424.
14. Hanke CW, Coleman WP III, Lillis PJ, Narins RS, Buening JA, Rosemark J, Guillotte R, Lusk K, Jacobs R, Coleman WP IV. Infusion rates and levels of premedication in tumescent liposuction. Dermatol Surg 1997; 23(12):1131–1134.
15. Hanke CW, Bernstein G, Bullock S. Safety of tumescent liposuction in 15,336 patients. J Dermatol Surg Oncol 1995; 21:459.
16. Asken S. Facial liposuction and microlipoinjection. J Dermatol Surg Oncol 1988; 14:297–305.
17. Chrisman BB. Liposuction with facelift surgery. Dermatol Clin 1990; 8:501–522.
18. Ostaad A, Kageyama N, Moy RL. Tumescent anesthesia with lidocaine dose of 55 mg/kg is safe for liposuction. Dermatol Surg 1996; 22:921–927.
19. American Academy of Dermatology. Guidelines of Care for Liposuction. Rev. ed. J Am Acad Dermatol 1001; 24:289
20. Narins RS. Liposuction surgery for a buffalo hump caused by Cushing's disease. J Am Acad Dermatol 1989; 21:307.
21. Lillis PJ, Coleman WP III. Liposuction for treatment of axillary hyperhidrosis. Dermatol Clin. 1990; 8:479–482.
22. Field LM, Novy FG III. Flap evaluation and mobilization by blunt liposuction cannula dissection to repair temple defect. J Dermatol Surg Oncol 1987; 13: 1302–1305.
23. Zocchi M. Ultrasonic liposculpting. Aesthetic Plast Surg 1992; 16:287–298.
24. Coleman WP III, Katz B, Bruck M, Narins RS, Lawrence N, Flynn TC, Coleman WP IV, Coleman KM. The efficacy of powered liposuction.
25. Coleman WP III. Powered liposuction. Dermatol Surg 2000; 26:315–318.
26. Gilliland MD, Coctes N. Tumescent liposuction complicated by pulmonary edema. Plast Reconstr Surg 1997; 99:215–219.

27. Klein JA. The two standards of care for tumescent liposuction. Dermatol Surg 1997; 23:1194–1195.
28. Coleman WP III, Hanke CW, Lillis P, Bernstein G, Narins RS. Does the location of surgery or the specialty of the physician affect malpractice claims in liposuction? Dermatol Surg 1999; 25:343.
29. Butterwick KJ, Goldman MP, Sriprachya-Anunt S. Lidocaine levels during the first 2 hours of infiltration of dilute anesthetic solution for tumescent liposuction: rapid versus slow delivery. Dermatol Surg 1999; 25:681–685.
30. Hanner H, Olbrisch RR. The treatment of type-I diabetes with insulin-induced lipohypertrophy by liposuction. Dtsch Med Wochenschr 1994; 119:414–417.
31. Brorson H, Svensson H. Complete reduction of lymphedema of the arm by liposuction after breast cancer. Scand J Plast Reconstr Surg Hand Surg 1997; 31:137.

2

Initiating the Practice of Liposuction

Timothy Corcoran Flynn
University of North Carolina
Chapel Hill, North Carolina, U.S.A.

Many dermatologic surgeons are quite skilled at liposuction. Dermatologic surgeons have pioneered techniques in the liposuction field [1], which has now been performed for close to 20 years in America. Liposuction is among the most common cosmetic surgical procedures performed in the United States, due largely in part to the excellent safety record and superior aesthetic results. With the advent of the tumescent technique, liposuction is now an elegant, satisfying procedure which effectively aspirates localized subcutaneous fat deposits. The cells that deposit excess calories are removed and are thus no longer capable of storing fat.

Patients now realize that localized areas of stubborn adiposity are not amenable to spot reduction. Excessive dieting to remove the genetically determined areas of excess fat often does not work [2]. Patients have become more interested in liposuction since the procedure is so effective and efficient and has helped so many. Many people inquire about liposuction after finding out that their friends or relatives have had a successful, long-lasting result.

The procedure is not complicated to learn yet takes a while to master. Teaching liposuction for almost 10 years has shown the author that while many dermatologic surgeons have a flair for the procedure possessing the finesse necessary to obtain a good result, other surgeons may find themselves not suited to the technique. Ill-suited individuals often approach the procedure too aggressively or perform the liposuction too quickly to obtain good outcomes. When performing liposuction a careful, thorough, and artistic approach is best used. When beginning liposuction, a graduated learning approach is best employed.

One of the best introductions to liposuction comes from attending forums on liposuction given by medical societies. The American Academy of Dermatology, the American Society for Dermatologic Surgery (ASDS), and the American Society for Cosmetic Surgery all hold sessions at their annual meetings on liposuction. Some of the best forums are presented at the American Society for Dermatologic Surgery's Annual Meeting. Large symposia on liposuction are held which detail basic concepts and expand on the latest developments. The dermatologic surgeon initiating a practice in liposuction would do well to begin with the large symposia at the ASDS annual meetings, where the basic concepts are presented. They also hold graduated "breakfast sessions" in beginning, intermediate, and advanced liposuction given by experts in the field. These sessions provide a more intimate forum in which to learn and allow for more open discussion and dialogue. Individuals of all degrees of experience and expertise interested in liposuction attend the breakfast sessions.

Individuals just starting to learn liposuction should study from liposuction textbooks (such as this one). Text study is essential for the liposuction surgeon to understand the science and the scholarly approach to the procedure. Texts allow reading about a subject in depth and are handy to have in the office. A text is fast, efficient, and concise.

Every dermatologic surgeon must maintain an active ongoing reading program in order to keep up with the latest literature. Good literature on liposuction is also available through special issues of medical periodicals. *Dermatologic Clinics* has had two excellent issues (Fig. 1) [3,4] on liposuction, the most recent of which was published in October 1999. *Dermatologic Surgery* [5] has also had issues devoted solely to liposuction. These issues allow for feature articles that discuss techniques as well as present the latest advanced information. Medical journals publish current liposuction articles. The journal most worth reading is *Dermatologic Surgery*, where current liposuction information is efficiently disseminated. The *Journal of the American Academy of Dermatology*, *Archives of Dermatology*, and *Plastic and Reconstructive Surgery* often contain articles of interest on liposuction. Practitioners of liposuction must be familiar with proper guidelines of care for liposuction. Both the American Society of Dermatologic Surgery as well as the American Academy of Dermatology have published guidelines of care for liposuction. Updated and revised on a regular basis, the most recent

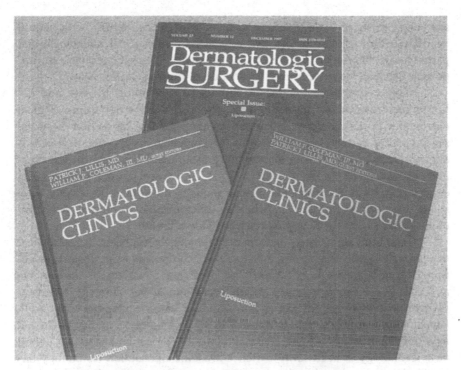

FIGURE 1 Special liposuction issues of medical periodicals. These special issues are "required reading" for any liposuction surgeon.

guidelines of care were published in the March 2000 issue of *Dermatologic Surgery* [6] and the September 2001 issue of the *Journal of American Academy of Dermatology* [7].

Perhaps the best instruction available appears in the form of individual "live surgery" postgraduate courses. These courses occur in a variety of settings around the country. The courses may be given by one individual expert in the field or may have participation by multiple faculty. Multiple surgeons at a course allows a variety of perspectives. These intimate courses have a great advantage in that attendees get an opportunity not only to receive didactic instruction in liposuction but also to get an opportunity to observe the surgery firsthand. Individual questions can be directly addressed. For example, the exact technique used in liposuction of the neck can be shown to the other attendees. Course instructors may have preferences for individual brands of equipment and types of cannulas, and most instructors are happy to share these opinions with their attendees. CME credit should be offered through any of the live courses. Certificates of attendance and participation should be provided to the attendees. These certificates are important because they document the attendees' training in liposuction.

Many young dermatologists have had the opportunity to learn liposuction in their residency. Training in liposuction is a portion of the core surgical curriculum in dermatology developed by the ASDS. Liposuction is an essential part of dermatologic training as recommended by the American Academy of Dermatology. Select dermatology programs have been offering residency training in liposuction since 1984. However, a variety of surgical experiences exist for residents. Some trainees unfortunately receive only some exposure to liposuction, whereas other residents perform their own cases under supervision, approximately twice a month.

Once individual study and course attendance has been accomplished, the dermatologic surgeon is ready to select equipment to perform liposuction. Practitioners must be aware that there are a variety of instruments available to perform liposuction. While many liposuction surgeons have their favorite instruments, most all of the standard instrumentation works well. Liposuction instrumentation is like any other technology: improvements and new developments occur every year. Practitioners must be aware that not all new technology is necessarily better. Ultrasonic liposuction technology has largely been abandoned by liposuction experts after studies showed no benefit over externally applied ultrasound [8] and "internal" ultrasonic cannulas were associated with an increased number of seromas and cutaneous burns [9].

With respect to instrumentation, blunt-tipped infusion needles as well as cannulas are useful. The beginning surgeon need not purchase a huge number of cannulas but rather can often start with two simple configurations such as a blunt-tipped dual-side port cannula and a more aggressive cannula design such as a triport or Mercedes design. Should liposuction surgeons wish to use the microcannula technique, there are a variety of sizes and varieties available. Many good aspiration pumps are available and easily produce 1 atm of negative pressure. Issues for the beginning surgeon to think about involve the amount of noise produced by the machine as well as size and ease of use. The beginning surgeon should also pay attention to collection canisters and should evaluate the tightness of the seal of these units. For both beginning and advanced liposuction surgeons the softer aspiration hoses are a pleasure to use. Those for whom liposuction is a greater portion of their practice may want to consider purchasing some of the newer technology that has proven to be an improvement, such as powered liposuction devices.

Beginning liposuction surgeons should carefully evaluate the space in which the liposuction is to be performed. Enough space to contain a mechanized procedure table and allow complete movement of the surgeon around the patient is essential. The surgeon must also evaluate tables, drapes, trays, and tubing used for liposuction. There must be adequate room for nursing personnel. Liposuction is a sterile procedure and sterile equipment must be used. The room should appear professional, neat, and as clean as possible. In short, proper ample space must be available for the comfort of both the patient and the surgeon (Fig. 2).

Once the equipment is obtained and the space organized it is important that the beginning liposuction surgeon review several critical aspects of the liposuction procedure. Proper cleaning and sterilization procedures for instruments must be in place in the office. Nursing personnel must be properly trained. The surgeon must ensure that they understand the proper preparation and use of tumescent anesthesia. Detailed, exact procedures for mixing the anesthetic solution must be followed, and it is imperative that certified individuals legally allowed to prepare medications mix the tumescent anesthesia. Liposuction surgeons must know the maximum dosage of lidocaine (currently ascertained to be 55 mg/kg body wt) and should be aware of signs of lidocaine toxicity. Checklists can be prepared for the office to ensure that the essential aspects of liposuction are understood and regularly reviewed by all personnel. Proper protocols must be followed.

The beginning liposuction surgeon must be careful about obtaining appropriate informed consent. Good informed consent both contains information about the procedure as well as carefully details potential risks and complications. Proper medical records must be kept, including careful records of tumescent anesthesia. Photography is an important component of any cosmetic procedure and the advent of digital photography has made documenting preoperative and postoperative pictures relatively inexpensive. Patient forms should be prepared for the liposuction patient. These include information about the procedure, preoperative instructions, and postoperative instructions. A "checklist" for the surgeon is helpful to ensure compliance to standards of care and minimize the potential for errors. It may be handy to show on the checklist medications which can interact with tumescent anesthesia. Orders for anesthesia should be written on an order form. A tumescent anesthesia record should be kept [9]. Before performing any cases of liposuction the surgeon must ensure that his or her malpractice insurance covers him or her for liposuction. There may be additional costs or riders that are necessary for those practitioners wishing to perform tumescent liposuction.

The first cases of liposuction performed by the surgeon may be done

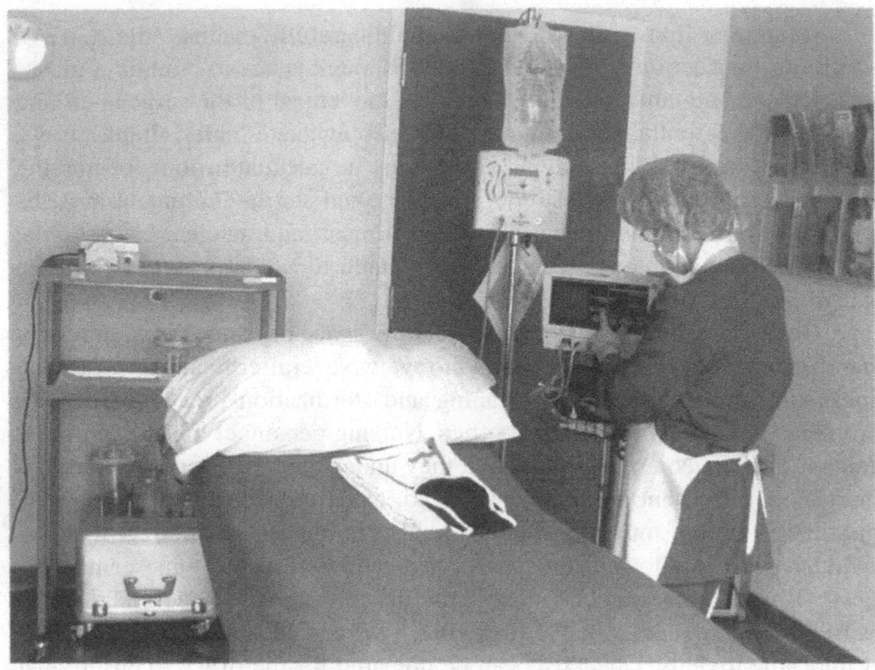

FIGURE 2 Liposuction procedure room. Patient comfort is assured with the large mechanized table. Adequate space is available for the surgeon and nurses. Cardiac monitoring equipment and a powered liposuction console mounted on the iv pole is seen.

on trusted individuals. These can range from members of the doctor's own staff to special cosmetically oriented patients. Full disclosure should be given to the doctor's first cases. The surgeon should simply explain that this is the first or second case of a procedure the surgeon is performing. Explaining to the patient how the physician has studied and learned about liposuction is informative and reassuring to the patient.

It is strongly advised that only one anatomic area of liposuction be done for the first cases. This should be a relatively simple area such as the outer thigh or lower abdomen. These areas are frequently associated with excellent results with minimal potential for complications. It is important to stick with these "simpler" areas. Do not perform liposuction on a difficult area (for example, the face) as one of the first cases. Difficult areas also may include pseudogynecomastia, calves, and the upper inner thighs.

Good postoperative care is essential for a good liposuction outcome (Fig. 3). Surgeons must understand the importance of leaving entry sites open to drain. Compression garments are employed to aid in drainage of the tumescent anesthesia. These garments are also comforting to the patient decreasing movement of the area treated. Many patients enjoy wearing the garments beyond the usual 2-week time period. Patients should be encouraged to resume regular movement postliposuction. This aids in drainage and minimizes the risk of deep venous thrombosis. They should return to their regular exercise program as soon as they feel comfortable.

Physicians initiating liposuction may want to carefully follow their first cases of liposuction. It is not unreasonable to have the first patients return to the clinic for follow-up on an every-other-day basis in order for the physician and his or her staff to learn of the typical postoperative course. It is very instructive for the liposuction surgeon to understand the drainage that will occur through incision sites left open following fat aspiration. It is also

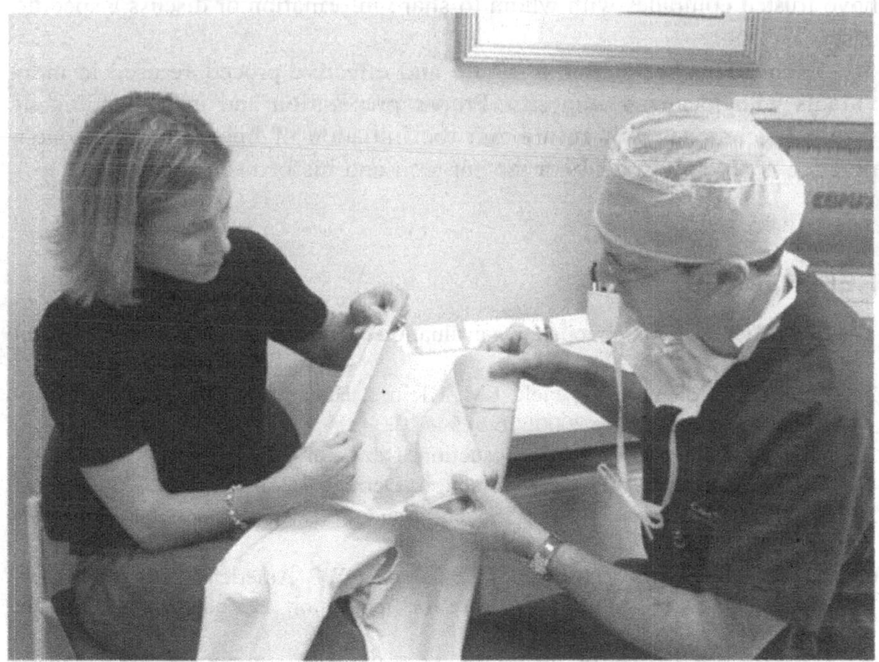

FIGURE 3 The surgeon emphasizes the importance of postoperative care to the patient. Note the compression garment.

important to recognize that the postoperative swelling and edema that occur during the first few days after liposuction will gradually lessen. The surgeon should realize that in selected cases there may be a firmness or wrinkled appearance to the edematous skin following tumescent liposuction. This will often resolve over time but may take months. Understanding the typical pattern of a normal postoperative course will assist the surgeon in caring for future patients.

Performing liposuction is exciting and gratifying. The beginning liposuction surgeon must have good training. This is obtained through exposure to liposuction at professional meetings, review of textbooks or special issues of journals devoted to liposuction, regular reading of the literature, and attendance at a live course prior to beginning liposuction in one's own practice. First cases should be done on simple areas such as the outer thigh and should be done on trusted individuals well known to the surgeon. As the surgeon performs more cases of liposuction they will continue to learn more about the procedure and develop finesse. The surgeon will also meet experts in the field and colleagues with liposuction experience. No physician should practice in a vacuum, and it is important that the liposuction surgeon have trusted comrades with whom to share information or discuss a specific case.

Tumescent liposuction is a safe and effective procedure used in individuals with localized adiposity. Proper preparation and understanding of surgical techniques will ensure that the initiation of liposuction into one's practice is rewarding for both the surgeon and his or her patients.

REFERENCES

1. Flynn TC, Narins R. Preoperative evaluation of the liposuction patient. Dermatol Clin 1999; 17:729–734.
2. Flynn TC, Coleman WP, Field LM, Klein J, Hanke CW. The history of liposuction. Dermatol Surg 2000; 26:515–520.
3. Lillis PJ, Coleman WP eds. Liposuction. Dermatol Clin 1990; 8:381–589.
4. Lillis PJ, Coleman WP eds. Liposuction. Dermatol Clin 1999; 17:723–915.
5. Coleman WP, Lawrence N eds. Special issue: liposuction. Dermatol Surg 1997; 23:1125–1226.
6. Lawrence N, Clark RE, Flynn TC, Coleman WP. American Society for Dermatologic Surgery guidelines of care for liposuction. Dermatol Surg 2000; 26: 265–269.
7. Coleman WP, Glogau RG, Klein JA, Moy RL, Narins RS, Chuang TY, Farmer ER, Lewis CW, Lowery BJ. Guidelines of care for liposuction. J Am Acad Dermatol 2001; 45:438–447.

8. Lawrence N, Cox SE. The efficacy of externally ultrasound assisted liposuction: a randomized controlled trial. Dermatol Surg 2000; 26:329–332.
9. Klein JA. Critique of ultrasonic liposuction. In: Klein JA, ed. Tumescent Technique: Tumescent Anesthesia and Microcannular Liposuction. St. Louis: Mosby, 2000:271–280.

3

The Surgical Suite for the Liposuction Surgeon

Gary D. Monheit
University of Alabama at Birmingham
Birmingham, Alabama, U.S.A.

In this day of outpatient surgery, scrutiny, and regulation, it behooves the surgeon to examine carefully the accepted standards of outpatient surgery and surgical facilities. The Accreditation Association of Ambulatory Healthcare can be helpful in guiding the surgeon in his or her design of an appropriate surgical facility for liposuction [1]. The liposuction procedure requires an operating room large enough for the surgeon and assistant to move around the table and nursing monitor and operate the bulky equipment. A minimal space is 15 × 15 ft, while many prefer 20 × 20 ft for maximal room.

The operating room walls should be smooth surfaced for easy cleaning. The floors need to be seamless for sanitizing and easy cleaning without risk of cracking. The floors and walls need to be disinfected and cleaned with surfaces that can be resistant to corrosion. This needs to be done on a regular basis. Excellent lighting from either high-intensity halogen lights or ceiling fluorescent lights can provide adequate visualization for the surgeon. Many liposuction surgeons prefer banks of fluorescent ceiling lights as they preserve the shadows needed to determine depth and contour. Many high-intensity halogen lights will "white out" all shadows in the evaluation of the curves, folds, depths, and contours needed for liposuction. An auxiliary power supply should be available in case of emergency power failure. This can be supplied by either a generator or battery system allowing sufficient power to maintain lighting and liposuction equipment—the aspirator and infiltrator—to complete the case. Ventilation should not only provide a comfortable environment but also must filter airborne contaminants below a level at which they would contribute to wound infection. Ideally, this should stand alone and not be recycled from the rest of the office but may be accomplished with fine particulate filters—high efficient particulate air.

During the planning stage, it is necessary to consider the needs of a location for electrical outlets, suction, foot-activated intercom system, and oxygen outlets. A floor-mounted electrical outlet should be in the center of the room where the operating table is placed. Careful planning of outlets for the walls, floor, and counters will depend on the equipment used needing electrical power. Most surgeons will need outlets for the monitoring equipment, aspirator, infiltrator, and lasers, if used.

Liposuction may be a prolonged procedure and performed under the tumescent technique means the patient will be awake; thus, he or she needs to be comfortable (Fig. 1). The aesthetics of the OR can allay anxiety of the

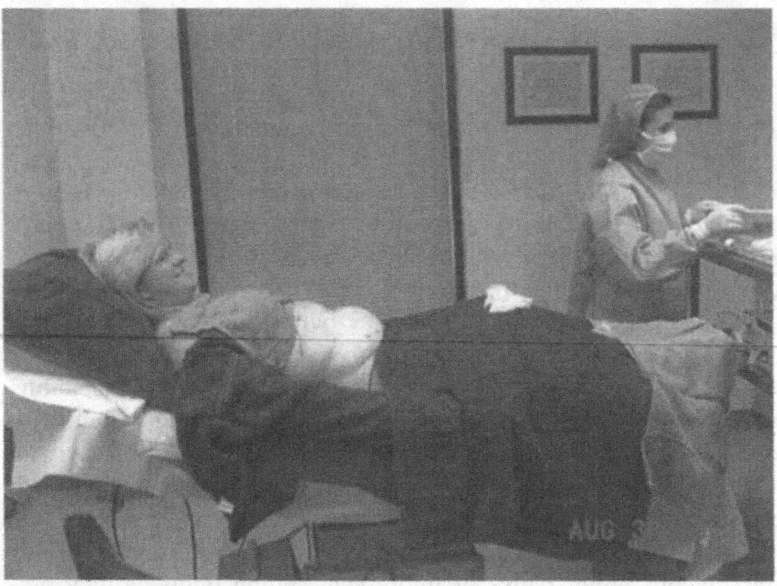

FIGURE 1 Liposuction patient on operating table in room large enough for staff and equipment. Sterile towels are placed under the disposable drapes and the nurse is gowned sterilely for the procedure.

awake or sedated patient to make the procedure a better experience. Soft, cool colors like blue and green in the operating room are preferred along with pleasing murals, windows, and artwork to distract from the procedure. The patient should not be in visual line of the monitoring equipment, flashing lights, aspirate material, or blood, as it would increase anxiety. Music, if it is chosen properly, can be a tranquilizing factor.

Equipment should be stored in sealed cabinets with glass doors so that needed supplies can be easily visualized and retrieved as needed. Separate shelves and drawers are designated for disposables, iv fluid, drugs, cannulae, and other equipment which must be kept covered in OR storage areas (Fig. 2).

The operating room must have a specific schedule for maintenance and cleaning. The OR should not be used as an extra examination or consultation room when not in use, as it would break the code of asepsis. Cleaning

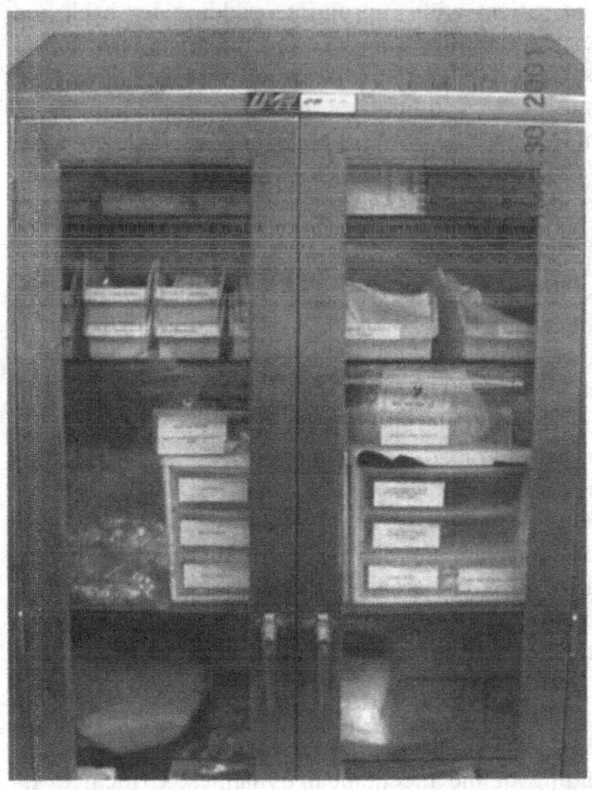

FIGURE 2 Operating room storage cabinets containing liposuction supplies.

techniques and sterilization methods vary but must conform to the postoperative infection rate, which should approach zero for this procedure. There is a variable pattern concerning the degree of sterilization for tumescent liposuction. Some surgeons perform clean rather than sterile surgery, using sterile instruments in a clean operating room environment. This author feels it is important to maintain strict sterility as an added precaution to prevent local wound infection, which can produce significant symptomatology and morbidity in this procedure.

The operating table must be comfortable for both patient and surgeon. It should be wide enough to support the patient for long procedures and allow the patient to turn in position for bilateral and even circumferential suctioning and yet narrow enough for the surgeon and assistant to assess the surgical area. The table should have full mechanical mobility for position changes in the various sections of the table during surgery. This should be foot-controlled so that strict sterility can be maintained. Because most tumescent liposuction procedures last from 1 to 4 hr, it is necessary to provide a comfortable table for the patient with appropriate padding for back and head support as well as vertical mobility to reduce the surgeon's back strain. Towel packs and pillows are used for patient support and positioning in order to access areas such as the hips, thighs, saddlebags, and medial thighs. Three molded Styrofoam wedges and hip supports are available to standardize positions during surgery. A layer of sterile towels placed over the cushions of the operating table and under the drapes helps absorb dripping fluids during the procedure.

Monitoring during liposuction surgery is within the standard of care, even during awake tumescent surgery. It is of critical importance when iv or intravenous sedation is used. Monitoring devices should include the electrocardiographic monitor, blood pressure and pulse monitor, and a pulse oxsymmetry monitor. A defibrillator, oxygen supply, suction for aspiration, and intubation material must be on hand along with emergency drugs and a staff fully trained with basic and/or advanced cardiac life support for unexpected emergencies (Fig. 3).

A recovery time after liposuction surgery is necessary to assure that the patient resumes full consciousness and physiologic homeostasis. Whether this takes place in a separate recovery area or the operating room itself, it should be maintained and provided for the patient's comfort and light nutrition. Only after the patient is fully awake and ambulatory and has taken fluids and light nutrition should he or she be discharged in the care of a companion.

Liposuction requires special instrumentation for which the surgeon should have an understanding of the mechanical dynamics. Critical to liposuction is the vacuum source, which creates negative pressure to suction

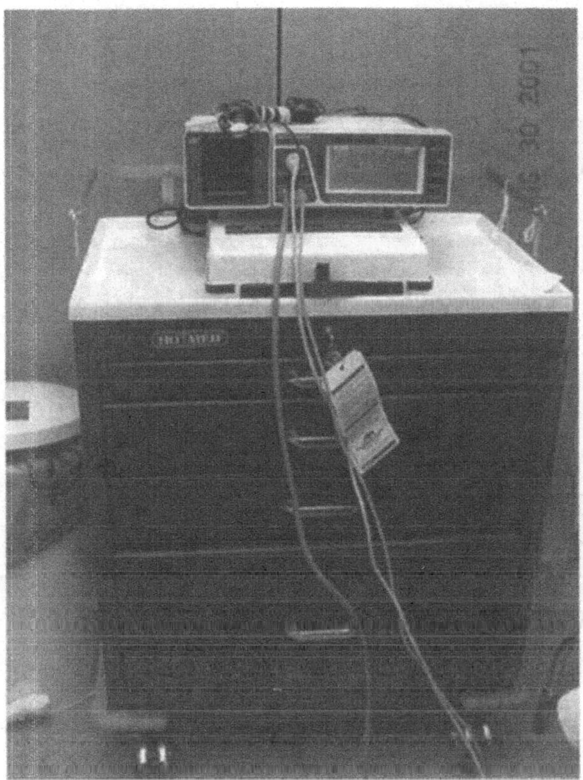

FIGURE 3 Monitoring equipment is kept at the head of the table on the crash cart and is monitored by the nurse.

adipose tissue (Fig. 4). This can be performed using either an electromechanical aspirator or manual syringe. Syringe liposuction can be used for small cases and has the advantages of being low cost, lightweight, and easy to transport. On the other hand, it can fatigue a surgeon in larger cases and may compromise results on specific areas.

Aspirators require a negative atmosphere system created by an air pump with a fat-collection canister. There are many systems on the market and most are adequate for liposuction. The following criteria are important in evaluating the appropriate system:

Closed system with collection system, overflow trap, and disposable air filter

Electric vacuum pumps with sufficient vacuum level for efficient uninterrupted suction

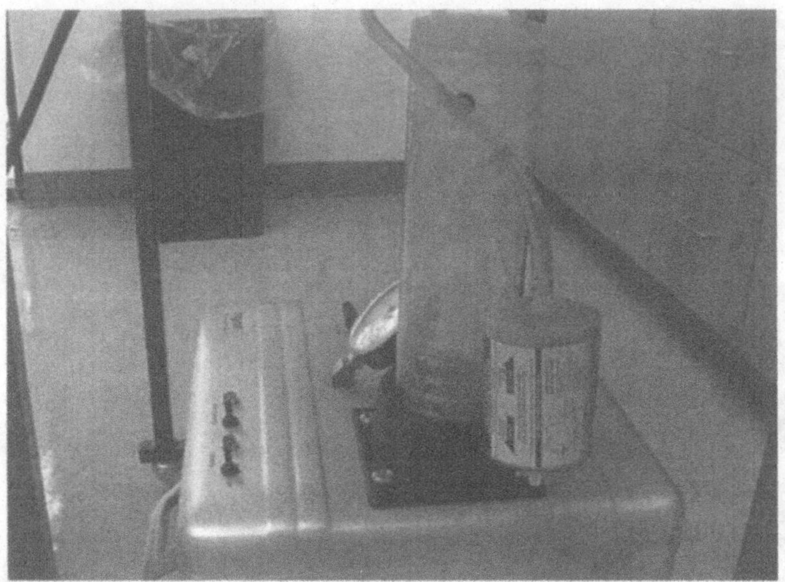

FIGURE 4 Aspiration pump with fillers and receptacle for fat.

Quiet operation
Durable yet light and compact

A minimal atmospheric pressure is needed for even flow of fat through cannulas and tubing. Doubling or tripling that pressure does not necessarily increase flow rates or efficiency of liposuction. Thus, a small quiet machine may be as effective as the more powerful, larger, more cumbersome, and noisy machines. The surgeon should have a reliable machine with appropriate backup equipment if there is pump or motor failure. Syringe suction instruments can suffice to finish a case but it is preferable for the busy liposuction surgeon to have a backup machine [2].

Cannulas are the stainless-steel tubes which penetrate the subcutaneous tissue to remove the fat through holes on the tip or diameter. The shape of the cannula, diameter of the lumen, placement of holes, and cannula size all determine the efficiency of the fat collected as well as the trauma and potential morbidity. Cannulas designed with holes near the tip are more aggressive and remove fat more efficiently. They, though, may cause more bleeding and potential trauma. Examples are the Cobra, Pinto, and Accelerator cannulas (Figs. 5a and 5b). Blunt-tipped cannulas with openings placed further back from the tip are gentler to tissue. These include the Klein, Fournier, standard, and spatula cannulas (Figs. 6a and 6b). The num-

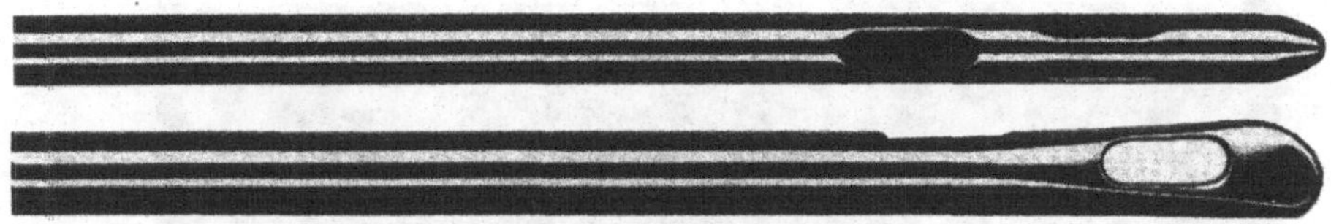

FIGURE 5 (a) Accelerator cannula. (b) Cobra cannula.

ber of holes around the cannula determine the rate of fat suction through the tubing. The safer cannulas are designed to place the holes on the ventral surface to prevent trauma to the overlying skin [3].

Cannula size is important for efficiency as well as trauma to the tissue. Early on, cannula diameter was commonly 8–10 mm and complications from troughing and trauma created irregularities on the skin surface. Gradually, cannula sizes decreased so that most liposuction surgeons rarely use a cannula larger than 4 mm. Microcannulas have an internal diameter of 2.2 mm or less, which is that of a 12-gauge hypodermic needle. These smaller cannulas are more delicate and cause less trauma to fibrous septae with less risk of contour irregularity or skin trauma. The microcannula, though, are more fragile and can fracture if not used delicately. Microcannulas are used exclusively with tumescent liposuction and create less trauma with less pain and better accuracy for superficial liposuction [4].

Anesthetic infiltration of tumescent fluid is accomplished either by manual syringes or a power pump infiltrator. To infiltrate larger areas, more tumescent fluid is needed and generally requires a mechanical assist to obtain a slow rate to create a hydro diffusion over the entire subcutaneous area for liposuction. The most efficient systems are the infiltration pumps that can deliver a variable flow rate by a speed control (Fig. 7). The infiltrator, thus, delivers the tumescent fluid through metallic, stainless-steel, blunt-tipped cannulae ranging in size from 12 to 18 gauge. The smaller the diameter, the less discomfort with infiltration. A 20-gauge spinal needle can deliver a slower rate of infiltration fluid in a comfortable manner. The surgeon, though, must be careful in that the needle is sharp and its cutting edge can

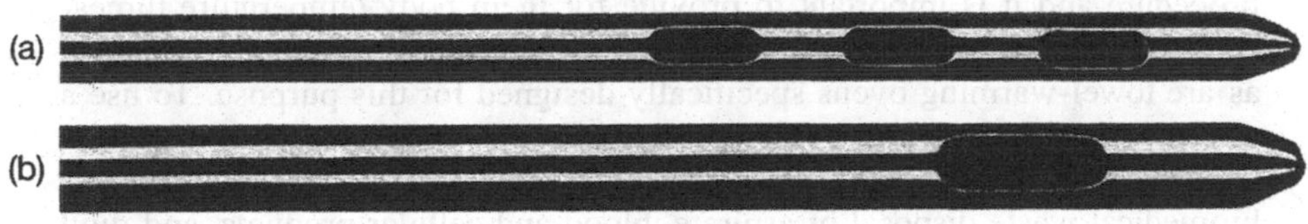

FIGURE 6 (a) Fournier cannula. (b) Standard cannula.

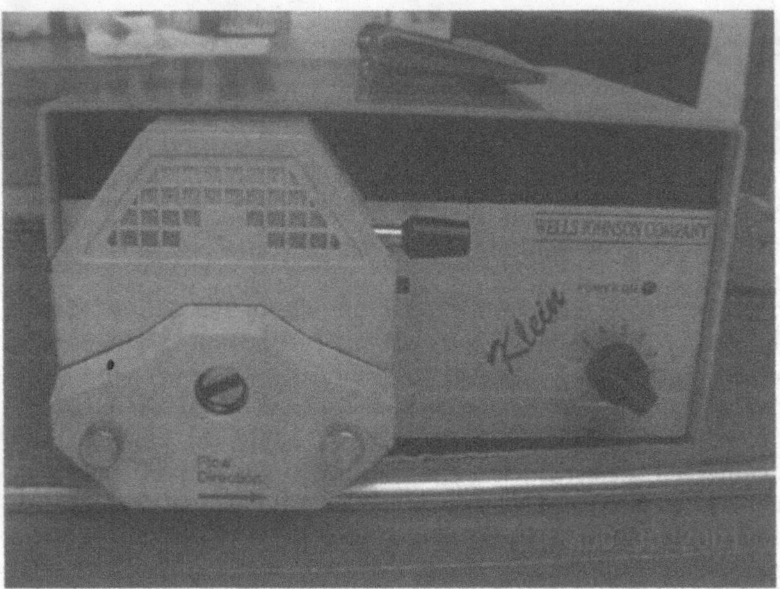

Figure 7 Infusion pump.

cause trauma to structures if not controlled carefully [4]. Other equipment used recently in liposuction include internal ultrasonic devices and power assisted liposuction cannulas. These innovations are discussed in other chapters considering these techniques.

The liposuction facility must be backed up with an appropriate sterilization area. The cleaning, rinsing, and sterilization of all cannulas and other surgical instruments should be performed under strict aseptic conditions. Brushes are needed to clean cannulas, both internally and externally, of adherent blood and tissue along the lumen. An ultrasonic cleaning device is also helpful. Instruments are then steam-autoclaved for sterilization. Other methods of chemical or cold sterilization are not effective enough in reducing bacterial content. Other devices such as aspirator tubing, infiltration tubing, syringes, collection canisters, collection bottles, and needles are single-use items and should be disposed. Patients become chilled during the procedure and it is important to provide for them body-temperature tumescent fluid and warm towels and blankets. Fluid warming baths are helpful as are towel-warming ovens specifically designed for this purpose. To use a microwave oven to warm iv or tumescent fluid is dangerous as it can overheat the fluid and burn the patient [5]. The surgeon is also responsible for biomedical waste disposal of aspirate, blood and cellular products, and fluid materials as per federal and state Occupational Safety and Health Administration standards. The sealed, plastic bottle aspirate containers can be discarded without opening and disposed of using an appropriate regulated waste remover such as that by Browning Ferris Industries.

Proper surgical attire is expected of all dermatologic and liposuction surgeons. Though some are more cavalier and wear street clothes, it is expected in this day and age of outpatient surgical scrutiny to dress appropriately. This includes wearing a cap, shoe covers, and scrubs, covered by fluid-resistant disposable surgical gowns. Eye protection is needed for both the surgeon and the operating team. Sterile surgical gloves are worn by the surgeon and his or her assistant to prevent contamination of the operating field. These standards are expected by our patients in the general population and are expected of us as surgeons.

Instrument and device tables and trays are of many types and descriptions. They must segregate the sterile from the unsterile areas and are commonly classified as the front and back tables. A multilevel liposuction stand designed by Dr. Jeff Klein is of practical use to separate instruments on each of its three levels. These include the following: (1) the top level—sterile tray, including infiltration and suction cannulas, sterile tubing, hexagonal nut to hold tubing on tray, syringes, blades, draping, and gauze (Fig. 8); (2) the middle level—infiltration pump, iv, and tumescent fluid bag hanging on the

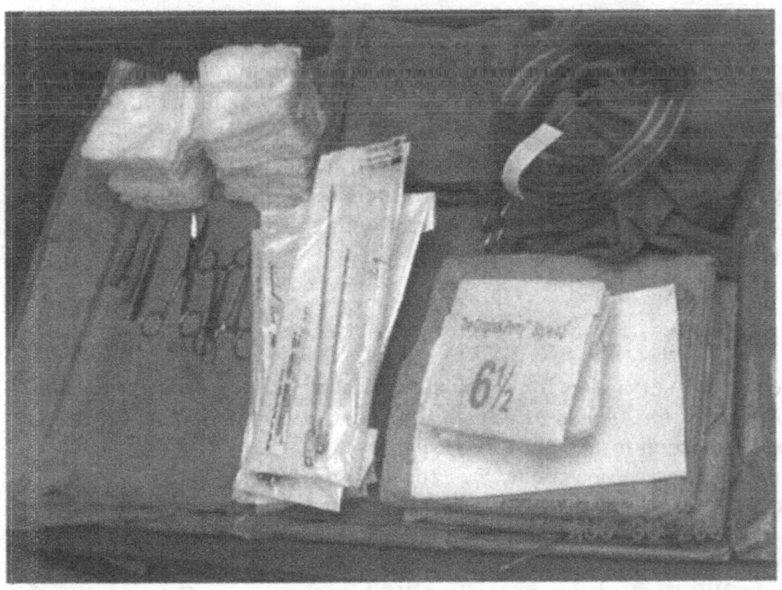

FIGURE 8 Sterile tray containing cannulas, instruments, tubing, and gauze packs.

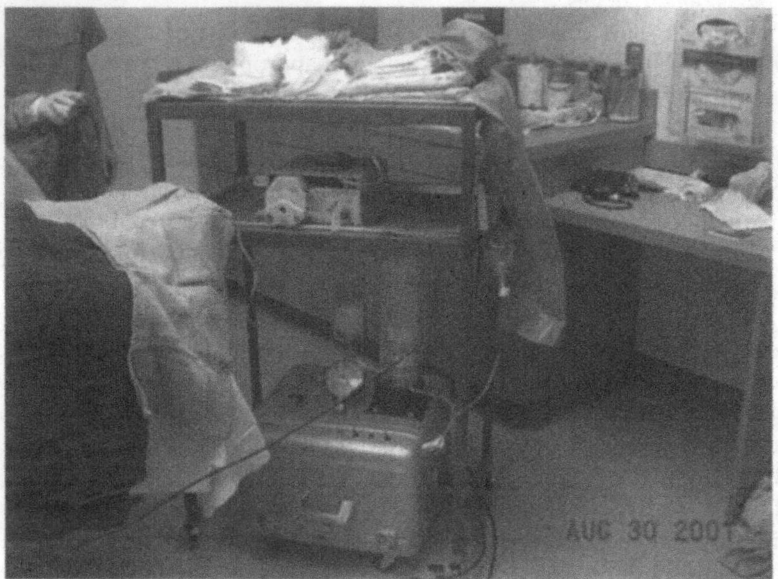

FIGURE 9 Equipment table with three layers separating the sterile upper tray, middle infusion pump, and lower aspiration machine and collection receptacle.

side; and (3) the lower level—liposuction aspirator pump with collection bottles. Other nonsterile tables are used for monitoring equipment, fluid mixing, storage, and so on (Fig. 9).

The liposuction surgeon thus has special needs and requirements as to operating room space, design, and instrumentation. To obtain best results, the surgeon should equip him- or herself with the necessary environment and tools.

REFERENCES

1. Accreditation Association for Ambulatory Healthcare Incorporated. *Accreditation Handbook for Ambulatory Healthcare*. 1996–1997 ed, Skokie, IL: Accreditation Association for Ambulatory Healthcare.
2. Klein JA. Tumescent technique. St. Louis: Mosby, 2000:222–235.
3. Cook W, Cook K. *Manual of Tumescent Liposculpture and Laser Cosmetic Surgery*. Philadelphia: Lippincott/Williams & Wilkins, 1999:2–11.
4. Klein JA. Tumescent Technique. St. Louis: Mosby, 2000:235–240
5. Coleman WP III, Letissier S, Hanke CW. Liposuction. In: Coleman WP, ed. Cosmetic Dermatologic Surgery. 187–195.

4
Tumescent Anesthesia

Carolyn I. Jacob
Northwestern University
Chicago, Illinois, U.S.A.

Michael S. Kaminer
Dartmouth Medical School
Chestnut Hill, Massachusetts, and
Yale University School of Medicine
New Haven, Connecticut, U.S.A.

Before the advent of tumescent anesthesia, liposuction was performed using general anesthesia. This form of sedation provided no hemostasis within the adipose layer and was fraught with complications such as hemmorrhage, hematoma formation, prolonged recovery time, disfiguring irregularities of the skin, and large volume fluid shifts. In many cases, blood transfusions and/or large volume intravenous fluids were necessary intra- and postoperatively.

In 1986 (published in 1987), Dr. Jeffrey Klein developed the tumescent anesthesia technique for liposuction surgery [1]. Using the principle of hypodermoclysis (the introduction of fluids into the subcutaneous tissues to replace loss of water and salt during illness or operation) Dr. Klein's concept of tumescent anesthesia has radically changed the way liposuction is performed today. By delivering large volumes of dilute lidocaine with epinephrine in buffered saline to the adipose layer, both local anesthesia and hemostasis can be achieved. This allows safe, painless removal of large quantities of fat with minimal blood loss. Goals of the tumescent technique include targeting anesthesia locally, expanding the adipose space, minimizing drug toxicity, and maximizing anesthetic efficacy (Table 1) [2].

TUMESCENT SOLUTION

The basic solution for tumescent anesthesia combines normal saline, lidocaine, epinephrine, sodium bicarbonate, and triamcinolone acetonide (Table 2) [3,4]. Other anesthetics, including bupivacaine, ropivacaine, and prilocaine, have all been used in performing tumescent anesthesia, but the gold standard is currently lidocaine [5]. Some surgeons choose to omit triamcinolone, which has been shown to decrease the inflammation and symptomatic soreness postoperatively [2]. Lactated Ringer's solution may be used instead of normal saline and has been reported to prolong the stability of epinephrine secondary to a more acidic pH of 6.3, but this higher acidity may make infusion more painful [6]. Sodium bicarbonate is used to buffer the acidity of epinephrine in order to decrease burning during infusion.

Not only does lidocaine provide anesthesia, but it also has been shown to be bacteriocidal for organisms isolated from the skin [7]. Concentrations of lidocaine greater than 0.5% provide a dose-dependent inhibition of bacterial growth, including gram-negative and gram-positive organisms [8]. In dilutions as low as 0.05%, lidocaine has been shown to be bacteriostatic for Staphylococcus aureus [9]. Sodium bicarbonate, in vitro, has been shown to augment this bacteriocidal activity of lidocaine [10]. Infection is a rare complication when tumescent anesthesia is used [11].

The concentration of lidocaine in the tumescent solution used can range from 0.05 to 0.125%. The higher concentration of lidocaine (0.125 or 0.1%) is used generally for more sensitive areas, such as the abdomen, lateral thighs, knees, inner thighs, periumbilical area, neck, flanks, and back [4,12].

TABLE 1 Goals of Tumescent Technique

Optimize biochemical and/or biomechanical drug efficacy
Target drug effects in local tissue compartments
Maximize drug concentration locally
Delay systemic drug absorption
Prolong local or systemic drug effects
Decreases systemic drug toxicity and increases the safe upper limit of drug dosage
Mechanically expand a targeted compartment
Benefit from augmented local hydrostatic pressure

Source: Ref. 2.

TABLE 2 Tumescent Anesthetic Solution Preparation

	Solution concentrations (%)			
Anesthetic	0.125	0.1	0.075	0.05
Normal saline 0.9%	1 liter	1 liter	1 liter	1 liter
Lidocaine (2%)	62.5 cc	50 cc	37.5 cc	25 cc
Epinephrine 1:1000	1 cc (1 mg) (final concentration 1:1,000,000)	1 cc	1 cc	1 cc
Sodium bicarbonate (8.45%)	12.5 cc (final solution, pH 7.4)	12.5 cc	12.5 cc	12.5 cc
Triamcinolone acetonide	1 cc (10 mg)	1 cc	1 cc	1 cc

Source: Ref. 3.

Some physicians choose to utilize only the 0.05% lidocaine formula for liposuction to decrease total lidocaine dosage and enable them to treat larger surface areas. However, 0.05% lidocaine is not as efficient as the 0.1% concentration at producing anesthesia. The authors have been using 0.075% lidocaine anesthesia in all body sites with excellent results. The 0.075% solution retains much of the anesthetic activity of the 0.1% solution, but with 25% less lidocaine, allowing larger areas to be treated in one session.

A dosage guideline of 35–50 mg/kg lidocaine, with a maximum of 55 mg/kg has been established empirically based on experience and patient side effects [4,13]. Dosages above 55 mg/kg have led to nausea and vomiting, but plasma levels in these cases did not reach toxic levels or exceed 3.5 μg/ml [14]. Lidocaine is lipophilic in nature, with a clearance rate of approximately 10 ml/kg/min. The clearance maximum (C_{max}) is 4–14 hr after infiltration [15]. Therefore the critical observation period for patients is within the first 14 hr after surgery. All patients should be accompanied by a relative or friend during this time period.

Lidocaine exists in both bound and unbound forms. In the bloodstream it binds to α1 acid glycoprotein [15]. This buffer is increased by surgery and smoking and decreased by oral hormones. Females on oral contraceptives or hormone replacement have been shown to have no increased risk of lidocaine toxicity, although theoretically they may have higher levels of unbound lidocaine present. The bioavailability of lidocaine is reduced 20% by the liposuction procedure alone [16]. Open drainage postoperatively facilitates a rapid reduction of lidocaine levels.

Lidocaine metabolism is slowed by concomitant use of drugs which inhibit the cytochrome P450 (CYP3A4) system (Table 3) [17–19]. Although no clear standard exists, it is prudent to consider temporarily discontinuing drugs which inhibit the CYP3A4 system if possible. Permission from the prescribing physician is essential. The withdrawal time period of the medications varies widely. If the medications cannot be discontinued, the lidocaine dosage should be adjusted downward accordingly or the patient should consider alternatives to surgery. Vitamin E and other herbal medications such as gingko biloba, garlic, ginger, and feverfew should be discontinued 1–2 weeks prior to surgery, as they may lead to increased bleeding [20]. In addition, older patients should have the lidocaine dosage decreased by 20% due to decreased cardiac output and subsequent decreased hepatic perfusion [15].

Epinephrine levels in the solution are usually kept at a constant. One milligram of 1:1,000 epinephrine added to a 1000-cc solution produces a concentration of 1:1,000,000. This concentration of epinephrine is most commonly used, but some surgeons have used concentrations of epinephrine as low as 1:2,000,000 with good results. Total dosage of epinephrine should be limited to a maximum of 5 mg.

Debate has occurred as to whether the tumescent anesthesia should be warmed prior to infusion. A double-blind randomized crossover study demonstrated that warming of local anesthetic solution for tumescent liposuction significantly reduces pain on infusion as perceived by the patient [21]. A randomized double-blind prospective trial of adult volunteers serving as their own controls showed that warmed buffered lidocaine was significantly less painful to infuse than plain lidocaine, buffered lidocaine, or warmed lidocaine [22].

TECHNIQUE

Tumescent anesthesia is delivered by blunt-tipped small-diameter cannulas (12–14 gauge) (Fig. 1). These are less traumatic than conventional sharp tipped needles and preserve the neurovascular structures [23]. They also minimize risk for penetrating deeper structures. In skilled hands, 18- to 20-gauge spinal needles can also be used for infusion. The authors choose this method for anesthetizing the lateral cheeks, jaw line, and jowls. Appropriate incision sites should be planned to account for the length of the liposuction cannula to be used, to provide adequate access to all treatment areas, and to facilitate draining of the tumescent fluid during the postoperative period. The surgeon can maximize the use of anatomic landmarks during this phase of the procedure, such as hiding an incision adjacent to the umbilicus, beneath the breasts, or within the lower abdomen/bikini line.

TABLE 3 Drugs Which Inhibit Cytochrome P450[a]

Generic name (Trade name)	Generic name (Trade name)
Acebutolol (Sectral)	Miconazole (Micatin)
Acetazolamide	Midazolam (Versed)
Alprazolam (Xanax)	Nadolol (Corzide)
Amiodarone (Cordarone)	Naringenin (grapefruit juice)
Anastrazole (Arimidex)	Nefazodone (Serzone)
Atenolol (Tenoretic)	Nelfinavir (Viracept)
Cannabinoids	Nevirapine (Viramune)
Carbamazepine (Tegretol)	Nicardipine (Cardene)
Cimetidine (Tagamet)	Nifedipine (Procardia)
Chloramphenicol	Omeprazole (Prilosec)
Clarithromycin (Biaxin)	Paroxetine (Paxil)
Cyclosporin (Neoral)	Pentoxifylline (Trental)
Danazol (Danocrine)	Pindolol
Dexamethasone (Decadron)	Propranolol (Inderal)
Diltiazem (Cardiazam)	Propofol (Diprivan)
Diazepam (Valium)	Quinidine (Quinaglute)
Erythromycin	Remacemide
Esmolol (Brevibloc)	Ritonavir (Norvir)
Fluconazole (Diflucan)	Saquinavir (Invirase)
Fluoxetine (Prozac)	Sertinadole
Fluvoxamine (Luvox)	Sertraline (Zoloft)
Norfluoxetine	Stiripentol
Flurazepam	Tetracycline (Achromycin, Sumycin)
Indinivir (Crixivan)	Terfenadine (Seldane; not available)
Isoniazid (Rifamate)	Thyroxine
Itraconazole (Sporanox)	Timolol (Blocadren, Cosopt, Timolide)
Ketoconazole (Nizoral)	Triazolam (Halcion)
Labetolol (Normodyne, Trandate)	Troglitazon (Rezulin)
Methadone	Troleandomycin (Tao)
Methylprednisolone (Solu-Medrol, Depo-Medrol)	Valproic Acid (Depakote)
	Verapamil (Calan)
Metroprolol (Toprol-XL)	Zafirlukast (Accolate)
Metronidazole (Flagyl)	Zileuton (Zyflo)
Mibefradil (Posicor)	

[a]Modified from Refs. 17–19.

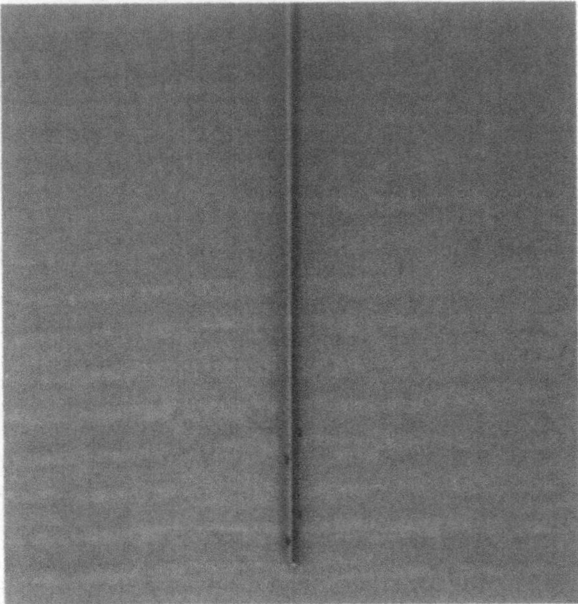

FIGURE 1 The sprinkler-tip tumescent anesthesia infusion cannula.

After marking the planned incision sites with a Sanford Sharpie fine-point permanent ink marker, the areas are anesthetized using a 30-gauge needle on a 3-mm syringe. Some physicians use buffered 1% lidocaine with epinephrine, but we prefer to use the same solution that will be used to provide tumescence. At each site, 3- to 4-mm incisions are made with a No. 11 blade, inserting the blade to an approximate 30% depth and at a 45° angle, with the sharp edge facing upward in order to avoid trauma to deeper tissues. A 1.5- to 2-mm punch biopsy tool is another alternative which may have the advantage of remaining patent longer than traditional incision sites to facilitate drainage [24]. When performed properly, the same incision sites are used for extraction of the adipose tissue and heal imperceptibly without the need for suturing. A blunt-tipped small-diameter infusion cannula is inserted, attached to the peristaltic motorized pump, pressurized infusion bag, or other delivery system (Fig. 2). The infusion rate may vary and is titrated to the comfort of the patient, most commonly less than 100 cc/min. More sensitive areas, such as the inner thighs, and small areas, like the neck and cheeks, require slower infusion as compared to the thick adipose of the abdomen. The rate of infusion may be increased proportionate to the amount of premedication given. Varying combinations of sedatives and analgesics

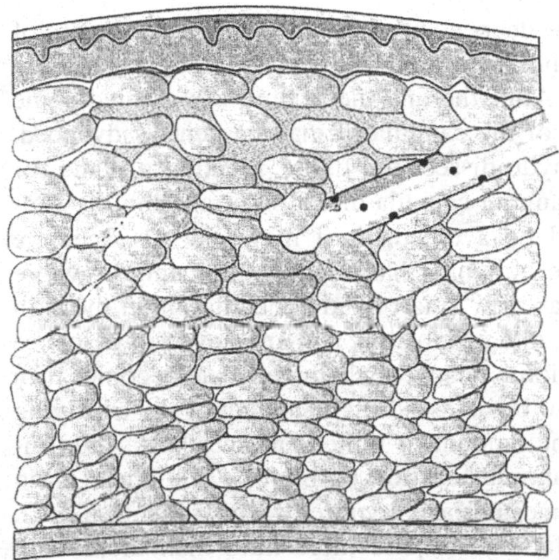

FIGURE 2 Infusion of subcutaneous tumescent anesthesia. The pink area represents anesthetic fluid hydrodissection and expansion of the adipose compartment.

are given (Table 4) [12]; however, each patient will respond to and metabolize medications at varying rates. Therefore, dosages and choice of medications used should be customized for each patient. The authors have had great success using 5–10 mg of oral diazepam 15–30 min preoperatively for comfort during liposuction.

It is best to anesthetize the areas using a fanned approach from each infusion site. This criss-crossing pattern will allow thorough anesthesia in a

TABLE 4 Commonly Used Sedatives and Analgesics

Name	Dosage
Diazepam (Valium)	5–15 mg po
Lorazepam (Ativan)	1–2 mg po
Triaxzolam (Halcion)	0.25 mg po
Hydroxyzine hydrochloride (Vistaril)	25–50 mg iv or im
Midazolam hydrochloride (Versed)	2.5–5 mg iv or im
Promethazine hydrochloride (Phenergan)	25 mg iv or im
Meperidine hydrochloride (Demerol)	25–50 mg iv or im

Source: Ref. 12.

horizontal plane. In addition the deeper and the more superficial layers of fat should be anesthetized in a similar fashion. Slow insertion of the cannula provides more patient comfort. After the anesthetic fluid has created some tumescence at the leading edge of the cannula, it may be gently advanced. The anesthetic fluid serves to hydrodissect the tissue, creating a plane for the cannula to move on [3]. Changing cannula direction or angling the cannula while in midstroke should be avoided, as it may lead to excessive discomfort. During infusion, the dominant hand guides the cannula, while the nondominant hand (known as the "smart hand") lies flat upon the skin and detects the cannula position, rate of infusion, and amount of tumescence (Fig. 3). The end-point for infusion is reached when the tissue becomes firm and indurated (Fig. 4). It can also be assessed by blanching of the overlying skin due to vasoconstriction. The amount of tumescent anesthesia fluid infiltrated will depend on the anatomic location (Table 5) [25]. There is no absolute rule as to how much anesthesia is required to fully treat an area. Areas with larger amounts of fat will require more fluid than those with small adipose layers. In addition, larger patients will require more anesthesia for a given area based on size alone. Care needs to be taken when anesthetizing critical areas such as the cheeks, as overfilling may lead to intraoral occlusion [26]. Adherence to the lidocaine maximum dosage of 55 mg/kg remains essential regardless of the body site treated.

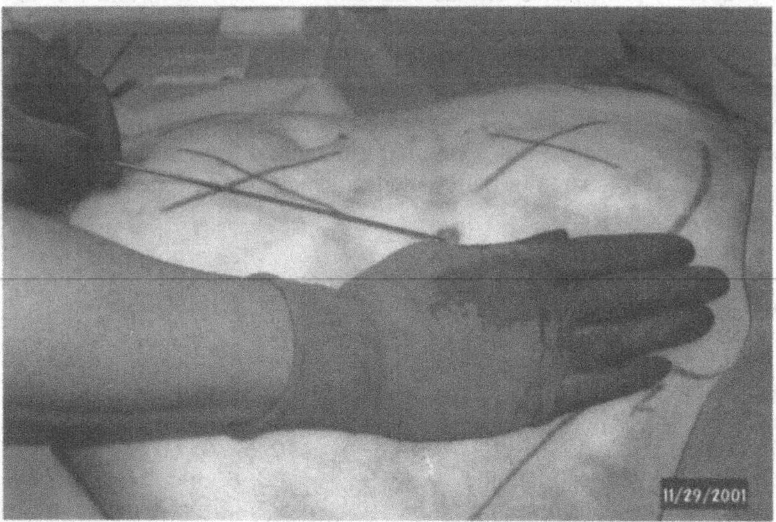

FIGURE 3 The "smart hand" is used to assess the tumescence. Note that the physician shown is left-hand dominant, therefore the smart hand is her right hand.

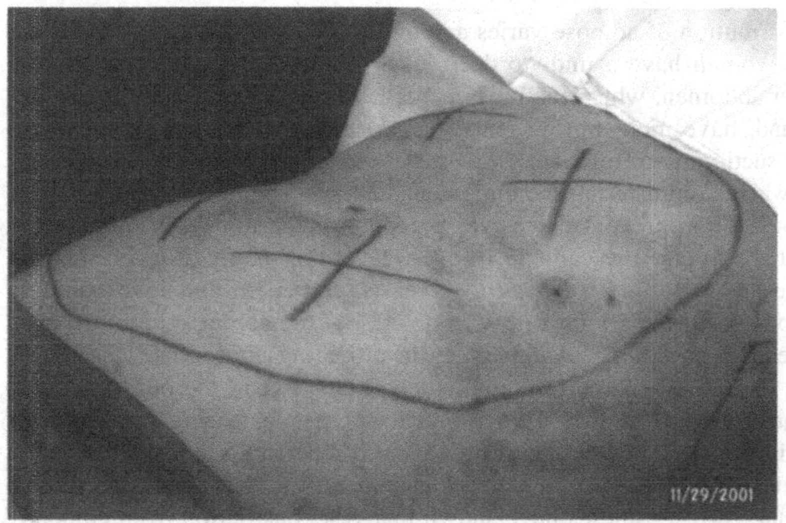

FIGURE 4 The tumesced abdomen.

TABLE 5 Approximate Volume of Anesthesia Used According to Body Site

Site	Volume (liters)
Neck	0.4
Arms	1.0/arm
Upper abdomen	0.75
Lower abdomen	1.0
Love handles	1.0/side
Flanks	0.75/side
Hips	0.75/side
Outer thighs	1.0/side
Inner thighs	0.75/side
Knees	0.5/side
Calves and ankles	1.0/side

Source: Ref. 25.

Distribution of adipose varies among body sites and between men and women. Women have a mid- to deep level of adipose tissue, especially in the lower abdomen, which requires deeper layers of anesthesia. Men, on the other hand, have more fibrous, superficial, subdermal fat that requires aggressive suctioning to remove. These differences must be taken into consideration when administering the tumescent solution. The fibrous bands within the adipose often prevent extensive spreading of the tumescent fluid, so it is essential to place the cannula in every level that is going to be treated. Sensitive areas in men, such as the breasts, abdomen, and love handles, should be anesthetized with full-strength (0.1%) tumescent solution to provide adequate anesthesia. Another key in providing appropriate anesthesia is to fill the tumesced areas approximately 2 cm beyond the borders of the diagrammed treatment area. This allows for proper feathering and blending into peripheral areas without risking patient discomfort.

After tumescence is completed it is necessary to wait for the anesthetic fluid to take effect. Studies have shown that vasoconstriction from epinephrine in the tumescent solution takes place in approximately 15 min [12]. This can be seen by blanching of the overlying skin. This is not, however, adequate time for anesthesia to occur. We have found that most sites require approximately 45 min from the start of tumescence to achieve complete anesthesia required for thorough adipose removal. Larger areas, such as the inner and outer thighs combined, may take longer.

When the anesthesia is completed, the removal of adipose may begin. Occasionally during the procedure, one may find sensitive underanesthetized areas, or "hot spots." This may be due to lack of appropriate layering of anesthesia, fibrous banding preventing spread of anesthesia, or feathering beyond the tumesced areas. If this occurs, it is appropriate to administer further anesthetic fluid and resume the suctioning in a different location until the anesthesia sets. Usually these hot spots can be treated within 10 min of adding the additional anesthesia.

DISCUSSION

Tumescent anesthesia has revolutionized the safety and efficacy of liposuction. Surgeons can and have performed small volume liposuction under strictly local, tumescent anesthesia in well-equipped, outpatient settings with an enviable safety record. The risks of fluid overload and excessive blood loss have all but vanished with the use of the tumescent-only anesthesia technique.

The proper dosage and administration of the tumescent fluid is essential to allow the physician to provide adequate yet thorough anesthesia. Studies have demonstrated and confirmed the safety of lidocaine dosages up to

55 mg/kg when tumescent anesthesia is used. For patients with complicating medical conditions or on medication which may interfere with lidocaine metabolism, lower doses of lidocaine are recommended.

In addition to its use for liposuction surgery, tumescent local anesthesia is extremely useful in other procedures where significant doses of lidocaine might be expected such as laser skin resurfacing, hair transplantation, and extensive reconstructions following Mohs Micrographic Surgery skin cancer removal. The versatility of low-concentration high-volume tumescent anesthesia has revolutionized the physician's approach to outpatient skin surgery, in particular liposuction.

REFERENCES

1. Klein JA. The tumescent technique for liposuction surgery. Am J Cosmet Surg 1987; 4:263–267.
2. Klein JA. Tumescent technique chronicles: local anesthesia, liposuction, and beyond. Dermatol Surg 1995; 21:449–457.
3. Narins RS, Coleman WP. Minimizing pain for liposuction anesthesia. Dermatol Surg 1997; 23:12:1137–1140.
4. Ostad A, Kageyama N, Moy R. Tumescent anesthesia with a lidocaine dose of 55mg/kg is safe for liposuction. Dermatol Surg 1995; 22:921–927.
5. Klein JA. Bupivicaine, prilocaine, and ropivacaine. In: Klein JA, ed. Tumescent Technique: Tumescent Anesthesia and Microcannular Liposuction. St. Louis: Mosby, 2000:179–183.
6. Fulton JE, Rahimi AD, Helton P. Modified tumescent liposuction. Dermatol Surg 1999; 25:755–766.
7. Miller MA, Shell WB. Antimicrobial properties of lidocaine on bacteria isolated from dermal lesions. Arch Dermatol 1985; 121:1157.
8. Parr AM, Zoutman DE, Davidson JSD. Antimicrobial activity of lidocaine against bacteria associated with nosocomial wound infection. Ann Plast Surg 1999; 43:239–245.
9. Kiak GA, Koontz FF, Chavez AJ. Lidocaine inhibits growth of Staphylococcus aureus in propofol. Anesthesiology 1992; 77:A407.
10. Thompson KD, Welykyj S, Massa MC. Antibacterial activity of lidocaine in combination with a bicarbonate buffer. J Dermatol Surg Oncol 1993; 19:216.
11. Klein JA. Antibacterial effects of tumescent lidocaine. Plast Reconstr Surg 1996; 104(6):1934–1936.
12. Hanke CW, Coleman WP III, Lillis PJ, Narins RS, Buenings JA, Rosemark J, Guillotte R, Lusk K, Jacobs R, Coleman WP IV. Infusion rates and levels of premedication in tumescent liposuction. Dermatol Surg 1997; 23:1131–1134.
13. Klein JA. Tumescent technique for regional anesthesia permits lidocaine doses of 35mg/kg for liposuction. J Dermatol Surg Oncol 1990; 16:248–263.
14. Klein JA. Anesthetic formulation of tumescent solutions. Dermatol Clin 1999; 12(4):751–7599.

15. Parish TD. A review: the pros and cons of tumescent anesthesia in cosmetic and reconstructive surgery. Am J Cosmet Surg 2001; 18(2):83–93.
16. Klein JA. Pharmacology of lidocaine. In: Klein JA, ed. Tumescent Technique: Tumescent Anesthesia and Microcannular Liposuction. St. Louis: Mosby, 2000: Chap. 17.
17. Shiffman M. Medication potentially causing lidocaine toxicity. Am J Cosmet Surg 1998; 15:227–229.
18. McEvoy GK, ed. AHFS Drug Information. Bethesda: American Hospital Formulary Service, 2000.
19. Gelman CR, Rumack BH, Hess AJ, eds. Drugdex System. Englewood, CO: Micromedex Inc., 2000.
20. Petry JJ. Surgically significant nutritional supplements. Plast Reconst Surg 1996; 97:233.
21. Kaplan B, Moy RL. Comparison of room temperature and warmed local anesthetic solution for tumescent liposuction: a randomized double-blind study. Dermatol Surg 1996; 22:707–709.
22. Colaric KB, Overton ST, Moore K. Pain reduction in lidocaine administration through buffering and warming. Am J Emerg Med 1998; 16:353–356.
23. Hunstad JP. Addressing difficult areas in body contouring with emphasis on combined tumescent and syringe techniques. Clin Plast Surg 1996; 23(1):57–80.
24. Klein JA. Post tumescent liposuction care. Open drainage and bimodal compression. Dermatol Clin 1999; 17(4):881–889.
25. Johnson DS, Lillis PJ, Kaminer MS. Liposuction. In: Kaminer MS, Dover JS, Arndt KA, eds. Atlas of Cosmetic Surgery. Philadelphia: WB Saunders, 2001: 202.
26. Jacob CI, Berkes BJ, Kaminer MS. Liposuction and surgical recontouring of the neck: A retrospective analysis. Dermatol Surg 2000; 26(7):625–632.

5

Liposuction: Consultation and Preoperative Considerations

Kimberly J. Butterwick
Dermatology Associates
La Jolla, California, U.S.A.

The popularity of liposuction has increased dramatically over the past decade as evidenced by statistics released by the American Academy of Cosmetic Surgery revealing a more than eightfold rise in the number of procedures performed from 1990 to 1999 [1]. The interest has grown due in large part to Klein's introduction of the tumescent technique, allowing this procedure to be performed less invasively under local anesthesia with minimal postoperative downtime and unparalleled patient safety [2,3]. Patients presenting to the office for a liposuction consult often have preconceived notions about the procedure, having heard both positive and negative reports through friends and the media [4,5]. Potential patients need education specifically regarding tumescent technique liposuction: the risks, benefits, and postoperative course, as well as a realistic appraisal of expected results. The surgeon utilizes the consultation visit to determine if the patient is mentally and physically healthy, has no contraindications to surgery, and has fatty deposits that are amenable to treatment. Once both the patient and the surgeon have adequate information, the decision to proceed can be made.

If the initial consultation is successful, a second visit is scheduled. The purpose of this second preoperative visit is to prepare for the day of surgery.

The recommended procedure is reviewed, a detailed history and physical examination are performed, and preoperative laboratory studies, prescriptions and photographs are obtained. All questions and concerns are reviewed in detail and consents are signed. The patient gains confidence in the surgeon and nursing staff by the organized and efficient process of the consultation and preoperative visits.

PATIENT SELECTION

The ideal patient is in excellent health, is not overweight, and has fatty deposits out of proportion to overall body shape. These areas are primarily genetic in origin, gender specific, and resistant to diet and exercise. Skin tone and elasticity are normal. The ideal patient is a reasonable person and has realistic expectations. The ideal age range is 30–55 years old, as this group in general is mature enough to undergo a procedure and free of underlying illness. Virtually any area in the body can now be treated with tumescent liposuction, from excessively full cheeks down to thick ankles. Additional non-cosmetic indications for liposuction include lipomas [6], angiolipomas [7], insulin-induced lipohypertrophy [8–10], post-surgical hematomas [11], axillary hyperhidrosis [12–14], chronic lymphedema [15], gynecomastia [16,17], and breast reduction [18,19].

The majority of patients vary from this ideal in some manner. The actual age of the patient is not as important as overall mental and physical health. We have performed liposuction on patients from 18 to 80 years old. Patients with mild controlled medical conditions such as diabetes or hypertension may safely undergo a limited procedure. Most patients are within 10–25 pounds of their ideal weight. However, some may be more than 20% heavier than their ideal weight yet have localized deposits of fat that would benefit from the procedure. Others may have a moderate degree of cellulite that will not improve with treatment yet may have significant underlying fatty deposits that would recontour dramatically. Older patients may have poor skin tone yet be more concerned about shape in clothing than skin laxity. They prefer the safety of tumescent liposuction to other more invasive options. These variations must be considered on an individual basis. The extent of the procedure will also determine the safety of the procedure and the ability of the patient to undergo the procedure.

Those prospective patients who are generally excluded are those with medical contraindications (Table 1), those with excessively loose skin, those with unrealistic expectations, and those who are emotionally or psychologically unstable (see also Table 5) [20,21]. The consultation and preoperative exam enable the physician to screen and choose patients who may vary from the ideal yet are suitable for the procedure.

Table 1 Medical Contraindications to Tumescent Liposculpture

Severe cardiovascular or renal disease
Severe coagulation disorders
Active hepatitis or chronic liver failure
Active cancer
Morbid obesity
Major immunosuppression
Pregnancy
History of malignant hyperthermia

CONSULTATION

Role of Consultant

In our practice, the surgeon is involved in several steps of the consultation process but a nurse consultant is also utilized. This not only saves the surgeon's time but also may enhance communication with the patient. The nurse selected for this consultant function should be personable, patient, and perceptive. It is helpful if he/she has had the procedure in order to answer questions in a personal and honest manner. Patients may feel more comfortable with the nurse than the surgeon and may reveal more information than might otherwise be obtained. For example, a patient may tell the nurse of a prior eating disorder and neglect to mention this to the surgeon.

Before the surgeon enters the room, several steps of the consultation are performed by the consultant (Table 2) and entered on the consultation form (Appendix 1):

1. Education about the procedure: The education process can be started before the patient enters the office by having an informational packet, brochure, or video mailed to the patient. Alterna-

Table 2 Role of the Consultant

Education
Health and medication history
Weight
Chief complaint
Review "before" and "after" photographs
Polaroid or digital photographs
Closing

tively, this material may be presented to the patient when they check in. The nurse-consultant then reviews information regarding the procedure and postoperative healing at length.

2. Health and medication screen: A health questionnaire is filled out by the patient in the waiting area. The consultant confirms the responses with the patient and records significant history on the consultation form. A detailed medication history is obtained, including vitamins and over-the-counter, and herbal formulations. Vital signs and weight are recorded. On occasion, previously undetected hypertension has been discovered.
3. Weight history: It is important to determine if the patient's weight has been stable over the past several years. The patient may find this discussion embarrassing with the surgeon but less so with the nurse. Diet and exercise habits are also reviewed. Counseling regarding diet after surgery and when to resume exercise after surgery is given.
4. Determination of the chief complaint/the patient's main area(s) of concern: The patient may be unsure which area is most problematic. They may be vague and want "everything from the neck down." A discussion of clothing size and fitting difficulties may help. Other patients may be afraid that the surgeon will suggest too many areas. The consultant asks if the patient would like the surgeon to suggest other potential treatment areas or to simply focus on the patient's main concern.
5. Review of before and after photographs: The consultant and patient review albums of "before" and "after" photographs with particular attention to those areas pertinent to the patient's concerns. It is important to show not only your best results and most attractive patients but the full spectrum of body types and results. The patient thereby gains a better idea of the type of results that can be reasonably expected. Photographs of patients who have had liposuction with subsequent weight loss or gain can also be shown. Photographs of the small liposuction incision sites can be reassuring as patients often fear scarring. Persistence of cellulite and striae can be demonstrated as well.
6. Polaroid or digital photographs of the patient: These images are used by the surgeon to clarify the recommended areas for treatment and to demonstrate expected results.

Role of Surgeon

The next part of the consultation involves direct interaction between the patient and the surgeon. It is an important time in which to establish rapport with the patient and develop reasonable confidence in one another in a short period of time. A few minutes can be devoted to social conversation to assess the patient's friendliness and social skills. Much of this process is a review of the information the consultant has gathered. One can look for consistency in the patient's answers to determine if the history is reliable. The patient's concerns and fears are revealed by observing the kinds of questions which are repeated. These fears need to be addressed in order for the patient to feel secure enough to undergo a procedure.

Medical and Surgical History

The surgeon must first verify the medical history to assure that there are no contraindications to surgery (Table 1). If the patient has one of these contraindications, there is no need to finish the consultation and raise the patient's hopes. Patients are preferably American Surgical Association (ASA) surgical risk Class I and sometimes Class II (Table 3) [22]. If there is an underlying medical condition, the primary care physician is later contacted for medical clearance once the patient has decided to have the procedure. It is important to screen for prior liver disease because adequate liver function is necessary for lidocaine metabolism [23]. Patients who are positive for hepatitis C but are otherwise healthy must be approached with caution due to potentially compromised immune and liver function. Similarly, HIV-positive patients who are otherwise healthy may have compromised liver function and unpredictable metabolism of lidocaine independent of antiviral therapy [24]. Patients who have undergone chemotherapy may have an altered ability to metabolize lidocaine even with normal liver function tests, as reported in one case of lidocaine toxicity which occurred up to 2 years after chemotherapy [25].

Screening for other conditions is also necessary. Immuonocompromised patients have an increased risk of infection and delayed wound healing and are poor candidates. Attention must also be given to identify risk factors for thromboembolism, including prior history of thrombophlebitis, thrombophilia or thromboembolism, high-dose estrogen therapy, obesity,

TABLE 3 ASA Surgical Risk Classifications

I. Normal healthy patients
II. Mild sytematic disease and no functional limitation
III. Moderate to severe disease that results in some functional limitation
IV. Severe systematic disease that is a constant threat to life and functionally incapacitating
V. Moribund and not expected to survive 24 hr with or without surgery

varicose veins, immobilization, and positive smoking history [26–28]. Such patients will require medical clearance before surgery. All allergies and intolerances need to be noted, including lidocaine, epinephrine, antibiotics, analgesics, soaps, ointments, and tape. An obstetric history is helpful in patients considering abdominal liposuction. Multiple pregnancies may signal weak abdominal musculature and the need for alternative procedures.

A surgical history is helpful to screen for poor wound healing, a tendency for keloids or hypertrophic scarring, infectious complications, and bleeding diatheses. A history of prior dental and cosmetic surgeries is included. This furthur screens for the patient's ability to tolerate procedures and postoperative pain. If the patient is excessively critical of prior procedures and surgeons, he or she may never be satisfied with another procedure. Patients who have undergone recent abdominal surgery should wait 6 months or longer before having a procedure in that area. Multiple abdominal surgeries may compromise results in that region through muscle laxity or adherent scarring.

Medications

A careful history of medication use is essential and includes prescription, over-the-counter, and herbal remedies. Anticoagulant therapy with warfarin is a contraindication for surgery. Medications containing aspirin and nonsteroidal anti-inflammatory agents are commonly discontinued 2 weeks prior to surgery to minimize intraoperative bleeding and bruising. A list of common medications containing these agents is given to the patient at the preoperative visit (Appendix 2). Some vitamins and herbal formulations should also be discontinued prior to surgery. These include vitamin E and the four Gs—ginko, ginseng, garlic, and ginger [29]. Feverfew used for migraines should also be avoided. These formulas affect clotting through different pathways and may increase bleeding.

Attention must also be given to medications that are metabolized by the liver's cytochrome P450 3A4(CYP34A) enzyme system as these potentially interfere with lidocaine metabolism [30–32]. These include some common antidepressants, antifungals, antivirals, and antibiotics (Table 4). Lidocaine is rapidly and almost exclusively eliminated by the P450 system [30]. Medications that are inhibitors of this enzyme may compete with lidocaine, leading to a potential rise in lidocaine blood levels. Toxic levels of lidocaine most likely due to such drug interactions have been reported [33]. Our patients are instructed to discontinue these medications 2 weeks prior to surgery after checking with the prescribing physician. Some may need to taper off over a longer period as recommended by their physician. For patients discontinuing antidepressant therapy, lorazepam (1 mg qhs) may be prescribed for 1 week prior to surgery. With this, patients have not had

TABLE 4 Medications Potentially Affecting Lidocaine Metabolism

Medication
Acebutolol
Alprazolam (Xanax)
Amiodarone (Cordarone)
Amitriptyline (Elavil)
Amprenavir (Agenerase)
Atenolol
Carbamazepine (Tegretol, atretol)
Chloramphenicol (Chloromycetin)
Cimetidine (Tagamet)
Clarithromycin (Biaxin)
Clomipramine (Anafranil)
Clozepine (Clozeril)
Cyclosporin (Neoral, Sandimmune)
Danazol (Danocrine)
Delavirdine (Rescriptor)
Dexamethasone (Decadron)
Diltiazam (Cardizem)
Divalproex (Depakote)
Efavirenz (Sustiva)
Erythromycin
Esmobolol (Brevibloc)
Ethinylestradiol
Felodipine (Plendil)
Flucanazole (Diflucan)
Fluoxetine (Prozac)
Flurazepam (Dalmane)
Fluvoxamine (Luvox)
Indimavir (Crixivan)
Isoniazid (Nydrazid, Rifanate, Rifater)
Itraconazole (Sporanox)
Ketoconazole (Nizoral)
Labetalol (Normodyne, Trandate)
Methadone (Dolophine)
Methylprednisolone (Medrol)
Metoprolol (Lopressor)
Metronidazole (Flagyl)
Miconazole (Monistat)
Midazolam (Versed)
Nadolol (Corgard, Corzide)
Nefazodone (Serzone)
Nelfinavir (Viracept)
Nicardipine (Cardene)
Nifedipine (Procardia, Adalat)
Paroxetine (Paxil)
Pimozide (Orap)
Pindolol (Visken)
Prednisone
Propafenone (Rythmol)
Propofol (Diprivan)
Propranolol (Inderal)
Quinidine
Quinaglute (Quinidex)
Ritonavir (Norvir)
Sertraline (Zoloft)
SSRI antidepressants
Tamoxifen (Nolvadex)
Tetracycline
Thyroxine
Timolol (Timolide, Timoptic)
Triazolam (Halcion)
Valproic Acid (Depakene)
Verapamil (Calan, Isoptin, Verelan)

difficulty tolerating the interruption in therapy. Alternatively, lower doses of lidocaine (<35 mg/kg) may be given for those patients unable to interrupt therapy. More than one treatment session may then be necessary.

Weight, Diet, and Exercise History

It is important that the patient's weight has been stable for several months prior to surgery. It is helpful to know the lowest and highest weight the patient has had in the past 5 years. Patients with patterns of progressive weight gain will most likely gain weight after surgery and have suboptimal results. Patients who have lost large amounts of fat in a short span of time will have very loose skin and are poor candidates for surgery (Fig. 1). Extreme fluctuations of weight or a reluctance to discuss weight may signal a history of an eating disorder. This needs to be explored with the patient.

Approximately 50% of liposuction patients are overweight according to some estimates [34], but are still excellent candidates for the procedure because of localized disproportionate fatty deposits. Many ask if they should diet before or after surgery. If the weight fluctuates by 10–20 pounds, it is best to perform liposuction at the high end of the weight range. The patient will then only improve when the weight fluctuates downward within that range. Some overweight patients may choose to use liposuction as a reward for losing part of the necessary weight. Others may choose to have liposuction first, as motivation, because they are frustrated by failed weight loss attempts in the past.

An exercise history will reveal the patient's commitment to health and his or her physical endurance. It is best to start sedentary patients on a program of walking prior to surgery and in the postoperative period, as this will speed recovery and optimize results. Some patients are professional

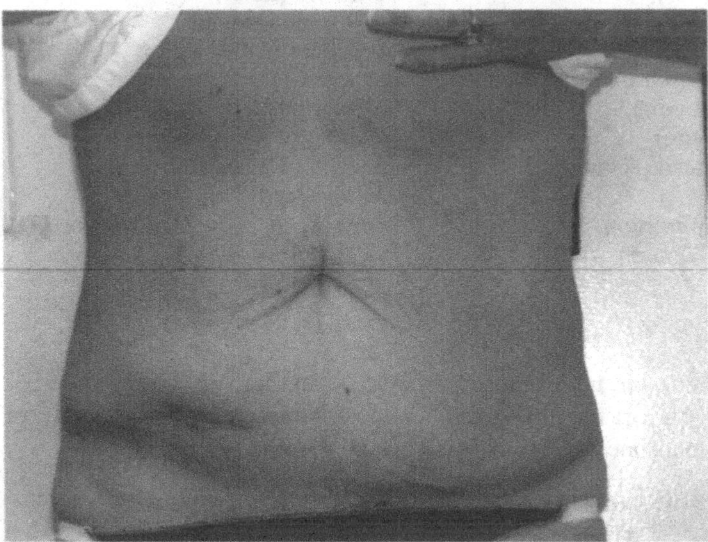

FIGURE 1 A patient with 80-pound weight loss in 1 year and excessively loose skin is a poor candidate for liposuction.

athletes or trainers or daily exercise enthusiasts and will need to be counseled as to how long to limit strenuous exercise and full range of motion.

This point in the consultation is an opportunity to emphasize the importance of weight maintenance postoperatively for optimal long-term results. Counseling regarding diet and exercise may be offered either through the office or an outside source. Although patients lose little weight with the procedure, the body-fat percentage is generally lower after liposuction and the basal metabolic rate (calories burned at rest) increases [35].

Psychosocial History

Patients must have realistic goals and appropriate reasons for undergoing treatment. Does the patient understand that this is not a technique for weight loss? Will the patient's body type and weight accommodate their goals? Are they pursuing treatment to please themselves or someone else? At times there is a controlling partner or a critical parent who is driving the request for treatment. Does the patient think liposuction will solve personal problems or emotional unrest? Patient maturity and ability to undergo a procedure are other factors to consider. A teenager who has never experienced surgical or medical procedures would most likely have difficulty conquering fears and tolerating the procedure. Certain personality traits and disorders have been suggested to correlate with dissatisfied patients (Table 5) [36–39].

A job history will help direct postoperative counseling. Someone with a sedentary job may return to work in 2 to 3 days. Others with physically demanding jobs undergoing more extensive liposuction may be most comfortable taking several days off.

Physical Examination

The physical examination of the potential areas to be treated typically begins with the patient's main area of concern. Although the entire body should be

Table 5 Traits of Potential Problem Patients

Unrealistic expectations
Highly critical of prior physicians or procedures
Perfectionists
Rude, demanding, and/or uncooperative to staff
Depressed, unhappy patients
Angry, hostile patients
Eating disorders
Body dysmorphic disorder

viewed, patients should be initially dressed in an examination gown and underclothing, and only the main area is viewed. Every attempt should be made to preserve dignity. Patients find this part of the consult most humiliating; they have often been concealing these bulges for years. A comment of empathy from the surgeon will put them at ease.

Patients should be standing and the dysmorphic bulge gently pinched between the thumb and forefinger to assess the volume of subcutaneous fat. Patients may be asked to contract muscles to better localize fat deposits, particularly in the abdomen and buttock/outer thigh areas. On occasion, the abdominal fat is primarily intra-abdominal or the outer thigh bulge is created by lax buttock muscles. Adjacent areas should then be examined. Overlying skin should be checked for tone, elasticity, striae, and cellulite. These irregularities should be pointed out to the patient during the examination. The patient needs clear understanding that these irregularities will not improve. Scars should be noted and palpated for adherence. Valsalva maneuvers will aide in checking for abdominal hernias.

The entire body should then be viewed for overall shape and symmetry. The spinal curvature should be examined for scoliosis or other deformities. Asymmetries are most likely skeletal or muscular in origin and should be brought to the patient's attention. There may be areas that are out of proportion adjacent to or distant from the patient's main area of concern. If treating only one area would cause aesthetic disproportion, it is appropriate to point that out to the patient. For example, if the patient's concern is the hip bulge and the outer thigh area also protrudes, treating only the hips would make the outer thigh appear larger and clothing would not fit well (Fig. 2). With the patient's permission, other distant areas that would benefit from the procedure may be suggested and examined at this time.

Recommendations for Surgery

The decision regarding which areas to treat can be made while reviewing the photographs taken by the consultant. The photographs effectively communicate irregularities and asymmetries, as well as posterior and lateral views, which are difficult for the patient to observe in a mirror. The decision depends not only on the body shape, but also on the patient's personal desires. A felt-tipped pen is used to draw on the photographs and demonstrate the expected change in contour (Fig. 3). Consideration needs to be given to how many areas can be safely treated at one time and how many procedures are required. If finances are a concern and only one procedure is feasible, those areas which will change most dramatically should be chosen. No single procedure should leave a body in greater disproportion, even if other procedures are planned. The overall goal is, of course, an optimal three-dimensional result for the patient.

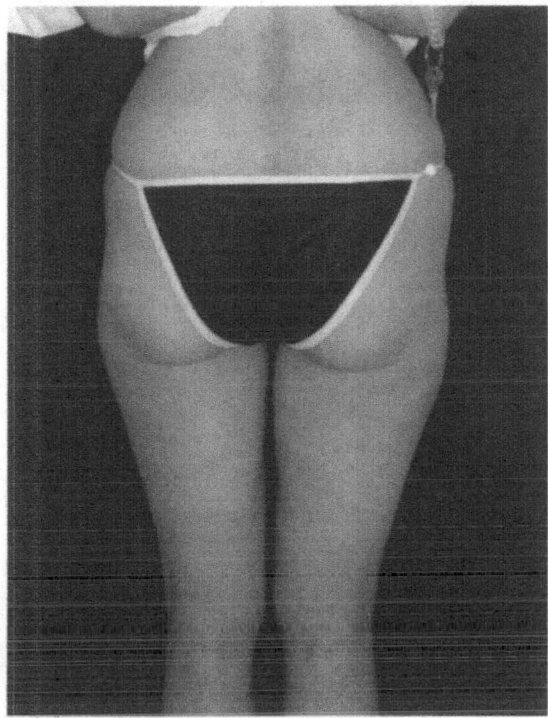

FIGURE 2 Patient's main concern is her large hips but liposuction of only that area would cause disproportion and make outer thighs appear larger.

Overview

At this point in the consultation, the surgeon has determined whether the patient is a suitable candidate for surgery. If the surgeon cannot achieve the patient's goals, the reasons must be explained, whether for health or physical restraints or limitations of the procedure. This can be difficult for unrealistic patients or those seeking perfection. However, most patients understand the explanation suggested by Jeff Klein, "I do not believe I have the skill to achieve the results that you desire, and therefore it would be unethical and inappropriate for me to attempt to do your liposuction surgery" [40].

Those patients who are appropriate candidates for surgery need more information in order to proceed. The consultant has educated them about the procedure and postoperative course, but this should be briefly reviewed by the surgeon. Although redundant, patients are comforted when the surgeon provides the same consistent information. The risks in general need to be discussed, but a detailed discussion of every risk can occur later at the

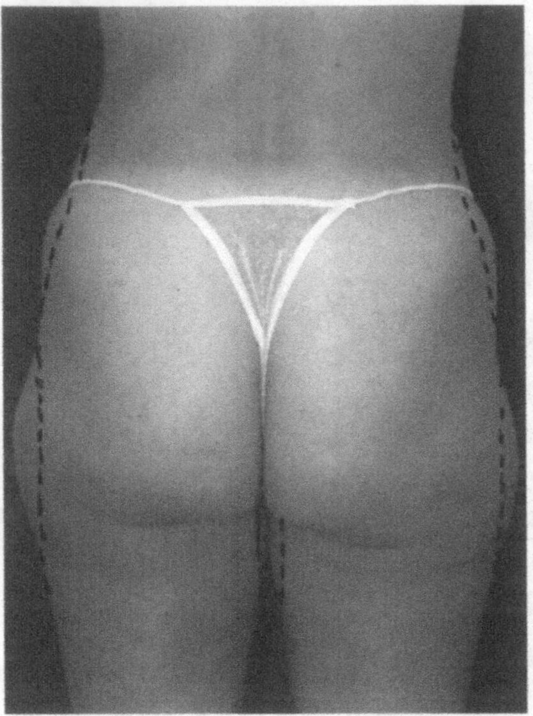

FIGURE 3 Patient's photograph taken at consultation with dotted line to demonstrate expected results.

preoperative exam. The risks and complications typically reviewed with the patient at the consultation include infection, temporary dysesthesia, prolonged induration, and the rare risk of thromboembolism. The potential for a touch-up procedure is discussed. The patient is given the informed consents to read thoroughly at home. The benefits have already been demonstrated by the photographs but any limitations should be underscored. The surgeon should emphasize improvement, not perfection, as the goal. Alternatives, both surgical and dietary are discussed. The patient is given the opportunity to have any further questions answered before this segment of the consultation is complete.

Closing the Consultation

After the patient dresses, the consultant reviews the proposed procedure. Since there may be confusion with terminology of anatomic areas, the areas to be treated are listed and drawn on the consultation diagram. The fees and payment arrangements are written on a fee quote and a copy is reviewed and given to the patient. The next steps, scheduling the procedure and a preoperative examination, can be done at this time or later for patients wanting more time to make a decision. The consultant has established a relationship with the patient and is a liaison for patients having questions or calling to schedule at a later date. Those patients calling with multiple questions may be invited for a second consultation with the surgeon. These types of patients usually become committed to the procedure once they feel thoroughly educated.

PREOPERATIVE EXAM

The purpose of the preoperative examination is to prepare for the day of surgery. Unlike the consultation, all patients coming for the preoperative exam have decided to have the procedure. They have been given the consents and information packets ahead of time, but surprisingly many patients prefer not to think about their procedure and do not read the information. This visit will assure that they are ready for their procedure.

In our office, the preoperative exam is performed by a trained nurse practitioner or registered nurse. The recommended procedure is reviewed. Next a detailed general history and physical exam is performed (Appendix 3). If the surgeon has noted unusual medical circumstances on the consultation form, these are addressed. For example, if the physician has noted that the patient is on Zoloft, the nurse practitioner will make sure the patient has contacted his or her therapist and is able to discontinue his or her medication. If the surgeon has indicated that he or she needs to speak directly with the patient's internist, he or she is given a reminder card with the phone number.

Particular attention is given to medications which affect clotting and should be avoided before surgery. The list of common agents is again presented to the patient (Appendix 2). Patients are further reminded to avoid alcohol, tobacco, and medications metabolized by the cytochrome P450 system. Any new medications prescribed since the consultation visit are identified. To reduce cardiac stimulation, thyroid replacement therapy (synthroid) and pseudoephedrine are stopped 3 days before the procedure. Caffeine is avoided on the morning of surgery. Appetite suppressants should also be discontinued gradually, 2 weeks prior to surgery, as per the prescribing physician.

Preoperative prescriptions are written: Duricef 500 mg bid × 7 days starting the day before surgery and Minocycline 100 mg qd × 7 days for penicillin allergic patients. Mephyton 5 mg bid × 10 days prior to surgery is also recommended to minimize bruising. Some patients are intolerant of mephyton (flushing and headaches) and are given arnica as an alternative [41]. For anxious patients, lorazepam 1 mg is prescribed for the night before and/or the morning of the procedure. Detailed preoperative and postoperative instructions in the patient's packet are reviewed verbally at this time (Appendices 4 and 5). In particular, patients need to be reminded that they cannot drive home and need to have someone stay with them the first 24 hr. Informed consents are reviewed point by point and signed by the patient (Appendix 6). If the patient has any unanswered questions regarding the consent, he or she will have the opportunity to discuss the issue with the physician. Informed consent typically includes the following elements: benefits expected, risks of the procedure, alternate treatment options, opportunity to discuss the procedure with the physician, and authorization for the physician to perform the procedure. Consents for laboratory studies, photographs, and observing physicians are also signed (Appendix 7).

Preoperative laboratory studies for most liposuction procedures include a complete blood cell count with differential and platelet count, chemistry panel, prothrombin and partial thromboplastin time, serum pregnancy test, and serologies for hepatitis B and C and HIV [42]. The results are reviewed by the surgeon preferably 2 weeks prior to surgery and any abnormalities are addressed. An electrocardiogram is ordered for patients over the age of 60. Preoperative photographs are obtained with every attempt to achieve consistent distance and background. Patients usually wear modesty panties or bathing suits for the photographs. Baseline measurements may be obtained at this time, including weight, percentage body fat, and circumferential measurements. These are later presented to the patient at the 3- to 6-month postoperative visit along with a preoperative photograph to reinforce the positive changes and the importance of a healthy lifestyle.

A final checklist (Appendix 8) and assurances are given to the patient. On the day of surgery, all that is needed is for the patient to arrive on time. The date, time, and directions to the surgicenter are provided.

SUMMARY

The consultation and preoperative examination are crucial for a successful liposuction practice. The professionalism and friendliness of the surgeon and staff will earn the patient's trust. It is a time to demonstrate competency, attention to detail, a caring attitude, and honesty. An organized, efficient, and consistent process will assure proper patient selection, optimal safety, and a procedure that is eagerly anticipated by the patient.

APPENDIX 1

Liposculpture Consultation

NAME: ____________________ AGE: ________ DATE: ____________

REFERRED BY: ______________________________

Summary of Pertinent Patient Information

VS: BP ______ P ______ T ______

Weight: ______________

Medications: ______________
(Include OTC)

Allergies: ______________

Medical History: ______________

Pregnancies: ______________

Previous surgery: ______________

Complications: ______________

Previous liposculpture: ______________

Tendency to bruise or bleed: ______________

Area(s) of Concern: ______________

Weight changes in past 5 years: ____

Current diet and exercise: ______________

Psychosocial:

☐ Pre- & post-op instructions and photos reviewed. Educational materials given to patient

R L L R

Assessment: ______________

Plan:

☐ Liposculpture of ______________

☐ Realistic benefits reviewed:

☐ Scars, skin irregularities and asymmetries noted: ______________

☐ General risks reviewed including infection, dysesthesia, induration and irregularities.

☐ Pre-op meds: Usual ☐

Changes: ______________

☐ Unusual medical/surgical circumstances:

☐ Fee quote

APPENDIX 2

Medication Precautions

INSTRUCTIONS TO FOLLOW BEFORE & AFTER YOUR SURGERY

- If you are on medication for arthritis, circulation, or anticoagulation (i.e., Baby Aspirin, Motrin, Naprosyn, Persantine or Coumadin), please inform us.
- For a two week period prior to and 5 days after the scheduled date of your surgery, please do not take any medication that contains aspirin or aspirin-related products such as ibuprofen (Motrin, Advil) as an ingredient. Aspirin has an effect on your blood's ability to clot and could increase your tendency to bleed at the time of surgery and during the post-operative period.
- If you have a cold or sinus condition, please be sure to avoid pseudoephedrine 3 days prior to surgery. Check bottle for ingredients.
- Please check the labels of all medications that you take, even those available without a prescription to make sure you are not taking any aspirin or aspirin-like substances.
- Please consult your physician before stopping any prescribed medication.

THE FOLLOWING IS A LIST OF COMMON MEDICATIONS & SUBSTANCES THAT CAN INCREASE TENDENCY TO BLEED:

Adprin
Advil
Alcohol
Aleve
Alka-Seltzer/Plus/cold
Anacin
Anaprox
Anaproxin
APC
Arthritis Pain Formula
Arthrotic
Ascriptin
Aspergum
Asprimax
Aspirin in any form (tablet, suppository, chewable)
Azdone
Backache maximum relief
Bayer Aspirin
Bayer
BC Powder
BC Sinus
Bufferin Tablets & Caplets
Buffex
Butalbital Compound
Cama Arthritis Pain Reliever
Celebrex
Cephalgesic
Cheracol Capsules
Clinoril
Congesprin
Cope
Coumadin
Damason P
Darvon, Darvon N with ASA
Daypro
Dipyridamole
Dolobid
Doan's caplets
Dristan
Easpirin
Ecotrin
Empirin, Empirin w/Codeine
Emprazil
Equagesic Tablets
Excedrin Tablets & Caplets
Femback
Feverfew
Feldene
Fiorinal, Fiorinal with Codeine
4 Way Cold Tablets
Garlic Capsules
Gelpirin Tablets
Genpril
Genprin
Ginger Tablets
Ginko biloba
Ginseng
Goody's Headache Powders
Halfprin
Haltran
Heartline
Ibuprofen
Indocin
Indomethacin
Lodine
Lortab ASA Tablet
Magnaprin
Meclomen
Medipren
Menadol
Meprobamate & Aspirin Tablets
Methocarbamol & Aspirin Tablets
Midol
Mobigesic
Momentum Muscular Backache Formula
Motrin
Nalfon
Naprosyn
Norgesic, Norgesic Forte Tablets
Norwich
Nuprin
Orudis
Oxycodone with Aspirin Tablets
Pamprin
PAC Analgesic Tablets
Percodan
Phenaphen
Ponstel
Propoxyphene
Quagisic
Rhinocaps
Robaxisal
Roxiprin Tablets
Rufin
Saleto Tablets
Scott-Tussin Cold Formula
Sine-Aid
Soma Compound w/Codeine
St. Joseph's Aspirin
Summit Extra Strength Caps
Talwin
Ticlid
Toradol
Trandate
Trental
Trigesic
Trilisate
Ursinus Inlay Tabs
Vanquish
Vick's Day Quil
Vioxx
Vitamin E
Voltaren
Zactrin
Zorprin

If you need pain medication, please take acetaminophen (Tylenol) or another non-aspirin medication. Tylenol or Anacin-3 are available at your local pharmacy without a prescription and have comparable pain relief potential to that of aspirin. If you are allergic to acetaminophen (Tylenol) or unable to take it for other reasons, please notify us so that we might arrange for a substitute.

APPENDIX 3

Preoperative History and Physical

PATIENT: ______ AGE: ______ SEX: ______ DATE: ______

CHIEF COMPLAINT/HISTORY OF PRESENT ILLNESS: ______

______

PAST MEDICAL AND SURGICAL HISTORY: ______

MEDICATIONS: ______

DRUG ALLERGIES: YES NO

FAMILY MEDICAL HISTORY: ______

______

SOCIAL HISTORY/HABITS: ☐ ALCOHOL USAGE ☐ SMOKES

Review of systems positive for:

- ☐ Fever bisters
- ☐ Migraine headaches
- ☐ Heart trouble
- ☐ Irregular heartbeat
- ☐ Abnormal EKG
- ☐ High blood pressure
- ☐ Asthma or lung problems
- ☐ Indigestion or ulcers
- ☐ Hepatitis or liver disease
- ☐ Abnormal hernias
- ☐ Malignant hyperthermia—patient
- ☐ Malignant hyperthermia—family
- ☐ Kidney problems
- ☐ Seizures or neurologic problems
- ☐ Psychiatric problems
- ☐ Diabetes or thyroid disease
- ☐ Lightheadedness or easy fainting
- ☐ Bleeding tendency or bruising
- ☐ Blood clots in legs, lungs or body
- ☐ Arthritis or back trouble
- ☐ Excessive scarring or abnormal healing
- ☐ Recurrent or chronic infections
- ☐ Reactions to anesthesia
- ☐ Bleeding tendencies
- ☐ Other (explain): ______
- ☐ None of the above

TEMP: ______ BP: ______ PULSE: ______ RESP: ______

PHYSICAL EXAMINATION:	NORMAL	ABNORMAL	FINDINGS
Skin	☐	☐	______
Heent	☐	☐	______
Heart	☐	☐	______
Lungs	☐	☐	______
Abdomen	☐	☐	______
Extremities	☐	☐	______
Neurological	☐	☐	______
Mental Status	☐	☐	______

BASELINE DATA:

WEIGHT: ______ PERCENT BODY FAT: ______

PERTINENT MEASUREMENTS: ______

DIAGNOSIS: ______

______

PLAN: ______

______

INFORMED CONSENT OBTAINED INCLUDING REVIEW OF BLEEDING PERFORATION INFECTION AND ADVERSE MEDICINE REACTION

DATE: ______ SIGNATURE: ______, M.D.

DATE: ______ SIGNATURE: ______, RN

APPENDIX 4

BEFORE Liposculpture Instruction Sheet

MEDICATIONS:

- Do not take products containing Aspirin, Ibuprofen (Advil or Motrin), Naprosyn (Aleve), Vitamin E, or any medication containing these drugs for 1 to 2 weeks before and after surgery as they will promote bleeding and bruising. You may take Tylenol for mild discomfort.
- Stop taking Synthroid or other medications for low thyroid 72 hours before the procedure.
- ANTIDEPRESSANTS; DO NOT TAKE ANTIDEPRESSANTS such as Zoloft for two weeks before surgery unless they have been pre-approved by your surgeon
- Other medications to avoid 1–2 weeks before surgery: decongestants with pseudoephedrine, diet pills and herbal formulas.
- Alcohol and tobacco—avoid for one week before and one week after surgery.
- Be sure to fill all prescriptions BEFORE surgery. Start Mephyton (VITAMIN K) 5 to 10 days before the procedure as directed and your antibiotic the night before.

CLEANSING AND CLOTHING:

- Please shower using Hibiclens the day before and the morning of surgery.
- Purchase additional absorbent padding: Super Kotex pads or Poise pads.
- There is usually quite a lot of drainage of slightly blood-tinged anesthetic solution after surgery that may stain clothing. We suggest you choose clothing that is machine washable, loose and comfortable in order to accommodate the bulky dressings that we place after surgery.
- WOMEN: Please choose a comfortable bra that you would not mind getting stained. MEN: Please choose jockey underwear or Speedo-type swim trunks (rather than boxers) which you will wear during the procedure.
- Please wear no unnecessary jewelry and no perfume, only the minimum of cosmetics (survival rations only), and no body moisturizers on the day of surgery (deodorant is okay). Do not bring valuables such as wallets and purses. Do not wear contact lenses.
- Because the operating room is relatively cool, you may be more comfortable wearing warm socks and/or mittens. You are welcome to bring them with you to wear during surgery.

OTHER PREPARATIONS:

- Arrange to have someone drive you home after surgery. It is suggested that someone stay with you the first night after surgery. Bring a towel to sit on in the car for the ride home.
- Protect your bed and chairs from drainage stains by covering them with towels placed over a plastic sheet. If you prefer, you may purchase plastic-lined disposable pads at any drug store.
- Music: We usually play soft music during the surgery. If you have any favorite CD's, please bring them with you. Be sure they are labeled with your name.
- Diet before surgery: If your surgery is scheduled in the morning, do not eat solid foods after midnight prior to surgery. If your surgery is scheduled in the afternoon, you may have a light breakfast but only clear liquids for lunch. Please avoid caffeine the day of surgery. We will provide you with juice and a snack after surgery.
- Please feel free to call our nurse with any questions.

APPENDIX 5

AFTER Liposculpture Instruction Sheet

ACTIVITIES:

- Plan to rest in bed immediately after surgery. Later in the day a short walk is permitted.
- The day after surgery you may resume normal light daily activities such as driving and walking.
- You may resume light exercise 3 to 4 days after surgery and vigorous physical activities (such as jogging and tennis) 2 to 3 weeks after surgery as tolerated. Resume exercise gradually.
- Depending on the extent of your surgery, you will feel well enough to return to a desk job within 1 to 3 days after surgery.

ELASTIC SUPPORT GARMENT:

- After liposculpture, elastic support garments are worn to promote drainage and prevent accumulation of fluid within the tunnels created by the removal of fat. You must wear these garments continuously (24 hours a day) except for showering for 3–7 days as instructed by your surgeon.
- If you have foam or tape in place, you must sponge bathe rather than shower. We will instruct you when and how to remove the foam or tape.

- After the first week it is suggested that a lighter elastic garment be worn 8 to 10 hours per day for one month. It offers support during movement and most patients prefer daytime use.

WOUND CARE AND DRAINAGE:

- A large amount of drainage from the small incisions is normal during the first 24 to 48 hours following liposculpture. The slightly blood-tinged fluid is residual anesthetic solution. In general, the more drainage there is, the less bruising and swelling there will be. Most drainage occurs the first 48 hours. You may have a small amount for up to one week.
- Beginning the day after surgery, wash the incisions with soap and water and apply antibiotic ointment twice daily.
- You should have some absorbent pads available (Kotex or Poise pads) so you can change your dressings as they become saturated.
- DO NOT cover the incisions with Band-Aids or occlude the drainage in any way.

DISCOMFORT AND BRUISING:

- The soreness is the worst about 24 hours after surgery and then improves almost daily.
- For relief of soreness and inflammation, take 2 extra-strength Tylenol every 4–6 hours while awake for the first 48 hours.
- If Tylenol is ineffective, you may take the prescription strength pain reliever we have given you (Vicodan, Darvocette, etc.).
- With the Tumescent Technique, most patients experience remarkably little bruising. Nevertheless, some patients have mild to moderate bruising, lasting 1–2 weeks.
- Swelling may actually increase 5–10 days after surgery and is treated with Advil or Aspirin.

MEDICATIONS:

- Take the full dose of oral antibiotics as prescribed.
- DO NOT TAKE ASPIRIN OR IBUPROFEN, OR MEDICATIONS THAT CONTAIN THESE DRUGS FOR 5 DAYS AFTER SURGERY, AS THEY CAN PROMOTE BLEEDING (SEE THE MEDICATION PRECAUTION SHEET).

BATHING:

- It is preferable to shower rather than bathe for 7 days after surgery.
- CAUTION: When garments are removed the first few days after surgery, patients may feel dizzy. Avoid this by removing the garments lying down,

then sit on the edge of the bed a few minutes, stand-up slowly. Lie back down after showering to redress.

- When showering, you may briefly get the incision sites wet. Afterwards, gently pat them dry and apply antibiotic ointment.
- Do not immerse in a bath, jacuzzi, swimming pool or the ocean until the incisions have healed completely (about 1 week).

DIET:

- After surgery, drinking generous amounts of fruit juices or water will prevent dehydration.
- Light foods are recommended for the first meal after surgery (sorry, no alcohol or caffeine). You may resume your usual diet in about 4 hours. Avoid salty foods (to minimize swelling) and high fiber foods (that may cause gas).

FOLLOW-UP APPOINTMENT:

- We will arrange a follow-up appointment for 24 to 48 hours after your procedure.
- Please make additional follow-up appointments for one week and two to three months after surgery.
- You are welcome to return to our office for follow-up visits at no charge if you have questions or concerns regarding your liposculpture and wish to be seen.
- Remember there will be some swelling for 6 weeks to 6 months. Don't expect the final result too soon!
- Please call our office with any urgent concerns at any time.

APPENDIX 6

Liposculpture Surgery Operative Consent Form

I CLEARLY UNDERSTAND AND ACCEPT THE FOLLOWING:

1. Reasonable expectations have been explained and discussed with me.
2. The goal of liposculpture surgery, as in any cosmetic procedure, is improvement—not perfection.
3. The surgery is purely elective. Alternative treatments have been explained to me.
4. The final result may not be apparent for 3 to 6 months post-operatively or longer.
5. In order to achieve the best possible result, a "touch-up" procedure *may* be required for which there will be a charge.

6. The surgical fee is for the operation itself and subsequent post-operative visits pertaining to the surgery.
7. Areas of "cottage cheese" texture (i.e., cellulite) will be changed little by liposculpture surgery.
8. Liposculpture surgery is a contouring procedure and is not performed for purposes of weight reduction.
9. Liposculpture will not help existing skin irregularities, scars or stretch-marks. It will not correct body irregularities due to bone or muscle asymmetry. Fat that is inside the abdomen will not improve.
10. There is no guarantee that the expected or anticipated results will be achieved.

ALTHOUGH COMPLICATIONS FOLLOWING LIPOSCULPTURE ARE INFREQUENT, I UNDERSTAND THAT THE FOLLOWING MAY OCCUR:

1. Skin irregularities, lumpiness, hardness and dimpling may appear post-operatively. Most of these problems disappear with time and massage, but localized irregularities may persist permanently. If loose skin is present in the treated area, it may or may not shrink to conform to the new contour.
2. Infection is rare, but should it occur, treatment with antibiotics and/or surgical drainage may be required.
3. Bleeding is rare. In rare instances it could require hospitalization and blood transfusion.
4. Numbness or increased sensitivity of the skin over treated areas may persist for months. It is possible that localized areas of numbness or increased sensitivity could be permanent.
5. Fluid accumulations are uncommon (seromas, hematomas) but may require drainage.
6. Objectionable scarring is rare because of the small size of the incisions used in liposuction surgery, but scar formation or pigmentation of scars is possible.
7. Dizziness may occur during the first day following liposuction surgery, particularly upon rising from a lying or sitting position. If this occurs, extreme caution must be exercised while walking. Do not attempt to drive a car if dizziness is present.

In addition to these possible complications, I am aware of the general risks inherent in all surgical procedures and anesthetic administrations. Although rare, examples of such complications include blood clots, infection, injury to other tissues, and allergic or toxic reactions to drugs. Any and all of the risks and complications can result in additional surgery, hospitalization, time off work and expense to myself.

By my signature, I certify that I understand the goals, limitations, and possible complications of liposculpture surgery. I have been given the opportunity to ask questions and my questions have been answered to my satisfaction. I have had sufficient opportunity to discuss the procedure with the physician. I understand that medicine is not an exact science and there can be no guarantee as to the exact outcome of this procedure. I hereby wish to proceed with Liposculpture Surgery by the Tumescent Technique and authorize my physician ______________________, to perform the procedure.

______________________	______________	________
Patient Signature	*Print Name*	*Date*
______________________	______________	________
Witness/DA Representative Signature	*Print Name, Title*	*Date*

APPENDIX 7

Other Consents

CONSENT FOR PHOTOGRAPHY

❑ With the understanding that care will be taken not to reveal my name, I consent to the taking of photographs/videos before, during and after the surgical procedure(s). These photographs/videos will be the property of my physician and may be used for medical, scientific, teaching, publication or promotional purposes. Exclusions, if any: ____________

CONSENT FOR OBSERVERS

❑ For the purpose of advancing medical knowlege. I consent the admittance of qualified observers to the operating room.

HTLV-III CONSENT FORM

❑ I have been informed that my blood will be tested in order to detect whether or not I have antibodies in my blood to the HTLV-III virus, which is the probable causative agent of the Acquired Immune Deficiency Syndrome (AIDS). I understand that the test is performed by withdrawing blood and using a substance to test the blood.

I have been informed that the test results in some cases may indicate that a person has antibodies to the virus when the person does not (false positive), or fail to detect that a person has antibodies (false negative). I also have been informed that a positive blood test result does not mean that I have AIDS and that in order to diagnose AIDS, other means must be used in conjunction with the blood test.

I have been informed that if I have any questions regarding the nature of the blood test, its expected benefits, its risks, and alternative tests, I may ask those questions before I decide to consent to the blood test.

By my signature below, I acknowledge that I have been given all of the information I desire concerning the blood test and release of results, and have had all of my questions answered. Further, I acknowledge that I have given consent for the performance of a blood test to detect antibodies to the HTLV-III virus.

The results of this test will be kept strictly confidential and will not be released by the Physician or any employee to a third party including, but not limited to, health reporting agencies, insurance companies and/or physicians without my expressed written consent.

______________________	______________________	__________
Patient Signature	*Print Name*	*Date*
______________________	______________________	__________
Witness/DA Representative Signature	*Print Name, Title*	*Date*

APPENDIX 8

Preoperative Checklist for Liposculpture

Thank you for scheduling your procedure with us. We look forward to caring for you & providing the best possible medical service & support.

YOUR PROCEDURE IS SCHEDULED ON ______________ AT THE FOLLOWING LOCATION:

____

YOUR SCHEDULED TIME TO ARRIVE IS: ______________________________

REMEMBER TO:

- ❑ Make sure that you have read and understand all of your pre-op and post-op instructions.
- ❑ Make sure you have arranged for a ride home following your procedure. You will need someone to stay with you for the first 24 hours.

- ❑ It is important that you follow your anesthesia instructions, especially if you are not to eat or drink before your procedure.
- ❑ Should you experience health changes (flu, fever, sore throat, etc.) 72 hours prior to your scheduled surgery, please contact your doctor. Health changes may necessitate the postponing of your surgery.
- ❑ Purchase Hibiclens soap, absorbent pads and plastic liners.
- ❑ Have any required labwork or diagnostic procedures (EKGs, eye exams, physicals, etc.) performed two weeks prior to surgery.
- ❑ Have all prescriptions filled. If you have any questions about your medication, please contact our office.
- ❑ Wear loose, comfortable clothing the day of surgery. Do not wear anything that must be pulled over your head.
- ❑ Avoid the medications on your instructions.

If you have any questions, contact us at the phone number listed above where you are scheduled for surgery.

On behalf of the physicians & staff, we wish you a speedy recovery!

REFERENCES

1. Leever N. Cosmetic surgery—a comparison of its growth in the 1990's. (compiled for the American Academy of Cosmetic Surgery; available at: www.cosmeticsurgery.org.)
2. Klein JA. Tumescent technique for regional anesthesia permits lidocaine doses of 35 mg/kg for liposuction. J Dermatol Surg Oncol 1990; 16:248–263.
3. Hanke CM, Bernstein G, Bullock S. Safety of tumescent liposuction in 15,336 patients: National survey results. Dermatol Surg 1995; 12(5):459–462.
4. Lasswell M. As she lay dying. Allure Magazine 1997; August:128–133.
5. Jerome R. A body to die for. People Magazine 2000; October.
6. Pinski KS, Roenigk HH Jr. Liposuction of lipomas. Dermatol Clin 1990; 8: 483–492.
7. Kaneko T, Tokushige H, Kimura N, Moriga S, Toda K. The treatment of multiple angiolipomas by liposuction surgery. Dermatol Surg Oncol 1994; 20:690–692.
8. Bodansky HJ. Treatment of insulin lipohypertrophy with liposuction. Diabetic Med 1992; 9:395–396.
9. Samdel F, Amland PF, Sandsmark M, Birkeland KI. Diabetic lipohypertrophy treated with suction-assisted lipectomy. J Intern Med 1993; 234:489–492.
10. Barak A, Har-Shai Y, Ullman Y. Insulin induced lipohypertrophy treated by liposuction. Ann Plast Surg 1996; 37:415–417.
11. Goldberg LH, Humphreys TR. Surgical pearls: using the liposuction cannulas/syringe apparatus for conservative evacuation of postoperative hematomas. J Am Acad Dermatol 1996; 34:1061–1062.

12. Lillis PJ, Coleman WP III. Liposuction for treatment of axillary hyperhidrosis. Dermatol Clin 1990; 8:479–482.
13. Payne CM, Doe PT. Liposuction for axillary hyperhidrosis. Clin Exp Dermatol 1998; 23:9–10.
14. Swinehart JM. Treatment of axillary hyperhidrosis: combination of the starch–iodine test in liposuction technique. Dermatol Surg 2000; 26(4):392–396.
15. Brorson H, Swensson H, Norrgren K, Thorsson O. Liposuction reduces arm lymphedema without significantly altering the already impaired lymph transport. Lymphology 1998; 31:156–172.
16. Dolsky RL. Gynecomastia: Treatment by liposuction subcutaneous mastectomy. Dermatol Clin 1990; 8:469–478.
17. Samdal F, Kleppe G, Amland PF. Surgical treatment of gynecomastia: five years experience with liposuction. Scand J Plast Reconstr Surg 1994; 28:123–130.
18. Gray LN. Liposuction breast reduction. Aesthetic Plast Surg 1998; 22:159–162.
19. Matarasso SL. Liposuction of the chest and back. Dermatol Clin 1999; 17:799–804.
20. Farmer ER. Draft guidelines of care for AAD member comment: 2000 guidelines/outcomes committee. Dermatol World October 2000.
21. Lawrence N, Clark R, Flynn TC, Coleman WP. American Society for Dermatology guidelines of care for liposuction. Dermatol Surg 2000; 26(3):265–269.
22. Morgan EG, Mikhail MS. ASA Classifications. In: Clinical Anesthesiology. 2nd ed. Old Tappan: Appleton and Lange, 1996:6–7.
23. Bargetzi MJ, Aoyama T, Gonzalez FJ, Meyer UA. Lidocaine metabolism in human liver microsomes by cytochrome P450111A4. Clin Pharmacol Ther 1989; 46:521–527.
24. Currier JS, Havlir DV. Complications of HIV disease and antiretroviral therapy. Int AIDS Society USA 2000; 2:16–20.
25. Kelley L. Lidotoxic at low lidocaine levels. World Congress on Liposuction, Detroit, MI, 2000.
26. Crandon AJ. Post-operative deep vein thrombosis: identifying high risk patients. Br Med J 1980; 281:343–347.
27. Weinmann EE, Salzman EE. Deep-vein thrombosis. N Engl J Med 1994; 331:1630–1638.
28. Goldman MP. Adverse sequelae and complications of venous hypertension. In: Sclerotherapy Treatment of Varicose and Telangiectatic Leg Veins. St. Louis: Mosby, 1991:32–60.
29. Cupp MJ. Herbal remedies: adverse effects and drug interactions. Am Fam Phy 1999; 59:1239–1244.
30. Klein JA. Cytochrome P450 3A4 and lidocaine metabolism. In: Klein JA. Tumescent Technique: Tumescent Anesthesia and Microcannular Liposuction. St. Louis: Mosby, 2000:131–141.
31. Shiffman MA. Medications potentially causing lidocaine toxicity. Am J Cosm Surg 1998; 15(3):227–228.

32. Cox SE. Liposuction council bulletin. Dermatol Surg 2001; 27:207–208.
33. Klein JA, Kassarjdian N. Lidocaine toxicity with tumescent liposuction. A case report of probable drug interactions. Dermatol Surg 1997; 23(12):1169–74.
34. Lawrence N, Coleman WP, Klein JA, Cox SE, Flynn TC, Butterwick K, Narins RS. Liposuction panel in liposuction: course 106. American Academy of Dermatology, March, 2001.
35. Butterwick KJ, Goldman MP. Body fat analysis before and after liposuction as a means of objectively quantifying response to treatment. American Society for Dermatological Surgery Annual Meeting, Nov 2000.
36. Alster TS. Preoperative patient considerations. In: Alster TS ed. Manual of Cutaneous Laser Techniques. 2nd ed. Philadelphia: Lippincott/Williams & Wilkins, 2000:13–32.
37. Zide BM. Four patients you love to hate. Plast Reconstr Surg 1998; 102(5): 1729–1784.
38. Phillips KA, McElroy SK, Keck PE Jr, Hudnon JI, Pope HG Jr. Body dysmorphic disorder: 30 cases of imagined ugliness. Am J Psychol 1993; 150: 302–308.
39. Phillips KA, Hollander E, Rasmussen SA, Aronowitz BR, DeCarnia C, Goodman WK. A severity rating scale for body dysmorphic disorder: development, reliability, and validity of a modified version of the Yale Brown Obsessive–Compulsive Scale. Psychopharmacol Bull 1997; 33:17–22.
40. Klein J. Surgical technique: Microcannular tumescent liposuction. In: Tumescent Technique: Tumescent Anesthesia and Microcannular Liposuction. St. Louis: Mosby, 2000:131–141.
41. Rohrich R, Fodor PB, Petry JJ, Vash P. Preoperative and postoperative management of the body contour patient: a panel discussion. Aesth Surg Quart 1996; Winter:218–221.
42. Flynn TC, Narins RS. Preoperative evaluation of the liposuction patient. Dermatol Clin 1999; 17:729–734.

6

Computer Imaging

Min-Wei Christine Lee
University of California, San Francisco, San Francisco, and
The East Bay Laser and Skin Care Center, Inc.
Walnut Creek, California, U.S.A.

Roy C. Grekin
University of California, San Francisco
San Francisco, California, U.S.A.

The advancement of digital photography and computer imaging has opened the door for creative new methods to document, display, and distribute the results of liposuction surgeries. Traditional photography that uses film has slowly been replaced by more flexible and easier digital solutions. Digital imaging allows the photographer to immediately view and evaluate photos, print as many copies as needed, and create interactive computer presentations. This chapter includes information on basic computer imaging principles, equipment commonly used, and an example on how to create a three dimensional (3D) representation of a liposuction patient that allows for the results to be seen from any desired viewpoint.

CREATING THE DIGITAL IMAGE

A digital image is made up of a complex grid of squares. Each of these squares, called pixels, has a specific color and brightness assigned to it. The density and number of pixels that form the digital image have a direct correlation to its quality and detail (Figs. 1a–1c). Digital images are described

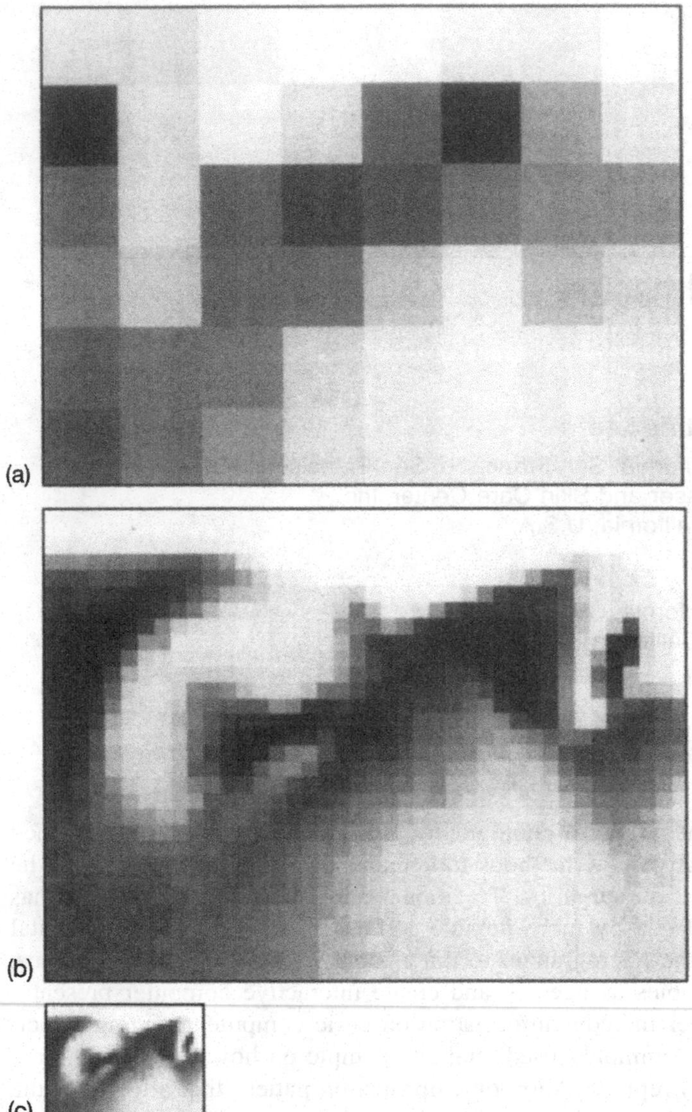

FIGURE 1 (a) This image consists of 48 individual squares (6 × 8). (b) This image consists of 1200 individual squares (30 × 40). It is the same size as Figure 1a, but has a higher ratio of pixels per inch. (c) This is the same image as Figure 1b. It also consists of 1200 individual squares, but the number of squares per inch is much higher. The result is a higher resolution image that reproduces at a smaller physical size.

by the density of pixels that make up the image. A low-resolution image might be described as 320 × 240 at 72 ppi (pixels per inch). This translates to an image that is formed by a grid that is 320 pixels wide and 240 pixels tall. The physical size of the image is determined by the number of pixels per inch. The low-resolution example just given would be 4.4 in. wide by 3.3 in. tall (320/72 = 4.4 and 240/72 = 3.3). A high-resolution image has a higher ratio in the number of pixels per inch, usually in the 200–300 ppi range. High-resolution images are used by publications for print work while low-resolution images are used for display on computer screens.

There are two basic ways to create digital photographic images. The first is to digitally scan a photographic print or slide that was taken with a standard film camera. This involves the use of a photo lab, the additional cost of prints, and extra time necessary for individually scanning the images. The second method, using a digital camera, saves considerable time and expense by keeping the entire process within the digital realm.

Traditional photographic methods use cameras that expose film to light. The light burns the visible image seen through the camera lens onto the film. The film is then taken to a photo reproduction lab where prints are produced. A digital camera uses a complex system of sensors that measure and record light. This information is recorded onto a memory card which is later transferred to a computer system where it can be displayed, edited, and printed.

DIGITAL EQUIPMENT

Camera

Which camera is best for documenting liposuction cases? The answer to this question is highly dependent on the intended usage of the images. A high-resolution-capable camera with easy-to-use features is the best solution for most practices. This type of camera allows for the most versatility in possible uses of the photo images taken. A camera that can capture a three megapixel image (i.e., 2048 × 1536 pixels) will take photos that can be printed with high-enough quality for most publication uses. Most cameras are equipped with the necessary auto focus, built-in auto flash, and light metering. All of the digital cameras on the market today come with a myriad of features and extras. Individual needs will determine which are important in the buying decision process. Some additional features that are offered include image stabilization, white point correction, multi-shot, digital video, low light compensation, and add-on lenses.

There are additional camera accessories that will improve the photographer's ability to take better and more consistent liposuction photos. A tripod will hold the camera steady and will ensure that a series of photos will be taken at the same height and distance. Purchasing a larger memory card (64–128 MB) for the camera will increase the number of photos that can be taken during one photo shoot. Digital cameras use batteries, and they use them up fast! Rechargeable batteries and a charging unit are necessary upgrades. Most cameras will also have an AC adapter option available that will allow you to power the camera from a wall jack.

Computers: Hardware, Software, and Accessories

Once the photos have been taken with a digital camera they will need to be transferred to a computer system to be fully utilized. Most cameras have the ability to transfer the digital images by directly connecting the camera to the computer. This method can be rather slow and cumbersome, so use of a digital card reader is usually preferred. A digital card reader acts much like a floppy disk drive for the digital memory cards that store the images taken by the digital cameras. To transfer files, the card is removed from the camera and inserted into the digital card reader. The contents of the memory card are then visible on the computer, where they can be copied into the appropriate folder or hard drive.

Almost all of today's present computer systems are capable of handling the requirements of digital imagery. At a minimum, it is necessary to have a color monitor capable of displaying the millions of colors that make up the photo images. Additional memory and hard disk space are the usual upgrades that most users opt for. At least one digital photo-editing software package that has the capability to crop, rotate, resize, and print the digital images is needed (i.e., Adobe Photoshop, available at www.adobe.com). As a practice's library of photo images increases, the need for a graphical database becomes paramount. The proper documentation and organization of these images can be handled with a graphical database program.

Printing of the images can be done with low-cost ink-jet printers on good photo-quality paper. The results are comparable to traditional photo prints with the added advantage being that as many prints as necessary can be created on demand. There are a number of manufacturers that offer photo-quality ink-jet printers. Once again, purchasing decisions will depend on specific needs.

As digital photo collections grow, the necessity of storing and archiving the images becomes obvious. Additional hard disk space may be needed to keep the images available for everyday use. Also, since disasters can always occur, a safe, reliable backup system is recommended. Copying the digital images onto CDs and storing them at a secondary location is standard practice.

Photo Rooms

Since most liposuction photos will be used in comparison situations, such as showing the "before" and "after" photos, taking photos in a controlled environment will minimize distractions and help focus the attention on the subject matter. It is preferable, if possible, to have a dedicated photo room available. To maintain the most consistent quality and settings, the best photo rooms should have no or heavily curtained windows, good-quality lighting, and a backdrop that is clear of distractions. A solid blue, white, or green backdrop is preferred. If a photo room is not an option, a portable curtain or backdrop can be purchased from a camera store.

USES FOR DIGITAL IMAGING TO DOCUMENT LIPOSUCTION CASES

Prints, Presentations, and Computer Display

Digital images of liposuction cases can be used in a multitude of ways. "Before" and "after" printouts can be made, images can be added to presentation materials, and web graphics are easily created.

Interactive Three-Dimensional Virtual Reality

One of the more effective and persuasive ways to display liposuction photos is through the use of 3D virtual reality (VR) on a computer screen (Fig. 2).

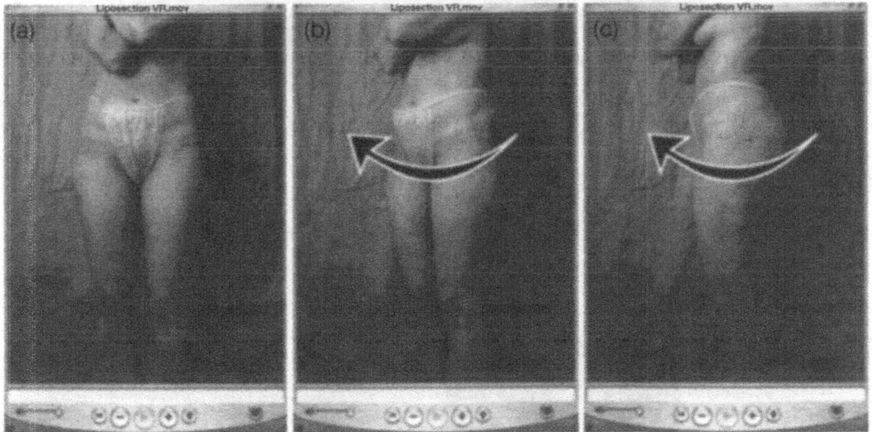

FIGURE 2 Examples of a 3D virtual reality movie of a liposuction case. The view of the figure is manipulated by mouse clicks in order to rotate it in the desired direction.

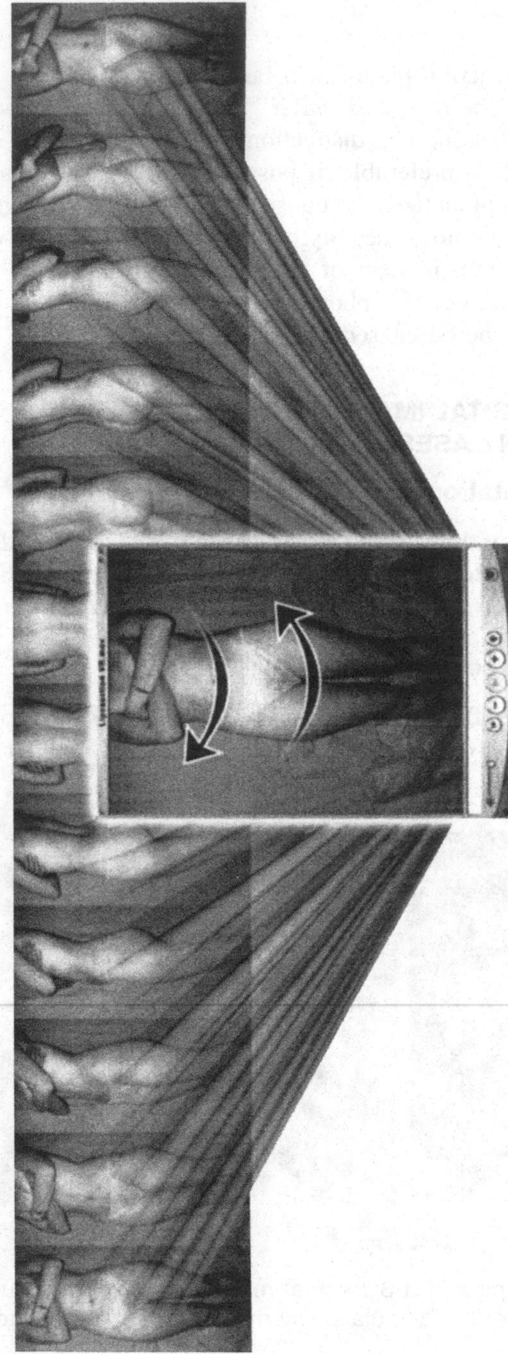

Figure 3 A series of photos of a patient are taken from a consistent viewpoint that differ from each other only by the angle at which the patient faces the camera. These photos are combined into a single VR movie file that allows for animatable interaction with the viewer.

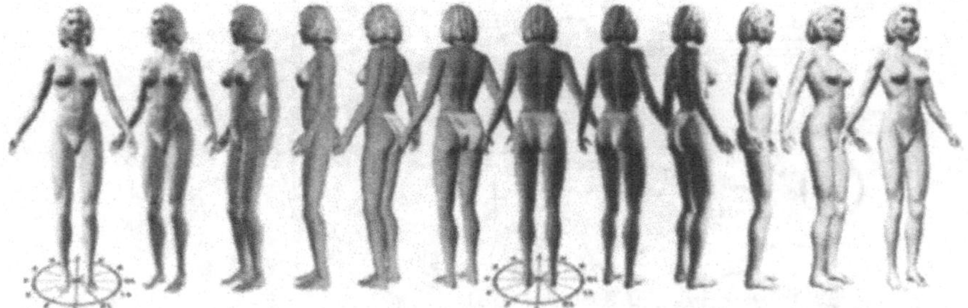

FIGURE 4 A full circle of photos needs to be taken to create a 3D VR file.

This allows a viewer to interactively manipulate the images on a computer screen in a manner that allows them to decide which angle of the patient they wish to examine and rotate the figure as needed.

In order to create a 3D interactive presentation, photos of the patient from multiple angles must be taken (Fig. 3). These photo images are then

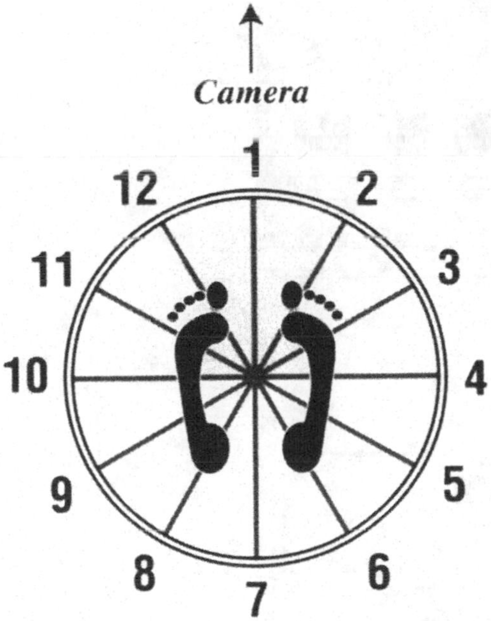

FIGURE 5 This is an example of a template to mark the angles for the patient to face. After each photo, the patient would turn and face the next number in order.

(a)

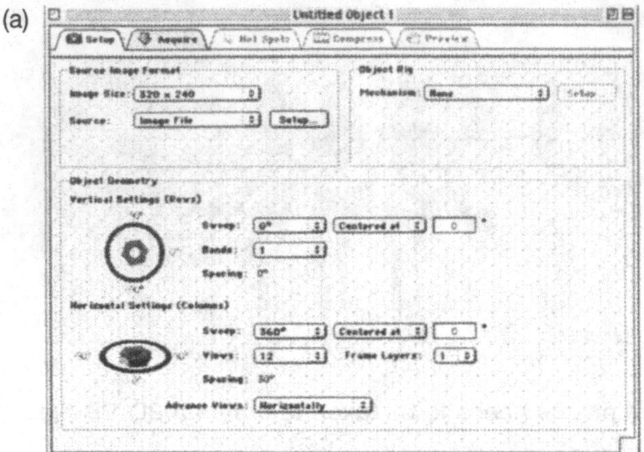

(b)

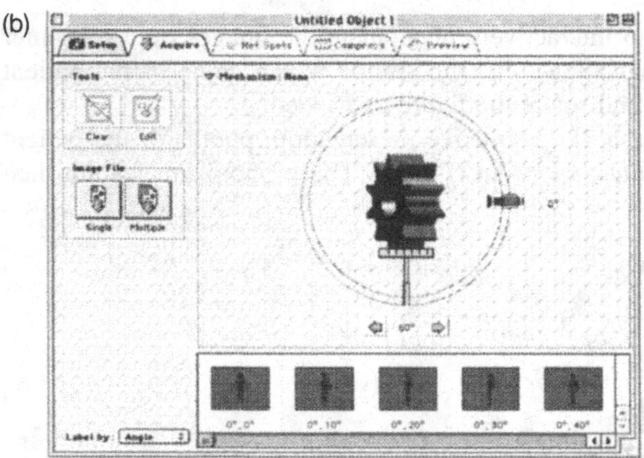

(c)

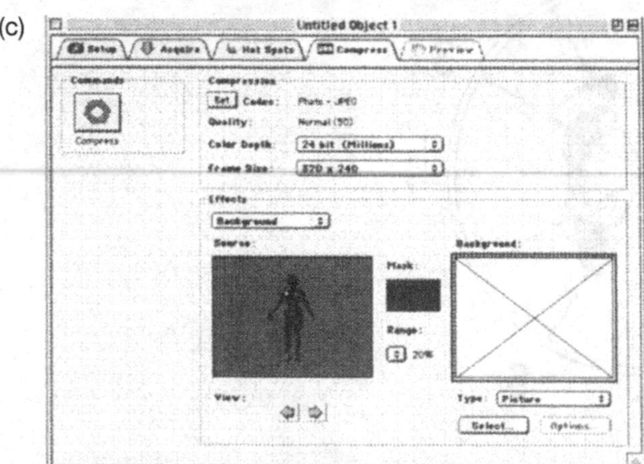

FIGURE 6 (a–c) Examples of the VR Object Worx screens and sample settings.

processed into a single file that can sequentially display each photograph. Finally, viewer interactive control is added.

The photographic images necessary to create a 3D interactive movie of a liposuction case can be created by taking a series of photographs of a patient at a set number of different angles. The initial position starts with the patient standing and facing directly towards the camera. A snapshot is taken and the patient is turned 30° to their right. Another photo is taken and the patient turns another 30° to their right. This process is repeated until a full circle and a total of 12 photos have been completed (Fig. 4). A more detailed 3D image can be created by having the patient rotate at smaller angle intervals and taking more photos. It is helpful to create a template for the patient to stand on that has the angles that they will be turning to marked (Fig. 5). Mounting the camera on a tripod will aid in maintaining the consistency of the look and quality of the photos taken.

Once the photo session is completed the images are transferred from the camera to a computer system. The images then are combined through software methods into single file, and interactive controls are added. There are a number of different companies offering software solutions to accomplish this process. For simplicity's sake, only one example is discussed here. VR Object Worx from VR Toolbox, Inc. (available at www.VRToolbox.com) is one software package that will import the series of 12 photos and export a 3D VR file. After the files are imported, they can be cropped and scaled for optimal look and playback performance. Users can put the desired settings into the appropriate entry fields (Fig. 6). Virtual reality and interactive controls are added in the same manner. The software combines all the photo images and interactive data into a single, new, self-contained VR object movie file in the Apple Quicktime format. More information on Quicktime and 3D VR files can be found at www.quicktime.com. All of the software and hardware solutions mentioned previously are available for both PC-compatible and Mac computer systems.

The self-contained, digital 3D VR liposuction movies can be interactively displayed directly on a computer screen or in conjunction with other presentation software such as Microsoft PowerPoint. They can be distributed on CDs, diskettes, or by e-mail and for greater visibility as part of interactive websites.

7

Photography for Liposuction Surgery

David J. Narins
New York University School of Medicine
New York, New York, U.S.A.

A medical photograph must be both of high technical quality and reproducible. Good photographs are a necessity in liposuction surgery. They are helpful in planning the procedure and for patient education and are indispensable for documenting the results of surgery. To evaluate the results of surgery, standardization of the photographic technique is necessary. The camera, lens, exposure, lighting, film, patient position, reproduction ratio, and background should be constants so that the changes between preoperative and postoperative photographs can be attributable only to the surgery. With basic equipment even a person with limited photographic knowledge can take high-quality, reproducible medical photographs in an office setting. It is especially imperative to take the care necessary to ensure good preoperative photographs, since there is only one opportunity to take them.

CAMERA

A 35-mm single lens reflex (SLR) camera is recommended for medical photography (Fig. 1). It can produce high-quality photographs with readily available slide film or either color or black-and-white print film. It is light enough to be easily portable and is reliable. Interchangeable lenses are available so that the best lens for a particular view can be chosen and lenses can be

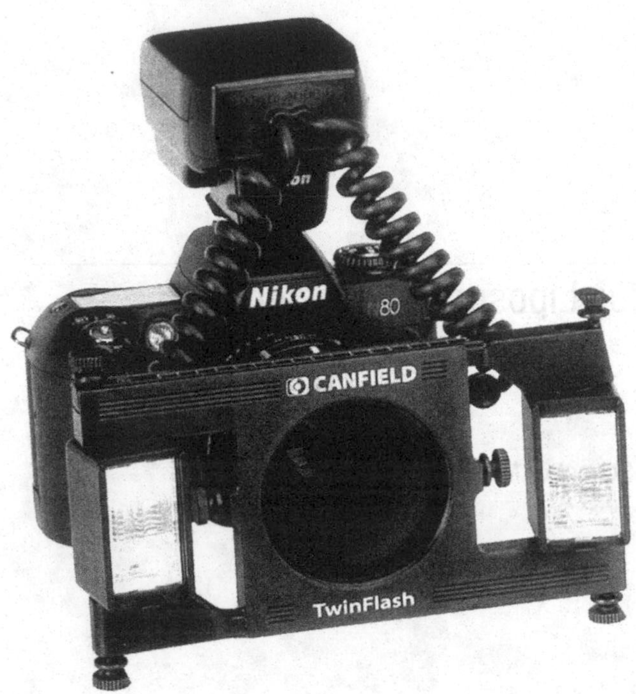

FIGURE 1 Canfield Clinical Systems' 35-mm Nikon N70 camera, with a 60-mm Slue macro lens and a CCS twin flash.

changed for various clinical situations. The what-you-see-is-what-you-get, through-the-lens (TTL) viewfinder enables the photographer to compose the photograph accurately. A camera that imprints the date on the film is preferable for pre- and postoperative photography in order to clearly document when a photograph was taken. This feature is built into some cameras; others require an accessory known as a "data back."

A Polaroid camera is also recommended if a digital camera (see below) is not being used. Preoperative Polaroid photographs provide a measure of insurance against having a roll of film lost and thus being left with no preoperative photographs at all. Instant photographs can also aid in preoperative planning and photographs taken after a patient has been marked for surgery will often demonstrate an asymmetry which might not be appreciated with the naked eye. Either a standard Polaroid camera with a close-focusing feature or the Polaroid Macro 5 SLR model (Fig. 2), which has five predetermined magnification ratios and a grid screen viewfinder for exact alignment and focuses using converging light beams, may be used.

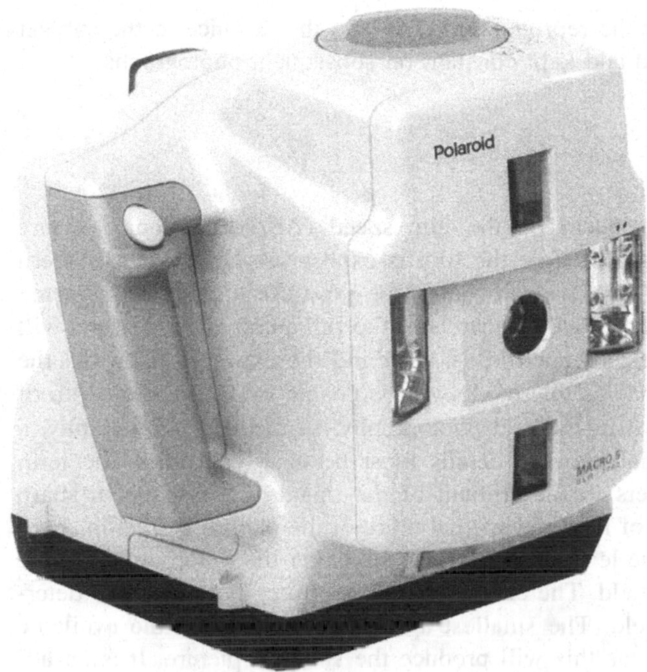

FIGURE 2 A Polaroid Macro 5 SLR Instant Camera.

The Macro 5 camera is ideally suited for taking high-quality instant photographs using Spectra film. If a digital camera is used the instantly available images can be used in the same fashion.

LENS

A lens should be selected with a focal length appropriate for the areas to be photographed. A 60-mm macro lens is ideal for most cases. The knee-to-shoulder view can be photographed in an average examining room. A medium-range telephoto lens (90–105 mm) is ideal for photographs of smaller areas such as the neck and jowls or arms or for fat-transfer procedures. The 105-mm macro lens has minimal distortion and a flat field, which is best for portraits or demonstrating smaller surgical areas. If only one lens is purchased, however, it should be a 60-mm macro since the camera-to-patient distance to take a knee-to-shoulder view with a 105-mm lens is 15 to 20 ft, which would be unwieldy in most office settings. The lens should have macrophotography (close-focusing) capability so that small areas can be photographed without accessory lenses. Macro lenses have adjustments on the focusing ring for the reproduction ratio and the distance to the subject so these can be noted and kept constant on subsequent photographs.

EXPOSURE

The exposure is dependent on the film speed (ASA), the lens aperture (f-stop), and the length of time the film is exposed to light. Most modern 35-mm TTL-metered cameras can control the exposure automatically during flash photography. Some cameras can be set to full automatic mode and will then control both the lens aperture (f-stop) and the exposure time, but the photographer who enables this mode will be unable to control the depth of field, which is critical in medical photography. In medical photography, a sharp image is crucial because details must be clearly visible. The term "depth of field" refers to the amount of the image that will be in sharp focus. Greater depth of field means that more of the picture will be in sharp focus. The smaller the lens aperture, (i.e., the larger the f-stop number), the greater the depth of field. The choice of lens aperture, therefore, will determine the depth of field. The smallest aperture possible with the available light should be used, as this will produce the sharpest picture. It is an advantage for the photographer to be able to choose the aperture manually. A TTL-metered flash automatically adjusts the length of time during which the film is exposed to light.

To determine the proper exposure, a test roll of film is taken. A limited number of views are usually sufficient to document a given procedure. One must determine camera setting for only three to four views to take all the photographs necessary. The camera is set at aperture priority. In this mode, the aperture (lens opening) is selected by the photographer and the camera automatically determines how long the shutter will remain open. For a test roll, one must take several photographs of each view at different apertures, recording the camera-to-patient distance (and consequent reproduction ratio) and the lens aperture (f-stop) for each exposure. Tables 1 and 2 show suggested f-stops for each of the four most common distances (reproduction ratios) for a 60- and 105-mm lens. Use these as starting-off points and take photographs one and two f-stops higher and one and two f-stops lower (called "*bracketing*") with your camera and lighting setup. (If using slide film, bracket the exposure by both $\frac{1}{2}$ and 1 f-stop.) From the five exposures for each distance, select from the properly exposed photographs the one that was taken with the smallest aperture. It is advisable to record the settings that correspond to the selected photographs to make a camera-setting table of your own for your camera and lighting set-up.

TABLE 1 Camera Settings for a 60-mm Lens (ASA 100 Film)[a]

Subject	Reproduction ratio	Distance from lens (in.)	Aperture
Full body	1:16	72	f4
Full face	1:10	25	f8
Half face	1:6	15	f11
Close-up	1:4	10	f16

[a]Take your own bracketed test photographs to determine settings for your camera and lighting.

LIGHTING

An electronic on-camera strobe light with automatic TTL exposure control is recommended. In the ideal lighting setup, the main lights are positioned at a 45° angle from the subject. A background light is positioned behind the patient to eliminate shadows, which would make the patient difficult to distinguish from the background shadow (Fig. 3). Slave flash units, which are triggered by the light from a flash on the camera (thus eliminating the need for interconnecting wires), can be used. The light intensity of the slave flash units is adjustable. Determine by trial and error how much light each slave unit should give; this setting can then be used for all future photographs. Such a setup will result in the most evenly lit, shadow-free photographs possible. However, the fact that both the main lights and the background lights are placed on stands at various positions relative to the patient makes it necessary either to have a dedicated photographic space or to spend a moderate amount of time setting up the room prior to taking pictures of each patient. A simpler setup, utilizing a single strobe flash unit on the

TABLE 2 Camera Settings for a 105-mm Lens (ASA 100 Film)[a]

Subject	Reproduction ratio	Distance from lens (in.)	Aperture
Full face	1:10	36	f5.6
Half face	1:6	24	f8
Close-up	1:4	16	f11

[a]Take your own bracketed test photographs to determine settings for your camera and lighting.

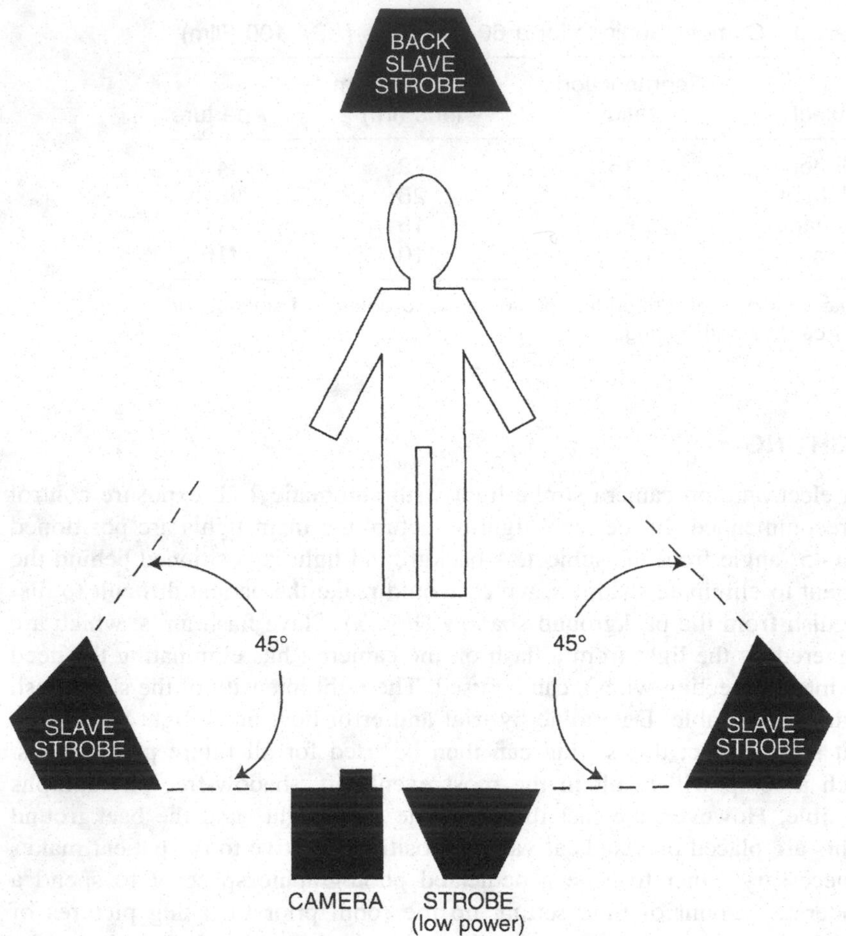

FIGURE 3 Photographic suite setup.

camera and one background light located directly behind the patient, can also result in photographs of excellent quality and is easy to set up (Fig. 4).

Either a ring flash or a unit that places the flash at the plane of the front of the lens should be used (Figs. 1 and 7) for close-up photography. If the flash is mounted on top of the camera, it will not illuminate the area being photographed when extreme close-ups are taken (i.e., where the camera is very close to the subject). A standard camera-mounted flash is more appropriate for body liposuction since the camera-to-patient distance is longer. The slave background flash should be set between $\frac{1}{4}$ and $\frac{1}{2}$ power so

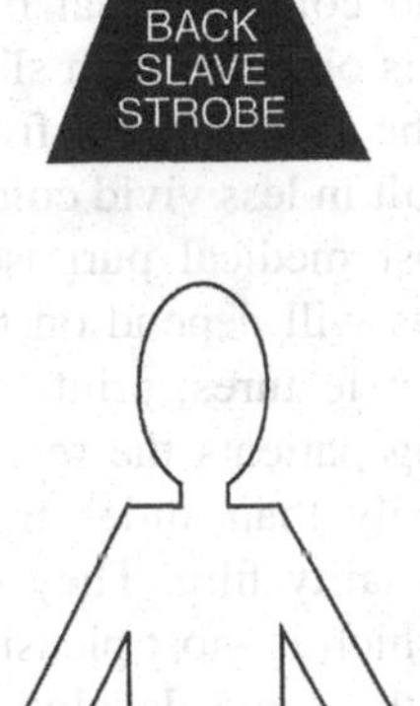

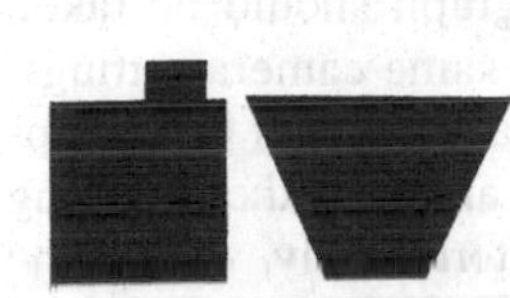

FIGURE 4 Simplified photographic suite setup.

that the background will not be overlit and will appear sky blue rather than an overexposed white or produce a halo effect around the subject. Setting the strobe at too weak a setting will result in shadows from the primary flash.

FILM

The "speed" of a film is a measure of its sensitivity to light. Film speed is measured by an ISO (formerly ASA or DIN) number. Slow film (i.e., film with a low ISO number) is less grainy than fast film and shows details better. Since patients are not moving and good lighting is obtained with electronic flash, slow (ISO 64 or 100) film can and should used. Daylight color film is used with strobe flash units to give proper color balance. Daylight film comes in two types: color negative film for prints and color reversal film for slides. The most vivid and accurate color rendition is obtained with slide film, since this is a one-step process. With print film, the print is made from a negative, thus involving a second step, which can result in less vivid colors and possible inconsistency from roll to roll. For most medical purposes, either will be acceptable. The choice of slides or prints will depend on the use to be made of the images. Slides are preferable for lectures; prints are easier to use for viewing in the office and for showing patients the results of surgery. Prints can be made from slides more easily than slides from prints. Kodak, Fuji, Agfa, and Ilford all make good-quality film. They reproduce skin tones differently, so you should decide which is most pleasing to you and stick with one brand. Always try to use the same developing laboratory to eliminate the variables inherent in differing processing techniques.

STANDARDIZATION OF VIEWS

Pre- and postoperative views must be identical so that the photographs will allow for accurate comparison and contrast. Therefore, the photographer must standardize the views to be taken. Each photograph should be taken at a predetermined distance from the patient with the same camera settings, so the exposure and image size will always be identical. This can be accomplished by having the patient stand at a fixed position and by either marking the floor to indicate the distance for each view or, alternatively, setting the distance on the macro lens and moving toward the patient until the image is in focus. The latter technique is called "*body focusing*."

For each procedure, there are certain views that best demonstrate the area being worked on. Frontal, oblique, lateral, and posterior views may be taken. A list should be created of the views and magnifications to be taken for any given procedure. Go through the list routinely during each photography session, taking all required photographs at each photo session. In this way, you will have comparison photographs at each stage of the procedure, preop, postop, and long-term. It is better to take too many photographs than too few. Unnecessary photographs can always be discarded, but one cannot go back in time to retake a photograph. Remember to be especially thorough when taking preoperative photographs, as these can never be retaken.

BACKGROUND

The background is a very important part of a medical photograph. A homogeneous background, free from distracting elements, is essential so that one can focus on the information being presented without being distracted by extraneous details. The color is also important. Sky blue is complementary to skin tones both in color and in black-and-white photography, giving good definition of the clinical area. A satisfactory background can be easily placed in any office. A wall or door can be painted with sky-blue matte paint, or background paper or felt material can be purchased in 4-ft-wide strips at photographic supply shops and hung from a wall. Several rooms can be prepared for photography, so that patients will not have to be moved to a dedicated photographic area for photographs and so that the backgrounds in all photographs documenting the clinical progress will be identical.

RECORD KEEPING

It is necessary to keep systematic records of photographs as they are taken and to be able to file them so they can be easily retrieved. A photographic logbook should be kept with the camera. Each roll should be numbered and there should be a line for each exposure on the roll. You should record the date, patient's name, procedure, and any other relevant notes for each photograph you take. To lessen the chance of losing a roll of film during processing, you should take a photograph of your name, address, and telephone number as the first exposure on the roll. In this way, if the film is mishandled at the laboratory, there will be some identification on the roll of film that would enable the photographs to be returned to you.

In addition to keeping the logbook, another aid in identifying and filing photographs is to take a photograph of a card with the patient's name, date, procedure, and any relevant notes before taking photographs of the patient (Fig. 5). Each photograph appearing on the roll until the photograph of the

Name: ....
Date: ....
Procedure ....
Notes:

Take a photo of a card with this information on it before taking a series of photographs of a patient. All photographs until the next identification photo will belong to that patient and can easily be identified and filed.

FIGURE 5 Archiving tip.

next name card will belong to that patient. This will make filing of the photographs easier.

ARCHIVING

Slides or prints can be stored either in the patient's chart or in a separate file. In either case, you should have a system that enables you to retrieve them easily. You should be able to reference them by patient's name and by procedure so you will be able get the picture you are looking for with a minimum amount of difficulty. As with all medical records, photographs must be stored in a secure place after office hours.

OTHER CAMERA SYSTEMS

If you do not presently own a suitable camera or are planning to upgrade your system and do not want to use a digital camera, you might consider the APS system. These cameras are almost identical to a 35-mm SLR camera in feel and use, but use a smaller, 24-mm film cassette. This cassette has practically foolproof drop-in loading, which eliminates incorrect loading and unexposed rolls of film. Film can easily be changed midroll if you have a need to switch from color print film to black-and-white for a particular situation. (There is, as yet, no slide film available in this format.) A Picture Quality Information Exchange feature stores exposure information on a magnetic layer on the film. This information can be used by the photofinisher to improve the quality of each print by making automatic frame-by-frame adjustments during printing. It also imprints the exposure factors (ISO, f-stop, and shutter speed) on the back of each print so you can change camera settings for future photographs if your results are not satisfactory. The cassette system is also ideal for archiving. Each cassette is numbered and this number is imprinted on the back of each print along with the date, frame number, and exposure factors. An "index print," showing a thumbnail view of each frame and the range of dates of exposure for the roll, allows you to quickly review the contents of each roll. Since the film is returned rerolled into the cassette, it can be filed safely for quick retrieval if copies of a print or a slide have to be made (Fig. 6). The index print, film cassette, and information on the back of each print share the same ID number to avoid confusion and help locate the proper negative quickly. The negatives are not handled and are thus less likely to become damaged or lost. The cassettes can also be scanned into a computer for incorporation into a presentation, letter, or e-mail. Thirty-five-millimeter slides, negatives, or prints can also be scanned into a computer with the appropriate scanner.

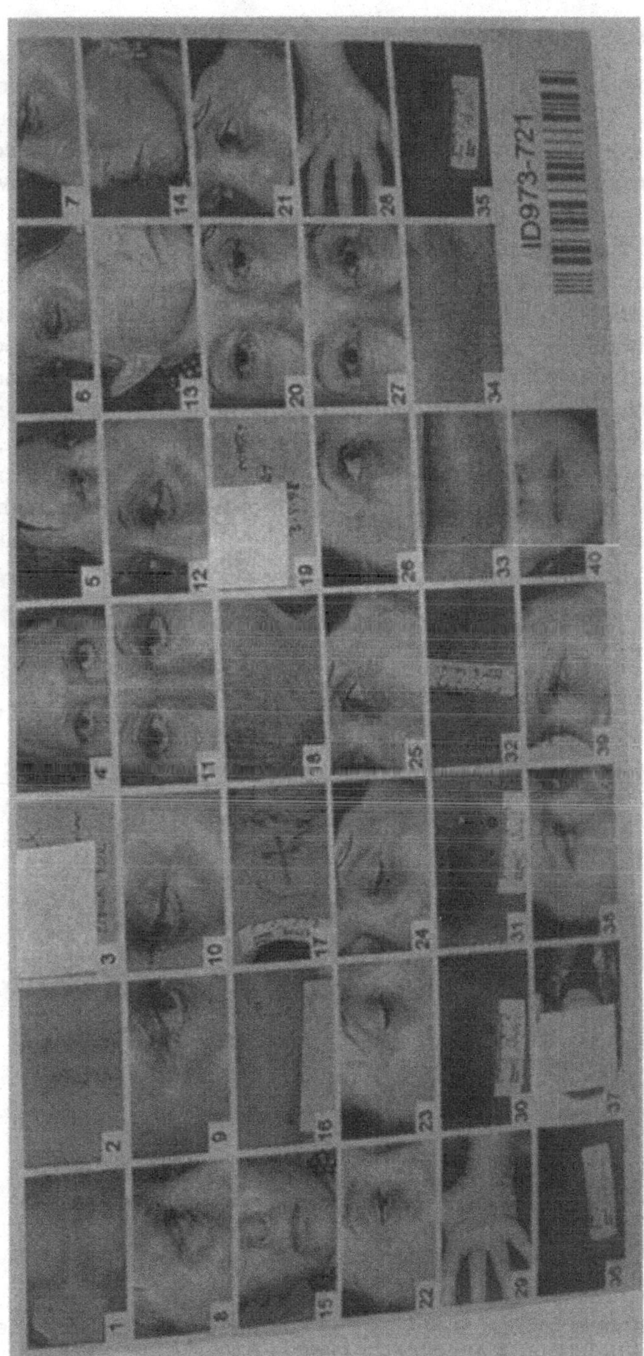

FIGURE 6 APS index print and film cassette storage.

DIGITAL PHOTOGRAPHY

Digital photography will probably be the standard within several years. Digital cameras will have the same impact on office photography that word processors have had on writing. Digital images are viewable immediately, do not require off-site processing, and can be easily filed and retrieved.

Digital cameras (Fig. 7) record images electrically and these images can be downloaded from the camera to a computer, where they can be stored. Computers are ideal for storing, manipulating, and retrieving photographic images. Images taken with a digital camera can be viewed and printed immediately without the need for processing. With the increasing processing power of computers and larger, less expensive storage media, large numbers of photographs can be stored and instantly cross-referenced and retrieved by searching for any information you have included with the image (e.g., name, date, diagnosis, and surgical procedure or any combination of criteria). Stored digital images are archival (they will not fade or degrade with time). Relatively inexpensive color printers can produce laboratory-quality archival

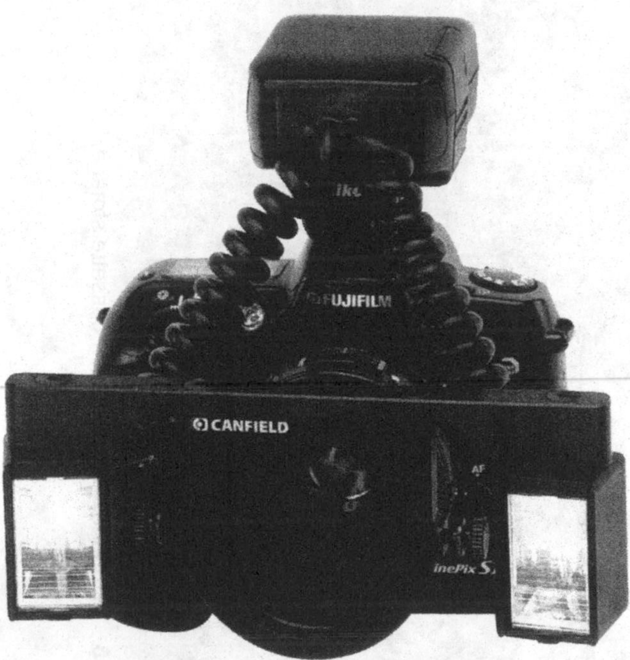

FIGURE 7 Canfield Clinical Systems' Fuji FinePix S1 Pro digital camera with a 60-mm macro lens and a CCS twin flash.

prints and the images can be included in correspondence or the patient's chart or e-mailed or incorporated into slides for presentations.

An electronic image is composed of many small dots called pixels (picture elements). In color digital photography, every pixel contains a red, blue, and green dot, each of which is energized at different intensities to produce different colors. The number of pixels in the width and the number of pixels in the height express the resolution of a digital image (e.g., 3040 × 2016 = 6 megapixels). The larger these numbers, the better the resolution. Higher resolution pictures require more memory for storage, fewer can be stored on the media in the camera, and they will take more time to download to the computer or to transmit.

Although many medical photographers are currently utilizing digital photography, there are several limitations that must be considered. To begin with, computers intimidate many people and others feel that they are unreliable for storing important clinical information. Downloading and filing the images is time consuming. At present, the equipment is still costly when compared to a 35-mm camera and the resolution (degree of sharpness) of even the best digital images is not as good as that of 35-mm film. The cost of equipment, however, is recouped since one no longer pays the costs of film and processing. For image quality, chemistry still has the edge over electronics, but this is narrowing. Top-quality photographic film can have 80 million pixels/in.^{2} while the best digital cameras (in 2002) have 6 million pixels/in.^{2} The latter is more than adequate for medical use and most images for documentation and presentation use can be taken at resolutions less than that. A 6-megapixel image uses 11 MB of memory. The storage media in present cameras suffice for only a small number of these high-resolution images. An additional limitation is that it is time consuming to download high-resolution images from the storage media to the computer. Six-megapixel images are not necessary for most clinical uses. Cameras can be set to take images at less than their maximum resolution to produce image files of smaller size. The files can be compressed to the JPEG (Joint Pictures Expert Group; .jpg) format; JPEG files are much smaller and therefore are superior in terms of saving disk space and download or transmission time. The degree of compression can be adjusted to produce a small file with little noticeable loss of image quality. Joint Pictures Expert Group images are more than adequate for most medical uses.

The factors in choosing a digital camera are the same as for a film camera. A single lens reflex digital camera will provide the photographer with the most control. There are good-quality range finder cameras that produce excellent-quality images, but the difficulties in precise focusing and determining the frame of the image make them unsatisfactory for taking standardized, reproducible photographs. The price of high-quality 6-megapixel single lens reflex cameras has come down to levels that are reasonable for medical use. These cameras function like their film counterparts and use the same lenses and accessories. One difference is that the chip that records the image is smaller than a 35-mm film negative, so the effective focal length of a lens for most interchangeable-lens digital cameras must be multiplied by 1.5. A 60-mm macro lens, therefore, functions like a 90-mm lens would on a 35-mm camera. This makes it excellent for portraits (e.g., necks, jowls, arms, and fat transfer), but would make the camera-to-patient distance for body liposuction a bit too long. This problem will, no doubt, be rectified and at present one camera, Contax, has a larger chip and its lenses have their true focal length. Other manufacturers will, no doubt, follow. The image quality and color rendition of these cameras are excellent.

The ability of computers to organize and provide almost instant access to photographic records will make digital photography the standard of the future. The cost of equipment is rapidly decreasing and the resolution of each new generation of cameras has improved. Storage capacity and ease and speed of inputting the images into the computer will improve, as will computer reliability.

As with any computer information, backing up photographs is essential. If photographs are not backed up they can be lost forever. A system must be in place to have all the photographic data backed up on a regular basis so it will be able to be retrieved if there is a computer crash. Each image is 500 to 1000 kb so the amount of data to be backed up is considerable. A second hard drive or tape backup system is necessary. It would be preferable to have the data available on two separate computers so if one crashes the other can still be used to view patient photographs while the first is being restored. If you store patient photographs on a computer and it crashes you will have lost access to all your photographs until the computer is working again or you have transferred the information to a backup computer. This can leave you unable to retrieve any photographic records.

There are many ways to store patient photographs on a computer. The simplest is to create a folder of patient photographs; subfolders for specific procedures; and, within those subfolders, folders for each patient. This has some imitations since the photographs will be stored in the orientation in which they were taken and some may be sideways or even upside down. Opening an image may require a photo-viewing program and can be time consuming and unwieldy. There are many photo-archiving programs commercially available. Some, which have been specifically designed for medical use, can make storing and retrieving more efficient. Two such programs are available through Canfield Scientific. One, PhotoFile, is a simple drag-and-drop program which is easily mastered and quick to use. Photographs can be retrieved by name, procedure, diagnosis, date, location, or other information you include when filing the images. A more advanced program, Mirror, requires a little more familiarity with computers and a longer learning curve, but has advantages for presentations and showing pre- and postoperative photographs. It is easier to print images and pre- and postoperative images can be adjusted to balance color and brightness for side-by-side comparison. This should not be necessary if you followed the instructions for planning photographs described earlier in this chapter.

This brings us to a controversial aspect of digital photography, the ease with which the images can be manipulated. It can be difficult to determine if a digitally created image has been electronically altered. Even relatively unsophisticated computer programs can edit images. This ability to manipulate images is purposely used in "morphing" programs, where the image can be changed to show a patient what can be expected after surgery by showing a digitally created "postoperative" view. Whether this is a good idea is debatable. Some say it is an educational tool and gives a patient a better understanding of what can and cannot be accomplished with surgery, while others say it can give a false expectation of postoperative appearance and can be construed as an implied warranty.

CONSENT AND LIABILITY ISSUES

As with all medical procedures, one must obtain consent to take photographs and a patient release to use them (Appendix 1). This is important if the photographs are intended to be used in publications or lectures and critical if they will be shown to other patients, used in advertising, or placed on a website for your practice. One should be careful never to show a photograph in which the patient is identifiable without specific consent for that use. Blacking out the eyes or part of the face is not adequate for disguising a patient's identity.

The legal parameters regarding electronic transmittal of patient information are just being developed. Patient's photographs and all clinical information sent by e-mail should be encrypted.

CONCLUSION

Taking a Photograph

1. Position the patient in front of the blue background.
2. Set up the slave background flash.
3. Set the camera for manual focus.
4. Set the camera for aperture priority.
5. Use a TTL-metered flash.

6. Set the distance (reproduction ratio) on the macro lens.
7. Move in until the image is in focus.
8. Take the photograph.

APPENDIX 1

Permission For Taking and Publication of Photographs and/or Videotapes

Patient: ____________________

1. I hereby consent that photographs, and/or videotapes may be taken of me or the named patient by Dr. __________ in connection with the medical care and treatment which I/the patient am/is receiving from Dr.__________.

2. Such photographs, videotapes, movies, histories, and/or audio recordings may be published, shown, exhibited or otherwise used by Dr. __________ for any purpose of medical education, knowledge, or research which Dr. __________may deem proper (including media publicity or other commercial trade purposes).

3. I understand that neither I/the patient nor members of my/the patient's family will be identified by name in connection with any public use of this material, and all care will be used to prevent such identification.

4. I grant this consent as a voluntary contribution and I waive any and all rights I may have to royalties or other compensation in connection with any such use.

Date ______________ Patient/Guardian Signature________________

Witness ______________ Relationship, if not patient ________________

Interpreter (if required)____________________

*The signature of the patient must be obtained unless the patient is an emancipated minor under the age of 18 or is otherwise incompetent to sign.
NOTE: THIS DOCUMENT MUST BE MADE PART OF THE PATIENT'S MEDICAL RECORD.

8

Abdomen, Hourglass Abdomen, Flanks, and Modified Abdominoplasty

Rhoda S. Narins
Dermatology Surgery and Laser Center
New York and White Plains, and
New York University Medical Center
New York, New York, U.S.A.

The shape of the abdomen plays an important role in a person's view of himself or herself as well as in how a person fits into their clothes. Many factors play a part in abdominal contour deformities, including local lipodystrophy, obesity, muscle laxity, fitness, previous surgery with resultant scars, skin laxity, age, previous pregnancies, hormone replacement therapy, menopause, and genetics. Various procedures may need to be employed ranging from liposuction alone to liposuction with scar undermining with or without skin excision to abdominoplasty with skin and muscle repair with or without umbilical translocation. The majority of patients can be treated by liposuction alone and both patients and surgeons, because of the ease of recovery and negligible morbidity, prefer that. Liposuction of the lower abdomen may be all that is necessary to treat a young, fit person, while liposuction of both the upper and lower abdomen is necessary for the best results in most people especially in those who are larger. Circumferential liposuction, "The Hourglass Abdomen" procedure is done in the patient who needs the upper and lower abdomen treated along with the waist, posterior waist, hips, and back to get a good result. Some patients need a miniabdominoplasty for loose skin or a complete abdominoplasty, which addresses both loose skin and muscle diastasis to achieve the desired result. This is a procedure that must be geared to the patient so an intensive evaluation and consultation are required.

I divide patients into five groups (Table 1). The first group consists of patients requiring liposuction of the lower abdomen only. This is usually a younger or an older but extremely fit patient (Figs. 1 and 2). This area responds very well to liposuction and the skin pulls back firmly. These patients are always happy. The second group consists of patients who need liposuction of the upper and lower abdomen. The lower abdomen always pulls back well and even a small or medium overhang or "apron" may disappear. Although the upper abdomen never pulls back as tightly as the lower abdomen, you can achieve excellent results, especially in the patient who is motivated to lose weight when necessary (Figs. 3 and 4). Many patients in this category think that they only need the lower abdomen done but this may lead to an unsightly upper abdominal bulge if they gain any weight at all or as they age. If a lot of fat is removed and the patient has large breasts prior to surgery they may get larger. Patients must be warned that this may happen as the fat equilibrates if they do not lose weight.

The third group consists of patients who need circumferential liposuction to get the best result (Figs. 5–9). The Hourglass Abdomen procedure addresses the waist, posterior waist, hips, and back as well as the upper and lower abdomen. If these other areas are not done and the patient does not lose weight, the fat removed from the abdomen equilibrates and may accumulate in these areas. The patient may still look "chunky" even though their abdomen is flat and need the same or even a larger clothing size. Sometimes the back has to be done all the way up to the axilla. This gives a more shapely look even if the roll does not totally disappear. Many patients have this type of shape due to heredity, but others are postmenopausal women or those on hormone replacement therapy, who often gain weight. In fact, many women (and men) between the ages of 45 and 55 lay down fat on the abdomen. This procedure also works well on men who also build up fat on the abdomen and flanks as they get older (Fig. 10). Men with a "beer belly" do not fare as well. The upper abdomen of a "beer belly" in men cannot be treated by liposuction as the fat is behind the muscle around the organs and not in the subcutaneous tissue. Weight loss helps in these cases while the liposuction works well on the lower abdomen and flanks. Occasionally women have this type of abdominal fat distribution, which is not amenable to liposuction as the fat is internal (Fig. 11).

The fourth group consists of patients with adipose deposits requiring liposuction and excision of flaccid skin; a miniabdominoplasty can be done along with liposuction for the best results. Skin can thin and stretch from

TABLE 1 Five Groups of Patients—Abdominal Liposuction

1. Liposuction: lower abdomen
2. Liposuction: upper and lower abdomen
3. Liposuction: Hourglass Abdomen
   Upper and lower abdomen, hips, waist, and back
4. Liposuction and skin excision: Miniabdominoplasty with or without umbilical translocation
5. Complete abdominoplasty

pregnancy, age, and repeated weight gain and loss. The fifth group consists of patients with muscle diastasis and loose skin who need abdominoplasty (Fig. 12). I do not address this last group in this chapter; I discuss the treatment of abdominal scars with each of the other four groups of patients.

CONSULTATION AND EVALUATION

The most important part of any cosmetic procedure is the consultation. Although the best results are always seen in the young slim patient with minimal fat deposits, gratifying results can be obtained in the realistic older,

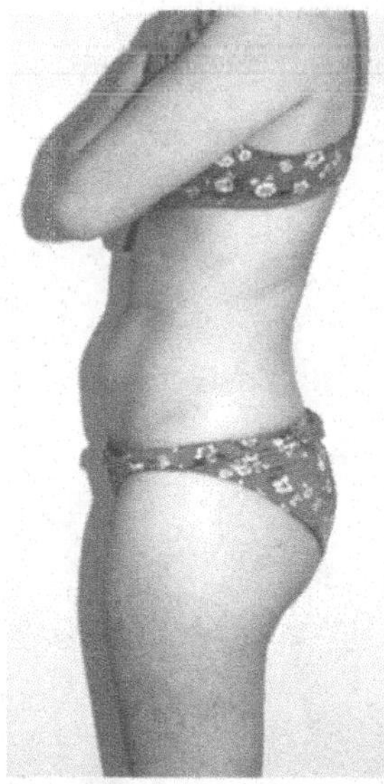

FIGURE 1 Abdomen patient before liposuction.

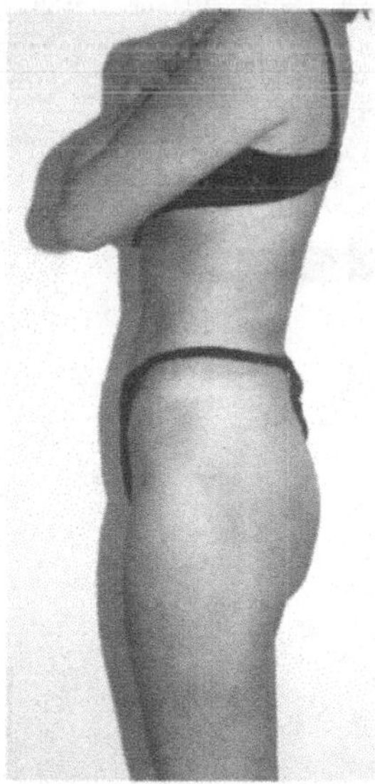

FIGURE 2 Abdomen patient after liposuction.

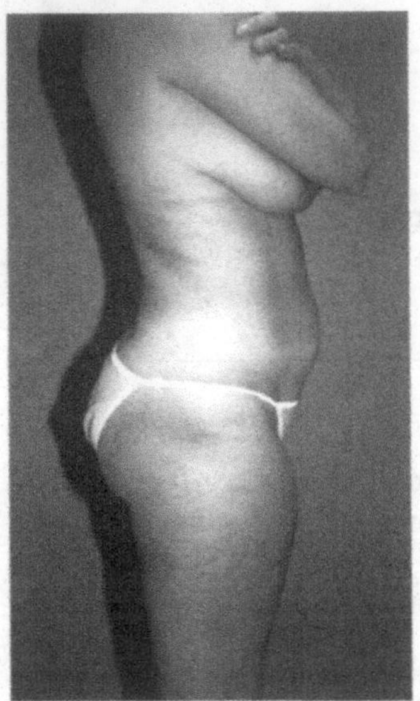

Figure 3 Abdomen patient 2 before liposuction.

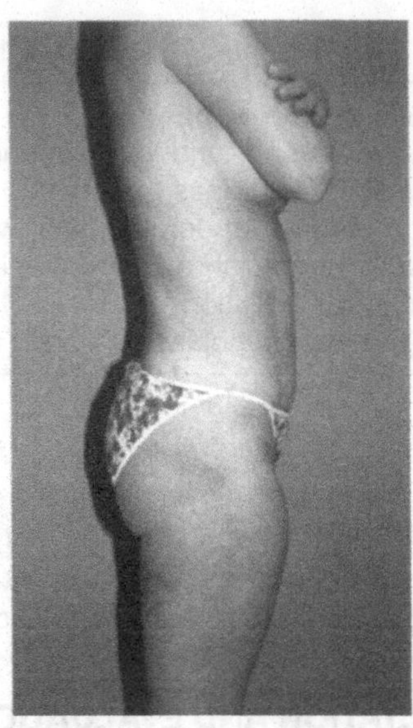

Figure 4 Abdomen patient 2 after liposuction.

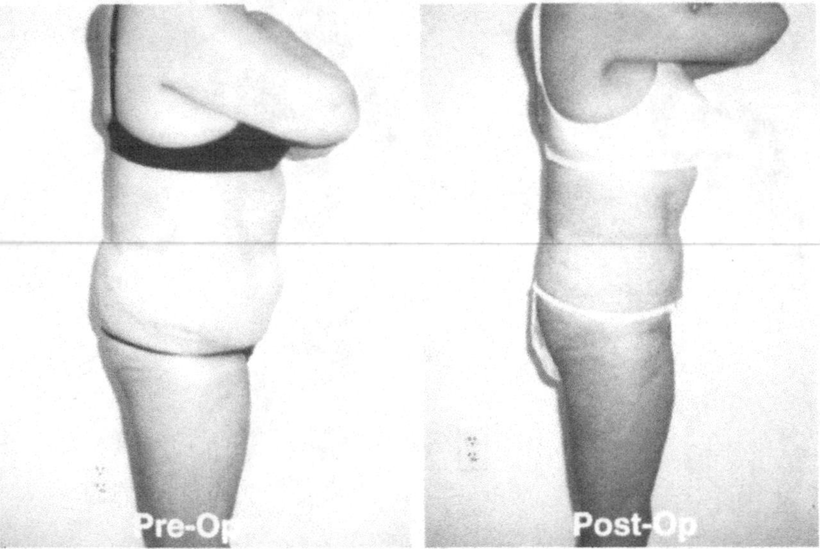

Figure 5 Hourglass abdomen before (left) and after liposuction (right).

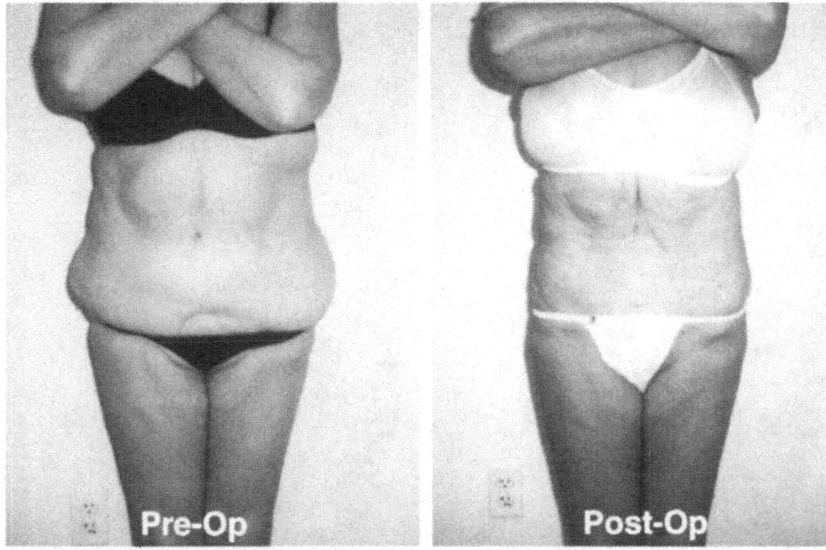

FIGURE 6 Hourglass abdomen before (left) and after liposuction (right).

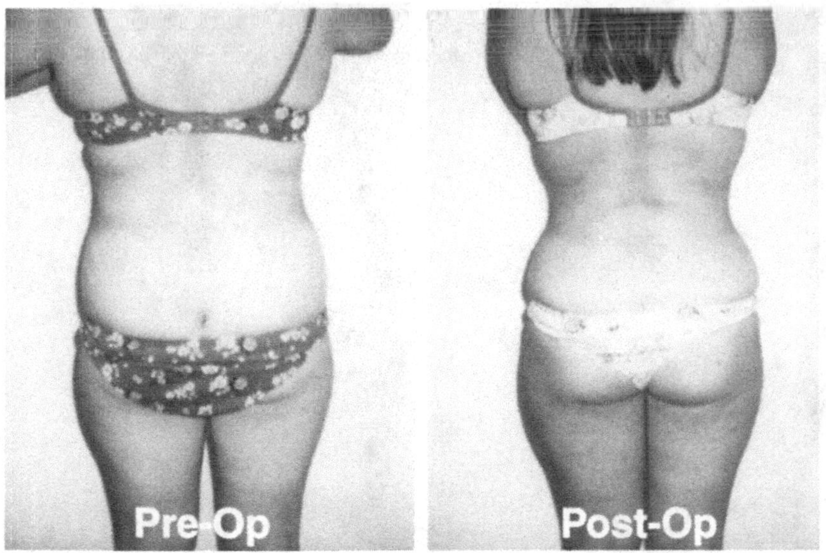

FIGURE 7 Hourglass abdomen before (left) and after liposuction (right).

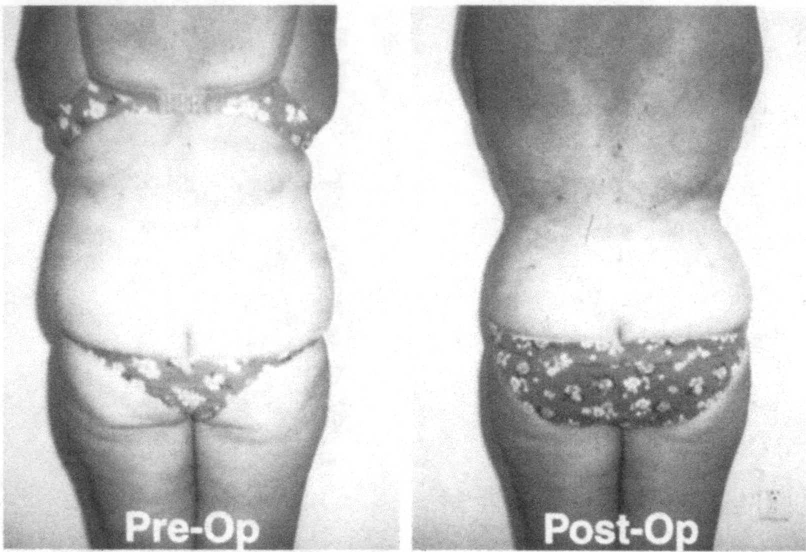

Figure 8 Hourglass abdomen before (left) and after liposuction (right).

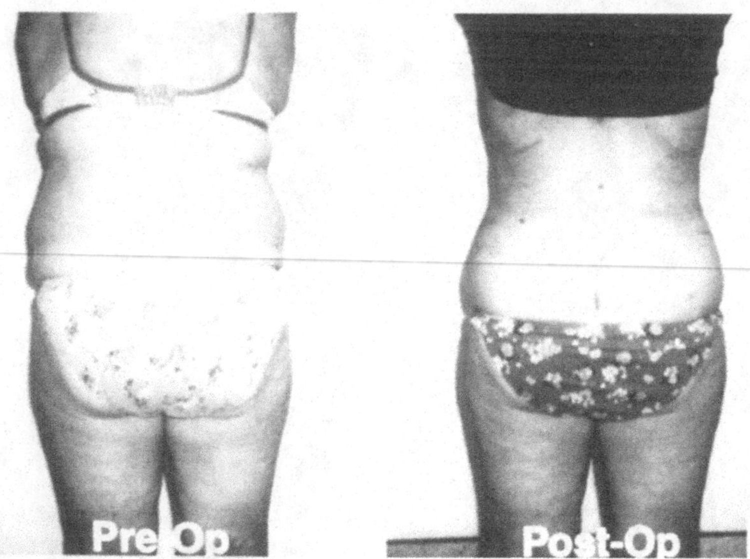

Figure 9 Hourglass abdomen before (left) and after liposuction (right).

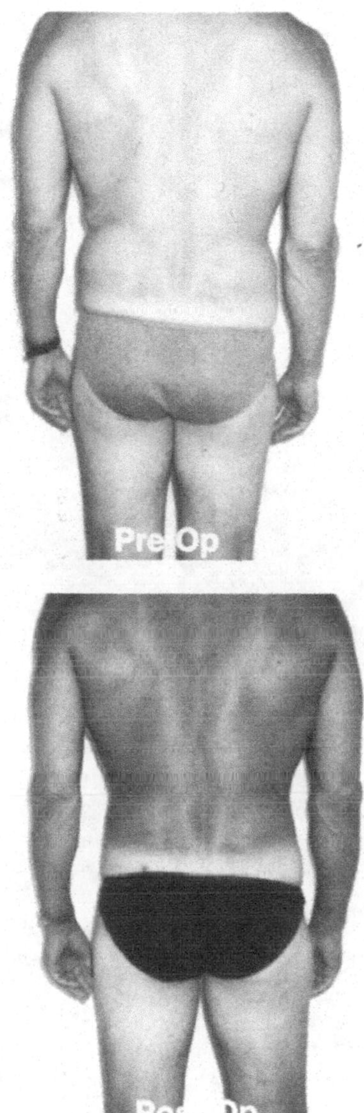

Figure 10 Male patient with "lovehandles" before (top) and after liposuction (bottom).

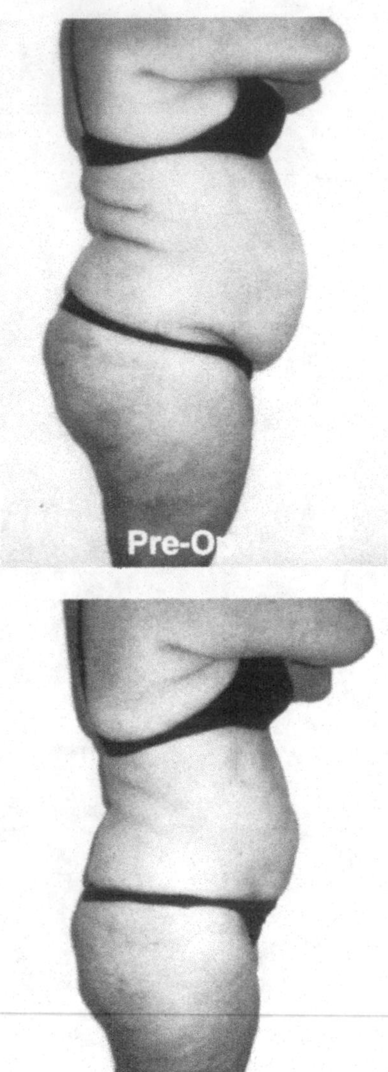

FIGURE 11 Large abdomen patient, fat behind muscles before (top) and after liposuction (bottom).

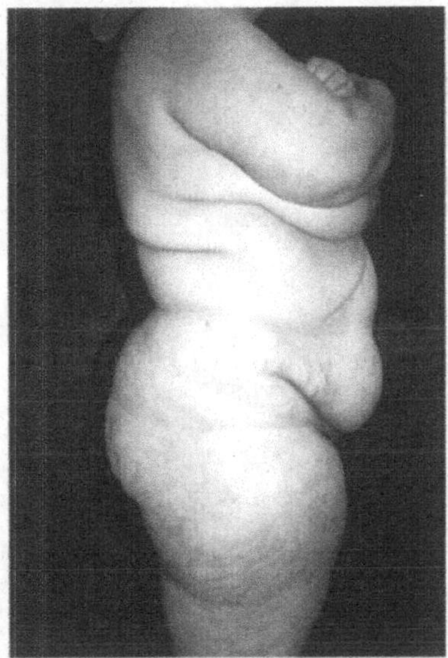

FIGURE 12 Abdomen patient, fat behind muscle.

larger patient (Fig. 13). During the consultation the patient must be evaluated not only to be put into one of the five groups previously listed, but also for hernias, goals, and mental outlook. This is the time to discuss the procedure and probable results in detail. The physician must explain which procedure should be done and why. The patient must be made aware of striae, which cannot be treated with liposuction, and scars as well as adipose deposits in the mons pubis so that they can be treated at the same time. They often hate the scars, which are bound down, allowing fat to build up on either side. Fat can hang over a Pfannenstiel C-section or hysterectomy incision. These unsightly lumps can often be seen in clothing and are very amenable to treatment during liposuction. It is important to know if the patient has had previous liposuction or laparoscopy as well as any other abdominal surgery because the fibrous tissue that may have developed postoperatively makes the liposuction more difficult to do.

PREOPERATIVE PROCEDURE

After discussing the benefits and limitations of the procedure as well as the risks, a Polaroid picture is taken for reference. It can also be used when discussing the expected results. The patient's medical history, including med-

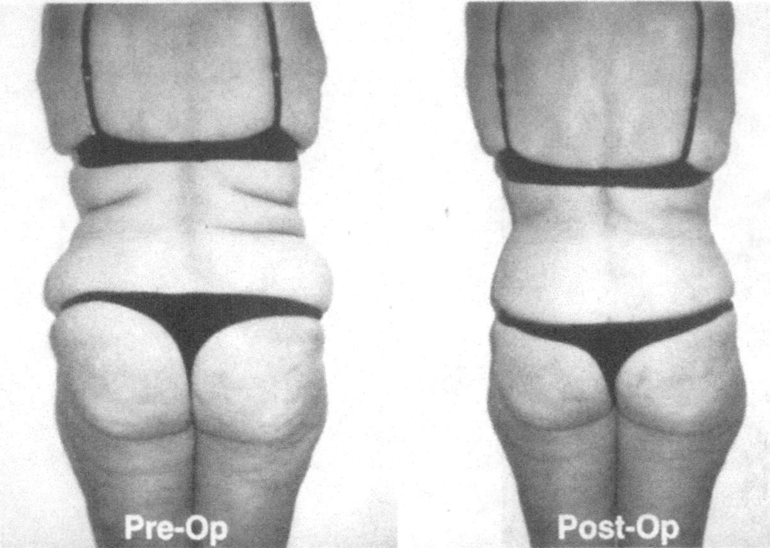

Figure 13 Hourglass abdomen before (left) and after liposuction (right).

ications, bleeding problems, allergies, recent weight gain or loss, previous surgery, and illness (including thrombophlebitis) is gone over at this time. The patient is given written information describing the tumescent technique of liposuction and is shown pictures of other patients who have had the planned procedure.

Once it has been determined that the patient is realistic and a good candidate for the surgery and the patient has decided to go ahead with the procedure, blood tests are done (Table 2). These include a complete blood cell count (CBC) with differential, Chem Screen 20, prothrombin and partial thromboplastin time tests, hepatitis C (Hep C) surface antibody test, hepatitis

Table 2 Preoperative Blood Tests

1. CBC with differential
2. Chem Screen 20
3. PT and PTT
4. Hep B surface antigen
5. Hep C surface antibody
6. HIV

B (Hep B) surface antigen test, and HIV tests. Tumescent liposuction requires the use of lidocaine, which is metabolized in the liver, so we do not do this procedure in patients with possible liver disease. Medical problems are evaluated individually and may require medical clearance. In our office, every patient over age 55 requires medical clearance with an electrocardiogram (EKG) and a note on the chart from their physician. Preoperative and postoperative instructions, including medications that must be avoided prior to surgery, are discussed at this time and copies are given to the patient (Table 3 and Appendices 1 and 2). We also decide if the fat is to be saved during the procedure so that the hand removal setup will be on the field if necessary. The patient is given a prescription for an antibiotic to start the day prior to surgery.

Most patients are very realistic about the results they can expect from tumescent liposuction and happy to be able to achieve them with such a safe procedure and minimal downtime. There are always those patients whom you can make perfect, those whom will show remarkable improvement, as well as those whom will show more subtle benefits such as looking better in clothing with very little scarring or morbidity. Liposuction is a very gratifying procedure for both the patient and the surgeon.

Preoperative Procedure on Day of Surgery

On the morning of surgery, vital signs are taken and on women a urine pregnancy test is done. Weight is measured to follow for future evaluation of results and to calculate the amount of lidocaine that may safely be used. Consent forms are gone over and signed (Appendix 3). Postoperative directions are gone over with the patient and a medical history is taken again. I perform a physical examination and fill out the medication sheet. I photo-

TABLE 3 Drug and Food Avoidance List

Avoid all products containing the following:
- Aspirin, salicylates, and/or salicylamides
- Nonsteroidal anti-inflammatory agents (NSAIS) such as ibuprofen, naproysyn, etc.
- Vitamin E or Coumadin

Avoid foods or supplements such as the following:
- Ginkgo biloba
- St. John's wort
- Ginger
- Ginseng

graph the patient with a Polaroid and occasionally a digital camera. The Polaroid shots are hung in the OR during surgery and kept on the chart to go over at postoperative visits.

Any questions the patient has are answered and the areas, including scars and any possible incisions, are marked (Figs. 14–16). This is done with the patient standing and then sitting. If skin is to be removed, the excision lines are marked at this time, sometimes using rhomboid templates made from X-ray film. A hep-lock is inserted and the patient is encouraged to go to the bathroom so that the bladder is empty prior to surgery as the amount of tumescent fluid injected may make the patient need to urinate and become uncomfortable during the surgery. The patient is then brought to the OR, where preoperative sedation is given.

Marking Incisions, Scars, and Skin Excision

If a patient with a small amount of fat involving just the lower abdomen is being done, I use three suprapubic incisions and two incisions in the lines emanating out from the navel, one on each side. These are also the incisions I use for a small upper and lower abdomen. If the abdomen is large or if I am also addressing the waist or hips, I will use two incisions, one on either side of the fat bulge on the lower and the upper abdomen, along with the

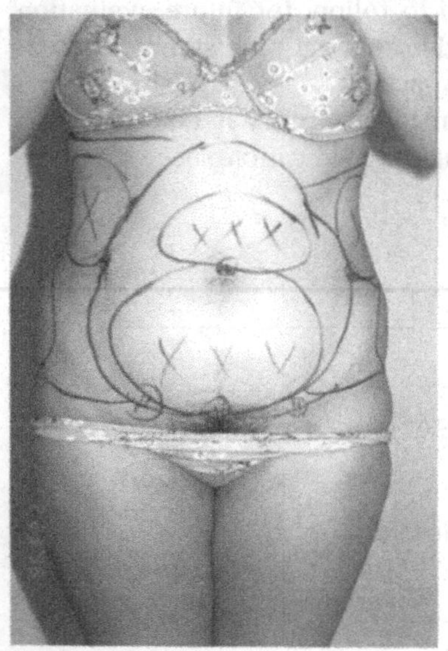

FIGURE 14 Markings for hourglass abdomen, front view.

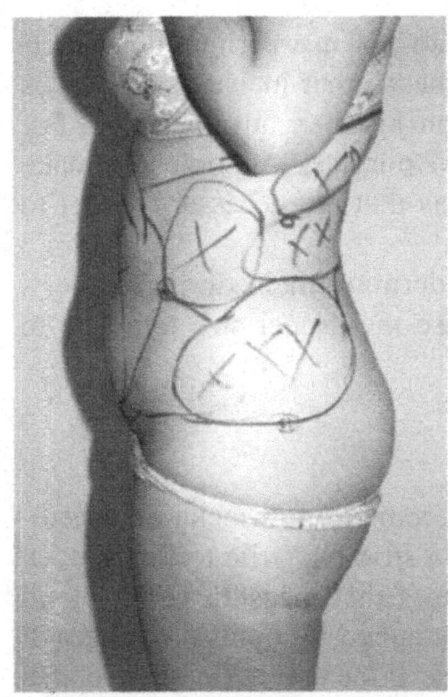

FIGURE 15 Markings for hourglass abdomen, side view.

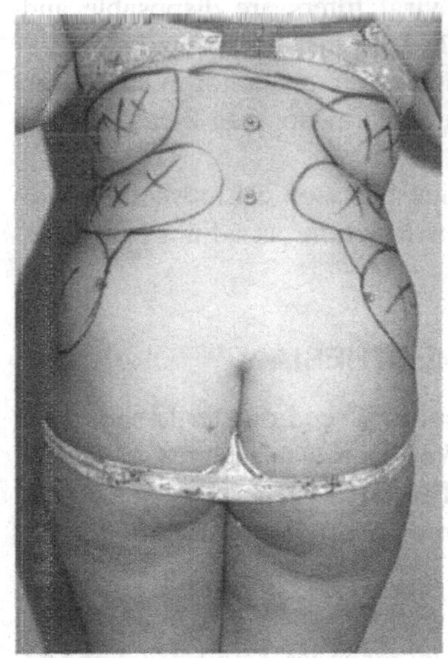

FIGURE 16 Markings for hourglass abdomen, back view.

three suprapubic incisions. In these cases, I do not use periumbilical incisions as I can reach the waist and hips from these other incisions as well as the abdomen. For the hips, I make an incision just beneath the bulge. For the back and the back of the waist for an Hourglass Abdomen, I make incisions over the spine and in any other areas that are necessary to get to the fat during surgery.

I also mark any scars so that I can undermine them during surgery. For skin excisions in the suprapubic area I use the proper size template to make the smallest possible excision.

EQUIPMENT

Our operating rooms are accredited by the Accreditation Association of Ambulatory Healthcare and surgery is done with a strictly sterile technique. All patients who have been sedated are on monitors that measure pulse, blood pressure, and EKG. In addition, patients are attached to a pulse oximeter. It is important to measure oxygen levels because lidocaine toxicity is related to decreased oxygen. The cannulas I use for the conventional liposuction include the Klein 10- and 12-gauge cannulas in three different lengths along with a 4-mm Lamprey and 3- to 4-mm Swann cannulas for larger areas, a 12-gauge Klein Capistrano cannula, and a 4-mm Scew cannula. I use a Toledo underminer to subcise scar tissue when necessary.

The aspiration machine has negative air pressure approaching 1 atm. The tubing, collection bags, canisters, and viral filters are disposable and comply with Occupational Safety and Health Administration standards.

In addition, I have backup aspirator machines, a generator in case there is a break in the electricity, and a syringe system so that I can always continue the case by hand.

In addition, I sometimes use a Lysonics Ultrasonic Liposuction Machine and/or a Xomed Powered Liposuction Machine as adjuncts to conventional liposuction.

SURGICAL PROCEDURE PRIOR TO ANESTHESIA

After being prepped with betadine, the patient is placed on sterile sheets on the OR table and drapes are put in place. We use a water-heated table pad under the drapes to keep the patient warm. The OR is generally cool, as the surgeon gets warm very quickly from the amount of energy used.

Anesthesia

For small areas I may use no sedation. For larger areas I will use 1 mg of catapres PO if the blood pressure is over 100/70, 5–10 mg of diazipam PO, and 50–75 mg meperidine, 25–50 mg promethazine, and 2.5–5 mg midazolam IM. On this regimen, the patient remains awake and comfortable during the procedure. The amount of sedation varies with the patient's weight, age, and medical history.

I use a three-step injection method [1]. I inject the incision areas with tumescent anesthetic solution using a syringe and 30-gauge needle. Using an 18-gauge spinal needle attached to the Klein infiltration machine on low (level 2 or 3), I inject a bolus of local tumescent anesthetic fluid directly under and through the incision site. Then I inject anesthetic solution radially out from the site. Next, I make the incision with a Nokor needle or no. 11 blade and insert the infiltrator through the already partially numbed areas with the machine still on low. The slower the rate of infiltration, the less the patient feels. I then inject tumescent anesthetic solution into all the areas using "showerhead" infiltrators and the Klein infiltration machine on level 6. The area is then rapidly and painlessly anesthetized.

Tumescent anesthesia, described by Jeffrey Klein, M.D., a dermatologic surgeon, has many benefits that make this procedure extremely safe with minimal recovery time (Table 4) (see Chapter 4 in this book) [2]. I generally use two concentrations of tumescent solution: .05 and .1% lidocaine both with 1/1,000,000 epinephrine (Tables 5 and 6). I try to use .1% lidocaine everywhere, but if I have to maximize the anesthesia because I am doing a three-dimensional or Hourglass Abdomen, then I will use .1%

Table 4 Benefits of Tumescent "Safe" Liposuction

Minimal blood loss	No transfusions necessary
Anesthesia long lasting	Minimal pain
General anesthesia not needed	Quicker recovery
Patient awake	Patient move into position needed
	Less thrombophlebitis/pulmonary embolism
	None of general anesthesia's risks
	Less risk of perforation of body cavities
	Patients feel better post-op
Surgery limited by safe amount of lidocaine	Fewer ancillary procedures (e.g., facelifts)
	Quicker recovery
	Shorter procedures
Tumescent solution antibacterial	Fewer infections
High volume solution	Provides fluid replacement
Infiltration of fluid into fat maximizes tissue	Smaller cannulas and smaller incisions

Table 5 .1% Lidocaine Tumescent Solution: .1% Lidocaine with 1/1,000,000 Epinephrine (1,000 mg Lidocaine)

950 cc Normal saline (0.9%)
50 cc Lidocaine (2%)
1 cc Epinephrine (1/1000)
12 cc Bicarbonate (8.4%)
1 cc Triamcinolone acetonide 10 mg/cc (optional)
Totals: 1,000 mg lidocaine
1/1,000,000 epinephrine

lidocaine in the abdomen and .05% in the other areas. I always leave myself some .1% lidocaine anesthetic solution to use if the patient feels any pain during surgery. I calculate the various options for the number of bags of tumescent anesthetic solution that I use based on the patient's weight and the safe number of milligrams of lidocaine that can be used (Table 7). These different concentrations are carefully marked with different-colored stickers. The final step is to inject 5–10 cc of 1% lidocaine directly into the most sensitive area around the umbilicus.

SURGICAL PROCEDURE

Liposuction surgery involves the removal of fat using long tubes—cannulas—inserted through small incisions in the skin made with a Nokor needle or no. 11 blade and attached to a suction aspiration machine. These cannulas are of varying lengths and widths and designs. The cannula tracks should

Table 6 .05% Lidocaine Tumescent Solution: .05% Lidocaine with 1/1,000,000 Epinephrine (500 mg Lidocaine)

950 cc Normal saline (.9%)
50 cc Lidocaine (1%)
1 cc Epinephrine (1/1,000)
12 cc Bicarbonate (8.4%)
1 cc Triamcinolone acetonide 10 mg/cc (optional)
Totals: 500 mg lidocaine
1/1,000,000 epinephrine

TABLE 7 Calculation of Safe Amount of Lidocaine

1. Calculate patient's weight in kilograms
   Weight in lb/2.2 = weight in kilograms
   For example: 160 lb/2.2 = 73 kg
2. Calculate safe amount of lidocaine assuming 50 mg lidocaine/kg body weight
   Weight kg × 50 mg/kg
   For example: 73 kg × 50 mg/kg = 3636 mg lidocaine
3. Round off to the nearest 500 mg
   For example: 3636 mg lidocaine to 3500 mg lidocaine
4. Calculate options for number of bags of solution
   For example: 3500 mg of lidocaine can be divided in several ways
   $3\frac{1}{2}$ bags of .1% lidocaine tumescent solution
   or
   3 bags of .1% lidocaine tumescent solution
   1 bag of .05% lidocaine tumescent solution
   or
   2 bags of .1% lidocaine tumescent solution
   3 bags .05% lidocaine tumescent solution
   or
   1 bag of .1% lidocaine tumescent solution
   5 bags of .05% lidocaine tumescent solution
   or
   7 bags of .05% lidocaine tumescent solution

criss-cross each other at multiple different levels to get the smoothest result. The smaller the cannula and the more superficial the cannula, the less the patient feels. The hand that does not hold the cannula, the guiding hand, tells you where the cannula is.

If I am collecting and/or saving fat for fat transfer, I do so by hand first using 10-cc syringes attached to a Coleman extractor. The next step, if the area is large or fibrous or if this is a secondary procedure, is to use the ultrasonic machine for 30 sec to 1 or 2 min with a 4-mm cannula on level 5. Sometimes I will use the powered liposuction machine instead of or after the ultrasonic machine. Most of the procedure (90% or more) is done with conventional liposuction. It is better to leave a little layer of fat under the skin for a smooth result. It is also important to make sure not to leave a donut of fat around the umbilicus but to make sure the entire area is even. The pubic area can also be treated at this time, if necessary, making sure to put a drainage incision at the lowest point and not to empty this area too aggressively.

When doing an Hourglass Abdomen, I start with the abdomen and then do each side. The final step is to have the patient prone and do the back areas. If I am releasing a scar, I use a Toledo underminer to detach the skin from the underlying tissue. If I am excising skin, I do so after the liposuction so that the skin is already undermined and only partially attached by some trabeculae to the underlying tissue. These can easily be cut without bleeding and the skin excised. The excision is then sutured with absorbable subcutaneous sutures bringing the lateral part of the rhomboid to the bottom and suturing from the sides toward the center. Then staples or a running suture of Ethilon or Prolene is used for skin closure and removed 2–3 weeks later. This technique enables the surgeon to make a smaller excision without dog-ears. The small gathers toward the center will smooth out with time. I do not suture the liposuction incisions.

IMMEDIATE POSTOPERATIVE CARE

After surgery the patient is cleaned and French tape is applied and left in place for 1 day to provide compression. In addition, a Klein leotard garment is worn until drainage stops. I think post-op compression not only makes the patient feel better as it stabilizes the skin, but also probably prevents hematomas and seromas. The patient is then moved to the post-op area and given something to eat and drink. Post-op directions are gone over again with the patient and whoever has come to accompany them home and a copy is given to the patient. A follow-up appointment is made for 1–3 days later. Unless there is a contraindication such as diabetes, I routinely give 2 cc of Celestone post-op and have patients continue antibiotics for 2–3 days after any drainage stops. Extra-strength acetaminophen is recommended for any discomfort the patient may have. Most patients need no medication for this problem.

Every patient is called that evening just to check on how they are doing.

POSTOPERATIVE CARE

Once drainage stops, the patient can switch to a panty girdle, bathing suit, or a "onesy" for compression. Again, compression feels good because it stabilizes the skin. Most patients wear the garment 24 hr/day for 2 weeks and then just during the day unless it feels better to wear it more often.

Patients generally return to work in 1–3 days and can start nonjarring noncontact sports the day after surgery if desired.

Patients are seen 1–3 days after surgery and at 1 week, 4 weeks, 3 months, and 6 months after surgery. Sometimes for various reasons we see them more often. Patients are weighed and repeat pictures are taken at the 3-month and 6-month visits. The lower abdomen may feel hard for 2–3 months. This is normal.

Liposuction is a debulking procedure with immediate results, but the subsequent formation of fibrous tissue that causes the skin to retract makes the final result even better (Fig. 17).

COMPLICATIONS

Tumescent liposuction is a very safe procedure with rare complications. Ecchymoses are uncommon and patients usually have only mild soreness post-op. Ecchymoses, if it does occur lasts only 3 weeks and mild dysesthesias, if they occur, can last 1–3 months. I have seen no hematomas or seroma. I have never had a patient need a transfusion. I have never had a patient develop thrombophlebitis or a pulmonary embolus and this is understandable as patients are awake and moving and walk in and out of the

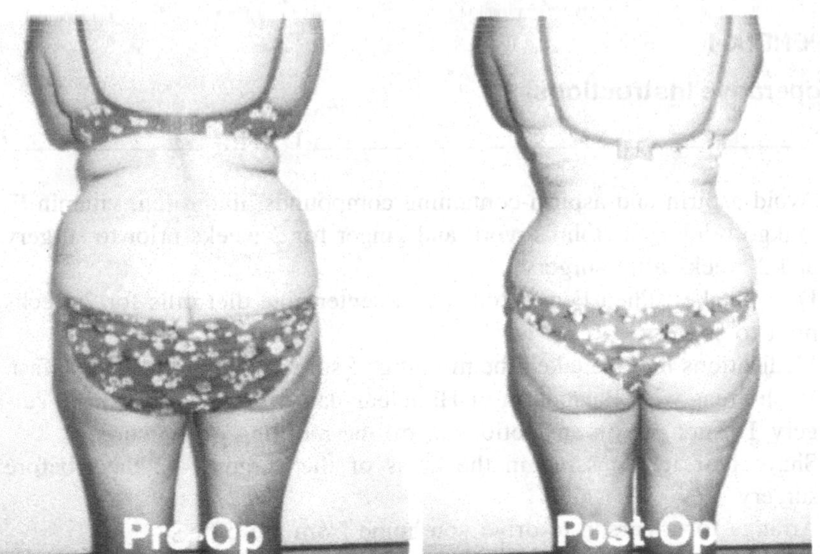

FIGURE 17 Hourglass abdomen before (left) and after liposuction (right).

OR. Patients with loose skin pre-op may get some waviness but this is not seen in patients with tight skin.

Small deposits of adipose tissue that may remain can easily be removed in 5–6 months with tiny cannulas using the aspiration machine or by hand with a 10-cc syringe. Most patients are thrilled with the results of the procedure. Sometimes patients who have excellent results are not happy. These patients should be weeded out at consultation. Occasionally a patient may gain weight post-op and it is important to have a weight record so you can point this out to them. Most dire complications are seen in hospitalized patients or in patients with general anesthesia where ancillary procedures are more likely to be done. In addition, it is difficult to perforate a patient who is awake.

SUMMARY

Tumescent liposuction of the abdomen using local anesthesia with or without release of scars, excision of excess skin, or concomitant liposuction of the waist, hips, and back provides wonderful improvement in body contour with minimal recovery time and negligible morbidity. Patients and surgeons are very happy with the results of the surgery.

APPENDIX 1

Preoperative Instructions

FOR: ______________________________ DATE: ____________

1. Avoid aspirin and aspirin-containing compounds, ibuprofen, vitamin E, ginkgo biloba, St. John's wort, and ginger for 2 weeks prior to surgery and 2 weeks after surgery.
2. Do not take "Phen-Fen," Redux or Phentermine diet pills for 2 weeks prior to surgery.
3. Medications may be taken the morning of surgery with a light breakfast.
4. Wash areas with Phisoderm or Hibiclens daily for 1 week prior to surgery. Do not put on any lotions or oil the morning of the surgery.
5. Shave hair if excessive in the areas of the surgery—2 days before surgery.
6. Arrange for a person to drive you home from the office.
7. Arrange for a person to stay with you overnight.
8. Start antibiotic as directed day before surgery.

9. Do not wear nail polish on the right index finger—if you have nail tips or acrylic nails, please remove them from the right index finger.
10. Wear loose comfortable clothing (e.g., sweatsuit—black or dark colored) that is easy to put on after surgery.
11. Wear slip-on shoes. (no laces or ties)
12. Bring girdle or binder in with you the day of the surgery.
13. Bring towels in with you the day of the surgery to put over car seats. Also bring a plastic bag to put directly over seat with towels on top to absorb fluid that is draining. Have both items ready on your bed as well.

APPENDIX 2

Postoperative Instructions

NAME: ______________________ DATE: ____________

1. ANTIBIOTIC: Please take all as directed.
2. PAIN MEDICATION: Pain is usually minimal and usually consists of soreness. It improves markedly over the first seven days. Extra-Strength Tylenol is generally all that is required. If you have pain unrelieved by Tylenol, please call the office.
3. MEDICATIONS TO AVOID: Do not take aspirin or non-steroidal anti-inflammatory medication such as ibuprofen for two weeks post-operatively.
4. OTHER MEDICATIONS: ______________________

   ____
5. DIET: Meals are not restricted. Please do not be concerned if there is weight gain in the first few days from the fluid injected. We prefer you stay on a low-fat diet. Please watch your weight. Try to stay 1–3 lbs. Lighter than your pre-op weight.
6. BATHING: Please sponge bathe until the tapes are removed. After that you may shower but replace the garment immediately after bathing. You may want to wash and dry the garment at the same time that you are showering. You can't take a bath for three weeks.
7. REMOVAL OF TAPES: Remove the tapes on ________________. Wet the tape in the shower. Let it stay wet for one hour and then take off tape while lying down. It is suggested that someone is with you while the tape is removed.
8. INCISIONS: Once tape is removed, grease incisions 1–2× daily for 4 weeks with Bacitracin ointment or Vaseline.

9. GARMENT: Your special garment or binder should be worn for 3–4 weeks. Please wear the garment 24 hours a day for 2 weeks following surgery, except when it is being washed. (After washing and drying the garment, put it back on with the seams on the outside). For the next 2 weeks the garment may be worn for 12–24 hours a day depending on your needs. The extent and location of your surgery will determine how long you need to wear the garment.
10. POSTOPERATIVE APPOINTMENTS: Please make an appointment 2 days post-operatively for a quick checkup. FOR FIRST POST-OP VISIT ONLY—please enter the office through the back door (to the left of the elevators) RING BELL, SPEAK INTO SPEAKER WHEN ANSWERED. At that time we will tell you when to come in for further follow-up.
11. DRAINAGE: Post-operative drainage occurs following surgery and can last 1–7 days. Place a large plastic bag or rubber mattress cover over mattress with towels on top to absorb the fluid that is draining. Although the fluid is red tinged, there is very little blood in it, most of it being injected local anesthetic and tissue fluid. If there is excessive bleeding or swelling or pain unrelieved by medication, please call the office immediately.
12. BRUISING: Mild bruising may occur for three weeks post-operatively.
13. NUMBNESS/SWELLING: Swelling will slowly disappear over 6 months. If mild numbness occurs it will usually disappear sooner. REMEMBER—ALTHOUGH YOU LOOK BETTER IMMEDIATELY FOLLOWING REMOVAL OF THE DRESSING, IT WILL TAKE 6 MONTHS TO SEE THE FINAL RESULT.
14. EFFECTS: Your skin may be flushed 1–3 days after surgery—this is normal.
15. DRIVING: You must wait 24 hours after surgery before driving.
16. RETURN TO WORK: Most patients can return to work within 1–2 days post-operatively.
17. EXERCISE: Patients can return to light non-jarring exercise as soon as they feel up to it. Jarring exercise, such as tennis, aerobics and running, can be resumed 3–4 weeks post-operatively depending on the extent and area of the surgery. A regular exercise program is encouraged.
18. QUESTIONS: If you have any questions, please call the office.

APPENDIX 3

Consent Form

I am aware that Dr. Narins has performed liposuction surgery since 1982. I have had the opportunity to ask questions about the procedure, its limitations and possible complications. By placing my initials next to the following items, I clearly understand and accept the following:

_____1. The goal of liposuction surgery, as in any cosmetic procedure, is improvement, not perfection.

_____2. The final result will not be apparent for 3–6 months post-operatively.

_____3. In order to achieve the best possible result, a "touch-up" may be required. There will be a charge for any "touch-up" operation performed.

_____4. Areas of "cottage cheese" texture, i.e. "cellulite" will be changed little by the liposuction surgery.

_____5. Liposuction surgery is a contouring procedure and is not performed for purposes of weight reduction.

_____6. Strict adherence to the post-operative regimen discussed by Dr. Narins (i.e. wearing an elastic garment for several weeks or months, exercise, diet and all other regimens discussed) is necessary in order to achieve the best possible results.

_____7. The surgical fee is paid for the operation itself and subsequent post-operative office visits. There is no guarantee that the expected or anticipated results will be achieved.

_____8. The goal of liposuction surgery, as in any cosmetic surgery, is to improve the appearance. It does not guarantee the reduction of any measurements, including the neck, waist and all other areas.

Although complications following liposuction surgery are infrequent, by placing my initials next to the following, I understand that they may occur:

_____1. Bleeding is rare, and in rare instances could require hospitalization and blood transfusion. It is possible that blood clots may form under the skin and require subsequent surgical drainage.

_____2. Skin irregularities, lumpiness, hardness and dimpling may appear post-operatively. Most of these problems disappear with time but localized skin firmness, lumpiness and /or irregularities may persist permanently. If loose skin is present in the treated areas, it may not shrink to conform to the new contour.

_____3. Infection is rare but, should it occur, treatment with antibiotics and/ or surgical drainage may be required.

_____4. Numbness or increased sensitivity of the skin over treated areas may persist for months. It is possible that localized areas of numbness or increased sensitivity could be permanent.

_____5. Objectionable scarring is rare because of the small size of the incisions used in liposuction surgery, but scar formation is possible.

_____6. Dizziness may occur during the first week following liposuction surgery, particularly upon rising from a lying or sitting position. If this occurs, extreme caution must be exercised while walking. Do not attempt to drive a car if dizziness is present.

_____7. Allergic or toxic responses to anesthetic are extremely rare, but possible.

_____8. In addition to these possible complications, I am aware of the general risks inherent in all surgical procedures and anesthetic administration.

_____9. I have not taken "Phen-Fen," Redux or Phentermine diet pills in the past 2 weeks.

My signature certifies that I have discussed the above material thoroughly with Dr. Narins and I understand the goals, limitations and possible complications of liposuction surgery, and I wish to proceed with the operation.

I hereby request, authorize, and give my consent to Dr. Rhoda S. Narins, to perform upon me:

____

____

____

(Please initial above each area) and whatever operations, treatments or technical procedures, may be deemed necessary or advisable in the diagnosis or treatment of my case. I further understand and agree that an associate of the stated doctor, under his/her supervision or control, may perform certain procedures. I also give permission to have such anesthetics administered as are deemed necessary or advisable.

I also give permission to use any of my x-rays or photographs in medical lectures or publications.

This particular operation which I am about to undergo has been explained to me in detail and I understand in general what is to be done, that there are calculated risks, and that the doctor has not made any guarantee whatsoever.

Because Dr. Narins is internationally known for her pioneering work in liposuction, visiting doctors from around the United States and other countries are frequent observers. I grant permission for any non-local visiting physician to observe the liposuction procedure.

____ ____________

Patient Signature Date

____ ____________

Witness Date

REFERENCES

1. Narins RS. Liposuction and anesthesia. Dermatol Clin 1990; 8(3):421–424.
2. Klein JA. The tumescent technique for liposuction surgery. Am J Cosmet Surg 1987; 4:263–267.

9
Violin: Hips, Outer Thighs, and Buttocks

Susan Ellen Cox
Cosmetic Surgery Center of North Carolina
Durham, North Carolina, U.S.A.

Females have a genetic predisposition to fat accumulation of the hips, outer thighs, and buttocks. The "violin"-shaped deformity describes the common pattern of fat overlying the iliac crest and the subtrochanteric area with an intervening gluteal depression. In anteroposterior view the contour mimics the shape of a violin. Liposuction can restore aesthetic balance to the disharmonious physique.

PATTERNS OF FAT DISTRIBUTION AND HORMONAL INFLUENCES

Localized predisposition to adiposities is dependent on regional differences in lipogenesis and lypolysis. The two most common patterns of fat distribution are gynecoid and android. Large thighs with trochanteric prominences, projecting buttocks, and enlargement of the hips characterize gynecoid, or peripheral, fat distribution. Android fat distribution is more commonly seen in men and is characterized by intra-abdominal fat. This pattern is not amenable to liposuction as the fat is often accumulated around the internal organs. Fat metabolism studies directly correlate with the clinical patterns. Adipocytes obtained from the abdominal and gluteal regions demonstrate four to five times greater lipolytic effect of noradrenaline than gluteal fat cells. The mechanism underlying regional differences is found at the receptor level. In the femoral region there is increased $\alpha 2$ receptor activity. Abdominal adipocytes showed a twofold greater increase in β-adrenergic density than did gluteal cells [1].

Obesity studies have been done to evaluate the mechanism behind increased gender-specific cardiovascular complications associated with visceral fat. In obesity, the catecholamine-induced rate of free fatty acid mobilization from visceral fat to the portal venous system is higher in men than in women. This is due to decreased function of the $\alpha 2$ receptor and increased function of the $\beta 3$-adenoceptors. Also, a larger fat-cell volume and increased ability of cyclic adenosine monophosphate to activate hormone-sensitive lipase was noticed in males [2].

In normal-weight females the hormone responsible for lipid synthesis lipoprotein lipase is higher at baseline in the gluteal/femoral (GF) region. These areas are larger and more sensitive to stimulation of lipogenesis by corticosteroids and estrogen. Early in pregnancy, lipogenesis of the GF region is stimulated. This creates a storage depot for fat, which can be mobilized in late pregnancy or during lactation. Femoral adiposities show a low sensitivity to the lipolytic effects of norepinephrine. However, in late pregnancy and during lactation, GF adiposities become sensitive to the lipolytic effects of norepinephrine. In starvation female abdominal lypolytic activity is increased; however, paradoxically, lipoprotein lipase and lipogenesis is increased in the GF region [3]. Therefore even when the female body is in a negative energy balance, fat in the GF region is preserved. It could be teleologically postulated that woman with the genetic predisposition to store fat in these areas were more likely to have progeny that survived during periods of starvation. Centuries of natural selection may have resulted in women with the common gynecoid fat distribution (Fig. 1) [4].

Another explanation for regional differences in mobilization of fat may be attributed to the fatty acid composition of specific areas [5]. Subcutaneous fat from the abdomen has a higher content of saturated fat when compared to fat from the outer thigh. The outer thigh subcutaneous fat has higher polyunsaturated fatty acid content. Adiposities having different fatty acid composition respond differently to caloric loss or excess [6].

PREOPERATIVE EVALUATION

Evaluation of the violin-shaped body requires addressing the cosmetic units of the hips, buttocks, and thighs. Isolated treatment of one area without addressing the others often produces suboptimal results. Additionally in some patients it may be difficult to separate treatment of the lateral thigh

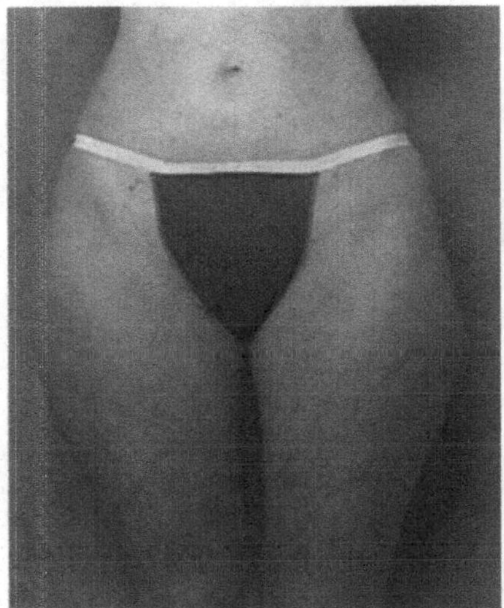

FIGURE 1 Gynecoid pattern of fat distribution.

from treatment of the anterior, posterior, and medial areas. More and more physicians are viewing liposuction as a three-dimensional contouring procedure [7–9]. Those patients with the typical violin shape will have a slim upper body with fullness of the hips, buttocks, and thighs. The thigh fullness in these patients is generally not isolated to the lateral region alone. It is often necessary to treat the thighs in two sessions to obtain a more slender appearance (Fig. 2). It is important to try and ascertain the degree of muscle mass that is contributing to the fullness. Patients with "large fullback thighs" should not be promised too much since the girth is secondary to large muscle mass and bone structure. Preoperatively the patient needs to understand the limitations that determine the degree of sculpting possible. The three limiting factors include musculature, skin elasticity, and cellulite [7].

The first limiting factor is the size of the quadriceps and hamstring muscles as these cannot be changed by liposuction. However, if the entire thigh is sculpted often thinning and balance can be achieved. Each section of the thigh contributes to the overall fullness and benefits from treatment. Additionally, weight loss and a program consisting of muscle-lengthening exercises such as yoga and swimming can aid in producing body-shape changes.

The second important factor, skin elasticity, has various etiologies. Poor skin tone may be due to sun damage and the aging process. Patients with inherited conditions of collagen such as Ehlers–Danlos or disorders of

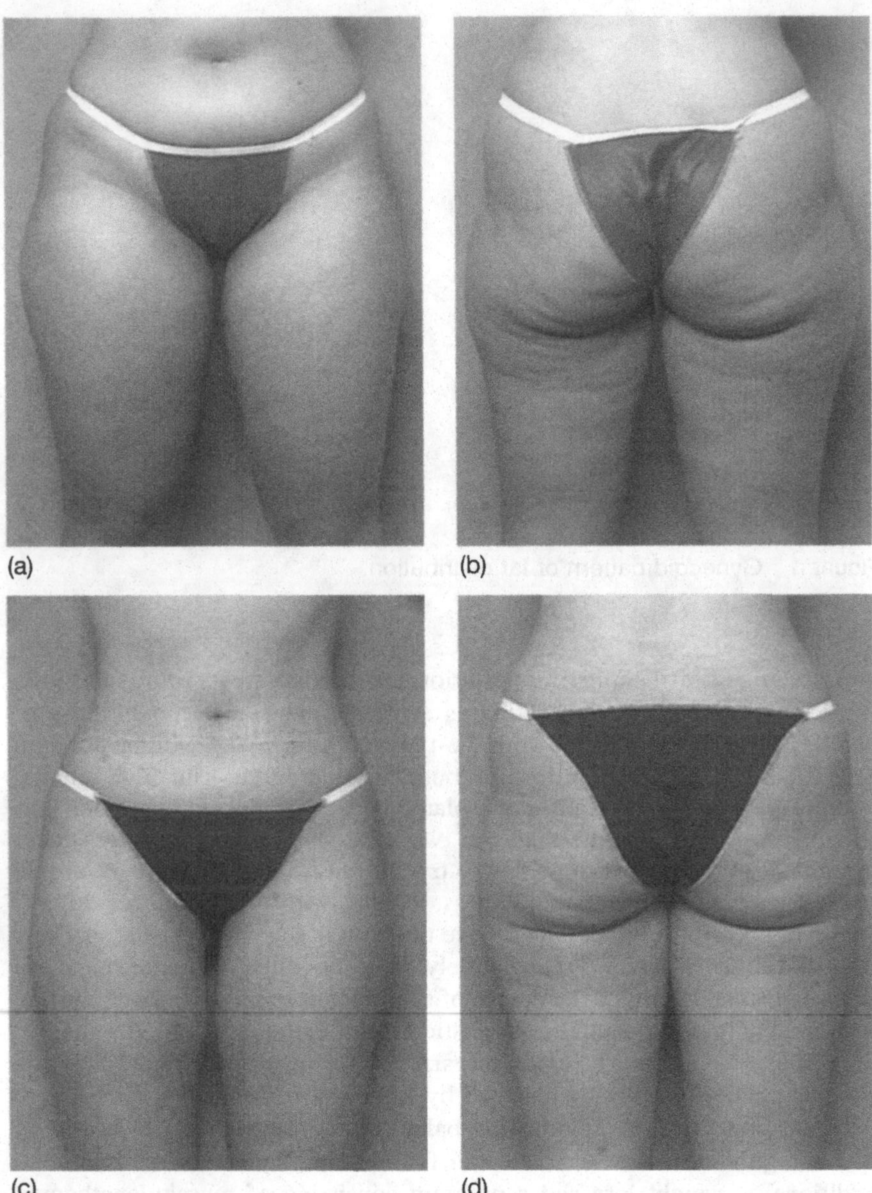

FIGURE 2 Circumferentially large thighs. Two liposuction procedures were required, the first session included the outer thighs, posterior thighs, and buttocks. The second session included the inner thighs, anterior thighs, and knees. (a and b) Preoperative anterior and posterior view. (c and d) Four months postoperation.

elastin such as cutis laxa should be identified [6]. Finally, patients who have had previous excessive weight gain and loss will be less likely to achieve good skin tightening.

The third factor is the presence of compartmentalized fat, or cellulite. Cellulite is mainly seen in the thigh and buttock regions of woman and affects 85% of postadolescent females. It is rarely seen in males and does not affect prepubertal females. Cellulite varies in degree from moderate to severe and it can be seen in normal or underweight individuals but excess weight accentuates the condition (Figs. 3a and 3b). Cellulite is thought to result from attachment of the skin to the underlying muscular fascia. It is a term used to describe irregularities of the skin with alternating areas of depression and protrusion [10]. Draelos et al. studied cellulite using ultrasound. She demonstrated projections of fat into the dermis and postulated that cellulite is a result of an inflammatory process involving the dermis and superficial fascia. Additionally an increase in dermal glycosaminoglycans has been reported in cellulite and this increase in water binding is picked up by ultrasound as low-density regions [11].

A variety of methods have been suggested for the treatment of cellulite. None have proven to be very successful. Recommendations include massage; endodermologie; weight loss; subcision of fibrous bands; dietary supplements; and creams, including retinoids, xanthine-based thigh creams, and herbal extracts [10,11]. Two of the more popular recent treatments include

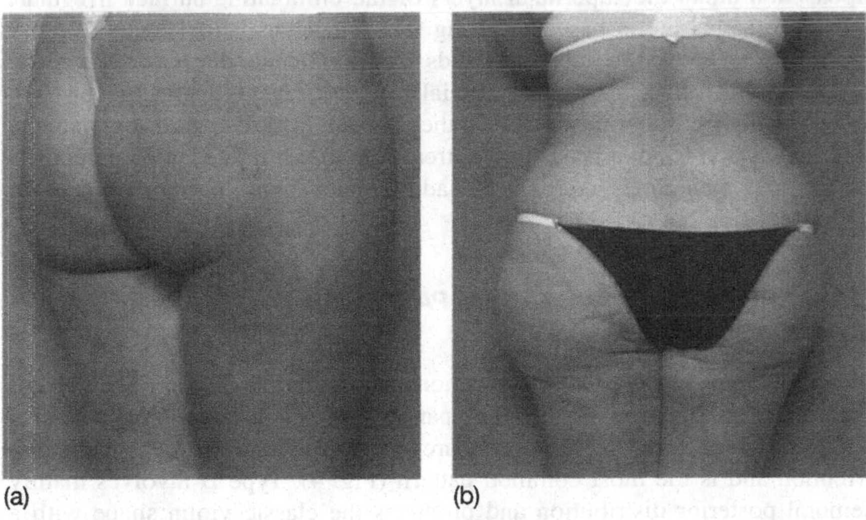

(a) (b)

FIGURE 3 (a) Minimal cellulite of outer thighs and buttocks in a thin individual. (b) Extensive cellulite in an overweight individual.

endodermologie and lymphatic drainage. Endodermologie (LPG, Ft. Lauderdale, FL) is a cellulite treatment based on the use of a patented machine which kneads the skin. The skin is sucked between rollers and kneaded. The company claims this improves the circulation, reduces tissue congestion, and enhances removal of waste products. The company is careful to state that it does not remove cellulite but reduces its appearance. An ongoing prospective study is evaluating liposuction followed by a 20-week course of endodermologie versus liposuction alone. Nine-month data show a 92% improvement in body contour and a 50% improvement in cellulite reductions with endodermologie. The second group showed no improvement in cellulite with 87% improvement in contour. Evaluation was based on photographic evaluation by four blinded physicians [12]. Lymphatic drainage or percussive therapy is a treatment that is emerging. Dr. Gregory Chernoff is conducting clinical trials using percussive therapy. A machine is used that oscillates in and out, up and down, and in a circular motion. The principle is based on driving lipophilic substances into the dermis. Chernoff plans to evaluate this by electron microscopic measurement of ions [13]. Long-term prospective studies validating the efficacy of many of the treatments for cellulite are lacking.

Physicians have varying opinions as to the success rate of treating cellulite with liposuction. Dr. William Cook finds the use of small cannulas near the surface attachment of the septal bands can release the depressed areas and improve the appearance [7]. Toledo et al. believe that superficial liposuction alters the superficial layers of fat, eliminating surface irregularities. The technique is based on using the Toledo dissector cannula with a forked tip to break the adherent bands in the reticular dermis followed by reinjection of a fine layer of superficial fat that prevents reattachment [14]. Occasionally liposuction can worsen the problem [15]. I stress to my patients that liposuction is not a procedure to treat cellulite. It treats regional deposits of fat, and sometimes there is the additional benefit of improvement of cellulite.

GASPAROTTI'S FOUR CLASSIC PATTERNS OF FAT ACCUMULATION

Gasparotti developed four classifications of commonly found "saddlebag" patterns. Classification of different patterns of fat distribution allows for subtle differences during the procedure. Type A is mainly trochanteric distribution and is the most common pattern (Fig. 4). Type B involves mainly femoral posterior distribution and produces the classic violin shape with a predominantly heavy buttock appearance (Fig. 5). Type C accounts for posterior inferior distribution (Fig. 6) and Type D is described as saddlebags

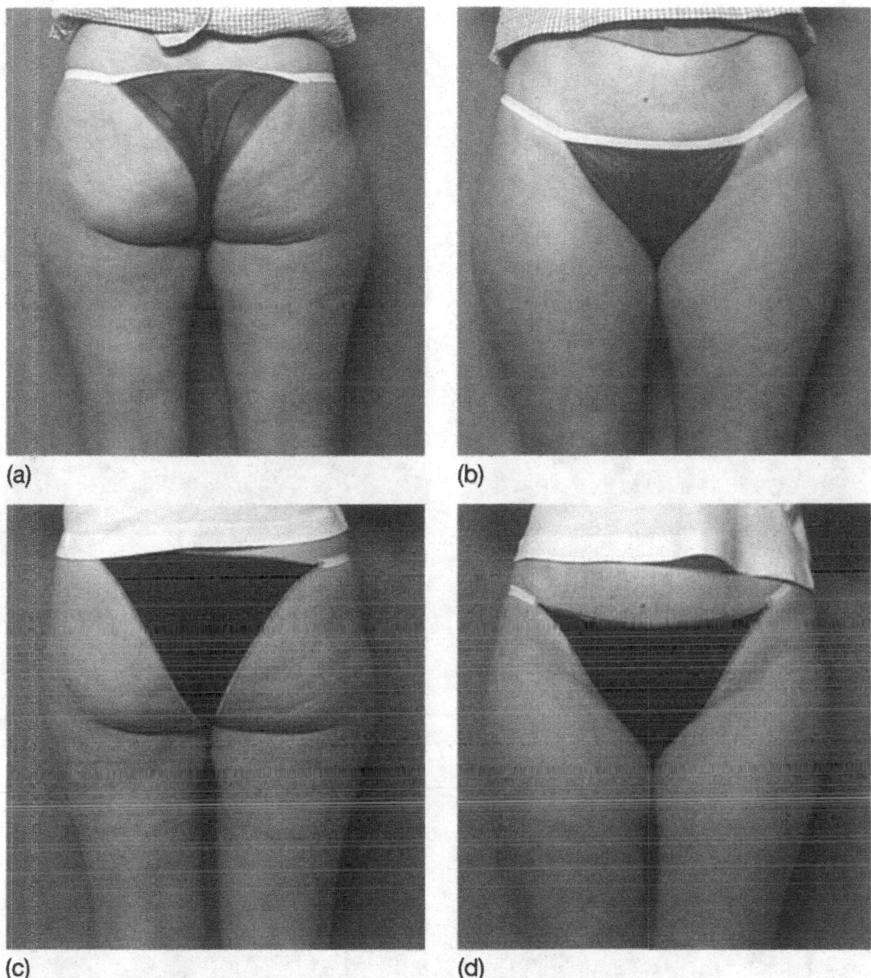

FIGURE 4 Type A saddlebag with mainly trochanteric distribution. (a and b) Preoperative. (c and d) Six weeks postoperative.

with sharp gluteal distribution (Fig. 7) [16]. Type A patients require removing more fat over the lateral femoral area and decreasing amounts peripherally. Type B (lateral femoral posterior) saddlebags require two points of greater aspiration laterally and posteriorly. In addition these patients often require more extensive sculpting of the buttock to achieve reduction of the buttock heaviness. Type C (posterior inferior) saddlebags can be viewed in a similar fashion to B but generally have less buttock involvement. For Type

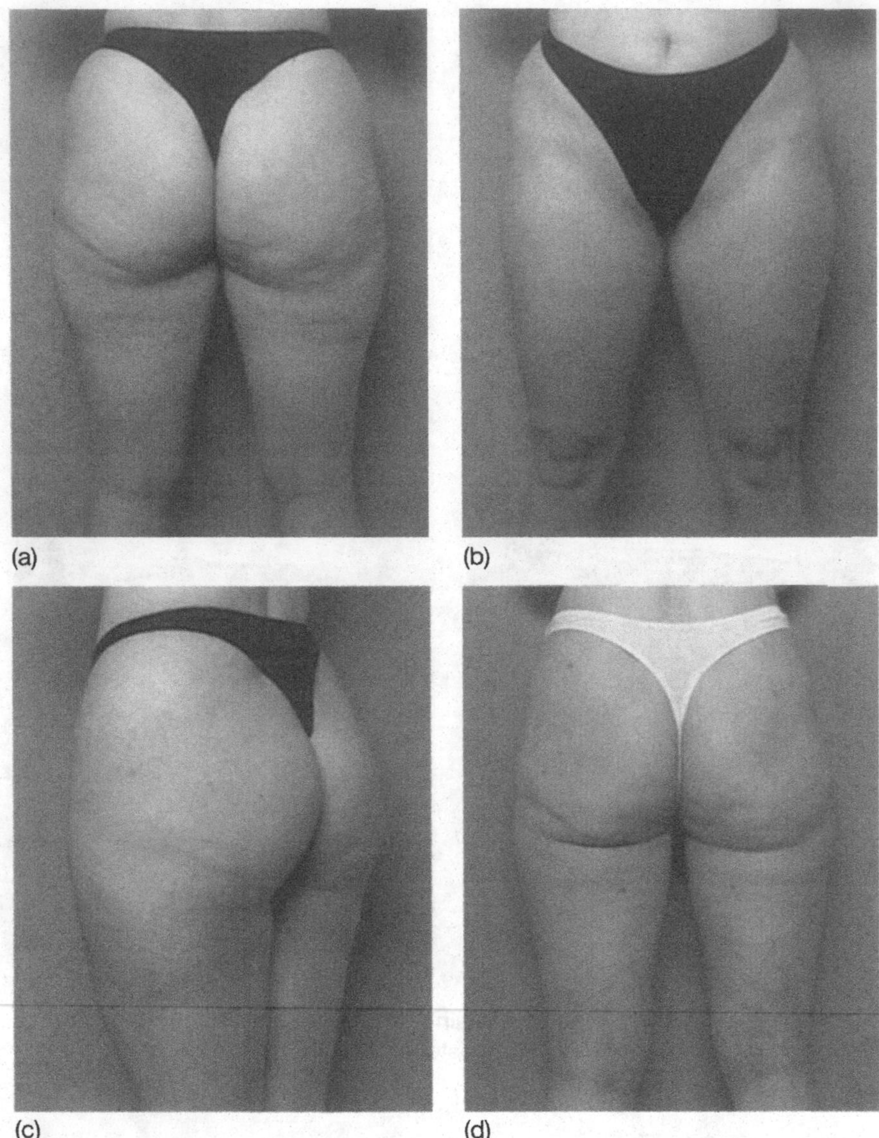

FIGURE 5 Type B saddlebag with mainly femoral posterior distribution. (a–c) Preoperative. (d–f) One year postoperative.

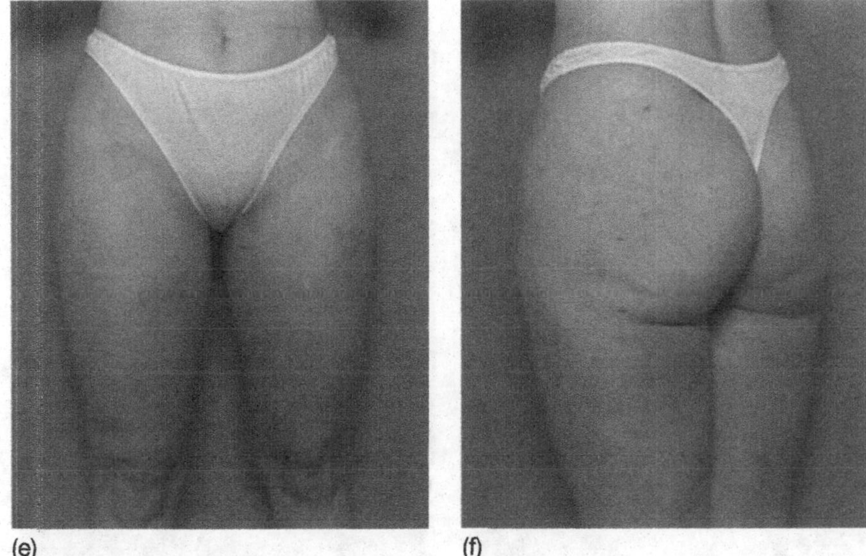

(e) (f)

FIGURE 5 Continued.

D saddlebags with a sharp gluteal fall, Gasparotti advocates careful aspiration superficially of the gluteal region decreasing toward the periphery to attain harmony of the lateral femoral and gluteal region [16]. This idea of more superficial liposuction in the gluteal region is contradictory to what is often taught. Many physicians recommend deep liposuctioning of the buttock to debulk it. Lifting of the cannula and sculpting with the natural curve can prevent flattening [7]. Others advocate a combination approach: deep and superficial liposuction in the upper one-third; deep liposuction in the middle third, where there is the greatest projection; and superficial suctioning of the curvature of the lower one-third with no violation of the infragluteal crease [17].

PHYSICAL EXAMINATION OF THE VIOLIN SHAPE: HIPS, LATERAL THIGHS, AND BUTTOCKS

The idealized female form as often displayed in the media and perpetuated through fashion presents a single smooth convex curve beginning at the waist, extending over the iliac crest and greater trochanter, and continuing to the knee [18]. The posterior view also presents a single smooth curve although in reality most women have a more pronounced gluteal recess. This plus the buttock heaviness accounts for the gluteal crease. The gluteal

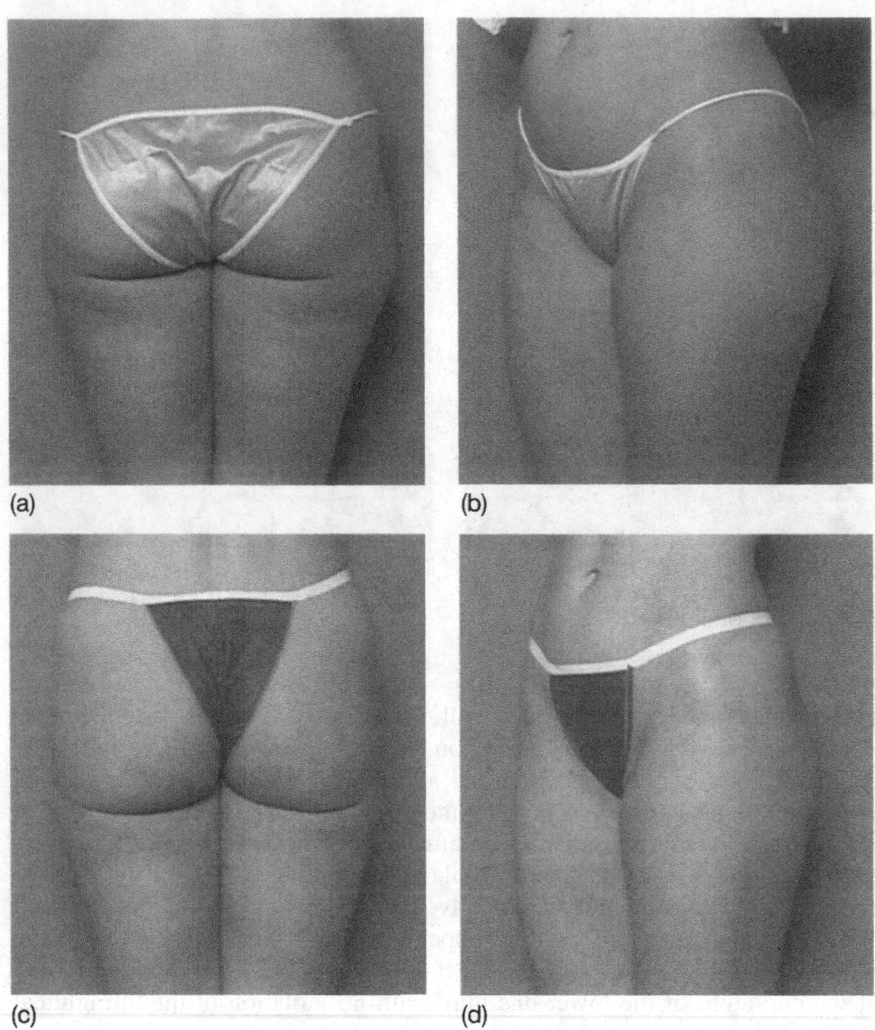

FIGURE 6 Type C saddlebag with posteror–inferior distribution. (a and b) Preoperative. (c and d) One year postoperative.

crease is variable in distance, extending from the midline and ending between one-third and two-thirds of the way to the lateral buttock. Some cultures idealize a fuller buttock with more projection from the lower back. Some gluteal fullness and rounding is important to maintain a youthful and desirable appearance.

The physical examination is always performed with the patient dis-

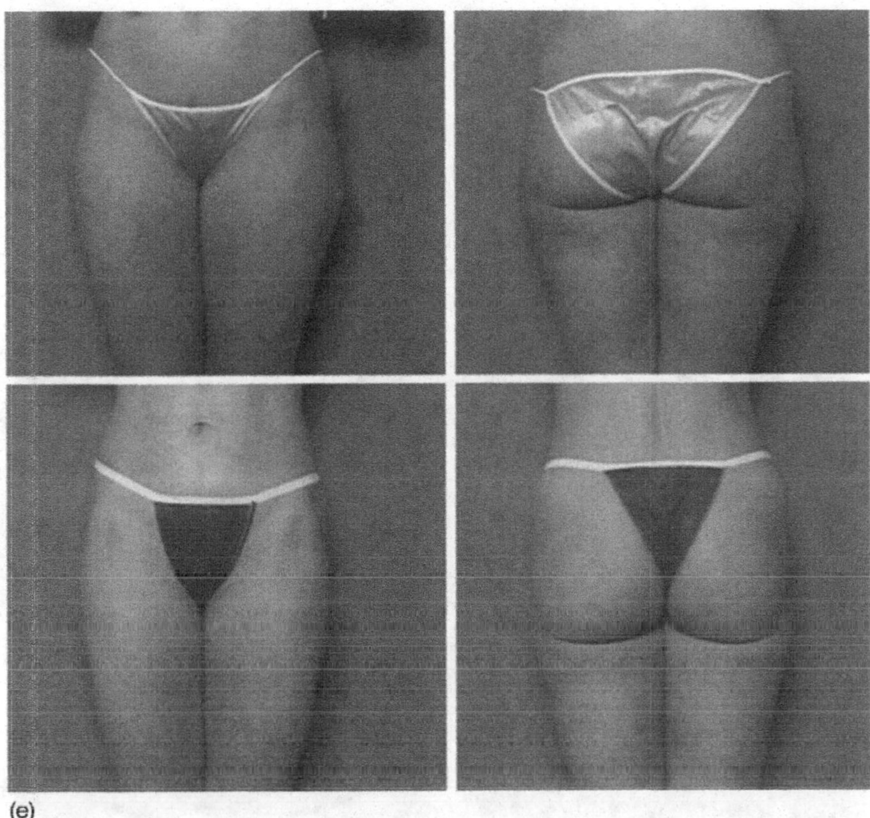

(e)

FIGURE 6 Continued. (e) Preoperative (upper) and one year postoperative (lower).

robed in the standing position. It is best to get the patient's input about her area of main concern. Defining the patient's realistic goals is crucial. Women often state that they want to be rid of the double bulge or "violin" deformity (Fig. 8). This is defined as fullness at the iliac crest area, fullness at the subtrochanteric area, and the intervening gluteal depression. Although a perfectly smooth, convex line along the lateral aspect of the thigh–hip area is the ideal, it may not be achievable or desirable for every woman [18]. Reduction rather than elimination of the double bulge is more realistic. Bodies that have disproportionately larger lower halves can be brought into balance with liposuction. It is crucial that the surgeon evaluates the cosmetic unit of the lateral and posterior flanks, buttocks, and thighs. Considering these interrelationships will permit uniform sculpting.

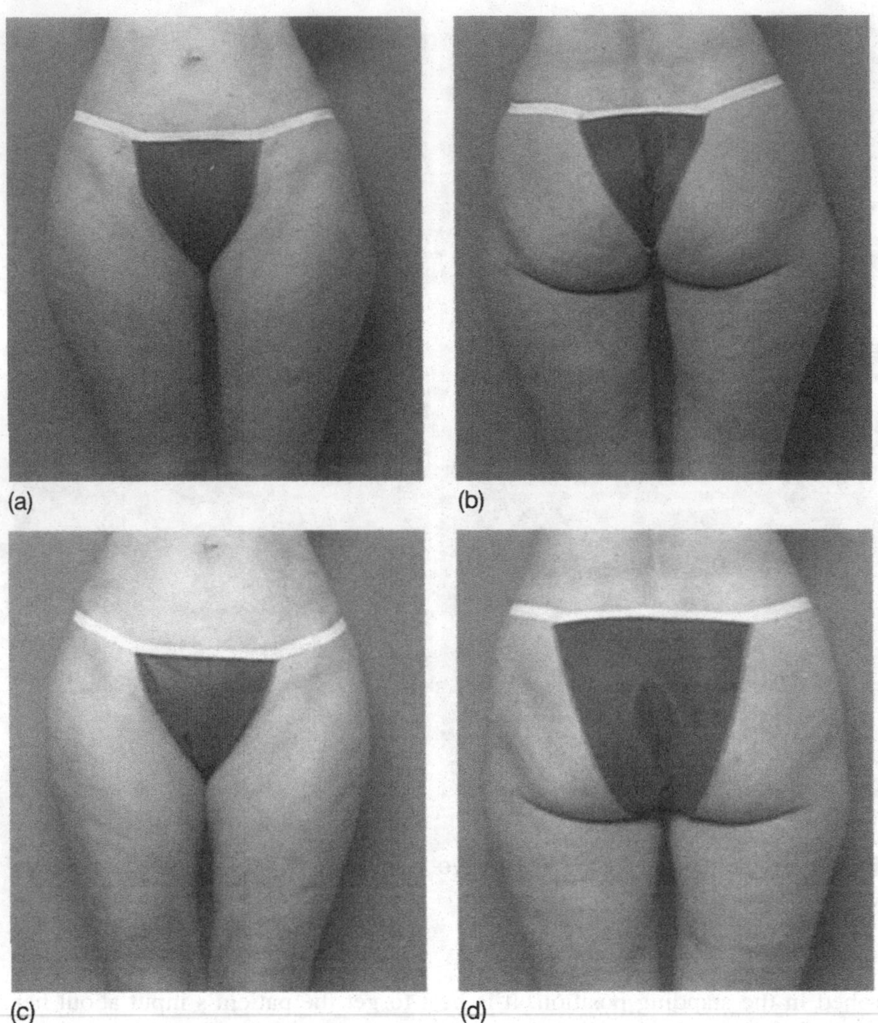

FIGURE 7 Type D saddlebag with sharp gluteal fall distribution. (a and b) Preoperative. (c and d) Six months postoperative.

Patients will usually point out the lateral thigh fullness. It is important to have the patient contract the buttock muscles forcefully to demonstrate the contribution of the lower lateral part of the buttocks to saddlebag formation. This maneuver will tend to flatten the outer thighs and force the fat medially and superiorly into the buttocks (Fig. 9). This allows the patient

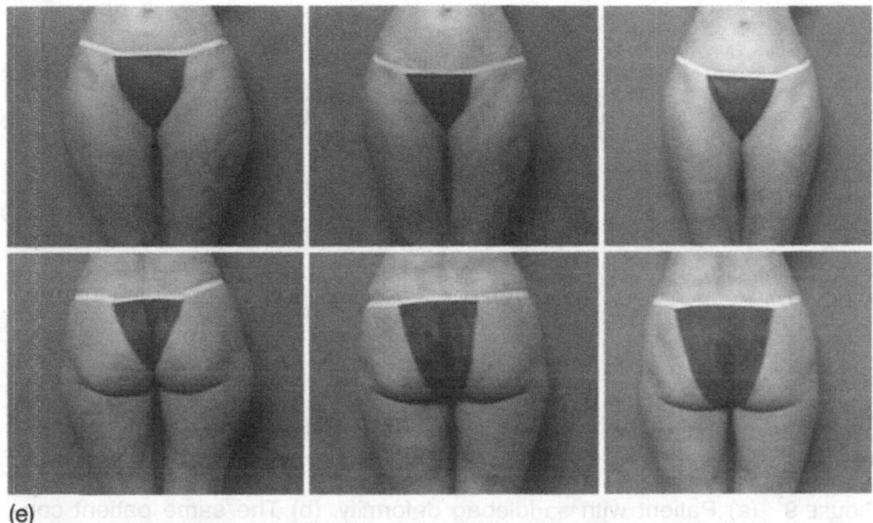

(e)

FIGURE 7 Continued. (e) Composite view preoperative (left), six weeks postoperative (middle), and one year postoperative (right).

to understand the importance of including liposuction of the lateral portion of the buttock to achieve the desired results.

The surgeon should evaluate the thighs and buttocks by palpation and inspection. Skeletal asymmetries such as scoliosis are noted first. Scoliosis will result in differences in the heights of the iliac crests and greater tro-

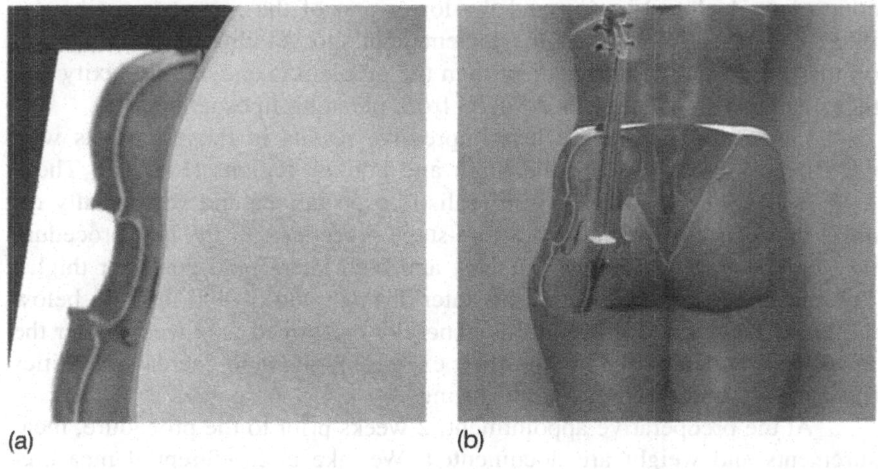

(a) (b)

FIGURE 8 (a and b) Double bulge or "violin deformity."

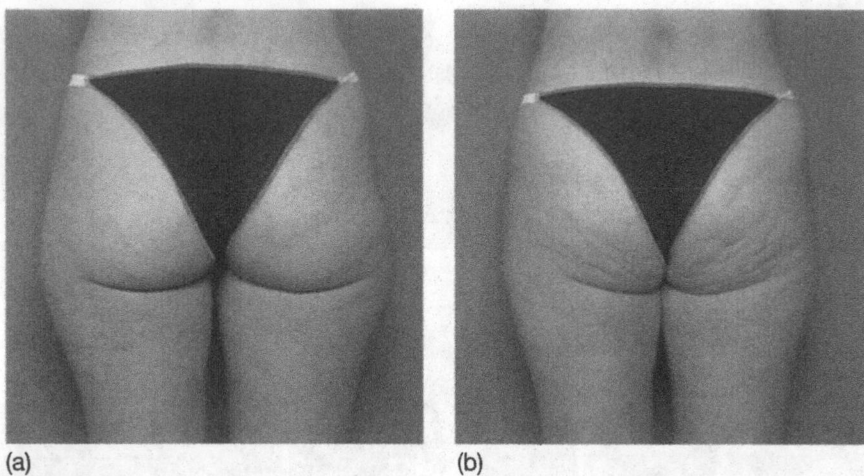

(a) (b)

FIGURE 9 (a) Patient with saddlebag deformity. (b) The same patient contracting the buttocks to help identify the lower lateral buttock contribution to saddlebag deformity.

chanter, which will result in asymmetry of the soft tissues (Fig. 10). Differences in extremities length will also produce asymmetries. Patients who have no underlying skeletal problems can also have asymmetries. Hypertrophy of one side of the buttock may be seen and should be brought to the patient's attention (Fig. 11). Gasparotti describes a technique for obtaining symmetry: "Where there is a difference in the height of the gluteal folds, the subgluteal part of the higher gluteus must be defatted deeply so it falls slightly. The contra lateral gluteal region and the lower part of the gluteus must be defatted superficially" [16]. If the patient points to cellulite or pulls upward on the skin to show improvement then the problem is one of skin laxity and these patients should be discouraged from pursuing liposuction.

Liposuction will yield less impressive results in those patients who have large muscle mass in the thigh and buttock regions (Fig. 12). These patients need to be counseled on realistic expectations and will usually require liposuction performed in a two-stage procedure. In the first procedure the surgeon treats the hips, buttocks, and both lateral and posterior thighs. The second session will target the anterior thigh and medial thigh to below the knee. The second procedure is generally performed 2–4 weeks after the first. These patients need to alter their exercise regimen to decrease activities that produce bulk such as weight lifting.

At the preoperative appointment, 2 weeks prior to the procedure, measurements and weight are documented. We take circumferential measure-

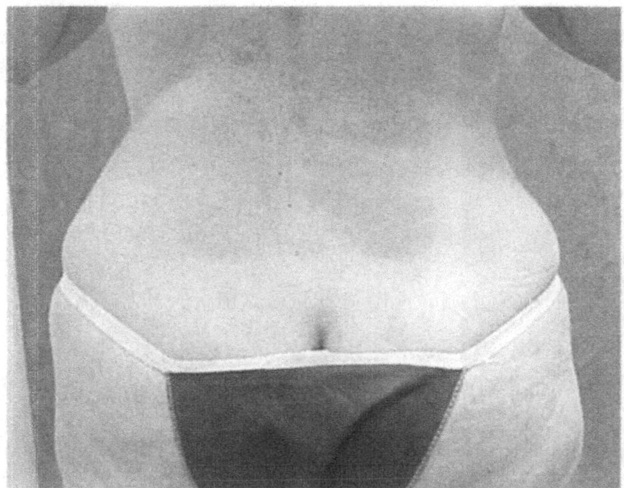

FIGURE 10 Scoliosis produces asymmetry. Note the elevation of the left hip and increased fullness on this side.

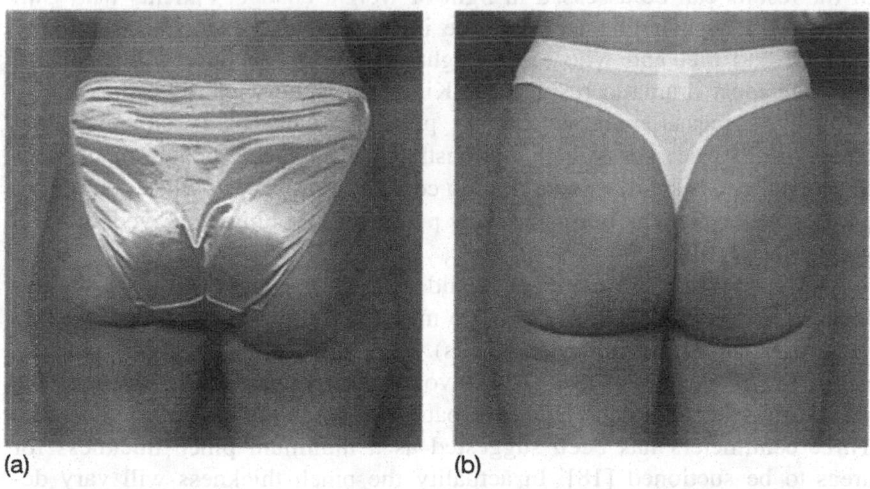

FIGURE 11 (a) Hypertrophy of the right side of the buttock and asymmetry of the infragluteal crease. (b) Postoperative correction of asymmetry.

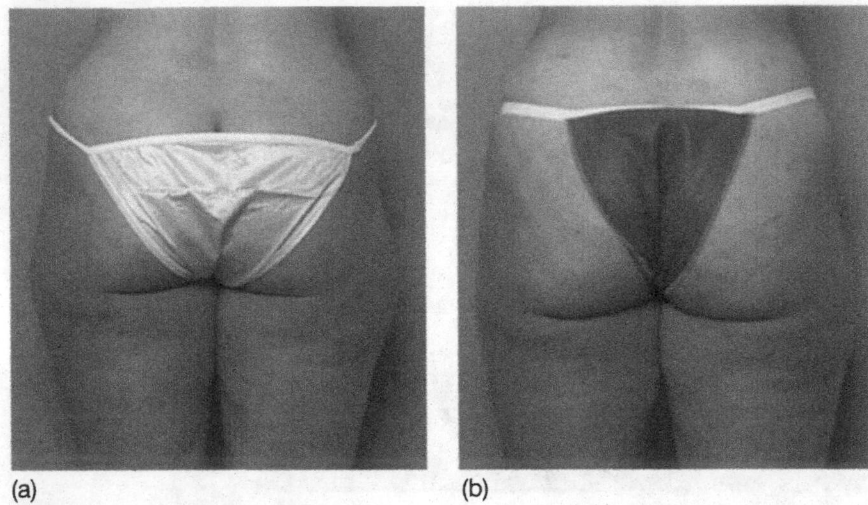

(a) (b)

FIGURE 12 (a) Preoperative view of a patient with large thigh muscle mass. (b) Postoperative appearance showing modest improvement after liposuction of the outer thigh, buttocks, and hips.

ments of each thigh and around the largest portion of the saddlebag with care to note the distance from the trochanteric depression. Measurements around the hips and buttocks are taken. Weight is recorded so that evaluation of the results can be assessed in light of weight change. Patients who gain weight will be negating some of the improvement. Patients who actively exercise and diet and who lose weight after the procedure will generally have the most dramatic results. Dr. Kimberly Butterwick advocates body-fat-analysis measurements pre- and postoperatively using calipers, float tanks, or other devices to help demonstrate a measurable benefit of liposuction to patients. She does note that no correlation was seen when comparing percentage change in body fat with percentage volume removed or with weight loss [19].

The physical examination should take into account the above issues (briefly, skin turgor, cellulite, muscle mass, asymmetries, scars, preexisting surface irregularities, and varicosities). I test for the thickness of subcutaneous fat by the pinch test. This involves three maneuvers: pinching the skin, lifting the skin, and having the patient contract the underlying muscles. Three centimeters has been suggested as a minimum pinch thickness for areas to be suctioned [18]. In actuality the pinch thickness will vary depending on the anatomic region. The outer thighs, buttocks, and hips are always thicker than the inner thighs or calves (Fig. 13). Lifting the skin

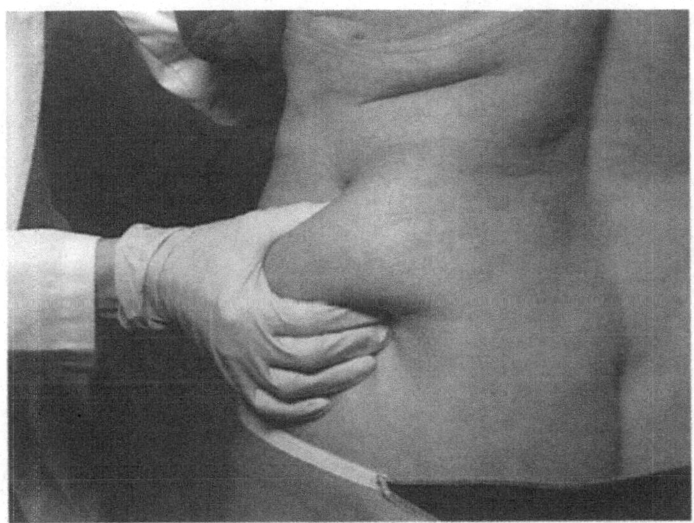

Figure 13 Pinch test is performed to determine if the patient will benefit from liposuction.

helps evaluate patients with poor skin turgor (Fig. 14) and muscle contraction, as discussed, evaluates the lateral thigh–buttock relationship. The preoperative assessment evaluates the entire region from all views (anterior, lateral, and posterior). The hips and lateral thighs are viewed as a framework for the buttocks area. The lateral gluteal depression or trochanteric depression is variable. This depression is caused by fascial connections from the superficial facial system to the deep muscle fascia. This landmark needs to be pointed out and discussed with the patient prior to surgery so that it is not later thought to be resultant of the surgery. This area should be marked appropriately and designated a zone not to be suctioned. Suctioning the hips and lateral thighs produces a tighter, more slender appearance of the buttocks.

The buttocks should be evaluated to determine the weight, protrusion, and ptosis present. In some ethnicities there may be greater posterior projection and muscle mass. A reduction in the size of the buttock is possible but often limited by the underlying muscle mass (Figs. 15a and 15b). Volume reduction of the buttock is important to relieve the downward and outward pressure that adds to lateral thigh protrusion.

The upper posterior thigh, or "banana fold" is a convexity from the inferior gluteal crease to the posterior thigh. This may be more prominent in some individuals. This deep fat acts like a pillar supporting the buttocks.

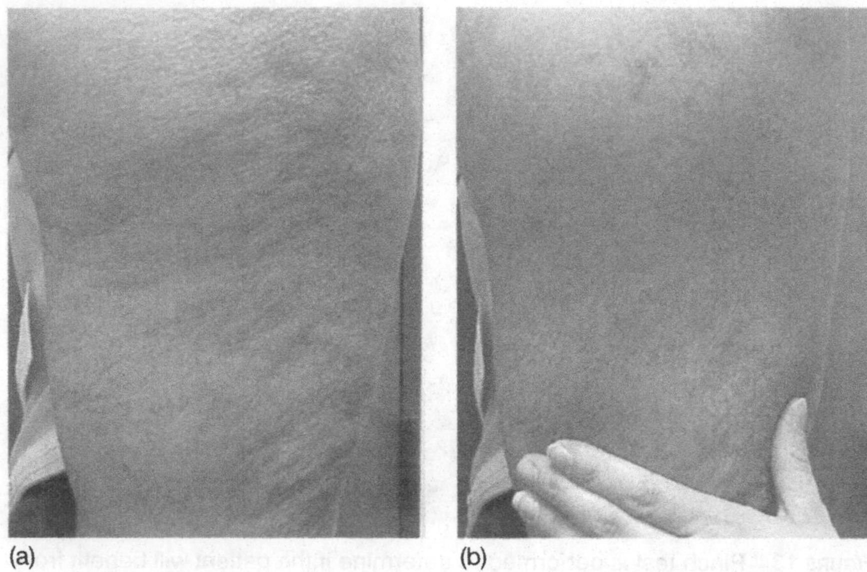

(a) (b)

FIGURE 14 (a) Skin laxity. (b) Stretching or lifting the skin helps identify poor skin turgor.

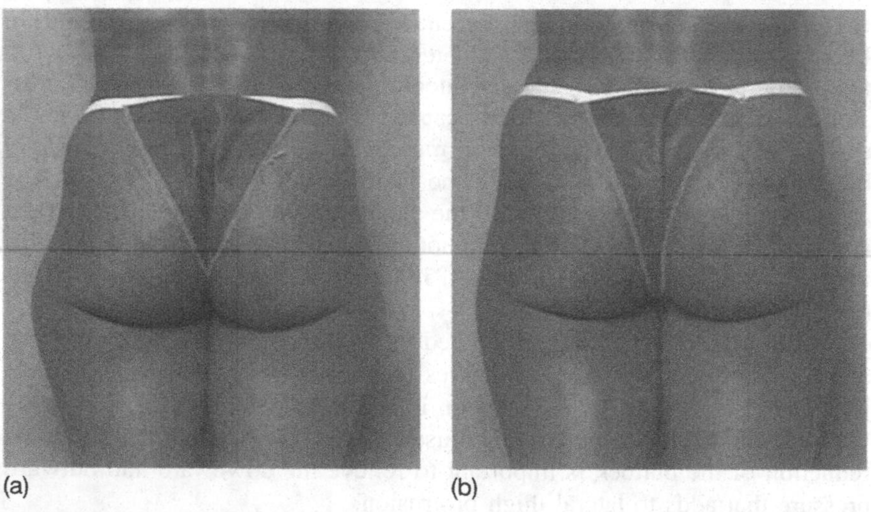

(a) (b)

FIGURE 15 (a) Preoperative African American female with posterior projection of the buttocks and significant muscle mass of the buttocks and thighs. (b) Six months postoperation.

Liposuctioning in this region should be avoided or done more superficially than in other areas so as not to disturb the infragluteal ligaments (Luschke's ligament) [17].

Patients to be selected for liposuction include those of normal weight to those moderately overweight. Patients with disproportionate fat deposits regardless of whether they are large or small can greatly benefit from liposuction.

INTRAOPERATIVE MARKINGS

Liposuction of the violin-shaped body requires contouring of the cosmetic unit consisting of the hips, buttocks, and lateral thigh. These areas should be marked and treated in a single session if possible. This will be dictated by safe usage of tumescent fluid; I limit myself to 55 mg/kg [20]. A contour map is drawn with the patient standing. I mark the areas with maximum fat excess by a series of concentric circles. The central circle represents the point of maximum projection. The outermost circles will also require thorough deep liposuction. A crisscross pattern is also marked from each incision site. Feathering is represented by straight lines at the outer edge of the furthest circle. Feathering is done by blending areas that have been liposuctioned with nonsuctioned areas. Areas to be avoided, such as the lateral gluteal depression, are marked with an "X" (Fig. 16). This landmark is best

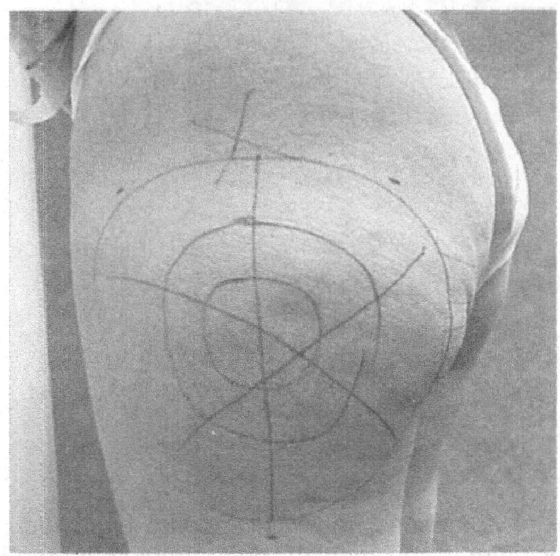

FIGURE 16 Preoperative outer thigh markings showing the lateral gluteal depression indicated by an "X."

identified by having the patient contract her buttocks. Incisions are made with a no. 11 blade and are no more than 3 mm in length. The incisions are carefully placed and asymmetry is desired in dark-skinned patients to prevent a "surgical appearance." One must take additional care with these patients to limit trauma to the skin, which increases the risk of postinflammatory hyperpigmentation. The number of incisions is determined by an effort to minimize scars and maximize smoothness and thorough liposuctioning of the area. Too few incisions will decrease the smoothness of the results and will produce a tunneling effect, or "waviness." Incisions that are too small or too few will increase trauma and friction to the skin.

I first mark the hips with incisions superior, posterior lateral, and inferior to the area outside the furthest circle. Incisions for the lateral thigh include two superior incisions, one inferior, and the fourth in the infragluteal crease (Fig. 17). An inferior incision allows for gravitational drainage of the tumescent fluid. Suctioning of the lateral thigh can be accessed through the infragluteal crease incision for blending with the posterior thigh and criss-crossing of the lateral thigh. It is crucial not to transect the infragluteal crease or disturb the superficial facial attachments when suctioning from these incisions. There is not a consensus on placement of incisions for the buttocks. Various suggestions include a single infragluteal midline incision [7]; three

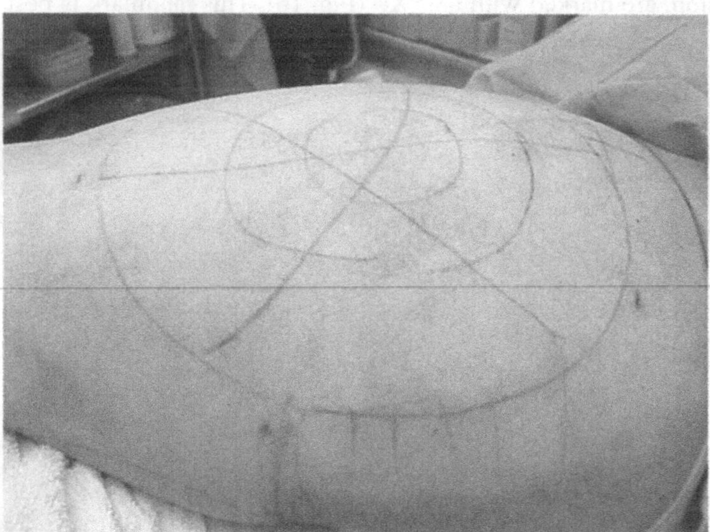

FIGURE 17 Outer thigh after being tumesced; the skin appears blanched. Note incision sites; two superior (lateral and medial), one infragluteal, and one inferior for drainage.

intragluteal incisions [21]; and, viewing the buttock as a clock placing three incisions on the left one at 11:00, 9:00, and 7:00 respectively and doing the same on the corresponding sites right (P. Lillis, personal communication, 1997).

INTRAOPERATIVE POSITIONING

The optimal position for liposuction of the hips is in the lateral decubitus. It is helpful to place a pillow between the knees to take pressure off the ileotibial band [7]. This facilitates the removal of the deeper fatty tissue.

Positioning for the thighs is also in the lateral decubitus position, but it is modified by the use of a midine wedge pillow (Fig. 18). The use of an intraoperative wedge allows the thighs to assume a position similar to standing. The pillow allows for proper positioning of the femur by rotating it anteriorly and medially and pointing the toes inward. An alternative to the use of the wedge is to have an assistant hold the leg at the knee and internally rotate and abduct the leg. This maneuver approximates standing so that oversuctioning does not occur. In order to not tire the assistant this can be done when suctioning over the greater trochanter (M. Kaminar, personal communication 2000). Both of these maneuvers accomplish the same goals:

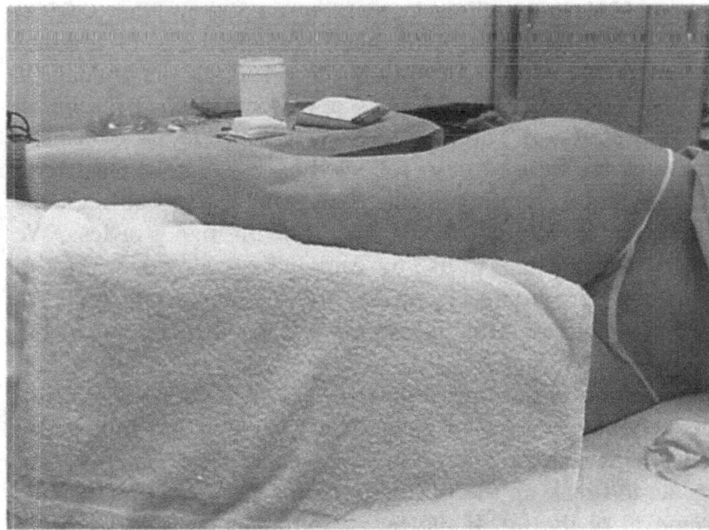

FIGURE 18 Positioning for liposuction of the outer thigh with the Midine pillow. This helps maintain the uppermost lateral thigh in an intraoperative posture that approximates anatomic position.

(1) to optimize the biomechanical positioning of the patient's thigh during surgery, (2) to produce superior aesthetic results for the lateral thigh, and (3) to allow the surgeon to remove the appropriate amount of fat without oversuctioning [22].

Positioning for the buttocks is in the prone position with a pillow under the pelvis to help facilitate deep suctioning in this location. It also helps maintain the natural curve to facilitate blending with the thighs.

PROCEDURE

After the patient has been marked he or she is sterilely prepped and draped. Standard monitoring is used, including blood pressure and pulse oximetry. Electrocardiogram is used in patients with cardiac history or in those over 65 years of age. An iv is placed and preoperative antibiotics are given. I generally use 1 g of Ancef unless the patient is penicillin allergic, in which case I will use either iv clindamycin or podoxycycline. Erythromycin and Ciprofloxicin are potent inhibitors of the cytochromeP450 system and should be avoided when using tumescent anesthesia. Patients generally receive 1 mg of polorazepam (Ativan) to help provide mild sedation and anxiolytic effects. Clonidine (0.1 mg) is used to counteract the tachycardic effect of the epinephrine in the tumescent fluid. Extensive discussions of tumescent fluid can be found elsewhere in this text and in Dr. Jeffrey Klein's textbook *Tumescent Technique* [22]. In my clinic I generally use 500 mg/liter (0.05%) or 750 mg/liter (0.075%) lidocaine, with dilute epinephrine at (1 mg/liter normal saline = 1:1 million). In addition 10 cc of sodium bicarbonate is used. This tumescent fluid is infiltrated using a 16- or 18-guage multipore infusion cannula into the entire subcutaneous layer with the aid of a peristaltic pump. The hips are infused first, followed by infusion of the lateral thighs and buttocks. Careful attention is paid to the total amount of lidocaine being infiltrated. The total amount infused should be 55 mg/kg or less. We calculate how many bags are safe to use for each individual patient prior to the procedure. A second procedure is scheduled if we cannot infuse all the areas that we planned to treat. After infusion we wait 30 min prior to beginning liposuction.

Suctioning is begun on the hips with removal of the deepest layer of fat first. I begin suctioning with a 14-gauge Klein cannula and follow this with a 12-gauge Klein cannula and/or a 3-mm accelerator cannula. The smaller cannulas act to break up the fibrofatty tissue and the 3-mm cannula provides easy removal of the fat. If the fat is fibrous or the area has been previously liposuctioned then the power liposuction instrumentation is helpful. It is also extremely helpful for sculpting and gaining definition of the waist and removal of fat from the back. I use the Xomed power liposuction instrumentation at 3000 rpm with a 2- or 3-mm accelerator cannula. I have found that larger cannulas increase the risk of seroma formation, possibly due to the effectively larger tunnels created by the vibratory movement. The tunnels for the most part should be vertical and parallel to the force of gravity. The exception is liposuctioning from the incision posterior mid-lateral aspect of the hip. It is important to feather into the waistline and anteriorly into the adjacent abdominal area. The inferior margin of the hip tapers off into a dell producing the violinlike appearance frequently seen in women. It is important not to oversuction the concavity. The end point for the hips is achieved both by visual inspection and by palpation of the skin fold thickness. Liposuction of the hips is one of the easiest areas to obtain an excellent result. The fat generally is relatively easy to remove and the elasticity of the skin in this region allows for a smooth contour. Touch-up procedures are rarely necessary in this location.

Following hip liposuction, one should proceed with liposuctioning of the outer thigh. With the patient properly positioned with a wedge support, described previously, contouring is begun in the deep plane with small cannulas. I start with the 14-gauge Klein followed by use of the 12-gauge Klein cannula and then gradually increasing the length (6 in. to 10 or 12 in.). Microcannulas produce a very even smooth contour. In very large individuals I will sometimes debulk using a 3-mm triport or accelerator cannula and fine-tune using the Klein instruments. Liposuctioning from the anterior and posterior lateral thigh incisions to the transverse tunnels is done systematically and parallel to the force of gravity. To effectively treat the deepest layers of fat, one hand picks up the tissue while the other advances the cannula. Multiple transverse tunnels should be established from all incision sites in a proximal-to-distal direction or vice versa. In most patients the majority of the fat is in the upper half of the lateral thigh; once deep suctioning has been performed one proceeds with suctioning the midplane depth. Dr. Kaminar finds that slightly suctioning superficial fat in the center thigh bulge helps to contour the area and eliminates the residual fullness sometimes seen after outer thigh deep liposuction that leaves a thin but visible layer of superficial fat. One is still well away from the dermis, but more superficial than in the other areas of the thigh. Klein cannulas are excellent for this purpose. It is important to suction from the infragluteal crease incision for blending with the posterior thigh and crisscrossing the lateral thigh. During the liposuction procedure there are various maneuvers to help assess the outer thigh's contour. One can push down on the buttock with the patient in the lateral decubitus position to see if additional fat is apparent. Alternatively the physician can abduct the patient's leg and bring it posterior—if no bulge appears then the area has been thoroughly treated (Fig. 19) (M. Kaminar, personal communication, 2000). Dr. Klein has the

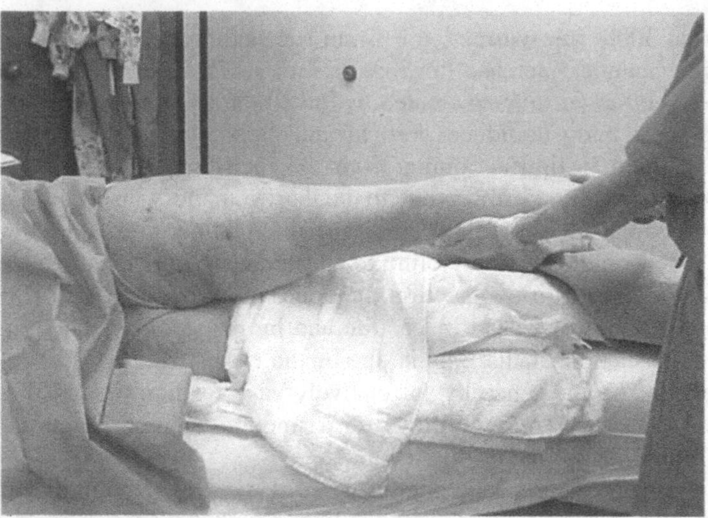

FIGURE 19 After liposuction abduction of the patients leg and posterior maneuvering helps the physician identify how thoroughly the area has been treated. The lateral thigh should appear flat.

patient straighten the leg and medially rotate the toe, pointing downward. This helps displace the trochanter anteriorly and flattens the area of the lateral thigh over the trochanter. The area should appear flat, but not concave [22].

The patient is now placed in the prone position for liposuctioning of the upper posterior thigh and buttocks. The posterior thigh should be treated with caution as this area acts as a fulcrum for the weight of the buttocks. This is one area where suctioning should be superficial. The cannula is always moved from superior to inferior or vice versa but never horizontally and never in a "windshield wiping" motion. One should avoid piercing the infragluteal ligament, as this may produce a dropped buttock and herniation of fat from the buttock to the posterior thigh (Figs. 20a and 20b).

Finally the buttock is liposuctioned. As previously mentioned, among physicians there are different incision sites used but the same principles are applied. Liposuctioning is performed in the middle to deep fat layers. One should avoid suctioning the most superficial 20 to 30% of the fat deposit so that dimpling is avoided. The goal of sculpting is to reduce the projection or heaviness of the buttock. A pillow can be inserted under the pelvis to elevate the buttocks and produce slight hip flexion. I begin sculpting from the lateral infragluteal incision with a 14-gauge Klein cannula in the deep plane. I then use a 12-gauge/10-in. Klein cannula for the majority of the

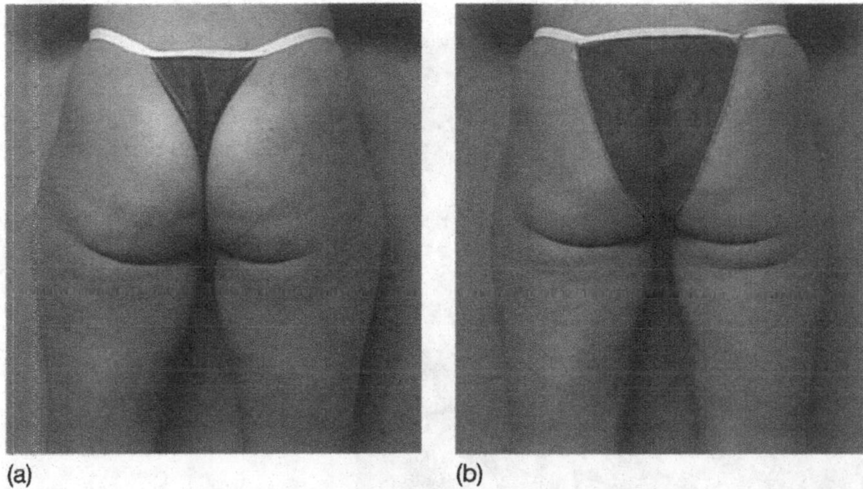

(a) (b)

FIGURE 20 (a) Patient with excessive fullness in the upper one-third of the posterior thigh. (b) After liposuction double fold occurred on the right side.

suctioning. I use long strokes from three incisions: infragluteal, superior lateral, and approximately 3 in. medially and lateral to the superior incision. A conservative approach is always warranted in this location. No more than 30–50% of the buttock fat should be removed by liposuction or ptosis may develop [22]. The central buttocks or inverted V-shaped area described by Fournier as the "Bermuda Triangle" may be cautiously liposuctioned using only the microcannular technique (Fig. 21).

PEARLS TO AVOID UNAESTHETIC RESULTS

1. Patients should be counseled to avoid weight gain after liposuction. Increased volumes of fat may appear in areas where they had not previously gained weight. Enlargement of the shoulders, arms, and breasts is common. It is important to educate patients that dietary intake must be decreased and exercise and energy output increased for the patient to achieve maximum benefit.
2. Patient surveys show that overresection leads to greatest dissatisfaction [23].
3. Women with very large outer thighs require a two-stage procedure. This will help the skin to retract gradually and adjust more smoothly to the reduced volume.
4. Keep fat extracted from the right and left side of the body in separate containers so that it is easy to compare sides.

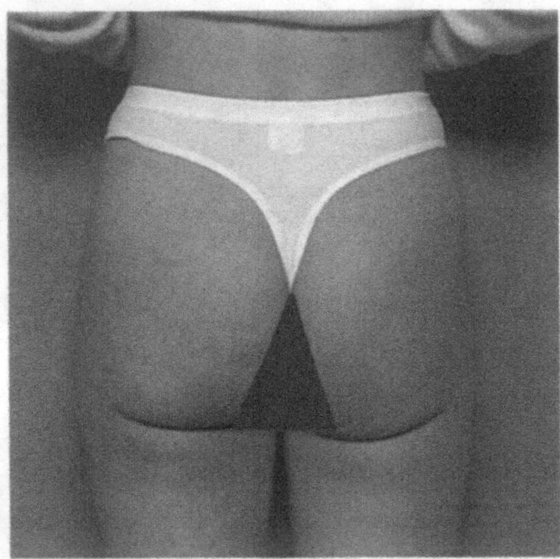

FIGURE 21 "Bermuda Triangle" describes an equilateral triangle with its base along the infragluteal crease and its apex at the lumbosacral junction.

5. Use small cannulas and multiple incision sites to achieve a criss-cross pattern and avoid contouring irregularities. Use a pistonlike motion.
6. Judge the end point by tactile and visual assessment of the contour. If the tunnel is "empty," blood or serous fluid will be extracted. Additional fat may be suctioned by entering the area from another incision with the patient positioned differently.

POST-OP INSTRUCTIONS

Directly after the procedure, the patient is cleansed and absorbent pads are placed over incision sites which are not sutured. The patient then is helped into his or her compression garment. This garment is worn 24 hr/day for 2 weeks and then 12 hr/day for an additional 2 weeks. The patient is instructed that drainage will occur for approximately 24–48 hr after the procedure. It is recommended that the patient rest for the first day. The second day the patient can expect to be sore and to experience some swelling and bruising. Most patients return to their normal routine within 1 to 2 days after surgery. Exercise is encouraged by the 7th postoperative day. Patients resume exercise gradually over the first 2 weeks. Most patients require little postoperative medication. We prescribe Darvocett N 100 or Tylenol depending on the amount of postoperative discomfort. Patients are reminded to finish their course of antibiotics and return to office for a follow-up in 1 week. A second follow-up visit will be scheduled for 6 weeks post-op. At that time measurements and photographs will be taken, and the patient will be able to appreciate their early postoperative improvement. A final visit is scheduled at 9 to 12 months post-op and at that time any refinements or additional areas are discussed.

REFERENCES

1. Wahrenberg H, Lonnqvist F, Arner P. Mechanisms underlying regional differences in lipolysis in human adipose tissue. J Clin Invest Aug 1989; 84(2):458–467.
2. Lonnqvist F, Thorne A, Large V, Arner P. Sex differences in visceral fat lipolysis and metabolic complications of obesity. Arterioscler Thromb Vasc Biol 1997; 17(7):1472–1480.
3. Skouge J. The biochemistry and development of adipose tissue and the pathophysiology of obesity as it relates to liposuction. In: Dermatologic Clinics. Vol. 8(3). W. B. Saunders Co. 1990:385–393.
4. Lawrence N, Coleman WP. Advances in Dermatology. Vol. 2. St. Louis: Mosby, 1996:10–35.
5. Phinney SD, Stern JS, Burke KE, Tang AB, Miller G, Holtman RT. Human subcutaneous adipose tissue shows site-specific differences in fatty acid composition. Am J Clin Nutr 1994; 60:725–729.
6. Flynn T, Narins R. Preoperative evaluation of the liposuction patient. In: Dermatologic Clinics. Vol. 17(4). W. B. Saunders, 1999:729–734.
7. Cook W, Cook K. Manual of Tumescent Liposculpture and Cosmetic Laser Surgery. 1st ed. Philadelphia: Lippincott/Williams & Wilkins 1999:89–138.
8. Narins R. Three-dimensional liposuction. American Academy of Dermatology, Orlando, FL, February, 1998.
9. Kaminar M. Liposuction. ASDS 26th Annual Meeting, Denver, CO, November, 2000.
10. Bernstein G. Liposuction of the thigh. In: Dermatologic Clinics. Vol. 17(4). Philadelphia: W. B. Saunders, 1999:849–863.
11. Draelos ZD, Draelos ZZ, Marenus KD et al. Cellulite etiology and purported treatment. Dermatol Surg 1997; 23:1177–1181.
12. Trenta GS. Combination therapy reduces the appearance of cellulite. Cosmetic Surg Times 2001; Jan–Feb:14.
13. Chernoff GW. Percussive therapy can fight cellulite as liposuction alternative. Cosmetic Surg Times. 2001; Jan–Feb:1 and 12.
14. Toledo CS. Cellulite. In: Superficial Liposculpture Manual of Technique. New York: Springer-Verlag, 1993:91–99.
15. Narins RS. Liposuction surgery of the lateral thigh. Dermatol Surg Oncol 1988; 10:1155–1161.

16. Gasparotti M, Lewis CM, Toledo LS. Technique. In: Superficial Liposculpture Manual of Technique. New York: Springer-Verlag, 1993:7–28, 101–106.
17. Lack EB. Contouring the female buttocks. In: Dermatologic Clinics. Vol. 17(4). Philadelphia: W. B. Saunders 1999:815–822.
18. Pitman GH. Liposuction and Aesthetic Surgery. St Louis: Quality Medical, 1993:337–411
19. Butterwick K, Goldman GP. Changes in body fat percentage following tumescent liposuction. ASDS 26th Annual Meeting, Denver, CO, November, 2000.
20. Ostad A, Kageyama N, Moy RL. Tumescent anaesthesia with a lidocaine dose of 55mg/kg is safe for liposuction. Dermatol Surg 1996; 22:921–927.
21. Butterwick K. Tumescent liposuction Foc 845. AAD Washington, DC, March, 2001.
22. Klein J. Tumescent liposuction. In: Tumescent Anaesthesia and Microcannular Liposuction. 1st ed. St. Louis: Mosby. 2000:325–341.
23. Dillerud E, Haheim LL. Longterm results of blunt suction lipectomy assissed by a patient questionnaire survey. Plat Reconstruct Surg 1993; 92(1):35–42.

10

Liposuction of the Medial Thigh, Knee, Calf, and Ankle

Kimberly J. Butterwick
Dermatology Associates
La Jolla, California, U.S.A.

Most of the areas in this chapter have been described as being "the most difficult" in liposuction surgery, yet are routinely done with gratifying results by many surgeons [1]. The challenge of treating these areas properly calls for some basic human virtues of patience, diligence, and determination. Humility is also a prerequisite, as heroic, bold measures will often cause defects.

Fatty deposits in medial thigh, knee, calf, and ankle are usually distinct areas in very thin patients but in the majority of patients, subcutaneous fat is contiguous from one area to the next and these areas are best considered together as one cosmetic unit. These four areas are not routinely treated at the same time because other areas of the body are requested more often by the patient. In our practice, the medial thigh and knee are often treated together along with other body areas in one session. The calf and ankle are treated together in a separate session. Over the past 2 years, 18% of our liposuction patients have undergone treatment of the medial thigh and knee in contrast to 1% who have undergone treatment of the ankle and calf [2].

MEDIAL THIGH AND KNEE

While the medial thigh is a difficult area in liposuction and is best performed by experienced surgeons, the knee is a relatively straightforward area and may be done by surgeons with basic experience [3]. These areas are requested by patients primarily for aesthetic reasons and sometimes functional reasons such as friction and chafing. In my experience, the minority of patients require liposuction of just one of these areas because they have a continuous layer from the upper medial thigh to the knee, which is best treated as one unit. In addition, as Klein points out, treating these areas together avoids the problem of a visible transition line from a treated area to a nontreated one [4].

Anatomy

A unique feature of the medial thigh fat is its soft, nonfibrous nature, which is the nemesis of liposuction surgeons. This softness actually makes the fat too easily extracted and defects can develop quickly. It also leads to difficulties in transitioning to neighboring areas of fat that have a more fibrous consistency and have a different feel by palpation or with a cannula. Another anatomic drawback of the medial thigh is the thin and inelastic nature of the skin. Skin laxity is common in this area due to aging processes or excessive weight loss. Skin retraction after liposuction of the medial thigh is notoriously poor compared to other areas [5].

The bulge of subcutaneous fat of the medial thigh is deepest and most prominent 2–8 cm from the perineal–thigh crease. The majority of fat is usually posterior, although in some patients a prominent anterior extension is visible (Fig. 1) [6]. There are variable extensions of fat to the adjacent anterior or posterior thighs. The subcutaneous fat tapers in the midthigh region and deepens again in the medial knee area.

The anterior muscles of the medial thigh are composed of the adductors (longus, brevis, and magnus), the pectineus, and the gracilis muscle. The sartorius muscle courses obliquely across the anterior femoral muscles from the anterior superior iliac spine and inserts on the medial aspect of the body of the tibia. This muscle forms one of the boundaries of the femoral triangle and is a natural boundary for the adipose tissue of the medial thigh. Posteriorly, the main muscle groups of the medial thigh are the semimembranosus and the semitendinosus. The only significant vessel in the subcutaneous fat in this region is the greater saphenous vein. This vessel ascends within the deep part of the superficial fascia on the anterior and medial aspect of the thigh accompanied by superficial lymphatic vessels. Just below the inguinal ligament, it penetrates the deep fascia at the fossa ovalis and

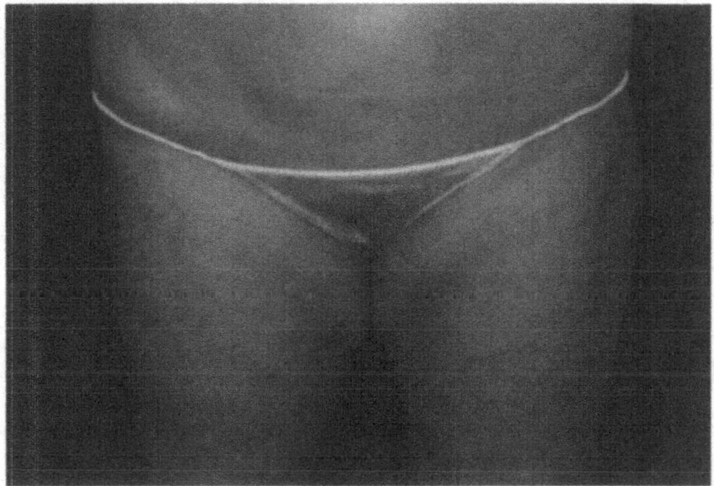

FIGURE 1 Prominent anterior extension of medial thigh fat.

enters the femoral vein. Tumescent liposuction has not been reported to injure this vessel.

The majority of the subcutaneous fat of the knee is well localized over the medial condyles of the tibia and femur. It is a dense, thick fat that changes little with weight loss or gain. This layer tapers proximally to a thinner zone of the midthigh region, at times extending over onto the medial portion of the anterior thigh. Extensions of this main fat pad usually course inferiorly and medial to the patella and at times are contiguous with an enlarged compartment of subcutaneous fat in the medial calf. Other fat pads in the knee area that are recognized and treated by liposuction surgeons include the lateral patellar component and discrete fibrofatty nodules in the patellar and infrapatellar area (Fig. 2) [2–4,6]. The suprapatellar fat zone is a fibrofatty region that may become ptotic and wrinkled with age and gravity. It cannot be treated aggressively due to poor skin retraction. In addition, the weight of the anterior thigh compartment rests on the suprapatellar region. If the suprapatellar fat pad is suctioned aggressively, ptosis of the anterior thigh may cause more sagging and creasing.

The shape of the knee is determined in large part by the underlying musculoskeletal structures, including the femoral condyles, the patella, and the condyles of the tibia. The large tendon of the quadriceps femoris encases the patella and inserts onto the tuberosity of the tibia. The vastus medialis of the quadriceps, the sartorius, and the gracilis muscles fill out the medial aspect of the knee. In athletes, particularly long-distance bike riders, the

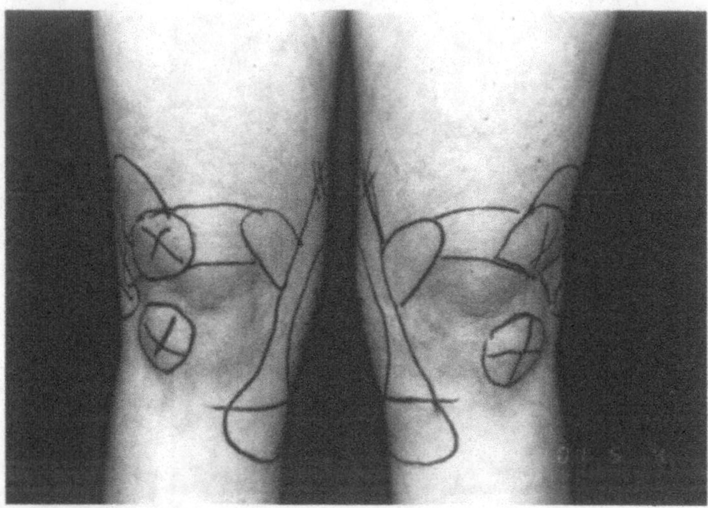

FIGURE 2 Fat pads in the knee area.

bulk of these muscles will enlarge the medial knee despite little subcutaneous fat. The greater saphenous vein is the only significant vessel in the subcutaneous fat and passes posteriorly over the medial condyles along with several small veins and lymphatics.

Aesthetic Considerations

The ideal medial thigh has a slight proximal fullness and tapers to a thin midthigh and knee (Fig. 3). There is subtle widening at the knee reflecting the underlying skeletal structure and a convexity just distal to the knee before the silhouette widens again in the midcalf. Patients tend to want as much space as possible between the medial thighs and sometimes prefer the medial thigh to be straight rather than curved.

The thigh should taper gradually into the knee with the medial aspect of the knee relatively flat. When one suctions the medial and lateral aspects of the knee, a rectangular shape of the thigh changes to a tapered, more graceful one (Figs. 4a and 4b). The ideal knee also includes a subtly tapered suprapatellar region with smooth skin and a convexity below the knee, corresponding to the natural shapeliness of the medial leg. The patellar and infrapatellar fat pads should be minimally visible.

The perfect inner thigh and knee are usually not obtainable due to naturally occurring flaws [7]. In many patients, there is subtle undulation of the medial thigh region prior to liposuction which is difficult and sometimes

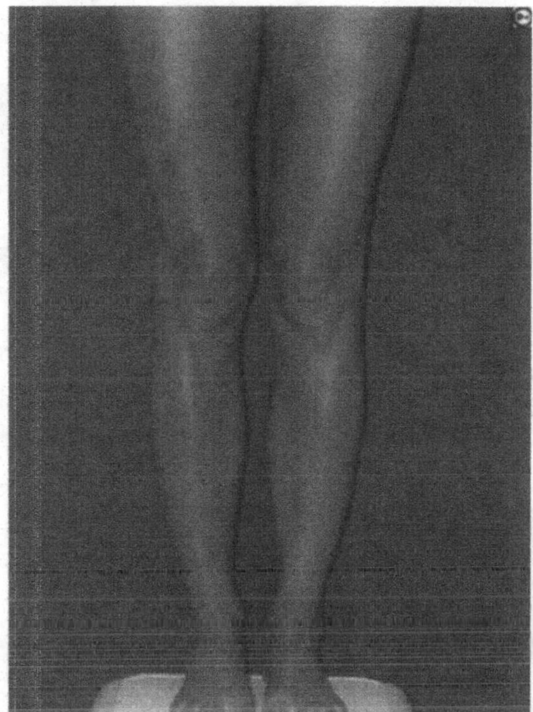

FIGURE 3 Ideal medial thigh and knee.

impossible to correct (Fig. 5). Klein has noted the frequent appearance of the medial thigh furrow, a subtle but often noticeable furrow which courses diagonally from the midinguinal area across the anterior thigh to the distal aspect of the medial thigh [4]. It is not seen in thin individuals and therefore does not represent underlying musculature. Liposuction is best performed above and below this line to diminish its appearance. Optimal results of the medial thigh liposuction are further limited by the degree of skin laxity, which will likely not improve with treatment. For example, after liposuction of the medial knee, an aesthetically pleasing contour can be achieved, but wrinkling in the suprapatellar region precludes aggressive liposuction and detracts from the final results.

Patient Selection and Evaluation

The typical patient seeking liposuction of the medial thigh area is female and has had persistance of this fatty deposit independent of weight changes. Larger patients complain of friction from the thighs rubbing. There may be

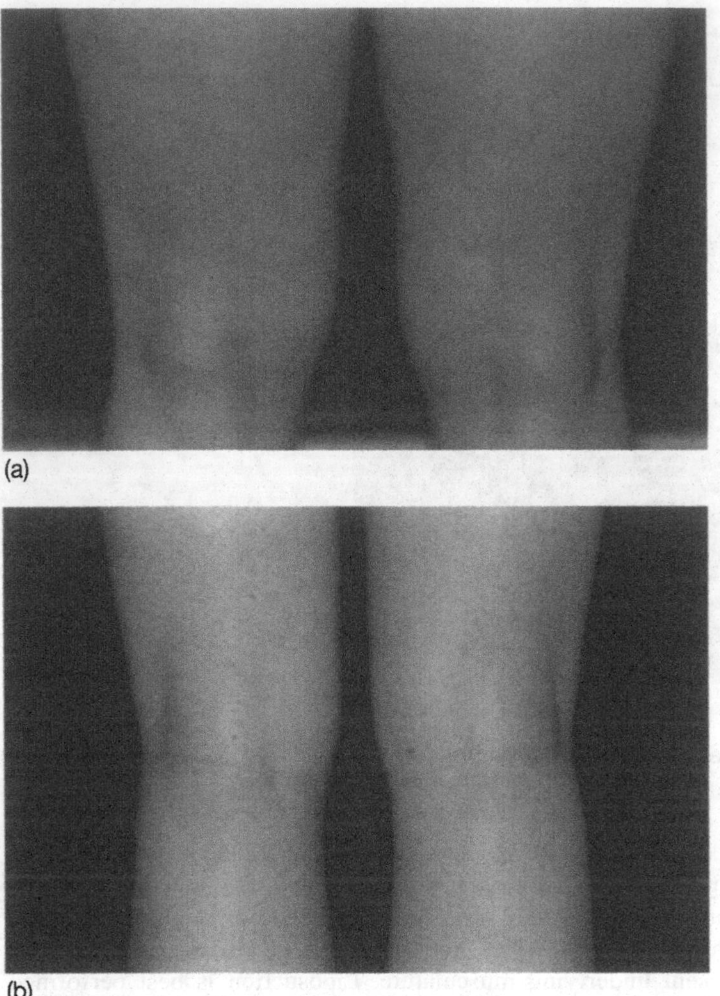

FIGURE 4 Retangular shape at the knee (a) changing to a tapered shape (b).

associated problems such as chafing in larger patients, hyperpigmentation, or even pseudoacanthosis nigricans in heavy individuals. Patients may stand in front of a mirror and pull the medial thigh tightly from behind in a practiced maneuver, indicating the degree of improvement that is desired. The patient has often not thought about the medial or lateral knee area and requests treatment of only the inner thigh. A Polaroid photograph taken at the consultation is useful to point out these deposits and the improved con-

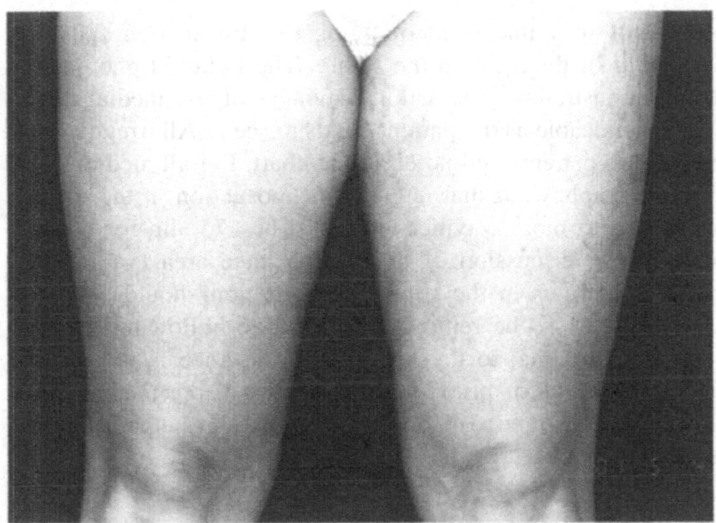

FIGURE 5 Subtle naturally occurring undulations of the left medial thigh region.

tour possible if they are removed. Patients in the 4th decade or older may have noticed some gravitational sagging of the medial knee and friction with walking or jogging. They may be particularly dissatisfied with the laxity of the suprapatellar region.

At the time of the consultation, the thigh should be examined for overall shape. The subcutaneous fat of the anterior or lateral thighs may contribute to an overall bulkiness of the leg which has not been noticed by the patient. There may be large muscle groups limiting the degree of tapering that can be reasonably achieved. The standard pinch test will determine the degree of subcutaneous fat present. A Polaroid photograph is taken and reviewed with the patient demonstrating disproportionate areas, subtle knee pockets of fat, and expected recontouring of the leg.

It is important to explore the patient's goals and expectations. Limitations depending on age, musculature, and skin laxity need to be clearly reviewed with the patient. A key element of the examination is assessing the quality of the skin in the medial thigh. If deep wrinkling and sagging of the skin are present, skin laxity could become worse after liposuction. These patients are poor candidates and the option of a medial thigh lift should be presented [8]. Some patients may choose to proceed with liposuction for contour changes and reduced friction in clothing, but it is important that they are aware of the limitations of the procedure regarding poor skin retraction. Patients may find it encouraging that liposuction does not preclude the possibility of thigh lift in the future. The Polaroid photograph is also helpful in demonstrating preexisting waviness of the medial thigh, which may be more noticeable as the patient bends to see it. All irregularities should be pointed out to patients and noted in the chart. For all medial thigh patients, it should be emphasized that aggressive liposuction in the medial thigh would likely lead to more waviness and it is best to aim for conservative improvement. The discussion of the medial knee area is relatively straightforward, but the limits in the suprapatellar region should again be reviewed. Patients should also be reminded of a subtle hollowing that appears after liposuction proximal to the knee while the knee is flexed 90°. Before and after photographs of prior patients treated in the medial thigh and knee areas will demonstrate realistic expectations and help set appropriate patient expectations.

Technique

There are many effective approaches to liposuction of the medial thigh and knee. Table 1 summarizes the positions, incision sites, and cannulas favored by various surgeons as described in the literature [1,4,6,7,9]. All recommend relatively nonaggressive cannulas for the medial thigh and more aggressive cannulas for the medial knee. I divide this region into three distinct areas: the upper medial thigh, the knee, and the midthigh. Liposuction is performed separately in each area and then they are blended together.

Marking the Patient

The patient is marked while standing with the surgeon seated. The anterior boundaries of the fat of the medial thigh and knee are marked first, with the usual topographic circles drawn to target the most prominent bulges (Fig. 6). If the medial thigh furrow is visible, it is negatively highlighted so as to avoid liposuction there. Cellulite and other irregularities of the skin are also marked. The middle third of the thigh is usually of relatively uniform thickness and straight vertical lines are drawn here to remind the surgeon to use vertical strokes and perform conservative liposuction in this region. Markings include the suprapatellar and lateral patellar extensions of the fat, as well as the small pockets overlying the patella. A horizontal line is drawn medially, inferior to the knee, as a reminder to enhance the natural convexity here. The patient is then turned to the posterior view and the concentric circles started anteriorly are completed posteriorly. For optimal results, it is important to adequately treat the farthest reaches of both the anterior and posterior projections.

TABLE 1 Various Techniques for Medial Thigh Liposuction

Author	Patient position	Incision sites	Cannulas
Bernstein	Lateral decubitus	Near infragluteal crease Inferior border, midline Anterior if needed	2–3-mm dual port spatula tip
Cook	Lateral decubitus	Infragluteal crease Lateral pubic	Klein Finesse (10- to 12-gauge) Cook (3- to 3.5-mm)
Klein	Lateral decubitus, supine if needed	Multiple along posterior diagonal border and one anterior thigh	Capistrano (14- to 16-gauge) Klein Finesse (12-gauge)
Narins	Lateral decubitus	Infragluteal fold Two in anterior groin	Klein Finesse (10- to 12-gauge) Accelerator (3- to 4-mm)
Pittman	Frog leg	Groin crease—4-cm medial to femoral pulse Inferior border, midline	2–4 mm

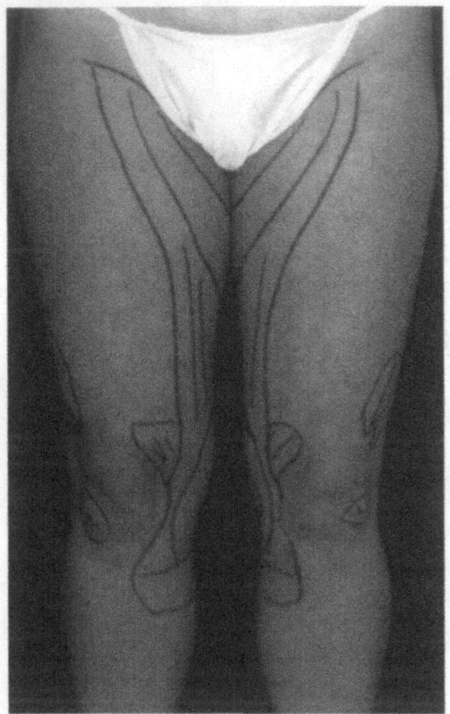

FIGURE 6 Markings of the medial thigh and knee.

Infiltration

I infiltrate with the patient in the lateral decubitus postion with the top leg flexed at the knee and hip and drawn forward to expose the opposite medial thigh. Infiltration is begun with 25-gauge spinal needles using standard tumescent solution containing 0.05–0.1% lidocaine with a 1:1,000,000 dilution of 0.65 ml of epinephrine and 10 meq/liter of sodium bicarbonate. The medial thigh and knee are sensitive areas and I have found that adequate anesthesia cannot be obtained with 0.05% lidocaine if only mild preoperative sedation is given. I therefore start by infiltrating 100–200 cc of 0.1% lidocaine solution in the medial thigh and knee. This is supplemented with 0.05% lidocaine solution to achieve maximum tumescence while staying within the safety guidelines for the maximum dose of lidocaine (55 mg/kg) [10,11]. Due to skin laxity of the upper inner thigh, tumescence may require more volume of fluid than an inexperienced surgeon might anticipate. The 20-gauge spinal needle may be utilized at a fast rate to accomplish this task rapidly [12]. I prefer infiltrating exclusively with spinal needles because incision sites are not necessary and the fluid does not leak out as readily. The patient stays dryer and warmer as the contralateral leg and other areas are being infiltrated.

Medial Thigh

Liposuction begins in the medial upper thigh with the patient in the lateral decubitus position and the top leg flexed high and placed on a covered foam cushion measuring 8 × 25 × 8 in. Two incision sites are placed posteriorly, one near the midinfragluteal crease and one placed 2–3 cm inferior and anterior to the first (Fig. 7a). These sites are hidden from the patient and allow cross-tunneling. Like others, I have found placing an incision site at the distal aspect of the upper thigh bulge or in the midthigh can result in a depression and therefore do not routinely place them there [1]. I start with a 14-gauge/9-in. Klein Finesse cannula in thin individuals and a 14-gauge Capistrano cannula in larger individuals. I work in the deep plane first from both incision sites and move back and forth, frequently checking that the medial thigh surface appears uniform. It is important to constantly monitor the progress of the suction to avoid overresection in any one area. I may then advance to a more aggressive cannula, such as a 2- to 3-mm eliminator or a 12-gauge Finesse, in larger individuals. I do not use aggressive cannulas in this region as a divot can develop quickly. The process is then repeated in the midplane of the subcutaneous fat with careful attention to leave a uniform blanket of superficial fat above the suctioned planes. The final end-point is determined by a uniform pinch test and visible flat surface of the medial thigh (Fig. 7b). Tunneling without suction is performed distally to the mid thigh area. This fat is more fibrous and feels thicker by palpation and with the cannula. Suction should be conservative in the lowermost border of the upper medial thigh, realizing that a pinch test will have a different feel in that area compared to the area immediately distal to it. Overresection at this transition border is the most common liposuction defect I have seen in patients presenting for correction (Fig. 8).

Medial Knee

I next perform liposuction of the medial knee with the patient remaining in the lateral decubitus position. One incision site is placed posteriorly, distal to the popliteal crease, through which most of the suction is performed. Incision sites placed within the crease are subject to too much movement and may not heal well [13]. The deep fat is resected first, usually with a 14-gauge/9 in. Capistrano cannula. The entire medial knee is treated initially with longer cannulas and then focused attention is given to the main medial bulge immediately adjacent to the medial condyles with a shorter cannula. This area is treated aggressively, suctioning first the deep fat, then the mid-

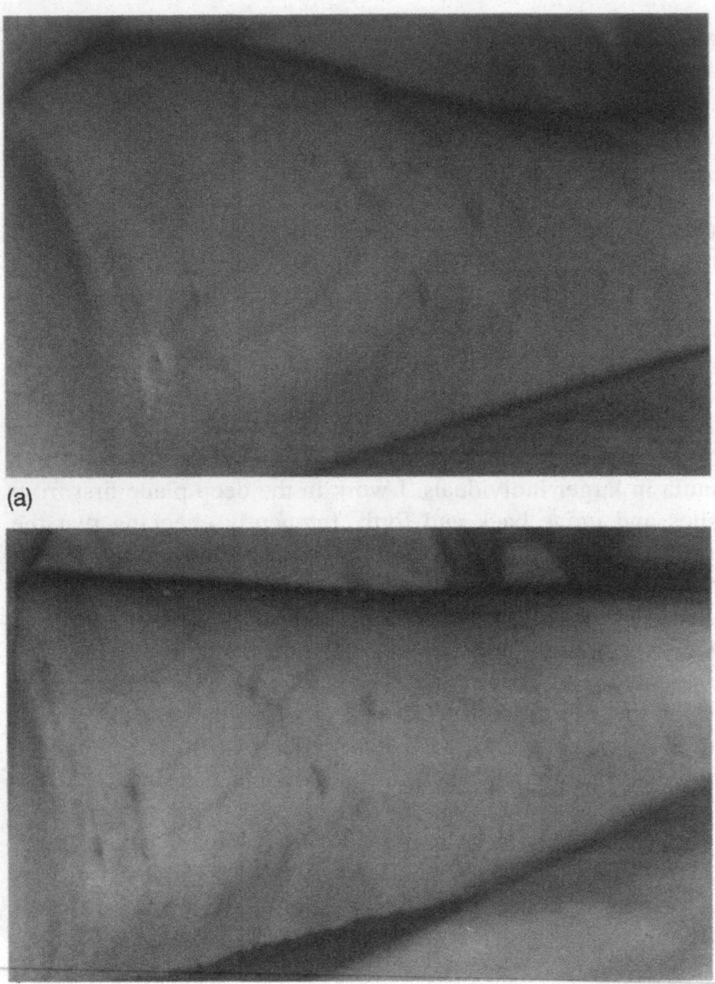

(a)

(b)

FIGURE 7 (a and b) Pre- and postoperative views of the upper medial thigh. Two primary incision sites at the upper posteromedial border. Two other sites added near completion for final smoothing. Cellulite marked inferiorly.

plane, and finally the superficial fat with a shorter, 6-in., Finesse cannula. When complete, the pinch test in this area is quite thin, measuring approximately 0.5 cm in thickness (Fig. 9). A second incision site placed approximately 2–3 cm superior to the medial popliteal crease is useful for cross-tunneling as well as for access to the middle third of the medial thigh. Less

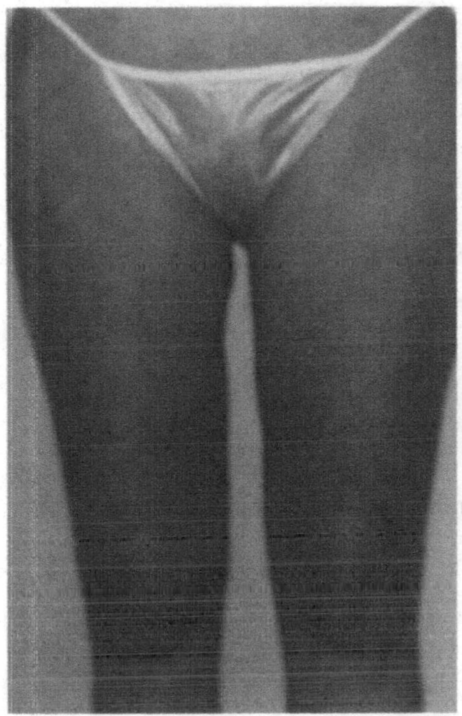

FIGURE 8 Overresection of the right leg at the transition from the upper inner thigh to the midthigh.

liposuction is performed through this incision, minimizing friction and promoting quick healing. The area inferior and medial to the patella is approached nearly as aggressively to achieve the natural indentation seen immediately distal to the medial knee protuberance. Blending into the medial calf is achieved with nonaggressive cannulas and little to no suctioning. Blending is also particularly important in the transition from the knee to the midthigh region. Overly aggressive liposuction in this area can result in permanent depressions (Fig. 10). If only treating the knee, I leave this area still containing some tumescent fluid slightly elevated above the flat surface and feather without suction into the midthigh.

Midthigh

I proceed next to suction the middle third of the medial thigh through the incisions made previously. Long smooth vertical strokes are made here with a 14- or 12-gauge Finesse cannula, staying in the midplane with care not to

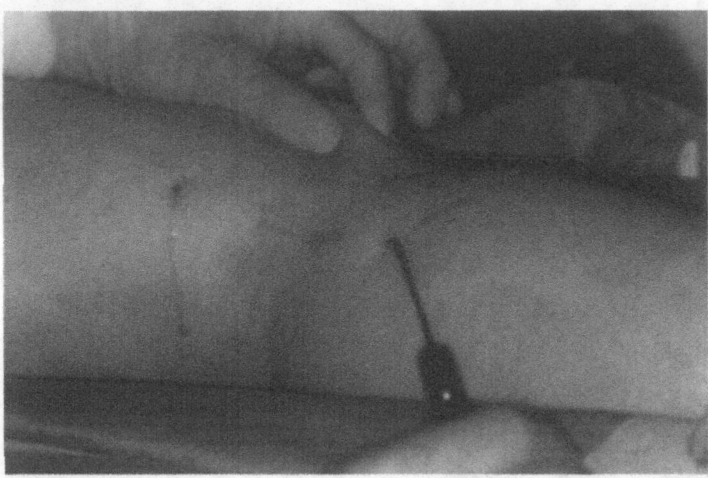

FIGURE 9 Pinch test of the medial knee with cannula appoximately 0.5 cm.

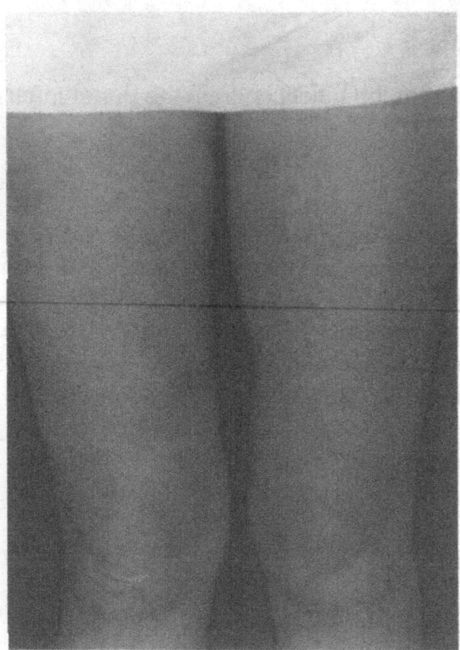

FIGURE 10 Defect at the transition from the left knee to the midthigh region.

overresect. A swan-neck cannula can facilitate liposuction from the knee incision in order to avoid lifting with the cannula and consequent trauma to the overlying skin. The foot section of the table can also be lowered so that better access is obtained and smooth, uninterrupted strokes may be performed (Kimberly Finder, personal communication). In this fashion, several small tunnels are created which smoothly decrease the diameter of this area. Conservative removal is the rule in the midmedial thigh, being careful to avoid superficial liposuction. Dimpling or waviness may result from excessive liposuction here [14]. The upper third of the medial thigh is further cross-tunneled from the knee incisions. Longer cannulas are utilized, with a 26-cm cannula or larger enabling a reach into the mid and anterior aspects of the upper medial thigh (Fig. 11).

The patient then turns to the contralateral side and the process is repeated. To ensure symmetry, amounts of supranatant fat are measured from each of the three areas and compared to the amounts taken from the side previously treated. Finally, the patient is placed in the supine position in order to reach the anterior compartments of subcutaneous fat with the legs slightly apart.

Anterior Portion of the Medial Thigh and Knee

I approach the anterior portion of the medial thigh through one incision site placed in the midanterior thigh 1–2 cm inferior to the inguinal crease. Incision sites have been recommended superior to the crease [6,9] but I have found the strokes from that site to be awkward. The incision site is small as cannulas 2 mm or smaller are used for this area. Although not hidden, sites here are minimally traumatized and they heal quickly without scarring.

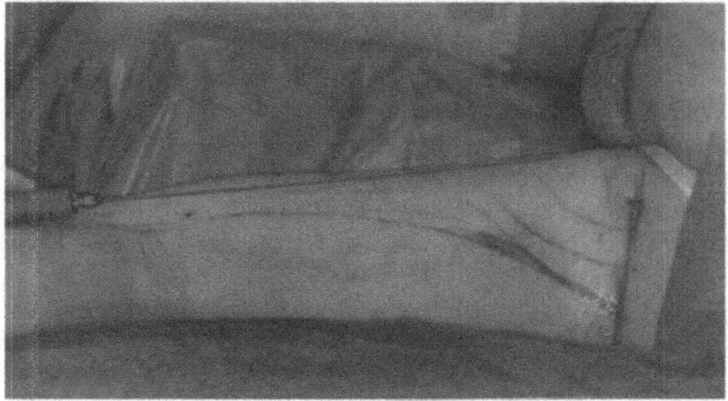

FIGURE 11 Long cannula (26 cm) useful for the midthigh and upper midthigh.

Most of the liposuction has already been completed from the lateral decubitus position. Limited suction is performed with a 14-gauge Finesse cannula or a 14-gauge Capistrano cannula in the midplane until the contour appears level with the anterior thigh. At times, a second, more medial, incision site is necessary to achieve this appearance. The leg can be rotated out slightly, but the frog leg position is avoided as the contour and skin twist unnaturally in this position and a defect could be created [4]. If any irregularity is noted and cannot be smoothed from these incision sites, a third incision site may be placed 5–10 cm below the inguinal crease and smoothing suction performed briefly. These sites take precedence over leaving an irregularity.

The anterior aspects of the subcutaneous fat of the knee are treated next. Incision sites may be placed in the medial and lateral knee rhytides, if present. Short 14-gauge/6-in. Finesse or Capistrano cannulas are used depending on the amount to be removed and the quality of the skin. If present, the lateral fat deposits proximal to the knee are treated through the lateral incision until a tapered appearance is achieved from the thigh to the knee. The medial incision is the approach used to crisscross back into the medial knee area as well as to feather up to the midthigh region. The medial bulge proximal to the knee should be tapered conservatively with feathering toward the anterior thigh. The suprapatellar area must be approached cautiously to avoid ptosis from the weight of the anterior thigh. The 14-gauge Finesse cannula is passed through the suprapatellar fat from the medial and lateral knee fold incisions into the deep and midplanes and conservative liposuction performed. Finally, the small pockets overlying the patellar region are treated through tiny distal incision sites. The 16-gauge Capistrano is my cannula of choice for these nodules; I grasp them with the left hand or immobilize them with traction and suction fairly aggressively. Very little fat is present and may not be measurable.

The anterior aspects of the midthigh fat are last to be treated. I utilize 14-gauge-diameter cannulas of longer lengths and suction through the medial knee fold incision and the anterior upper thigh incisions. Suction here is again conservative with care to blend to adjacent areas. A 2- to 3-mm Eliminator/Accelerator swan-neck cannula can also be utilized from the distal incision for final smoothing of this area all the way to the proximal inner thigh. When the contralateral side is treated, an attempt is made to place the incision sites asymmetrically from the first side for aesthetic purposes [15].

Postoperative Care

Immediately postoperatively, the area is cleansed, incision sites are left open, and absorbent padding is applied. Tubular elastic netting (Surgilast) holds the pads in position and an ankle-length support garment is placed on the patient. Care is taken to pull the garment proximally to the crural fold to avoid pressure from the edge of the garment more distally. Poor drainage and defects may result if the garment edge slips distally and puts undo pressure in the middle of the treated area [16]. Early ambulation is encouraged and patients may return to normal activities in 2–3 days. After 1 week of compression 24 hr/day, the patient may wear the ankle length garment or compression stockings during the day (20–30 mmHg) for 1 month. Patients are seen at 24 hr post-op for a dressing change, at 1 week post-op, and at 6–8 weeks postoperation. At the last visit it behooves the surgeon to present a preoperative photograph. Preexisting skin irregularities are long forgotten by the patient. If necessary, touch-up procedures are performed 6 months or longer postliposuction.

Complications

Occasionally patients may note pedal edema 1–3 days postoperatively, particularly if below-the-knee rather than ankle-length garments are applied. Leg elevation, compression hosiery, and ambulation correct this problem in days. Skin irregularities and defects are the most common complications of medial thigh liposuction, particularly with superficial liposuction (Fig. 12).

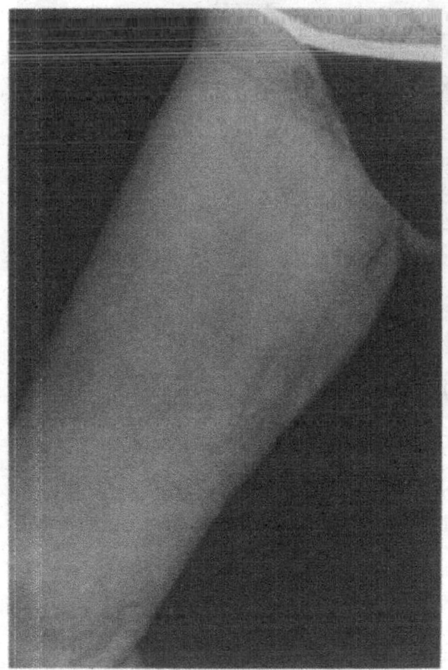

FIGURE 12 Skin irregularity due to superficial liposuction of the medial thigh.

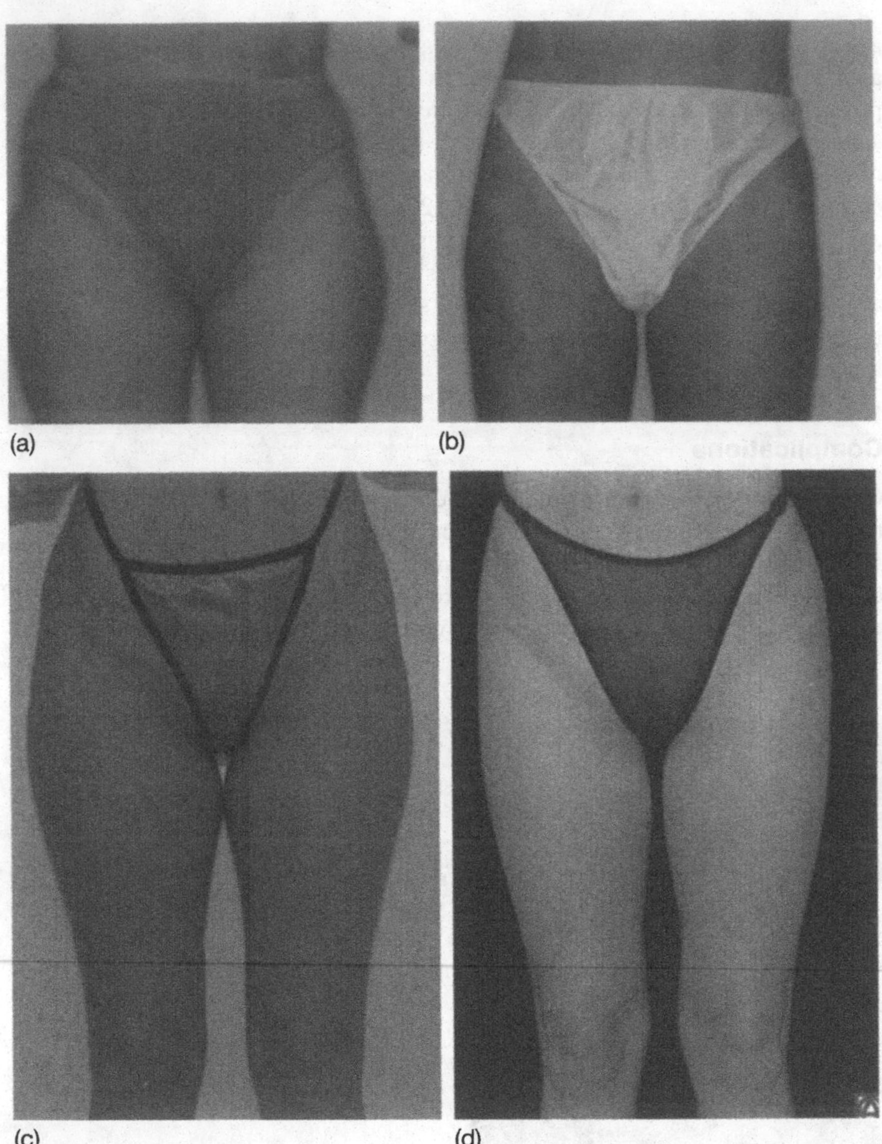

FIGURE 13 (a and b) Before and after liposuction of inner and outer thigh with 5-lb weight loss. (c and d) Before and after liposuction of inner and outer thigh with 5-lb weight gain.

Problem areas include the transition of the upper medial thigh to the midthigh and the transition from the medial knee to the medial midthigh area and the suprapatellar area. Excessively superficial liposuction of the medial thigh can injure the dermal plexus and cause the mottled reticulated pattern known as erythema ab liporasperation [4]. Defects most likely due to slippage from the garment have been reported [16]. No other complications unique to this area of liposuction have been reported.

Summary

The medial thigh, midthigh, and knee are usually considered one cosmetic unit in the majority of patients. Yet they are best treated as three distinct areas which are then blended together. Attention must be given to both posterior and anterior extensions of these fatty deposits, as well as at the transition zones of the three regions to avoid defects. Skin retraction is poor on the inner thigh and suprapatellar region and a smoothing layer of fat must be left behind in these areas. Both the surgeon and the patient need to understand these limitations. In contrast, skin retraction is excellent at the inner knee and aggressive liposuction is appropriate. Shaping and recontouring about the medial and lateral knee gives an overall slenderization of the leg. The inner thigh and knee are excellent areas for recontouring with careful liposuction and attention to detail (Figs. 13a–13d).

CALVES AND ANKLES

History

The history of liposuction of the calves and ankles unfortunately begins with a tragic and oft-quoted case from the 1920s: A ballerina required amputation after undergoing blunt curettage to remove ankle fat by French surgeon Dujarrier [3,17,18]. The next report came decades later when Shrudde reported his 13-year experience in treating ankle fat using a sharp curette [19]. He demonstrated good results, although 4 of 15 patients had skin necrosis. Skin necrosis was also reported in another case of ankle curettage in the early 1980s [20].

Illouz described his experience in body contouring using a slightly hypotonic solution to soften fat and blunt cannulas in over 3000 cases in 1983 [21]. The ankles were treated in 12% of the cases with "successful correction" and "minimal complications." Illouz warned, as have many surgeons to follow, of the difficulty in treating the ankles due to the small margin for error [17,22]. Multiple reasons for the difficulty in treating these areas have been suggested (Table 2) [23,24].

TABLE 2 Problems Unique to Liposuction of the Calf and Ankle

Consists of only one layer of fat
Relatively subtle results due to small quantities
Lack of well defined bulges in many cases
Curved contours make access difficult
Visible incision sites
Prolonged healing
Inappropriate patient expectations

Despite these caveats, surgeons in the 1990s began to express more enthusiasm in performing liposuction of the calves and ankles [18, 23–25]. The tumescent technique subsequently led to smaller cannula size and fewer complications [26]. In addition, the benefits of a nearly circumferential approach were recognized [23,24,27]. Proper management of the postoperative edema and management of patient expectations further contributed to increasing satisfaction with performing liposuction of these areas [22]. Nevertheless, these areas are generally requested less often than other areas. Watanabe noted that calf and ankle liposuction is performed in 20% of all his liposuction cases in Japan, a higher rate than that reported in Europe and the United States where the reported frequency of treating these areas ranges from 1 to 12% [18,21,24]. With experience and careful technique, this can be a most gratifying area for the surgeon in that there is often the opportunity to truly sculpt.

Anatomy

A unique feature of the calf and ankle region is that the fat is composed of only one layer [25]. It lacks the superficial and deep components seen in other areas. The fat in this region is primarily genetic in origin and is relatively independent of body weight. Patients may display only localized adiposity over the medial and lateral malleoli or have circumferential adiposity of the entire lower extremity from the knee down, sparing only the pretibial and Achille's tendon regions.

The musculature of the calf and ankle largely determine the shape of the potential silhouette. The medial and lateral heads of the gastrocnemius muscle combine and join the distal and more anterior soleus muscle to form the conjoined Achilles tendon. Hypertrophy of these muscles will limit the degree of slenderization possible. At the ankle, the laterally located peroneus brevis and the medially located flexor digitorum longus may be enlarged and limit potential results [17]. The anterior–posterior (A-P) diameter of the ankle is primarily determined by the tibia and the Achille's tendon [24]. In most cases, the A-P diameter is essentially impossible to reduce.

The subcutaneous fat in this region contains few significant structures. The greater and lesser saphenous vein course through the subcutaneous fat but all major arteries and nerves are beneath the fascia. Varicose veins may be present. Some surgeons recommend removal of these veins at least 3 months prior to liposuction [17]. We often proceed with the liposuction despite asymptomatic mild varicosities noting, like Lillis, that these thick-walled veins are easily "pushed out of the way" and are not problematic. [3].

Aesthetic Considerations

What features comprise a beautiful calf and ankle? Figure 14 demonstrates one concept, with a narrowing distal to the knee, a natural fullness overlying the gastrocnemius and tapering to a narrow ankle. Ideally, very little adipose tissue is present medially or laterally to the Achille's tendon. Most women do not want a straight leg devoid of shape nor an excessively muscular,

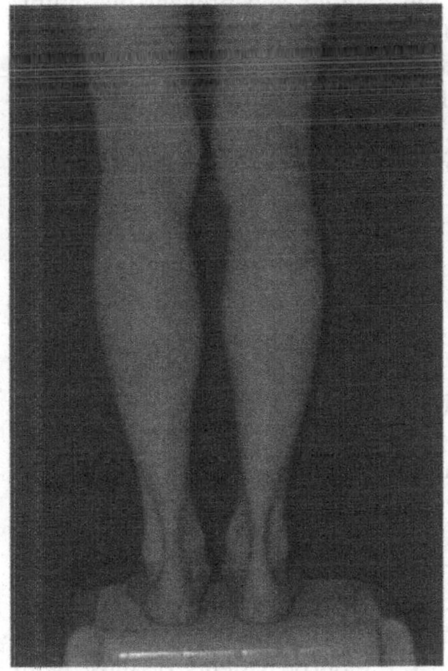

FIGURE 14 Ideal calf and ankle.

masculine leg. Aesthetic consideration should also be given to the size of the upper thigh, so that the upper and lower leg are proportionate. At times the medial knee and/or medial thigh should be treated simultaneously.

Watanabe has provided his perspective regarding the aesthetics of this region [25]. He recommends suctioning more from the lateral rather than medial aspects of the leg to avoid a concave shape of the medial leg. He suggests there is a relative softness of the medial aspect of the calf and relative ease of removal, necessitating more attention to the lateral calf. I have found this attention to the lateral leg essentially smoothes a bowed appearance of many lower legs, yet preserves a shapeliness medially.

Accentuation of muscle definition has also been recommended [17, 22]. Undesired adiposity often obscures the lower border of the gastrocnemius. Specific attention to this area will give a more tapered, defined look to the leg. Mladick also places emphasis in this "transition zone" in which the calf muscles taper and, in contrast to Watanabe, recommends more attention to the medial rather than lateral fat compartments [28]. Lillis no longer deliberately enhances this muscle border, but rather prefers a uniform, aggressive suctioning of the entire leg to a final muscular appearance [3]. I enhance the muscle border only in those individuals with small, straight musculature who need a shapelier leg and leave a softening layer of fat below a large gastrocnemius to blend the contour and prevent masculinization of the leg. Attention to the medial versus lateral portion of the calf will vary depending on the shape of the patient's leg.

Further aesthetic concerns include deliberate contouring medial and lateral to the Achilles tendon to maximize definition (Fig. 15) [22,25]. Patients have also requested attention to small pads extending down to the medial foot.

Patient Selection and Evaluation

The typical patient pursuing liposuction in this area is female and has been troubled by large calves or ankles since teenage years. She often has had to conceal the problem with long pants, long skirts, or boots. Usually clothing sizes present little difficulty, but sometimes pants and or boots are too tight at the calf due to the disproportion.

Younger patients are the best candidates for this procedure because of good skin tone and lack of circulatory problems. The preoperative history should screen for a history of phlebitis, deep vein thrombosis, lymphedema, pitting edema, circulatory insufficiency, or cellulitis. Any of these conditions could potentially impair healing and lead to increased complications [29–31]. Medical clearance is necessary in these instances. Although skin retraction is generally good in this area [32], elderly patients or those with poor skin elasticity are not good candidates.

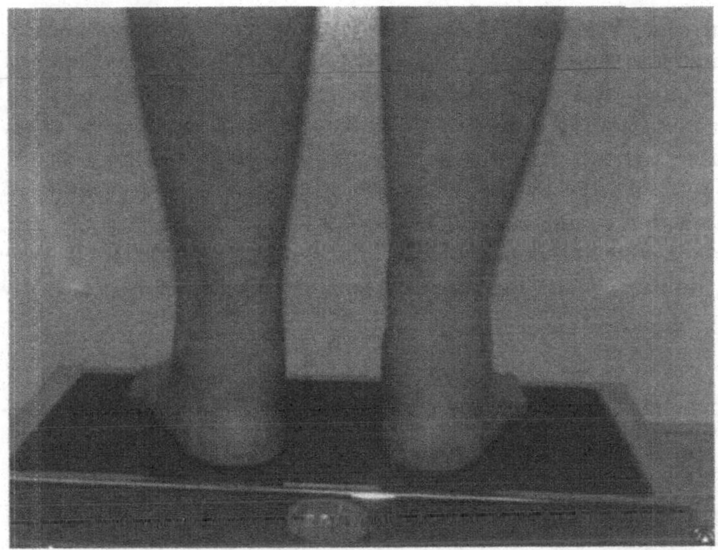

FIGURE 15 Fat pads on either side of the Achilles tendon obscuring definition.

Evaluation of the patient is done with the patient standing flat footed on a step stool. The entire leg is examined in all views. One can usually visually determine whether the problem is localized or diffuse. Asymmetries, scars, and any other irregularities are noted. The patient then stands on tip toe to view the size and border of the gastrocnemius and determine the amount of subcutaneous fat relative to the musculature. A standard pinch test is routinely performed. However, due to the tightness of the skin and musculature in this region, it can be difficult to pinch up the fat while the patient is standing. I follow Klein's recommendations that the standing patient bend one knee on a chair to soften the calf musculature of that leg and facilitate the pinch [26]. Others prefer to perform the pinch test with the patient in the standing position [3], sitting with the legs dangling [28] or in the supine position [25]. A minimum pinch of 1.5 cm for the ankles and 2–3 cm for the calves has been suggested in order to warrant liposuction in this area [17,25].

If the examination determines that the area is suitable for treatment, an open discussion should follow regarding the patient's expectations and desires. Does the patient want a tapered leg without defined musculature or a more athletic appearance that enhances musculature? It must be explained that this preference can only be partially accommodated because the size of the underlying musculature will ultimately determine the outcome possible.

Will the patient with large musculature be happy with modest improvement? All patients should be shown before and after photographs of other patients to gain an appreciation of realistic attainable goals. In addition, the post-operative course is relatively prolonged in the calf and ankle area. It is important to assess if the patient will be compliant with wearing support hose for prolonged periods and be adequately mature to wait out postoperative edema until final results are evident months later. The key to the patient's satisfaction with liposuction of this area is to clearly define the expected results, limitations and the expected postoperative recovery period.

Technique

Marking the patient is done with the patient in the standing position on a stepstool and the surgeon in a low seat so that the areas to be treated are close to eye level. The majority of fat is located posteriorly and the patient initially faces away from the surgeon. Some surgeons first mark the inferior border of the gastrocnemius muscle while the patient is standing on her toes. [17,22] Rohrich recommends having the patient pivot and flex her toes to confirm the markings in this region with movement [33]. Others do not routinely mark this muscle mass [3,25]. I first outline the most prominent areas of fat accumulation in the calf area and medial and lateral ankles (Fig. 16). Areas that require special attention are then outlined, such as the area medial and lateral to the Achilles tendon and the inferior gastrocnemius and lateral calf areas. Some surgeons include marking areas that contain very little subcutaneous fat and are generally not suctioned, namely the pretibial region and Achilles tendon [3,17,25]. Many further divide the lower leg into segments or quadrants by marking vertical midlines anteriorly and posteriorly as intraoperative reference lines to guide even removal [3,17,28].

Not surprisingly, there is considerable variation in technique among liposuction surgeons when treating the calves and ankles regarding preferred position, anesthesia, incision sites, cannulae, end points, and postoperative care (Table 3) [3,17,22,26,28]. The goal in this area is not only to reduce size circumferentially but also to reshape the leg in an even and thorough manner. Because of the small amount of subcutaneous fat and rounded contours, this is a relatively difficult area and all surgeons recommend nonaggressive cannulas, crisscross tunneling, and careful technique. This should be performed only by surgeons with advanced experience in other areas. Small depressions and grooving can appear intraoperatively rather rapidly so it is important to constantly check the area being treated and approach it from multiple angles.

My preferred technique is as follows. Patients are in the prone position during infiltration and for three-quarters of the suctioning. A pillow or towel

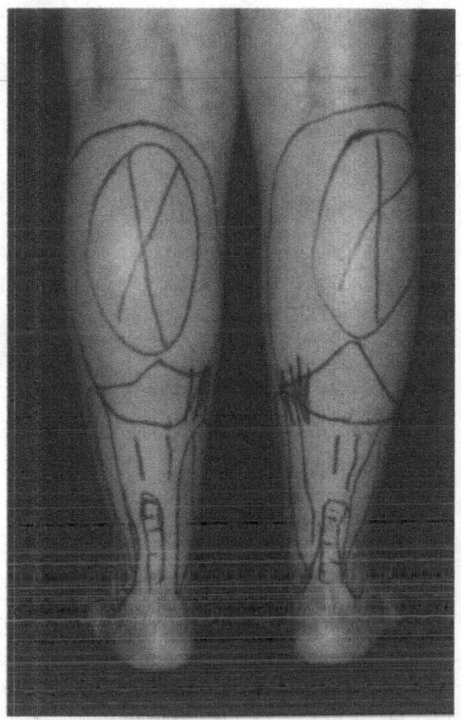

FIGURE 16 Markings of the calf and posterior aspects of the ankles.

roll is placed in the pretibial region to raise the ankles for better access. Standard tumescent anesthesia is infiltrated with the classic Klein technique, starting with 25-gauge spinal needles and then 20-gauge spinal needles. The spinal needles allow placement around contours and small recesses more easily and comfortably than longer infusion cannulae. A minimum of 150–200 cc of 0.1% lidocaine per leg is necessary for adequate anesthesia although more solution is necessary for the desired maximum tumescence. If other areas are being treated and maximum total doses of lidocaine are being approached, 0.05% lidocaine can then be utilized. The tumescent solution may cause more dramatic vasoconstriction here than seen in other areas and may be alarming the first time it is seen, but it is of no clinical consequence [3].

I start with four incision sites, two at the posterior medial and lateral ankles and two at the posterior medial and lateral knee. I begin by suctioning at the ankle with a 14-gauge/9-cm Klein Finesse cannula in the midplane of the subcutaneous fat. Suctioning is performed parallel to the leg's long

TABLE 3 Various Techniques for the Calves and Ankles

Author	Patient position	Incision sites/legs	Cannulas
Cook	Prone, pillow under pretibial area	Six medial/lateral Ankle Mid calf Superior calf	Klein Finesse 12-gauge (4- to 10 in.) Cook (3-mm)
Klein	Lateral decubitus Prone rarely	Multiple	Klein microcannulas (14- to 16-gauge)
Lillis	Lateral decubitus and prone	Six medial/lateral Ankle Mid calf Superior calf	Accelerator (3-mm)
Mladick	Supine, frog leg and lateral decubitus	Four ankle Medial/lateral Anterior/posterior malleoli Two midleg medial/lateral Two medial/lateral superior calf	Byron (2- to 4-mm) Curved and convex Accelerator
Pittman	Lateral decubitus	Six medial/lateral Ankle Mid calf Superior calf	2.4- to 3.7-mm, not specified

axis with some criss-crossing between the medial and lateral sites. Next the 14-gauge Capistrano cannula is utilized with long smooth strokes in the middle and deep planes with care to avoid the superficial fat with this more aggressive cannula. The fat is then approached through the proximal incision sites just below the knee with the same cannula. Usually it is difficult to remove fat adequately and thoroughly without one or two more incision sites immediately distal to the border of the gastrocnemius muscle. Suctioning can be performed both upward and downward from these midcalf incisions. Because these incision sites seem to heal more slowly and visibly, I try to minimize friction and the amount of suctioning performed through them by debulking the calf and ankle through the other incisions. I next utilize a 2-mm curved Accelerator/Eliminator cannula through all the incision sites to assure thorough removal. This cannula enables one to reach the pockets around either side of the Achilles tendon and the border of the gastrocnemius muscle from a proximal incision site (Fig. 17). The foot can be raised or the foot section of the table can be lowered for ease of approach. My cannula handle always has an opening requiring occlusion with the thumb for suctioning. Excessive suction and grooving through the entry site is easily avoided by raising the thumb.

Nearly 75% of the suctioning is performed from the prone position but the most anterior aspects of the subcutaneous deposits cannot be reached from this position. The patient is then turned to the lateral decubitus position with the top leg forward. Nonaggressive crisscross suctioning of the lateral and anterior calf and ankle on one side and the medial and anterior calf and ankle on the opposite leg is then performed with the Finesse 14-gauge can-

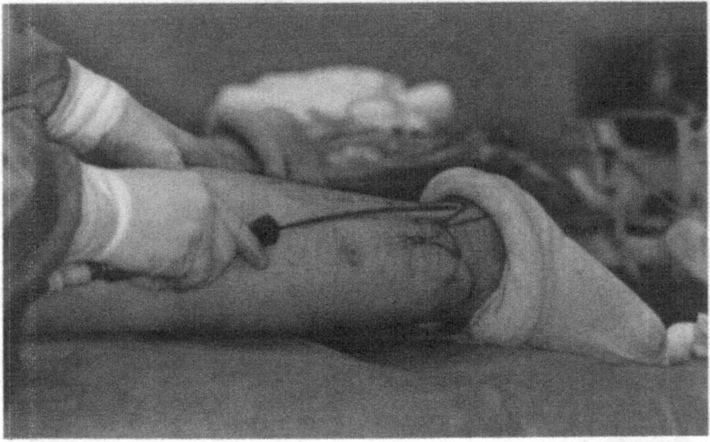

FIGURE 17 Curved cannula for improved access of the calf and ankle.

nula and the 2-mm curved cannula. The lateral calf may be thinned more than the medial calf depending on the desired postoperative shape. The patient then turns to the contralateral side and the process is repeated. A final look for symmetry and shape is done with the patient back in the prone position. The endpoint is assessed visually and by palpation. Additionally, a cannula is passed through incision sites and lifted up to check for evenness. Anterior edges of the treated sites are feathered with this cannula without suction. A superficial layer of subdermal fat is always desired even by the most aggressive surgeons [3]. Final pinch test recommendations range from 3–7 mm for the ankle to 3–15 mm on the calf (Fig. 18) [3,23,25]. At this point, subtle refinement may be done via tiny incision sites and a 16-gauge Capistrano cannula for small unusual deposits such as anterior ankle or small foot deposits.

It serves the surgeon just gaining experience in this area to heed advice from experienced surgeons. Since there is only one plane of subcutaneous fat, it can be difficult to discern when one is too superficial. Both Watanabe and Mladick suggest pretunneling first without suction at the level of the most superficial plane desired [23,25]. Subsequent liposuction can then be carried out deep to this pretunneled plane and superficial defects will be avoided. Watanabe further recommends feathering at the end of the procedure without suction with a three-holed cannula passed against the subdermal blanket of fat. To assure symmetry, Pitman measures the amounts removed from each of the four quadrants of the leg and suggests equalizing

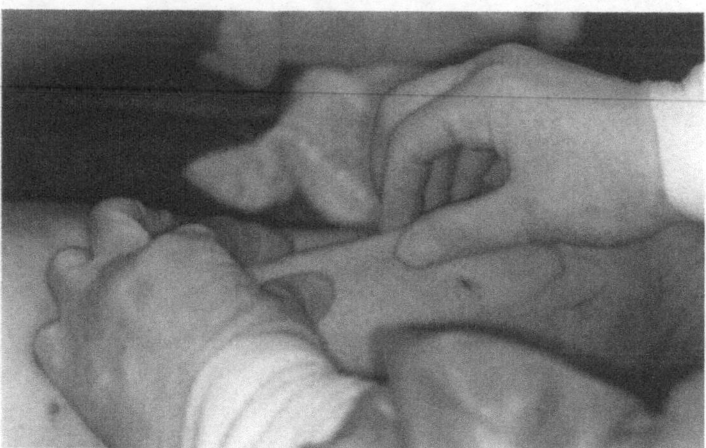

FIGURE 18 Pinch test at ankle.

the amounts from the quadrants of the opposite leg [17]. Mladick has devised both convex and concave Accelerator cannulas for access of hard-to-reach areas [28].

Postoperative Care

Postoperative compression is more important in this area than any other area of liposuction due to potential dependent edema and inherent risks of infection or venous thrombosis. Various regimens are recommended for postoperative compression.

In our practice, immediately postoperatively, incision sites are left open and patients are placed in light support hose of 15–20 mmHg. These hose have a loose mesh and allow drainage through them. Absorbent padding is applied over these hose and held in place with tubular elastic netting. Finally, an ankle length support garment is applied over the absorbent padding. Patients are instructed to elevate the legs the first 24 hr but are permitted to ambulate in the house. Bed rest is not necessary. There may be some sharp discomfort with the first few steps each day but this resolves with just a few more steps. Normally acetominophen provides adequate pain relief. Patients are seen the next day and measured for higher compression stockings of 30–40 mmHg. However, these stockings are painful to take on and off the first few days so they are not worn until postoperative tenderness and drainage subsides in 2–3 days. Compression stockings with zippers for ease of placement are also available [3]. Patients are advised to wear the support hose continuously for 1 week and then during the day for 6–8 weeks or longer. When there is less edema, the lighter support hose may be worn 3–4 weeks into the recovery period.

Postoperative activity is gradually resumed. Patients may return to work 2 or 3 days postoperatively but should avoid prolonged standing. Walking is encouraged during the first postoperative month. High-impact exercise is limited by discomfort and generally cannot be resumed for 1 month. When possible, patients should elevate their legs at intervals during the day. Prolonged edema has not been a problem when patients follow these instructions. Postoperative intermittent compression boots have been recommended by some [28,33] and could be helpful in a rare patient with an unusual degree of edema.

Patients may see impressive results 24 hr postoperatively only to be partially obscured by postoperative edema at the ankle or foot for 4–6 weeks. Final results may not be seen for 6 months or longer. Serial circumferential measurements may be taken at 1, 3, and 6 months out to demonstrate ongoing improvement to the patient (Figs. 19a and 19b).

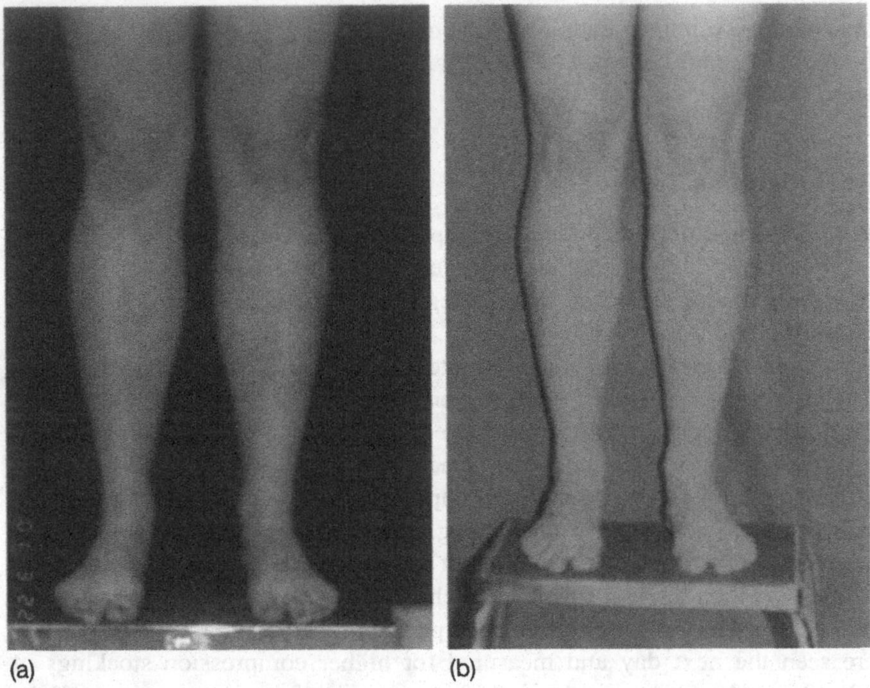

(a) (b)

FIGURE 19 (a and b) Pre- and post-op of calf at 1 month showing only subtle change in the silhouette; the circumference has decreased 3 cm at the midcalf level. Continued improvement will be seen over the next five months.

Complications

Complications are rare with good technique, attention to detail, and narrow cannulas. Postoperative edema is expected to some degree and may be noticeable, particularly of the ankle or foot, at the end of the day for a few months. Irregularities of the skin are the most reported complication and are difficult to correct. A touch-up procedure for undercorrection is easier to perform than treating a divot from overcorrection, so conservative removal is best when starting out in this region. Prolonged postinflammatory hyperpigmentation of the incision sites is not uncommon. I place these incisions as posterior as possible, away from the patient's view, and avoid excessive friction of the midcalf incisions. Patients with Fitzpatrick type III–VI skin should be advised of this probability and expect a longer time for the incisions to fade. Pigmentation resulting from bruising has been a reported complication, but has not been a problem in our practice nor has it been reported to result in permanent staining [25]. Other complications have been noted

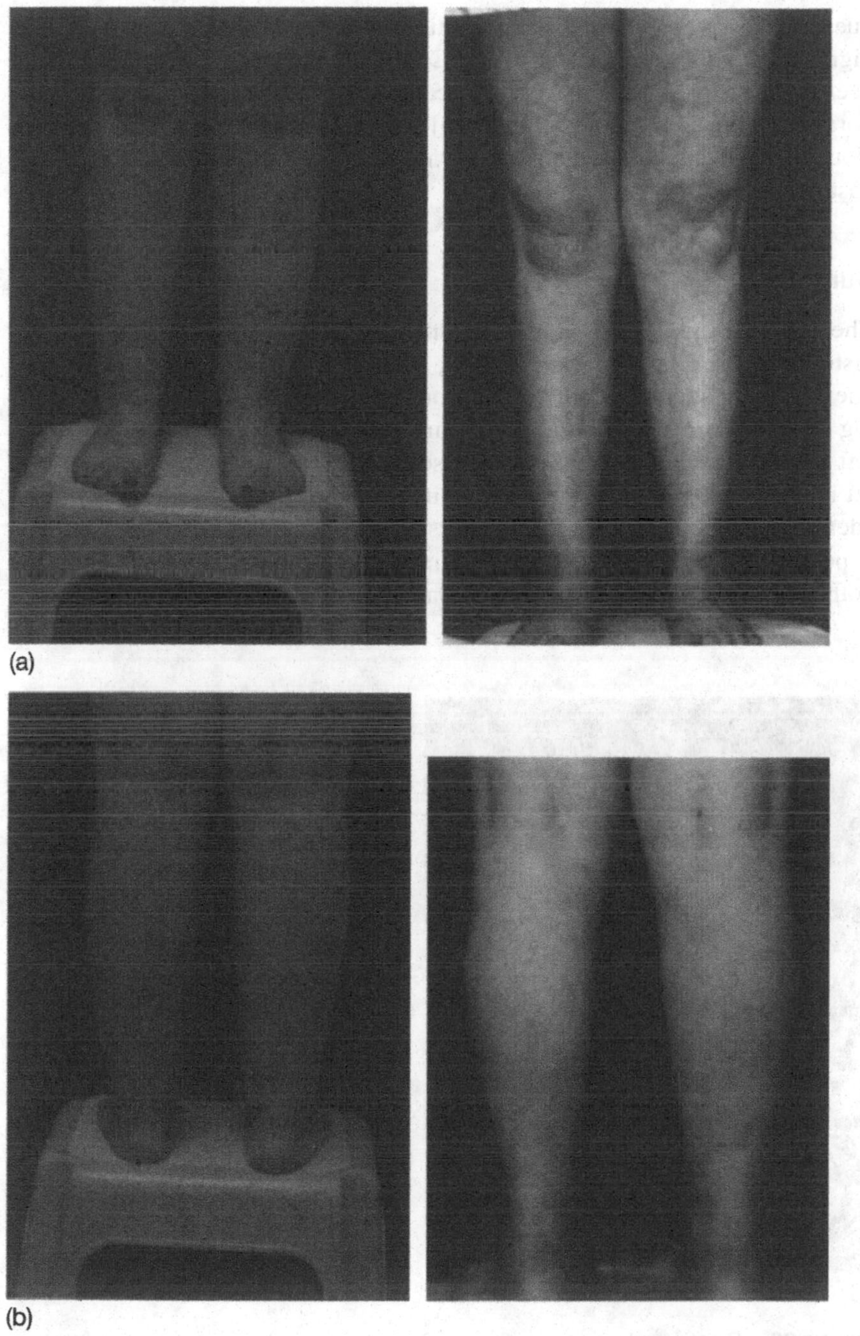

(a)

(b)

Figure 20 (a–c) "Before" and "after" views of calf and ankle.

due to excessively superficial liposuction of the ankle, including increased pigmentation and telangiectasia [24]. Complications of liposuction that have been seen in other areas have also occurred in this region, including temporary numbness [23] and seromas [3]. Serious complications such as skin sloughing or venous thrombosis have not been reported in this area in the past 10 years.

Summary

The calf and ankle areas are more difficult to treat because there are no distinct bulges to flatten, the working surface is curved, and there is only one relatively small layer of fat. Thorough, focused, nonaggressive suctioning is recommended with care to assure that a blanket of subdermal fat is left behind. Reshaping is possible to some degree by leaving more or less fat in some areas. Skin retraction is quite good in this area but postoperative edema prolongs the postoperative course. With proper preparation of patient expectations, results for the calf and ankle areas can be quite rewarding for both the patient and surgeon (Figs. 20a–20c).

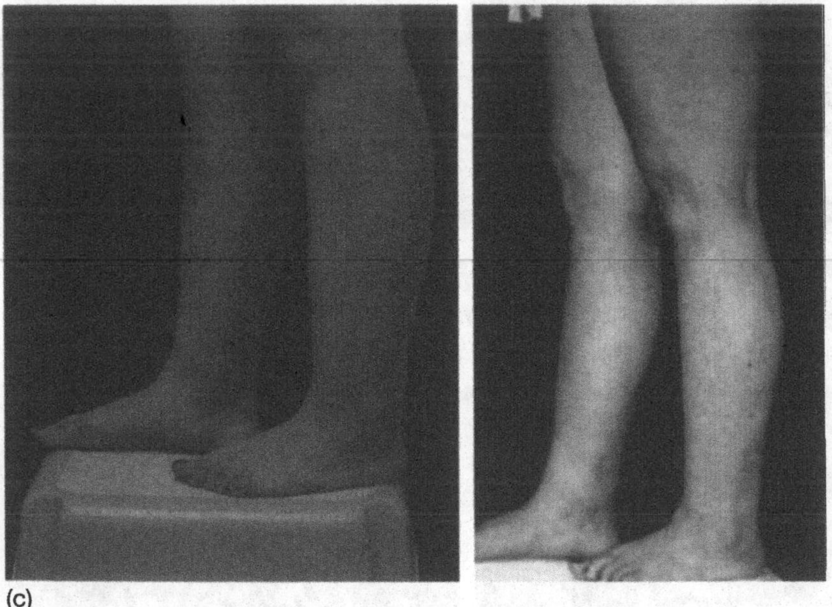

(c)

Figure 20 Continued.

REFERENCES

1. Narins RS. Liposuction surgery. In: Roenigk and Roenigk's Dermatologic Surgery Principles and Practice. 2d ed. New York: Marcel-Dekker, 1996:1269–1291.
2. Butterwick KB, Amiri S, Goldman MP. Touch-up procedures following tumescent liposuction: a two year retrospective study of 945 cases. 32nd Annual Clinical and Scientific meeting of the American Society for Dermatologic Surgery, November, 2000.
3. Lillis PJ. Liposuction of the knees, calves and ankles. Dermatol Clin 1999; 17(4):865–879.
4. Klein JA. Medial thighs, knees and anterior thighs. In: Tumescent Technique Tumescent Anesthesia and Microcannular Liposuction. St. Louis: Mosby, 2000: 357–371.
5. Lillis PJ. Liposuction: How aggressive should it be? Tumescent Liposuction Council Bulletin. Dermatol Surg 1996; 22:973–978.
6. Cook WR, Cook KK. Liposculpture of the anterior thighs, medial thighs and knees: surgical procedures, postoperative considerations, results. In: Manual of Tumescent Liposculpture and Laser Cosmetic Surgery Philadelphia: Lippin cott/Williams & Wilkins, 1999:127–138.
7. Bernstein G. Liposuction of the thigh. Dermatol Clin 1999; 17(4):849–863.
8. Lockwood T. Medial thigh surgery: surgical strategies. Aesthet Surg Q 1996; 16(2):94–96.
9. Pittman GH. Thighs and buttocks. In: Liposuction and Aesthetic Surgery. St. Louis; Quality Medical, 1993:337–413.
10. Ostad A, Kageyama N, Moy RL. Tumescent anesthesia with a lidocaine dose of 55 mg/kg is safe for liposuction. Dermatol Surg 1996; 22:921–927.
11. Coleman WP, Hanke CW, Glogau RG. Does the specialty of the physician affect fatality rates in liposuction?: a comparison of specialty specific data. Dermatol Surg 26:611–615.
12. Butterwick K, Goldman MP, Sriprachya-anunt S. Lidocaine levels during the first two hours of infiltration of dilute anesthetic solution for tumescent liposuction: rapid versus slow delivery. Dermatol Surg 1999; 25:681–685.
13. Tobin HA. Liposuction surgery of the knees. Am J Cosmet Surg 1988; 5(1): 45–48.
14. Collins PS. The methodology of liposuction surgery. Dermatol Clin 1990; 8(3): 395–400.
15. Brandy N. The use of asymmetrical incisions in liposuction. Am J Cosmet Surg 1997; 14:459–462.
16. Scarborough DA, Bisaccia E. Post-liposuction skin depression. Cosmet Dermatol 1999; January:22.
17. Pitman GH. Knees, calves and ankles. In: Liposuction and Aesthetic Surgery. St. Louis: Quality Medical, 1993;413–445.
18. Ersek RA, Salisbury AV. Circumferential liposuction of knees, calves and ankles. Plast Reconstr Surg 1996; 98(5):880–883.

19. Schrudde J. Liphexheresis (liposuctions) for body contouring. Clin Plast Surg 1984; 11:445–447.
20. Pflug M. Complications of suction for lipectomy. Plast Reconst Surg 1982; 69: 562.
21. Illouz YG. Body contouring by lipolysis: a 5-year experience with over 3000 cases. Plast Reconstr Surg 1993; 72(5):591–597.
22. Cook WR, Cook KK. Liposculpture of the calves and ankles: Preoperative evaluation, surgical procedure, postoperative care. In: Manual of Tumescent Liposculpture and Laser Cosmetic Surgery. Philadelphia: Lippincott/Williams & Wilkins, 1999:139–142.
23. Mladick, RA. Lipoplasty of the calves and ankles. Plast Reconstr Surg 1990; 86(1):84–93.
24. Reed LS. Lipoplasty of the calves and ankles. Clin Plast Surg 1989; 16(2): 365–369.
25. Watanabe K. Circumferential liposuction of calves and ankles. Aesth Plast Surg 1990; 14:259–269.
26. Klein J. Female legs and ankles. In: Tumescent Technique Tumescent Anesthesia and Microcannular Liposuction. St. Louis: Mosby, 2000:440–443.
27. Elam ME. Knee, calf, ankle liposuction. Am J Cosmet Surg 1985; 2(4):5–6.
28. Mladick RA. Advances in liposuction contouring of calves and ankles. Plast Reconstr Surg 1999; 104(3):823–831.
29. Lawrence N, Clark RE, Flynn TC, Coleman WP III. Editorial: American Society for Dermatologic Surgery guidelines of care for liposuction. Dermatol Surg 2000; 26:265–269.
30. Farmer ER. Draft guidelines of care for AAD member comment: 2000 guidelines/outcomes committee. Dermatol World 2000; October.
31. Jackson RF, Carniol PJ, Crockett CH Jr, Dolsky RL, Hanke CW, Lack EB, Leventhal MS, McMenamin PG. 2000 guidelines for liposuction surgery: The American Academy of Cosmetic Surgery. Am J Cosmet Surg 2000; 17(2): 79–84.
32. Lillis PJ. Liposuction of the arms, calves and ankles. Dermatol Surg 1997; 23: 1161–1168.
33. Rohrich RJ. Discussion: Advances in liposuction contouring of calves and ankles. Am J Cosmet Surg 1985; 104(3):832–833.

11

Liposuction of the Arms and Back

Lisa M. Donofrio
Yale University School of Medicine
New Haven, Connecticut, U.S.A.

Liposuction of the arms and back presents an interesting challenge to even the most experienced of liposuction surgeons. The circumferential requirements of arm liposuction allow a truly artistic sculpting of the area and the fibrous nature of the back makes liposuction of this area a technical challenge.

ANATOMY

Anatomic considerations for liposuction of the arms and back are relatively few. Liposuction of both these areas takes place in the immediate subcutaneous fat plane. The musculature that lies deep to the fat plane is protected from blunt injury by the muscular aponeurosis. The important nerves of the brachial plexus are covered by the fibrous axillary sheath that lies deep to the biceps, the coraco-brachialis, and pectoralis muscles. In the fat compartment of the arm and forearm there are only sensory cutaneous nerves and cutaneous veins with the exception of the ulnar nerve, which courses subfascially on the medial head of the triceps to the posterior medial epicondyle of the humerus, where it is palpable. The cephalic vein arises at the level of the clavicle, starting deep to the fascia of the deltoid and pectoralis muscles, and courses inferiorly on the anteriolateral aspect of the arm coming superficial a third of the way down the arm. At the level of the antecubital fossa the basilic vein becomes subcutaneous, dividing into the median cubital vein [1].

PATIENT SELECTION

Patients with more fat than skin excess in the arm area are good candidates for liposuction. This can be assessed by pinching the skin over the area of the triceps and comparing it with skin over the forearms and volar upper arm. The skin should be pliant and devoid of severe actinic damage, stria, and senile purpura to ensure good postoperative tissue contraction. However, even large hanging fat deposits can respond with adequate skin retraction to aggressive thorough liposuction [2]. If there is any doubt in the surgeon's mind as to postoperative skin contraction this as well as the alternative procedure of excisional brachioplasty should be discussed with the patient [3]. In the author's experience any suction of excess adiposity can result in an improved contour and possibly a smaller brachioplasty incision if needed in the future (Fig. 1).

PREPARATION

A thorough patient medical history is taken before procedure. A patient with a history of deep vein thrombosis, pulmonary embolus, or documented allergic reactions to lidocaine are in most instances not a candidate for liposuction. Preoperative lab tests always include a chemistry panel, complete blood count with platelets, and prothrombin and partial thromboplastin times. The surgeon may also desire hepatitis and human immunodeficiency viral screens as additional tests. Before the procedure patients are told to stop all nonsteroidal anti-inflammatory drugs as well as vitamin E, ginko biloba, ginseng, and St. John's wort. The author also prefers to have female patients discontinue both oral contraceptives and serotonin reuptake inhibitors for 1 week before the procedure. Cephalexin at a dose of 500 mg twice a day is started the day before the procedure and continued for 6 days afterward. Penicillin-allergic patients are given 500 mg of ciprofloxacin twice a day instead. Figure 2 illustrates the most helpful positions for photodocumentation of the arms and back. These should be taken with the patient undressed with standardized background and lighting. If the baseline photographs are performed on the day of the procedure they should be done first before the patient is premedicated or washed. Skin preparation is accomplished with sterile water and a chlorhexadine wash, being thorough in covering all the areas that are to be suctioned. Using a sterile marking pen, the fatty deposits on the arms and back are circled using positional change

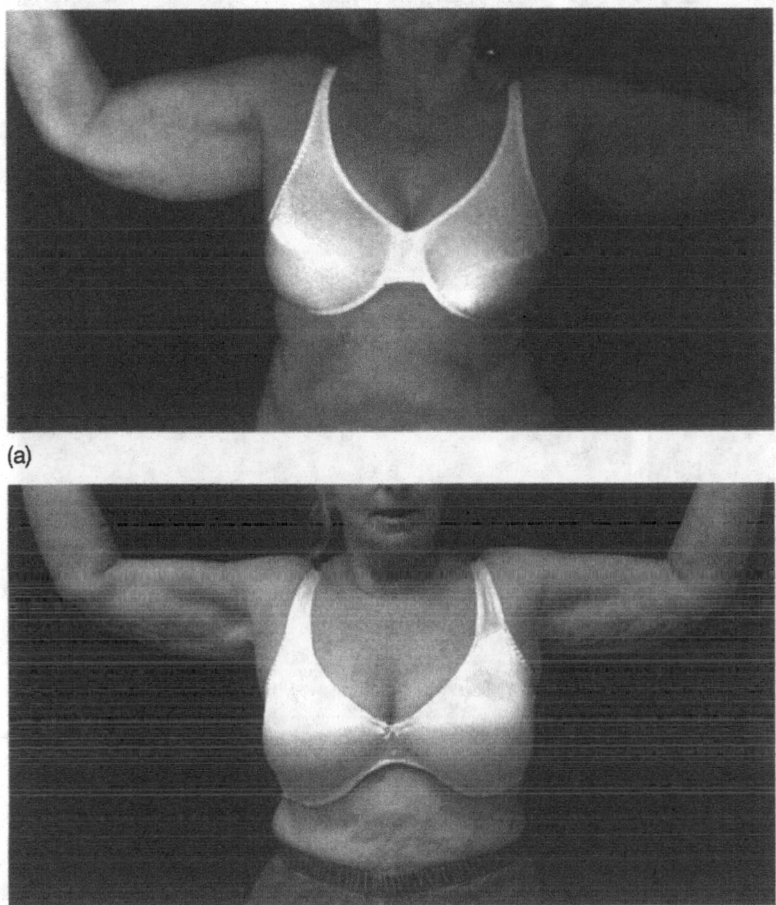

(a)

(b)

FIGURE 1 Excellent skin contraction with mild textural irregularity (a) before and (b) after liposuction of 1000 cc from each arm.

and skin pinching to help elucidate the areas (Fig. 3). Occasionally in the female patient it is necessary to elucidate certain bulges that occur from the margins of the bra line. This can be done with the patient dressed in a snug bra before washing. Careful attention is paid to drawing taper zones between fatty areas so that the postoperative result is blended and seamless. At this point the patient may desire premedication. One to two milligrams of Ativan by mouth gives adequate anxiety relief and somnolence in 20–30 min. After the administration of oral sedation the patient is laid on a sterilely draped

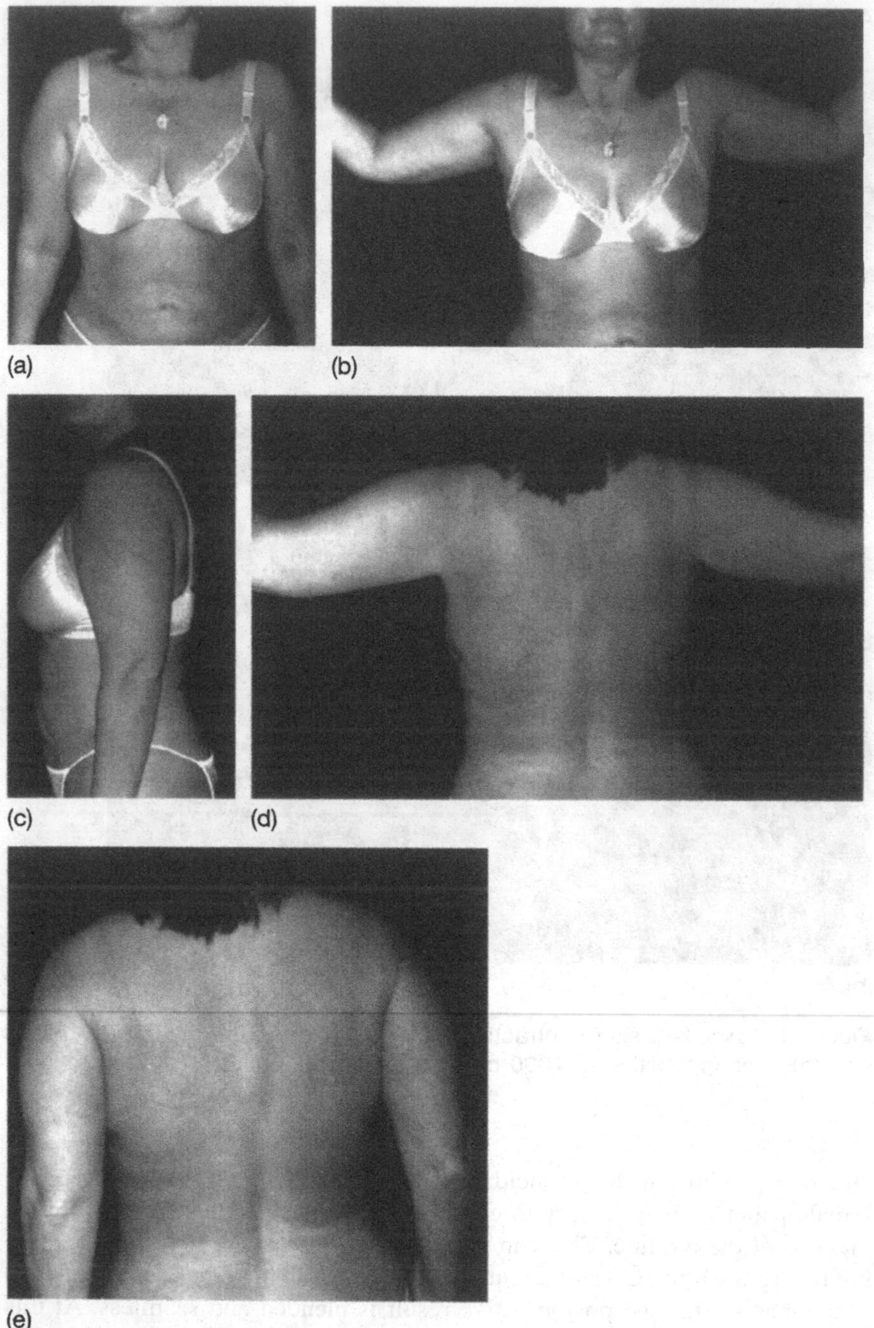

FIGURE 2 Poses for photodocumentation of arms and back: (a) frontal arms at rest, (b) frontal arms out to side, (c) lateral arms at rest, (d) posterior arms out to side, and (e) posterior arms at rest.

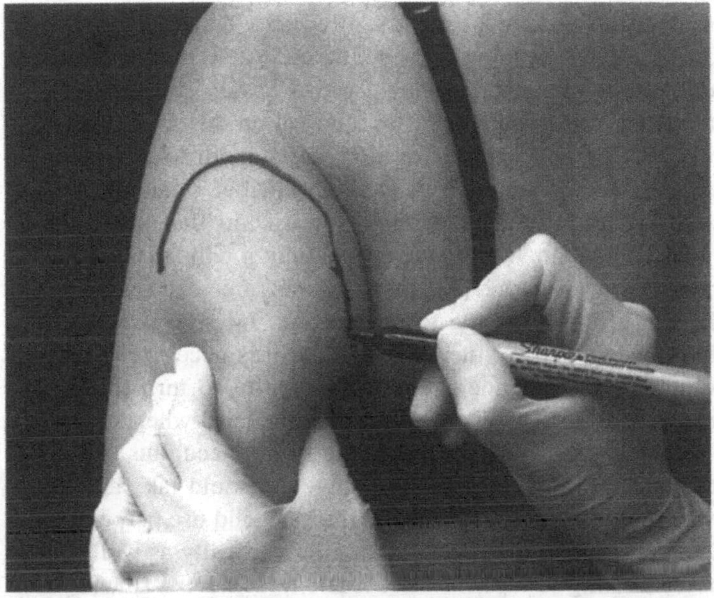

Figure 3 The pinch test is helpful in determining areas to be suctioned.

procedure table and hooked up to pulse oximetry and cardiac monitoring. The cardiac rhythm as well as baseline vitals signs are evaluated before the administration of local anesthesia.

TECHNIQUE

Local anesthesia is administered via the tumescent technique [4]. Standard Klein tumescent solution at a strength of 0.05% xylocaine with 1:2,000,000 epinephrine is infiltrated through a 16- to 18-gauge spinal needle or 2-mm multiholed cannula with the assistance of an infusion pump. The end point is turgidity and complete filling of the tissues. Expected tumescent volumes vary but range from 1 to 2 liters per arm and 2 to 4 liters for the back. Safe lidocaine dosing is achieved by keeping the total under 55 mg/kg [5]. Fibrous areas of the back may require a lower pump setting or tumescing by hand due to increased discomfort for the patient when an infusion pump is used. Adequate anesthesia and hemostasis is achieved by 20 min post-infusion.

Cannula selection is extremely important for suction of the arms and back. The fibrous tissue present in the back requires that the cannula be strong and short to prevent bending or breaking and of a small diameter to prevent ridging. A small-diameter cannula is also absolutely necessary to prevent textural change and ensure even fat removal on the arms. However, a longer cannula may be preferable here to create smooth long strokes on the vertical axis. The author prefers a 2- or 3-mm diameter cannula for use on the back and a 2-mm diameter cannula for use on the arms. Newer multiport cannulas enable smooth copius fat extraction and may reduce injury to the fibrous tissue network [6]. Incision sites are made with a 1.5-mm punch. These heal up with little to no scarring. Incision sites for suctioning should be made wherever the surgeon feels it is necessary to access the fat in a complete, even manner. It is often helpful to turn the patient from side to side as well as to extend the arm over the head when suctioning this area (Fig. 4). For the back, suctioning in the lateral decubitus and prone positions are the most helpful (Fig. 5). The surgeon should take advantage of the thick, forgiving tissue of the dermis on the back and use perpendicular incision sites and cross-hatched strokes, suctioning vertically as well as horizontally and remembering to taper at the borders to achieve a smooth transition into nonsuctioned areas. The arms are somewhat more restrictive in the direction of suction strokes. Due to the thin translucent nature of the volar skin of the arm, suctioning in this area should be with small cannulas staying at a depth of at least 0.5 cm below the dermis in vertical direction only. A vertical stroke direction should also be used on the posterior arm but the suction can take place higher up to the subcutaneous junction. A pinch test determines if suctioning of fat has been done evenly and completely. It is necessary to taper onto the shoulder since its thick fibrous fat is prone to ridging.

Incision sites are left open to facilitate drainage [7]. With the patient lying supine the arms are extended upward while compression tape is applied (Fig. 6). The direction of skin pull should be toward the axillae and posteriorly with the tape applied in strips on the posterior lateral and medial aspect of the arm avoiding circumferential "tourniquet" like application. After taping, the arms and back are wrapped loosely with absorbent dressings and a front closure compression garment that covers the suctioned areas is applied. The compression garment and the tape is worn for 3 days post-op and then over the course of the following 2 weeks as desired for comfort. In patients with poor skin tone where post-op skin contraction is a concern, it may be desirable to extend use of the garment and tape to 1 week. Follow-up takes place 2 weeks after the procedure and at 2 months. Postoperative photographs are taken when skin contraction appears to be complete, which can be anywhere from 2 to 8 months.

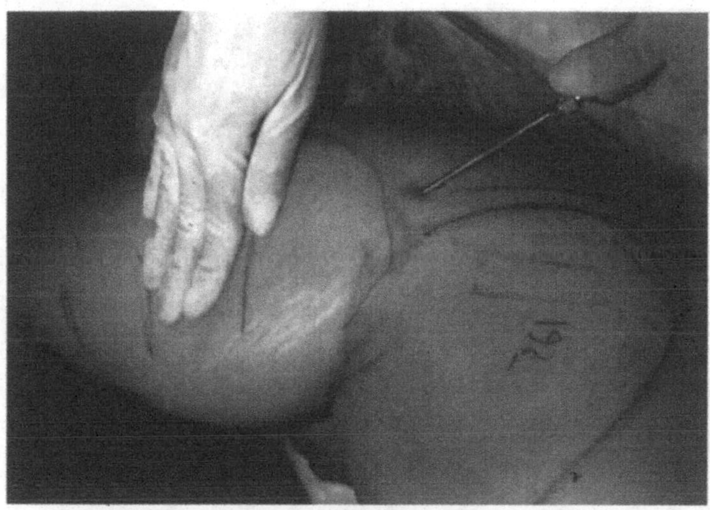

(a)

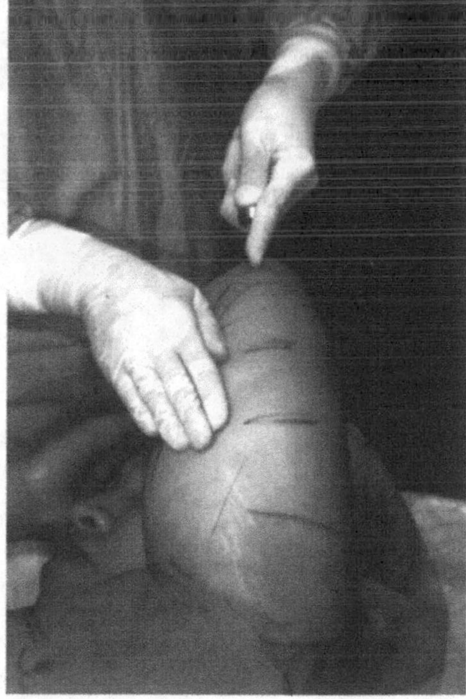

(b)

Figure 4 Positions for arm suctioning: (a) lateral decubitus arm extended over head posterior entry site and (b) supine arm extended over head lower posterior arm entry site.

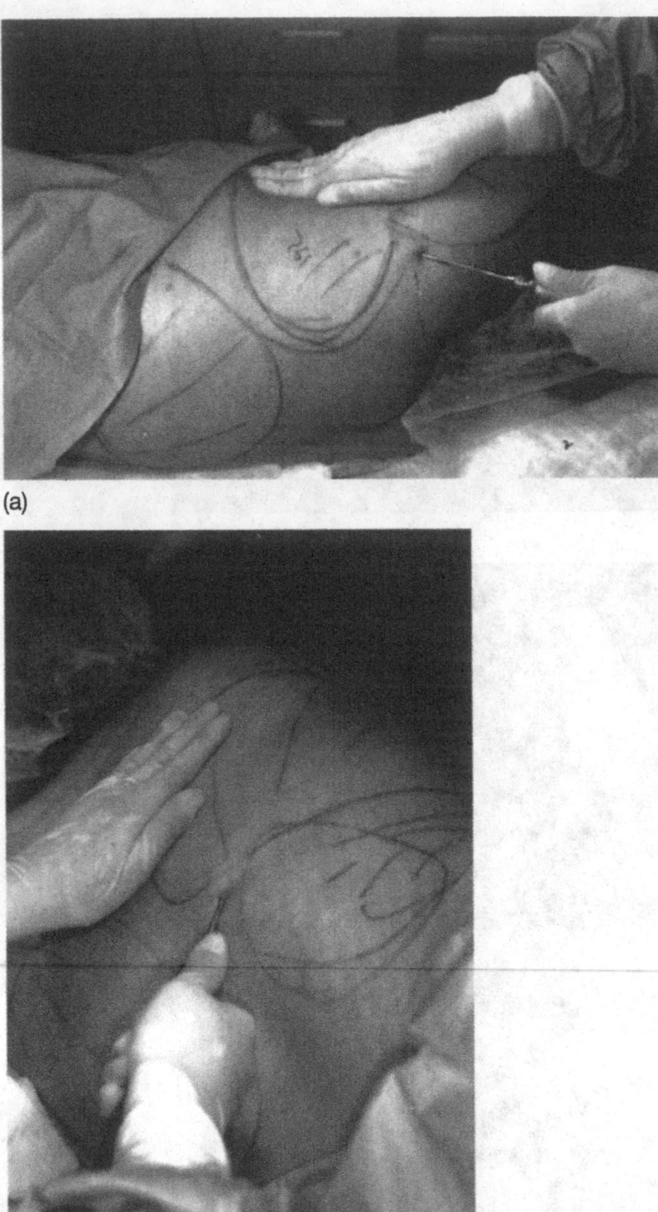

(a)

(b)

Figure 5 Positions for back suctioning: (a) lateral decubitus arm extended over head posterior entry site and (b) prone midback entry side.

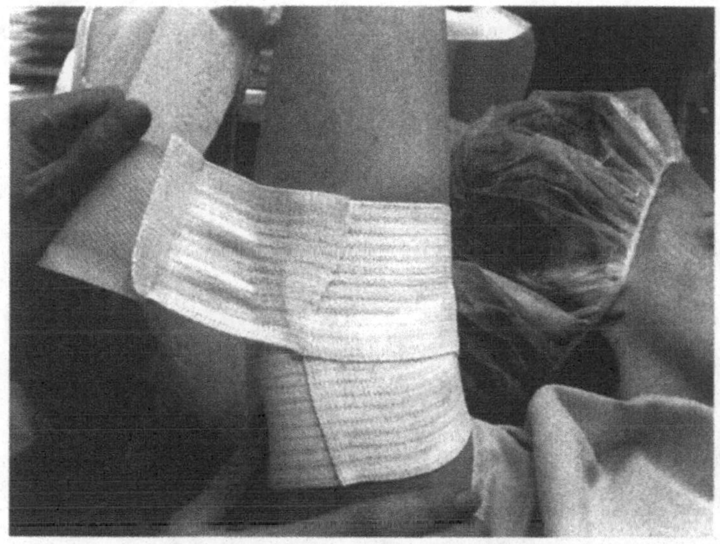

FIGURE 6 The application of tape postoperatively.

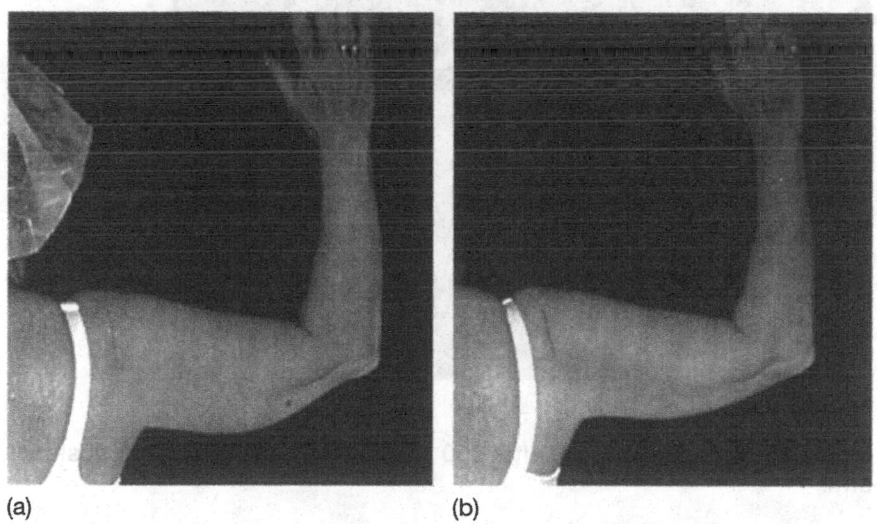

(a) (b)

FIGURE 7 (a) Before and (b) after 200 cc of fat was suctioned from arm.

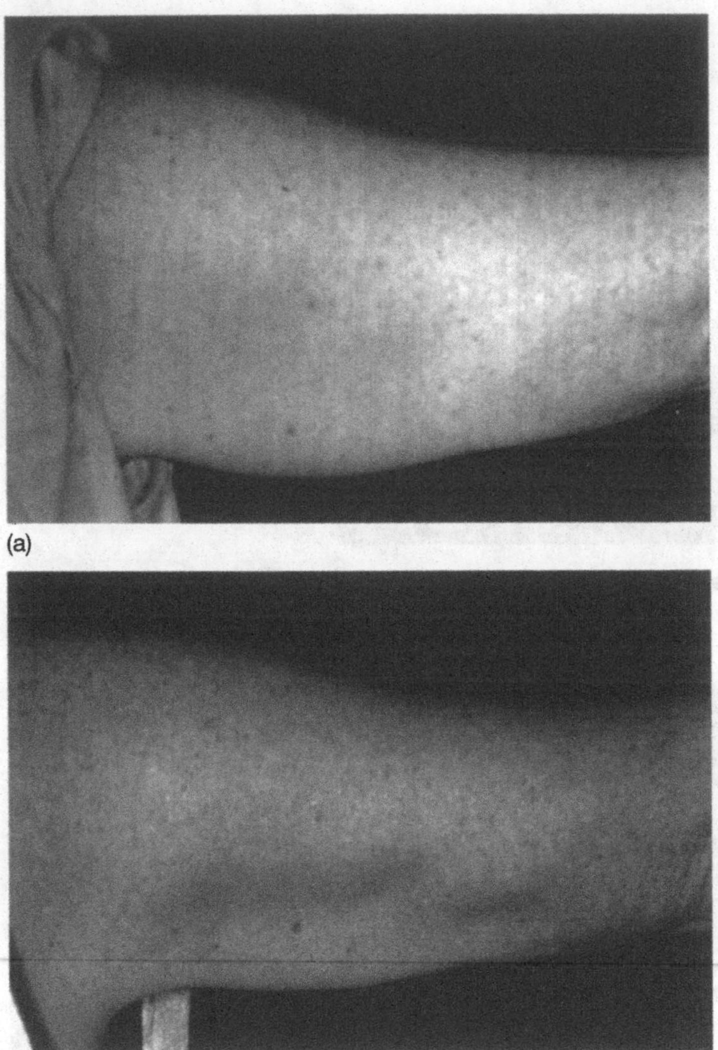

(a)

(b)

FIGURE 8 (a) Before and (b) after 350 cc of fat was suctioned from posterior arm.

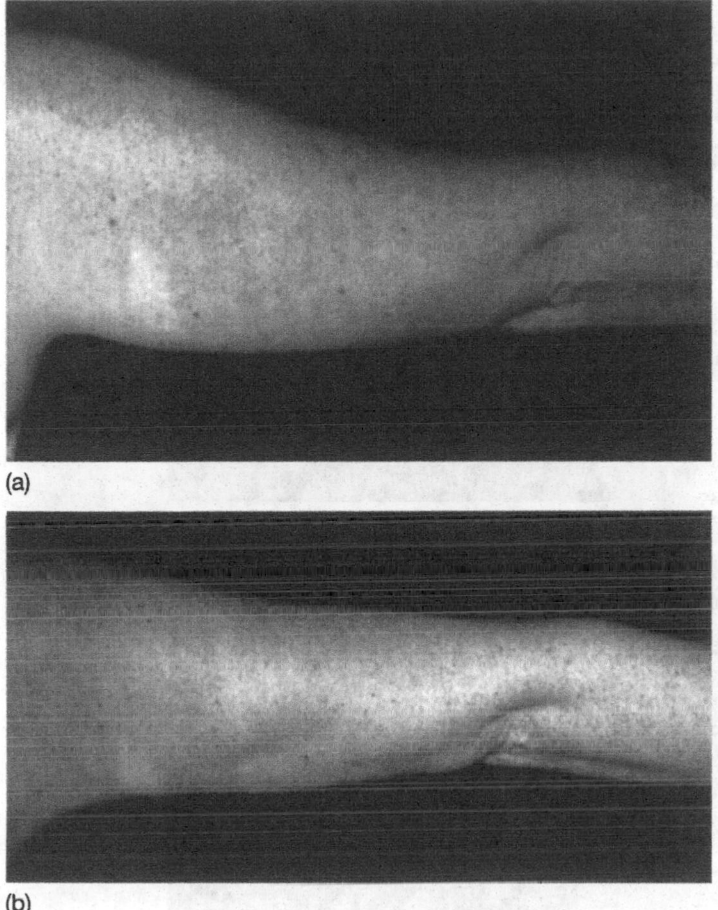

(a)

(b)

FIGURE 9 (a) Before and (b) after 250 cc of fat was suctioned from posterior arm.

COMPLICATIONS

Complications are similar to those seen with tumescent liposuction in other body areas [8]. Common and expected sequela include ecchymosis, edema, discomfort, and temporary paresthesias. However, recovery from arm liposuction is relatively easy for the patient with very little pain or swelling. The back may require a longer convalescence, especially if the procedure proved to be aggressive and the back was particularly fibrous. Patients who have large volumes suctioned from the arms or have lax skin tone should

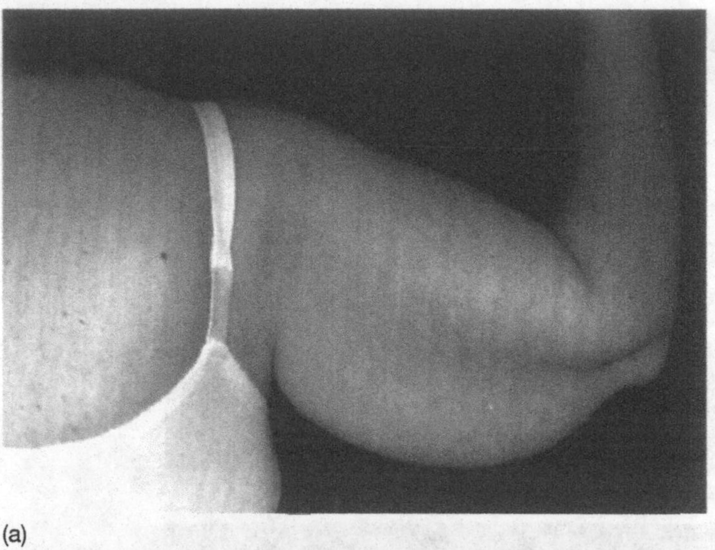

(a)

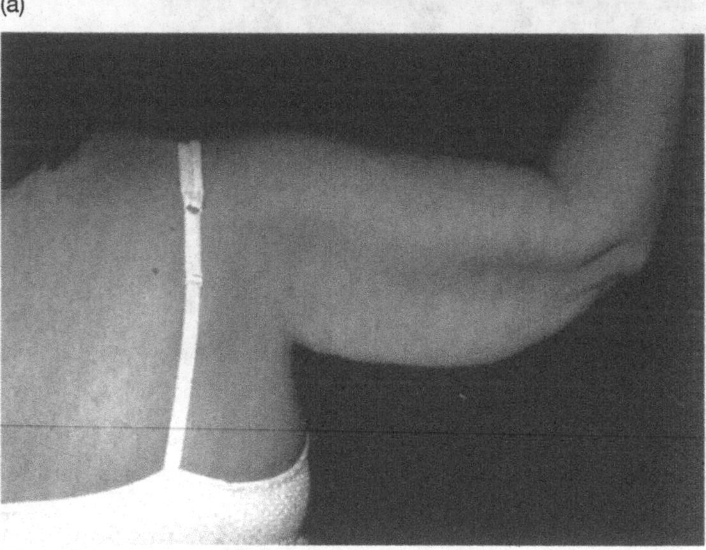

(b)

FIGURE 10 (a) Before and (b) after 600 cc of fat was suctioned from arm.

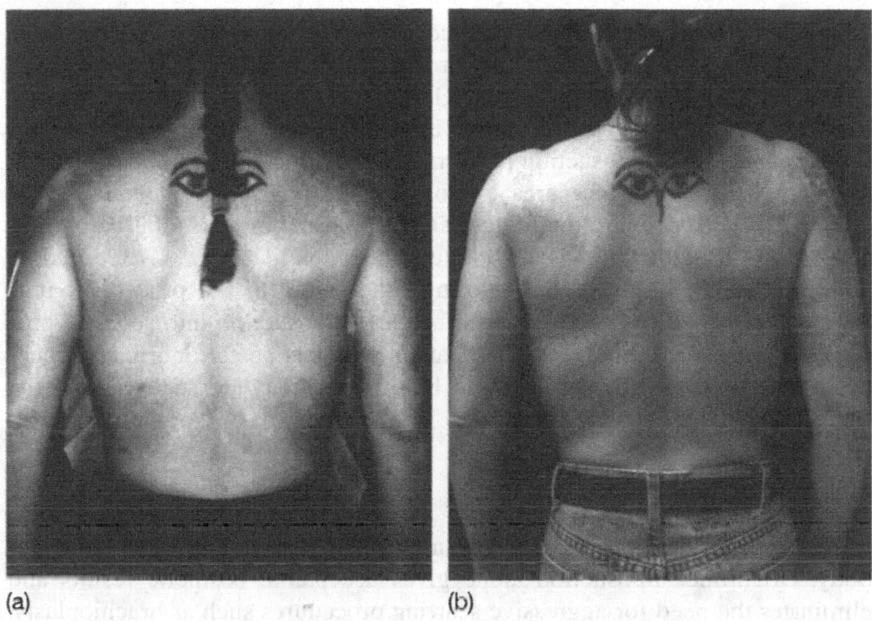

(a) (b)

FIGURE 11 Increased definition of musculature (a) before and (b) after 400 cc of fat was suctioned from upper back and arms.

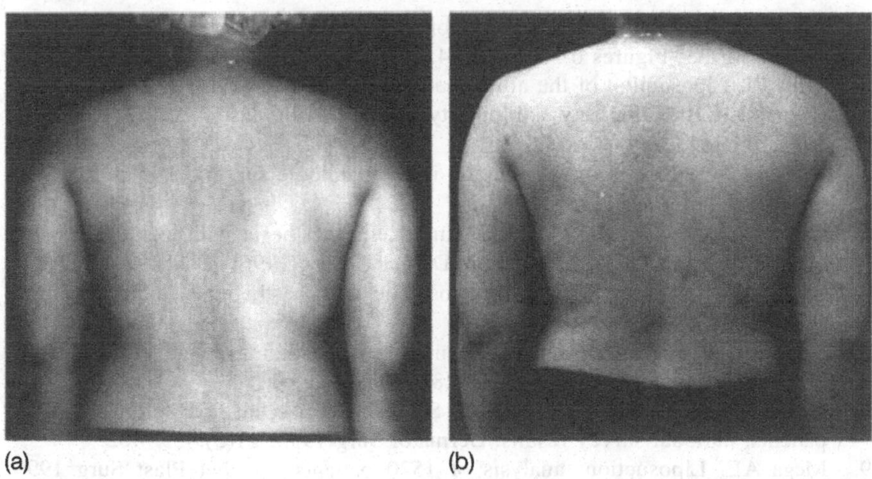

(a) (b)

FIGURE 12 (a) Before and (b) after 590 cc was suctioned from back and posterior arms.

be reassured that complete skin contraction can take 8 months. Similar healing times are expected when firm fibrosis is encountered postoperatively in the back. Textural irregularities, though uncommon when small cannulas are used, are possible as is postoperative infection (Fig. 7). The surgeon should limit the amount of liposuction performed at any one sitting to minimize the amount of diffuse surface area trauma and the possibility of serious side effects [9]. Performing circumferential arm liposuction and total back liposuction on the same day, even if the total lidocaine dose is not exceeded, is not recommended and may compromise the safety of the procedure. It is always preferable to divide large-surface-area liposuction into separate procedures; however, a relatively small patient with just posterior arm and upper back fat should have no problems if both these areas are suctioned on the same visit.

CONCLUSION

Liposuction of the arms and back is an excellent way to recontour the upper body. Oftentimes liposuction alone gives acceptable cosmetic results and eliminates the need for aggressive scarring procedures such as brachioplasty. Arm liposuction results are best when young patients with a greater excess of fat over skin are selected, but even poor candidates often achieve some improvement with complete and adequate suctioning (Figs. 8–12).

REFERENCES

1. Anderson JE. Grant's Atlas of Anatomy. 8th ed. Baltimore, MD: Williams & Wilkins, 1983: Figures 6-35 and 6-64.
2. Lillis PJ. Liposuction of the arms. Dermatol Clin 1999; 17(4):783–797.
3. Regnault P. Brachioplasty, axilloplasty, and pre-axilloplasty. Aesthet Plast Surg 1983; 7(1):31–36.
4. Klein JA. Anesthesia for liposuction in dermatologic surgery. J Dermatol Surg Oncol 1988; 14(10):1124–1132.
5. Ostad A, Kageyama N, Moy RL. Tumescent anesthesia with a lidocaine dose of 55 mg/kg is safe for liposuction. Dermatol Surg 1996; 22(11):921–927.
6. Sattler G. European Society for Cosmetic and Aesthetic Medicine, Cannes, France, 2000.
7. Klein JA. Post-tumescent liposuction care: open drainage and bimodal compression. Dermatol Clin 1999; 17(4):881–889 and viii.
8. Hanke CW, Bernstein G, Bullock S. Safety of tumescent liposuction in 15,336 patients: national survey results. Dermatol Surg 1995; 21(5):459–462.
9. Mega AE. Liposuction: analysis of 1520 patients. Aesthet Plast Surg 1999; 23(1):16–22.

12

Surgical Approaches to the Aging Neck

Carolyn I. Jacob
Northwestern University
Chicago, Illinois, U.S.A.

Michael S. Kaminer
Dartmouth Medical School
Chestnut Hill, Massachusetts, and
Yale University School of Medicine
New Haven, Connecticut, U.S.A.

INTRODUCTION

With the advent of tumescent liposuction, many advances in cosmetic surgery have occurred. Liposuction of excess adipose tissue from the submental area, jowls, and neck, along with cold steel surgery, have become attractive alternatives to the face-lift for cervicomental aesthetic surgery. Effects of time, sun damage, and gravity can include increased deposition of fatty tissue in the submental area, sagging jowls, and neck skin redundancy with or without banding of the platysma muscle. This often gives the appearance of excessive weight gain or aging to an otherwise healthy person. The traditional approach to these patients has been face-lift surgery, but with the introduction of tumescent anesthesia, neck liposuction has evolved as a safe procedure to enhance the appearance of the neck and jawline in such individuals. Many variations and additions to neck liposuction have been employed. These include concomitant simple platysma plication; the Corset Platysma repair; simple platysma plication with carbon dioxide resurfacing of the platysma and dermis (Weekend Alternative to the Facelift) [1]; and a combination of neck liposuction, platysma plication, and subcutaneous musculoaponeurotic system (SMAS) plication.

Platysma repair can improve refinement of the cervicomental angle in addition to eliminating visible bands. The etiology of platysmal bands is speculated to be due to stretching and loss of contractility of skin and fat overlying the anterior platysma, plus stretching of the overlying SMAS, which normally retracts the muscle [2]. Both of these contractility failures are exacerbated with overuse of the muscles and advancing age. An alternative treatment for early and mild platysma muscle banding is Botulinum toxin A (BTX-A) (Allergan Inc., Irvine, CA) injections into the vertical platysma bands. Although quite useful in some patients, BTX-A injections provide temporary (3- to 12-month) improvement and will not help some patients.

Those patients with excessive sagging of the jowls and cheeks or poor skin elasticity will benefit from concomitant SMAS plication and skin excision with repositioning. For patients with severe elastosis of the face with sagging skin at the temporal and malar areas, a full face-lift may be appropriate. However, many patients have aging changes limited to the lower cheek and jowl which can be greatly improved via SMAS plication and skin excision alone. The advantage of this safe, less invasive, and less time-consuming procedure, performed under local anesthesia, is that it eliminates the risks of intravenous or general anesthesia and gives excellent results with reduced morbidity.

PATIENT EVALUATION

Choosing appropriate candidates for neck liposuction is essential and perhaps one of the most important determinants of the postoperative result. Several analyses of cervicomental esthetics have been performed and show that patients with ideal neck proportions have cervicomental angles between 90° and 135° [3–7]. The ideal position of the hyoid bone was found to be at the C3–C4 level and at a location equal to or higher than the menton (the most inferior point on the mandibular symphysis in the midsagittal plane) [8]. These details should be considered when selecting patients for neck liposuction, as additional procedures may need to be employed for maximum results. For example, those patients with relatively low set hyoid bones are less likely to achieve a sharp cervicomental angle because their underlying anatomy will not support it. Hyoid position is an important landmark for muscular attachments and thus is an important determinant of neck angles and contour. Optimal candidates include those patients with full jowls but otherwise good skin elasticity, patients with high-set hyoid bones, and those with submental fat pads palpable by pinch techniques.

Several maneuvers can be performed to assess submental fat; the patient is asked to clench his or her teeth, which will tighten the platysma muscle and define the fat as pre- or retroplatysmal fat. Preplatysmal fat can be suctioned through a small submental incision, but retroplatysmal fat must be excised directly. Asking the patient to place his or her tongue up against the hard palate will also help the surgeon to identify fat location. The surgeon should also release the skin as part of a snap test to determine skin elasticity. If the skin feels loose and does not recoil quickly, then liposuction alone is unlikely to provide maximal benefit. This type of patient may be a good candidate for a partial superficial muscular aponeurotic system plication. The clenched teeth test is also useful to evaluate the platysma location and banding as nondecussating platysma muscle fibers become evident. Patients with prominent platysmal banding should be given the option for platysma repair at the time of liposuction as this will maximize final results.

The surgeon should also evaluate submandibular gland position. Many patients have ptotic submandibular glands which appear as a subcutaneous fullness bilaterally along the inferior midportion of the mandibular ramus. This ptotic gland can resemble jowls and is important to identify preoperatively. Platysma repair over these glands can improve this ptosis in some patients.

Gender may play a role in patient selection as well. We have found that male neck skin takes longer to retract and redrape after neck liposuction as compared with female neck skin. Whether this is due to differences in hormones, skin thickness, or volume of fat removed remains unclear. As with all patients, postoperative skin retraction may be suboptimal if preoperative skin elasticity is poor.

LIPOSUCTION TECHNIQUE

The process of neck liposuction involves first marking the mandibular border, jowls, submental fat pad, anterior borders of the sternocleidomastoid (SCM) muscle, left and right platysmal bands (if present), and the thyroid cartilage. This is done with the patient in a seated position (Fig. 1). Care must be taken to identify the jowl bilaterally as it will extend slightly below the mandibular ramus. The superior extents of the jowl should be marked as well. These landmarks help to delineate the areas for liposuction, and the top of the "T" placed at the level of the thryroid cartilage marks the distal extent for plication of the platysma, if necessary. Preoperative marking is essential to define landmarks which will be otherwise distorted after tumescence.

The procedure is performed in a well-equipped ambulatory surgery setting, with appropriate sterile technique and nursing staff assistance (Table

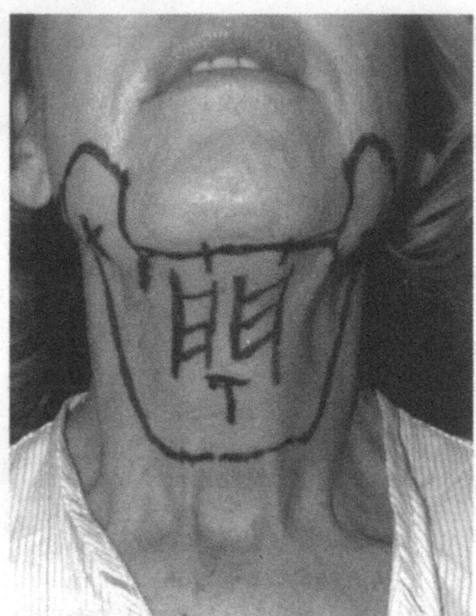

FIGURE 1 Preoperative patient markings.

1). The patient's face, neck, and upper shoulders are cleansed thoroughly with povidine iodine and sterile towels are wrapped around the head. After the patient is prepped and draped in sterile fashion, a small amount of local full-strength (0.1% lidocaine) tumescent anesthesia is administered in the submental crease. With a No. 11 blade, a small 2- to 3-mm incision site is made in the anesthetized area. The patient's head is gently extended back with the chin raised. A small-diameter, 6-in. sprinkler-tipped infusion cannula is used to carefully deliver full-strength tumescent solution through the submental incision into the immediate subdermal adipose compartment. Before and after tumescence, the patient is asked to purse the lips and clench the lower teeth to check the functioning of the marginal mandibular nerves. A 20-gauge, $3\frac{1}{2}$-in. spinal needle (Becton–Dickinson and Co., Franklin Lakes, NJ) is used to create infusion points at the lateral cheeks. Tumescent

TABLE 1 Neck Liposuction Instruments

1. 3-mm, 6-in. spatula-tipped cannula (Bernsco Surgical Supply, Inc., Seattle, WA)
2. 2-mm, 3-in. spatula-tip cannula (Wells Johnson, Tuscon, AZ)
3. 4-mm closed neck dissector (Byron Medical, Tuscon, AZ)

solution is infused into the subcutaneous cheek and jowl areas bilaterally. Caution must be exercised during this buccal infiltration as overzealous filling can potentially lead to intraoral airway occlusion. A total of 400–500 cc of tumescent anesthesia is required to anesthetize the average patient's neck and jowls.

After tumescent anesthesia is complete and allowed to take effect over a 45-min time period, a 3-mm spatula-tipped liposuction cannula is used to gently debulk the submental, anterior, and lateral neck adipose tissue via machine suctioning through the submental incision (Aspirator III, Wells Johnson, Tuscon, AZ) (Fig. 2). This is fine-tuned by suctioning using a 2-mm, 3- to 4-in. spatula-tipped cannula attached to either machine suction or a 5-cc syringe (Fig. 3). The syringe method of suction has been evaluated by several surgeons and found to be a precise and controlled method for adipose removal [9,10]. Caution must be used to keep the cannula in the middle to superficial fat and to stay medial to the anterior border of the sternocleidomastoid muscle. This helps to avoid injury to large veins in the area (Fig. 4). Suctioning is then continued with the 2-mm spatula-tipped

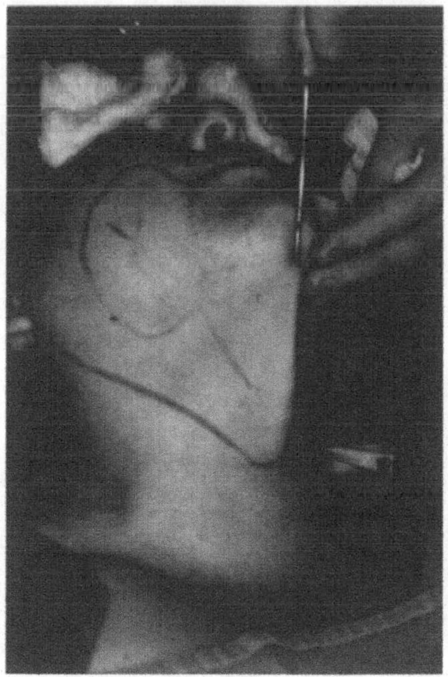

FIGURE 2 Superficial machine liposuctioning. Note placement of left hand along jawline to identify the marginal mandibular nerve location.

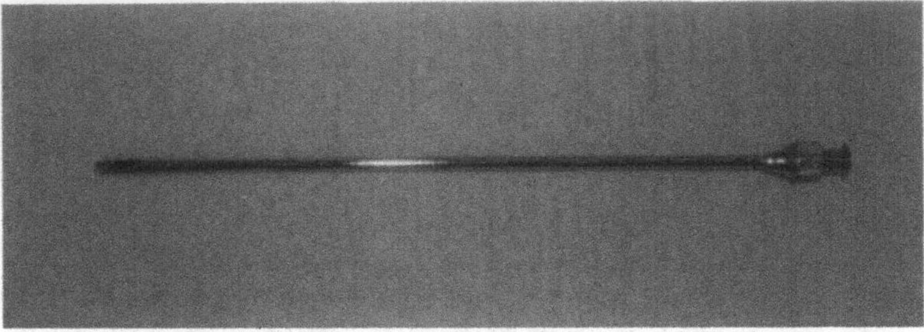

FIGURE 3 A 3-in., 2-mm spatula cannula.

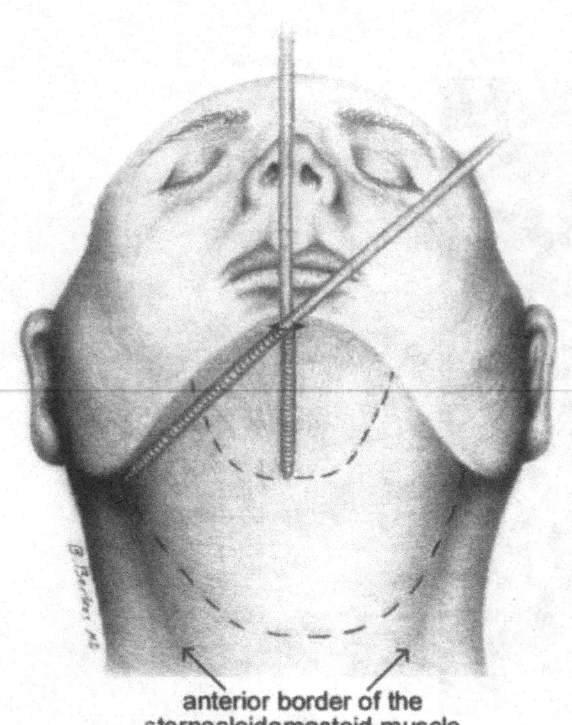

FIGURE 4 Lateral borders of the sternocleidomastoid muscles of the neck.

cannula through No. 11 blade stab incision sites placed along the lateral portion of the cheek, lateral to each jowl. Head extension and lateral rotation provides appropriate positioning for suctioning the cheek, jowl, lateral neck, and jawline. The midplane of jowl suctioning is first identified with syringe-assisted hand suctioning, followed by gentle contouring of the jowl and jawline via machine-assisted liposuction. During suctioning, the operator's free hand is used to identify the mandibular rim and the skin is lifted upward by the cannula motion to prevent injury to the marginal mandibular nerve. It is important to note that while the patient's head is extended and laterally rotated, the marginal mandibular nerve may drop as much as two finger-breadths below the mandible, become more superficial, and pose a greater risk for nerve injury (Fig. 5). Care is taken to stay in a middle to superficial adipose plane.

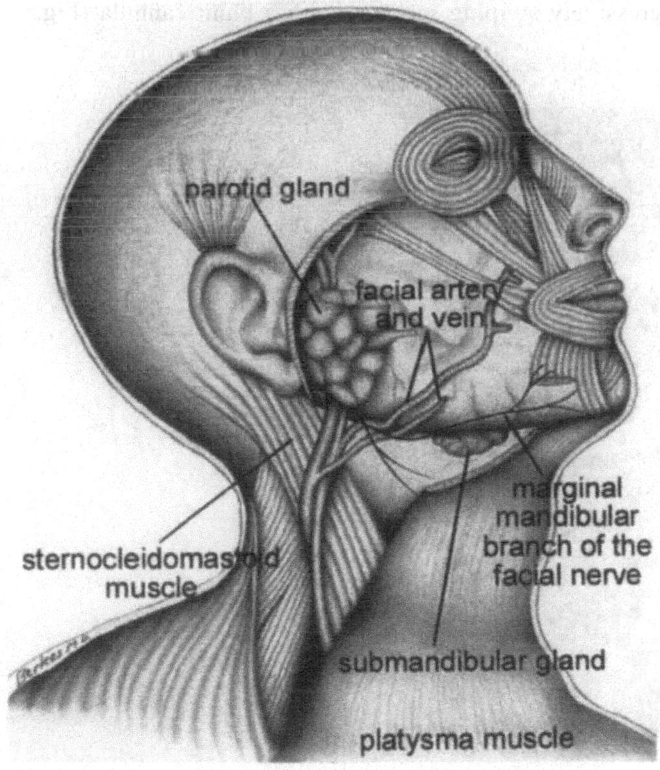

FIGURE 5 Location of the marginal mandibular nerve.

At times it can be helpful to turn the cannula opening upward toward the dermis, particularly in the submental region. While contouring the cheeks and jowls, one must avoid aggressive suctioning of the medial and superior cheeks as this can result in unwanted dimpling or hollowing. This is most likely to occur at the junction of the buccinator and masseter muscles where the parotid duct travels through the buccinator to the oral mucosa. Labiomandibular tethering near the depressor anguli oris may require gentle blunt dissection with the cannula to allow adequate adipose removal and contouring of the jowls. Removal of neck adipose extending to the medial border of the sternocleidomastoid muscles bilaterally and to the thyroid cartilage inferiorly is necessary if the surgeon will be performing a platysma repair. After contouring is achieved, a 4-mm closed neck dissector (Byron Medical, Tuscon, AZ) is used to release the superficial submental and anterior neck septae via the submental incision (Fig. 6). It is essential to release these tethering fibrous bands to allow smooth redraping of the neck skin. The sharp V-shaped notch of the dissector allows a more thorough and gentle approach than aggressively swiping the area with a blunt cannula (Fig. 7).

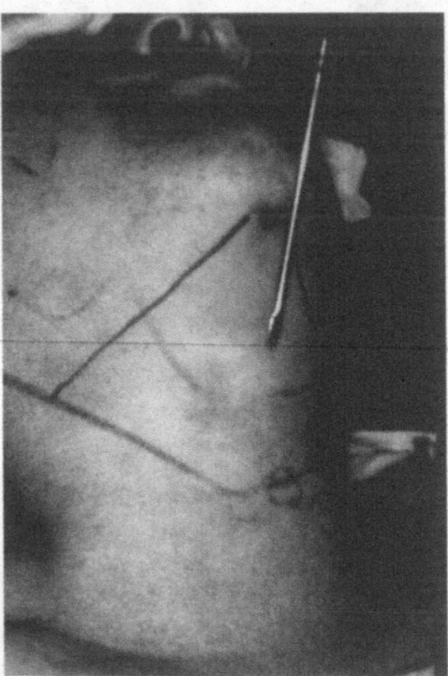

FIGURE 6 Lines delineate lateral extent of undermining and fibrous band release with Byron closed neck dissector.

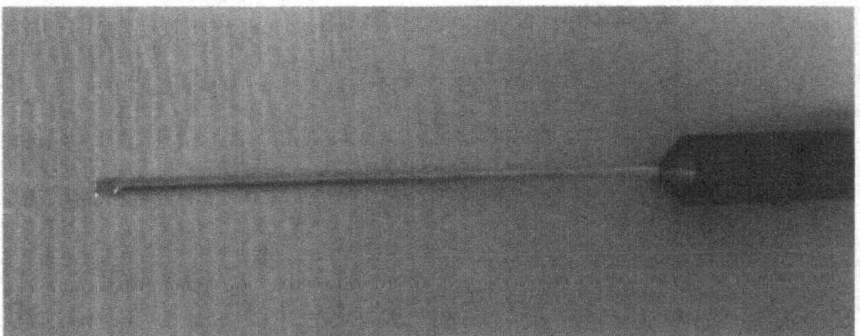

Figure 7 Byron closed neck dissector.

Gentle rasping of the underside of the dermis may also facilitate tightening and adherence of the skin to the underlying muscle. A cannula may then be used in a side-to-side motion to check for full release of the fibrous bands.

ADDITIONAL PROCEDURES: PLATYSMA REPAIR AND SUBCUTANEOUS MUSCULOAPONEUROTIC SYSTEM PLICATION

In patients who lack decussation of the platysma (crossing of the medial fibers of the platysma), or who have laxity of the muscle fibers, plication can be performed (Fig. 8). Current methods of platysma repair include bilateral platysma plication, midline platysma plication with transection of distal fibers, and necklift with skin excision [11–13]. The corset platysmaplasty, originally described by Joel Feldman, M.D., is an extremely effective and comprehensive anterior approach to platysma tightening and correction of submandibular ptosis (Table 2) [11,14].

Simple Midline Platysma Repair with Transection

Following liposuction, a 3-cm ellipse is removed encompassing the submental incision site. Gentle lifting of the submental skin for platysmal visualization is performed with a deaver retractor. After diligent hemostasis using an electrocautery pen equipped with a 13-cm straight electrode extension adapter (Surgistat, Valley Labs, Boulder, CO), the platysmal bands are identified using long metzenbaum scissors and forceps. Platysma repair is performed by approximating the medial portions of the left and right platysmal bands with CV-4 Goretex (W. L. Gore & Co., St. Louis, MO) or similar buried sutures. Other authors have used 4-0 polyglactin 910 (Vicryl, Ethicon, Inc., Somerville, NJ) or polyglycolic acid (Dexon, Davis & Geck, Wayne, NJ) sutures with similar results [14,15]. The platysma repair is con-

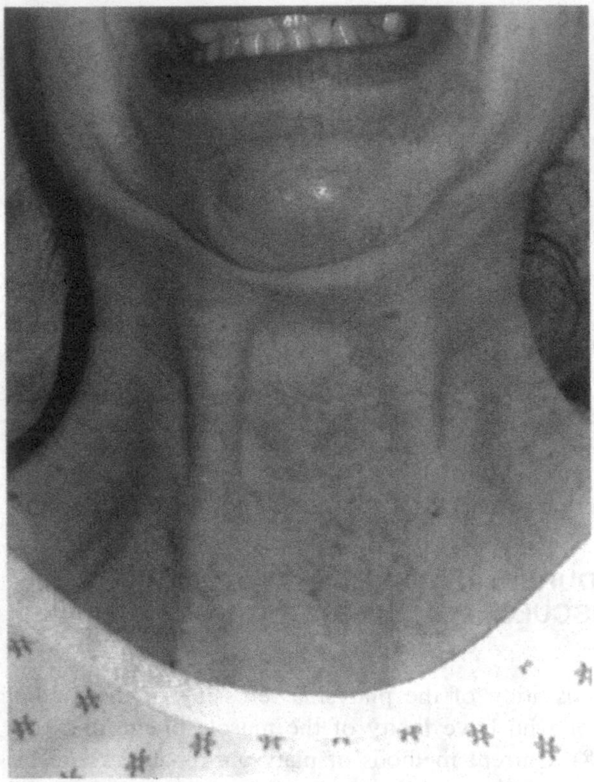

FIGURE 8 Demonstration of nondecussated platysmal bands.

TABLE 2 Corset Platysma Repair Instruments

1. Neck liposuction instruments as above
2. Surgical loupes and fiber-optic headlight (SurgiTel Systems, Ann Arbor, MI)
3. Deaver retractor (Sklar Instruments, Westchester, PA)
4. Long Metzenbaum scissors (Sklar Instruments, Westchester, PA)
5. 7-in. DeBakey atraumatic tissue forceps (Sklar Instruments, Westchester, PA)
6. 7-in. Webster smooth needle holder (Sklar Instruments, Westchester, PA)
7. Electrocautery pencil with 13-cm straight electrode extension adapter (Surgistat, Valley Labs, Boulder, CO)

tinued inferiorly to just above the level of the thyroid cartilage. Electrosection is then used to transect the distal portion of the platysma bilaterally from the proximal midline bundle. The skin incision is closed with 5-0 polyglactin 910 and 6-0 polypropylene sutures. The small incision sites on the cheeks and jawline are left for drainage purposes and heal secondarily.

The Corset Platysma Repair

The Corset Platysma repair is performed following liposuction of the neck and is begun by creating a 3-cm elliptical incision enveloping the submental crease incision. Surgical loupes (SurgiTel Systems, Ann Arbor, MI) and a fiber-optic headlight are essential to obtain an adequate visual field. A Deaver retractor (Sklar Instruments, Westchester, PA) is used to retract the skin (Fig. 9) and the medial bands of the platysma are identified and isolated via blunt dissection using long Metzenbaum scissors (Sklar Instruments, Westchester, PA). Hemostasis is achieved and any further platysma-dermal tethers are removed via electrocautery. The retroplatysmal space is then accessed through a small incision in the fascia overlying the platysma. If excess retroplatysmal fat is present superior to the hyoid bone, a small amount (approximately 3 cc) is excised after careful dissection of the superficial

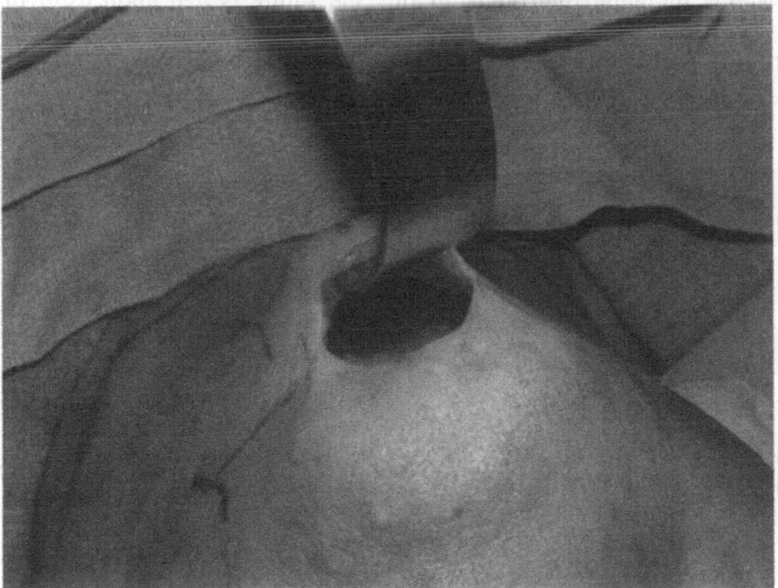

FIGURE 9 Visualization of the platysma using a Deaver retractor.

fascia (Fig. 10). Care is taken to identify, divide, and coagulate any prominent veins when necessary as they may lie in the fat deep to the fascia and the medial platysma edges. The medial borders of the split platysma bands are then identified with blunt and sharp dissection to produce clearly defined borders for suturing the muscle together. Hemostasis is then confirmed. A running 4-0 mersilene (Ethicon, Inc., Somerville, NJ) or clear nylon suture is used, and with a 7-in. needle holder, a running suture is started at the superior portion of the split platysma bands. Seven-inch DeBakey atraumatic tissue forceps (Sklar Instruments, Westchester, PA) are used to gently grasp the medial edges of the platysma bands, and suturing is continued inferiorly in a running locked fashion as the edges of the right and left platysma muscle are approximated. The running suture proceeds inferiorly toward the thyroid cartilage, making sure that adequate sections (approximately 1 cm) of platysma and overlying fascia are incorporated into each bite. Upon reaching the level of the thyroid cartilage, the running suture is continued in a running reverse direction proximally while plicating the more lateral borders of the platysma muscle over the now sutured medial fibers (Fig. 11). This is the corset portion of the repair, and the double-layer plication creates a smooth surface to the midline plication as well as superb muscular apposition and tightening. This "overplication" produces firm tightening of the anterior platysma and sharpening of the cervicomental angle as well as the jawline. Upon reaching the submental incision site, the suture is tied upon itself in buried knot fashion. During the overplication corset phase of the repair, there is a gratifying part of the procedure where the platysma literally falls onto

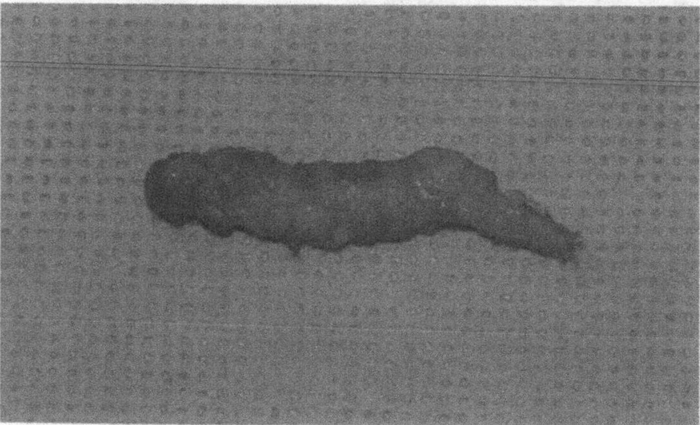

FIGURE 10 Retroplatysmal fat.

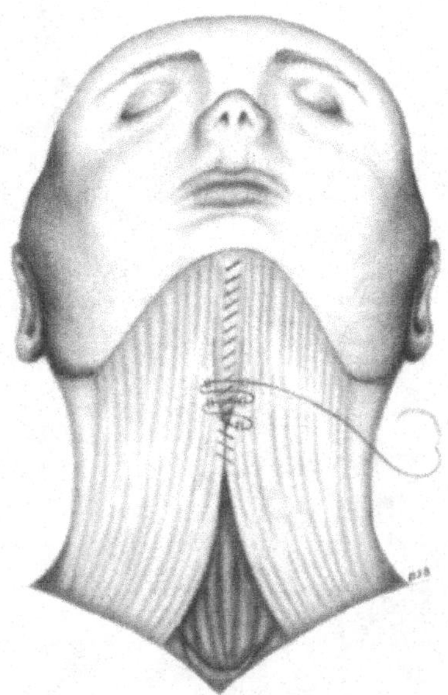

FIGURE 11 The reverse running suture of the corset platysmaplasty

the underlying hyoid bone as the muscular tightening causes the muscle to assume its natural shape on the neck.

Some patients have prominent submandibular glands due to ptosis of the glands inferior to the jawline. These patients benefit from an oblique plication performed on the left and right submandibular area to further tighten the platysma muscle and elevate the ptotic submandibular gland. These lateral platysma bands and associated muscle laxity are less clearly identified, and the lateral positioning makes the approach to their repair challenging through the small submental incision. On each side, small oblique running sutures are placed to a length of 5–8 cm with 4-0 mersilene. A locked running suture is first placed from proximal to distal and then a running "baseball-type" stitch is performed as the suture is continued from distal to proximal (Fig. 12). The suture is then tied upon itself. Finally, in the original description by Feldman, two interlocking sling sutures are performed, one from the right submental platysma fibers to the left mastoid process, and one through the left submental platysma fibers to the right mastoid process. The sutures are interlocked in the submental position. We have not found this portion of the procedure to be necessary in the majority of patients, but it may benefit those patients with extreme platysma laxity or ptotic submandibular glands.

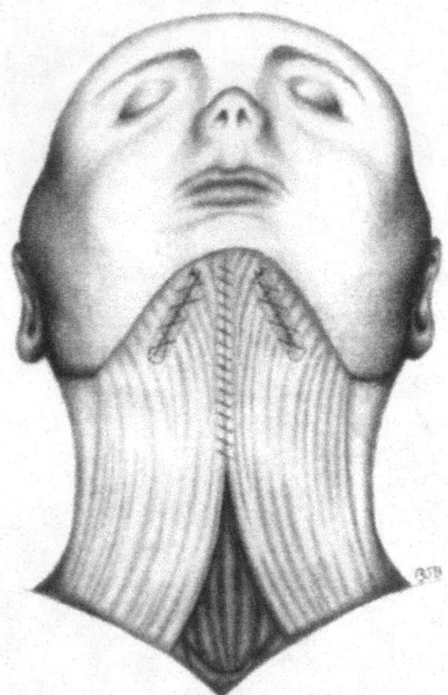

Figure 12 Plication over the lateral submental platysma.

Redraping of the neck and jawline skin occasionally requires further release of the lateral platysma-dermal bands to avoid puckering of the skin at the lateral neckline. Occasionally redundant skin occurs submentally after the plication. Excision of this skin at the level of the submental incision can be performed if the superfluous skin is substantial. Closure of the submental incision is accomplished with 5-0 polyglactin 910 and 6-0 polypropylene sutures.

Superficial Muscular Aponeurotic System Plication

In patients with excessive sagging of the jowl and jawline skin, or advanced age and poor skin elasticity, a subcutaneous musculoaponeurotic system plication can be performed. Following liposuction and repair of the platysma muscle, lidocaine (1% with 1:100,000 epinephrine) is locally injected along the planned incision line to an area 3 cm anterior to the ear (in the lateral cheek area in the region to be undermined), as well as in the postauricular sulcus. An incision is made along the inner rim of the tragus (similar to standard face-lift incision in this area) [16] and extended inferiorly anterior to and under the ear lobe and then superiorly along the posterior ear sulcus to approximately one-third to one-half the length of the ear. Undermining 3 cm anteriorly from the incision in the midsubcutaneous plane allows visualization of the SMAS. Suture plication of the SMAS is performed in a superior-lateral direction and the skin is redraped. Subcutaneous musculoaponeurotic system plication is intended to tighten the musculature along the jawline and upper neck. A total of 7–10 sutures are used, with plication extending down from the pretragal region, anterior to the earlobe, and along approximately 3–5 cm of the superior aspect of the SCM muscle. It is essential to place buried knot plication sutures along vectors that optimize jawline definition and enhancement. Redundant pre- and postauricular skin is excised and the edges are reapproximated with 5-0 polyglactin 910 and 6-0 polypropylene sutures.

Postoperatively, conventional bandages, a Reston foam support (Reston, 3M Medical-Surgical Division, St. Paul, MN), and a five-tabbed compression neck liposuction garment (Flex support compression garments, Universal facial garment, Wells Johnson, Co., Tuscon, AZ) are applied and left in place for 24 hr. The foam is then removed, and the patient is instructed to wear a two-tabbed garment (Facial, Chin, Neck Supporter, Cosmetic Surgery Suppliers, Tucker, GA) layered with a chin strap support garment (The Wrap, Byron Medical, Tuscon, AZ) daily for 1 week and then at least 8 hr a day for the following 3–4 weeks. The use of double-layered postoperative compression garments appears to enhance skin redraping and jawline contouring. Final cosmetic results occur several weeks to months postoperatively, as mild edema requires time to resolve, and skin retraction may be slower in the aging neck (Figs. 13a, 13b, 14a, 14b, 15a, and 15b).

DISCUSSION

The neck can be a challenging anatomic region to rejuvenate, and complications are a legitimate concern. There are inherent risks of tumescent neck liposuction which include bleeding (intraoperative and postoperative), seroma formation, injury to the marginal mandibular nerve, and vertical band formation with poor skin retraction. But, with careful patient selection, neck recontouring can be performed in a safe and efficient manner.

Important measures for maximizing results in neck liposuction include using small (2- to 3-mm) cannulas, combining hand and machine suctioning, creating sufficient numbers of entry sites for thorough suctioning, releasing submental fibrous subcutaneous bands, and having the patient wear appropriate postoperative garments. Despite proper postoperative care, some patients will develop soft vertical bands or small submental nodules which resolve with time (usually 6–12 months). Resolution of these may be hastened with the use of ultrasound massage.

Neck liposuction, either alone or in combination with platysma repair and in some cases SMAS plication, can produce excellent recontouring of

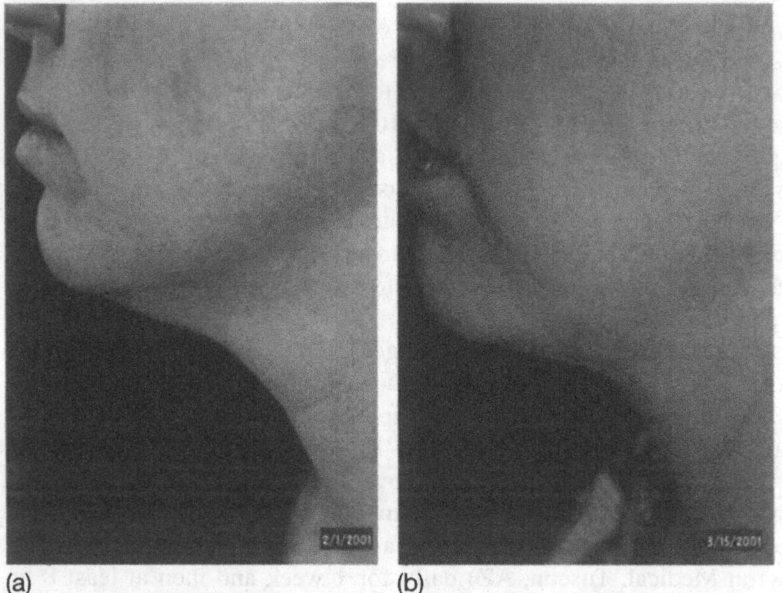

FIGURE 13 (a) Patient 1 preoperatively, side view. (b) Patient 2 postoperatively, side view 2 months after liposuction.

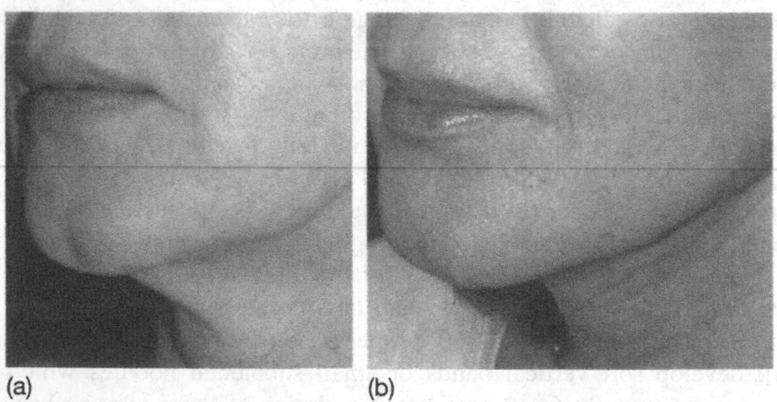

FIGURE 14 (a) Patient 2 preoperatively, side view. (b) Patient 2 postoperatively, side view 2 months after liposuction and platysmaplasty. Note softening of jowls as well as improved contours of the cervicomental angle.

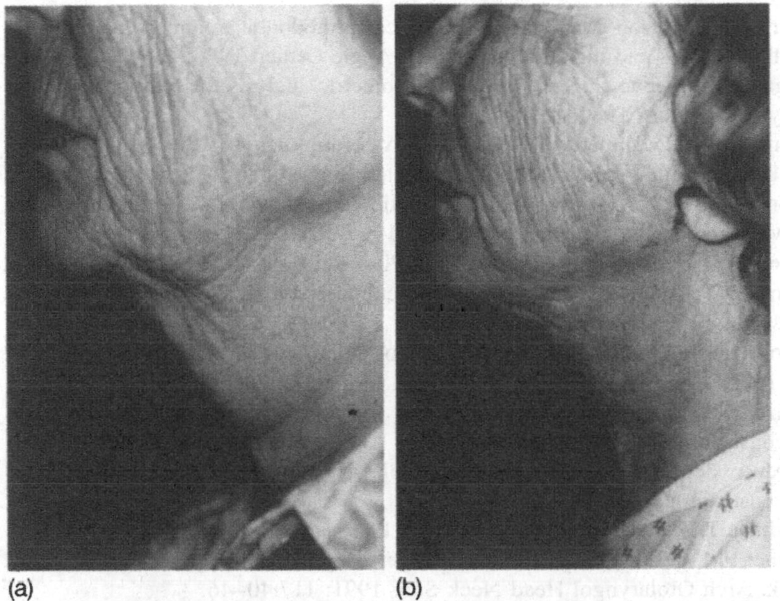

(a) (b)

Figure 15 (a) Patient 3 preoperatively, side view. (b) Patient 3 side view, 3 weeks postoperative. Liposuction with platysmaplasty and SMAS plication. Although this is a relatively short follow-up, this photo shows the immediate skin tightening achieved with this technique.

the aging or obese neck and jawline. The goals of these procedures are to define the cervicomental angle and jawline. It is important to educate patients regarding duration of healing, as results will continue to improve over several months as the skin tightens and redrapes over the neck. By carefully utilizing these complimentary procedures in one surgical session, the surgeon can safely and effectively improve neck contours.

REFERENCES

1. Cook Jr. WR, Johnson DS. Advanced techniques in liposuction. Semin Cutan Med Surg 1999; 18(2):139–148.
2. Webster RC, Smith RC, Smith KF. Face lift, part 2: etiology of platysma cording and its relationship to treatment. Head Neck Surg 1983; 6(1):590–595.
3. Marino H, Galeano EJ, Gondolfo EA. Plastic correction of double chin: importance of the position of the hyoid bone. Plast Reconstr Surg 1960; 31:45.
4. Ellenbogen R, Karlin J. Visual criteria for success in restoring the youthful neck. Plast Reconstr Surg 1980; 66:826.

5. Worms F, Isaacson R, Speidel T. Surgical orthodontic treatment planning—profile analysis and mandibular surgery. Angle Orthod 1976; 46:1.
6. Legan H, Burstone C. Soft tissue cephalometric analysis for orthognathic surgery. J Oral Surg 1980; 38:744.
7. Sommerville JM, Sperry TP, BeGole EA. Morphology of the submental and neck region. Int J Adult Orthod Orthognath Surg 1988; 3:97.
8. Moreno A, Bell WH, Zhi-Hao Y. Esthetic contour analysis of the submental cervical region. J Oral Maxillofac Surg 1994; 52:704–713.
9. Toledo LS. Syringe liposculpture. Clin Plast Surg 1996; 23:683–693.
10. Hunstad JP. Tumescent and syringe liposculpture: a logical partnership. Aesthet Plast Surg 1995; 19:321–337.
11. Jacob CI, Berkes BJ, Kaminer MS. Liposuction and surgical recontouring of the neck: a retrospective analysis. Derm Surg 2000; 26(7):635–632.
12. Knize DM. Limited incision submental lipectomy and platysmaplasty. Plast Reconst Surg 1998; 101:473–481.
13. Cardoso de Castro C. The changing role of platysma in face lifting. Plast Reconstr Surg 2000; 105(2):764–775.
14. Feldman JJ. Corset platysmaplasty. Clin Plast Surg 1992; 19(2):369–382.
15. Kamer FM, Lefkoff LA. Submental surgery: a graduated approach to the aging neck. Arch Otolaryngol Head Neck Surg 1991; 117:40–46.
16. Alt TH. Facelift surgery. In: Elson ML, ed. Evaluation and Treatment of the Aging Face. New York: Springer-Verlag, 1995:110–168.

13

Gynecomastia—Dynamic Technique

Michael Bermant
Bermant Plastic and Cosmetic Surgery, Richmond, Virginia, U.S.A.

DEFINITION/INTRODUCTION

Gynecomastia is a commonly occurring condition of the male chest found in up to 60% of the male population. In most cases, it is a self-limiting problem resolving spontaneously. Tools for male breast surgery include liposuction, excision, skin reduction, nipple reduction, and fat sculpture. A gynecomastia surgeon needs to be comfortable with all of these tools, using each to its maximal advantage. This is not a good operation for liposuction alone or a significant number of patients will end up unhappy.

WHAT IS A "NORMAL" MALE CHEST?

Artists and culture have constructed an image of the male chest that sometimes is idealized beyond the reach of an average man. Each man's self-image of what "looks male" is different. Exposing the male chest in public is a natural part of interaction whether on the beach or in sports. Many fine cloths drape over the skin, exposing the shape of the chest.

The normal male chest is a contour of skin, fat, and muscle over the framework of bones and cartilage. The shape of the pectoral muscles in front and the spread of the shoulder girdle muscles on the side define a masculine look. A natural thin layer of fat provides a gliding buffer between the skin and underlying structures. A good-looking chest should move well. Static images just do not show tissue interaction. Contour issues, distortions, and scars can disturb a refined look. As the skin is tightened with the arms drawn back, firmer tissues between the muscle and the skin protrude.

The male breast is formed by skin, fat, gland, and muscle. Most men have a small amount of gland under the nipple areola region (Fig. 1). It does not take much fat and gland to distort the "male" outline. With more fat and gland, a mound can exist under the areola, projecting more and more like a female breast. The excess can be great enough to start draping from the chest to create an inframammary crease.

Femalelike breasts on the male body can be embarrassing. Kids can be cruel. Peer pressure can affect emotional well-being. Someone bothered by his breasts will often try to avoid exposure and try to camouflage them.

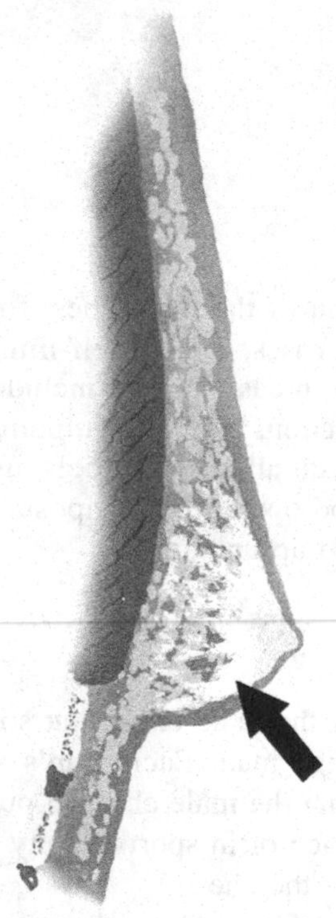

FIGURE 1 Male glandular tissue is often located under the nipple and areola with fingers of denser gland tissue extending into the fat.

Heavy fabric, extra layers of clothing, and elastic compression are some of the tools men use to hide breasts. Many will just avoid interactions where chests are bared and thin clothing that exposes their contour.

THE MALE CHEST WITH GYNECOMASTIA

Skin

Skin can be stretched to different degrees. With small breast growth, there is little extra skin and it will easily redistribute after surgery. Areola size enlarged with underlying tissue actually decreases when that tissue is removed. The true nature of how much the skin will adjust is just not predictable. Younger skin tends to adjust much better than that of an older man. Loose creepy skin does not shrink well. Tissue already loose from major weight loss can get looser with further breast gland/fat reduction.

Massive male breasts can have too much skin. Skin excess can result in a submammary fold. Only so much loose tissue will redistribute after surgery. After a certain point, a skin reduction as in female breast reductions is necessary.

The doughnut periareola skin excision camouflages the scar in the only prominent male breast feature. If too much skin is present, short vertical scar techniques can limit scar visibility to a certain degree. However, any scar beyond the areola just does not look good on the male chest. The male chest hair pattern can radically change with any significant skin reduction.

Fat

The normal male chest has a thin layer of fat between the skin and the underlying structures. There tends to be a slightly thicker fat layer at the lower pole of the male breast that gently adds a slight roundness to the chest abdominal interface. This band concentrates under the areola and tapers toward the axilla. With weight gain, this area can build up, creating breasts of fat alone. Dieting and exercise can affect the fat, but have little influence on the shape of tissues.

Muscle

When muscular tissues define a man's chest, the look is purely "male." As these muscles are built through exercise programs, what ever is on top is just pushed forward. Watching the chest move dynamically, small gland and fat collections under the areola disrupt a "cut" look.

In the aging male chest, muscles tend to lose their bulk with resulting sagging. Male chest contouring will not help the muscular aspect of this problem. Bodybuilding has a much better chance of helping with this condition. However, localized fat and gland may then become more prominent.

Bone/Cartilage

The shape of the ribs and sternum also influence the male chest. A pectus excavatum deformity with a depressed sternum can accentuate the breasts. This depression will not be improved with fat/gland contour surgery. Demonstrating this aspect to the patient before surgery helps avoid confusion about what surgery will offer.

Gland

The gland of the breast, even in the male chest, is normally under the areola and continues into the nipple. It may be a dense mass, fingers of thick glandular tissues extending into fat, or a combination. The variation is quite remarkable and can approach what is found in a female breast.

There are many factors that can influence gland growth. The most common is an often transient increase during puberty. In most cases, this resolves without treatment. Medical problems, endocrine conditions, medications, and drugs can cause male breast growth. A stimulated gland enlarges and becomes sensitive, sore, tender, and sometimes has a discharge.

PATIENT SELECTION

Gynecomastia chest contouring is elective surgery and a patient should be in good general health. Breast growth should be stabilized. If a patient reports that the breasts are still enlarging, investigate the cause of the stimulation. Since surgery does not remove the entire gland, failure to correct the underlying cause or stop the stimulating factor often results in failure. Medical or endocrine evaluation may be indicated before surgery.

Teenagers with transient growth will do better without surgery. If the growth resolves on its own, a little patience may be better than even the best surgical scar. Each patient needs to be individually evaluated. Very large breasts and significant emotional stress may warrant an operation that may need revision.

Although male breast cancer is rare, a surgeon undertaking male chest sculpture must be able to evaluate the breast for cancer. A good history and physical examination of every patient is essential before any surgical undertaking. Any suspicions should result in the appropriate laboratory testing. Biopsy for suspicious male breast mass requires a different technique less likely to spread potential cancer.

Since fat will be left behind, surgery is not a good solution for someone who wants to lose weight. Someone who eats more calories than he uses can have new breast growth. Once fat cells are removed, they are gone. However, remaining fat cells can put on more fat. Weight loss is a coarse tool. Where fat comes off during weight loss is unpredictable. Surgical chest contouring is better after achieving weight goals.

A patient and family must have reasonable expectations about this surgery. A thorough discussion of risks, benefits, and alternative methods of care is essential for a patient to make an informed choice.

DOCUMENTATION

A meticulous patient history and physical are important to document the patient's well-being before surgery. Recording details about the gland, fat, muscle, skin, and chest boney structure help define the problem to be treated. Document the patient's concerns, the discussion of risks, benefits, and alternate methods of care.

Photographic

Capturing potentially small male chest problems can be difficult. Consistent lighting, camera lens focal length, and distance from the subject are critical. Slight variations in shadows and angles will distort results. While movies are best for documenting the movement of tissues, storage and retrieval of these recordings is not simple. Static views can incorporate reproducible actions and documentation. Standard photographic views (Fig. 2A) of the male chest should extend from the lower neck to the upper abdominal region and include the following views.

Still-Image Camera Oriented Horizontally

For the frontal chest, the following positions should be documented:

- arms at the side
- arms extended straight over the head
- arms on the hips pectoral muscles relaxed
- arms on the hips pectoral muscles tensed

From the front oblique position (with the breast meridian parallel to the photograph plane), the arm further from the camera should be bent behind the back with the other arm resting against the side, including the following views:

- left
- right

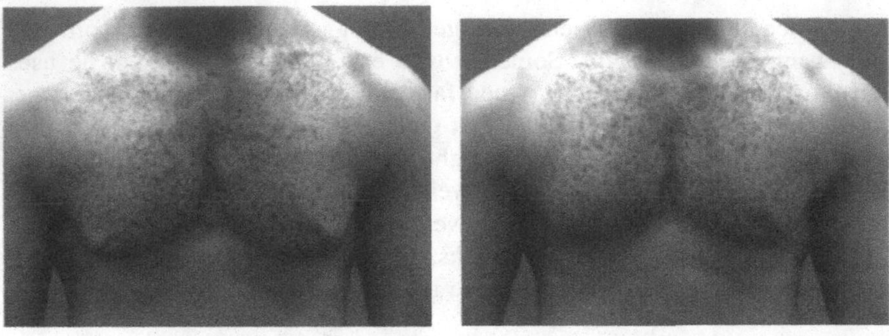

Frontal Image Arms Down

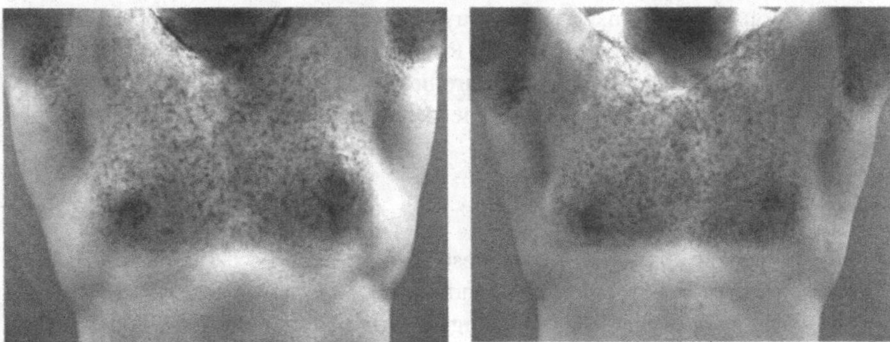

Frontal Image Arms Elevated

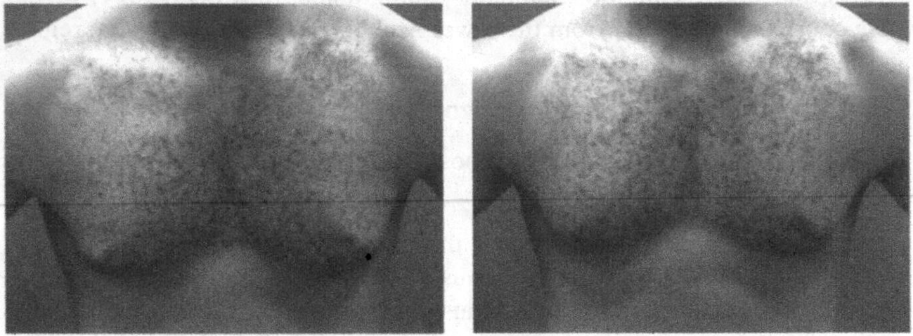

Frontal Image Arms on Hips Chest Muscles Relaxed

FIGURE 2A A standard series of photographs can show subtle deformities and problems on animation. This is a 26-year-old black male before and 10 weeks after excision gland, fat flap, and liposuction of chest. Notice how the contour problems show in varying degrees with the different views. All images were taken in the exact same lighting.

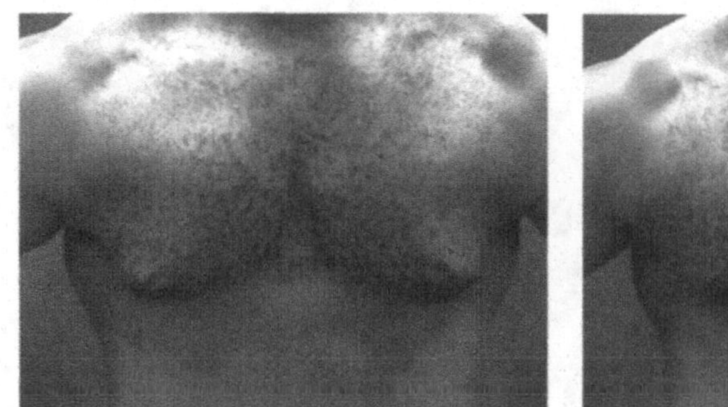

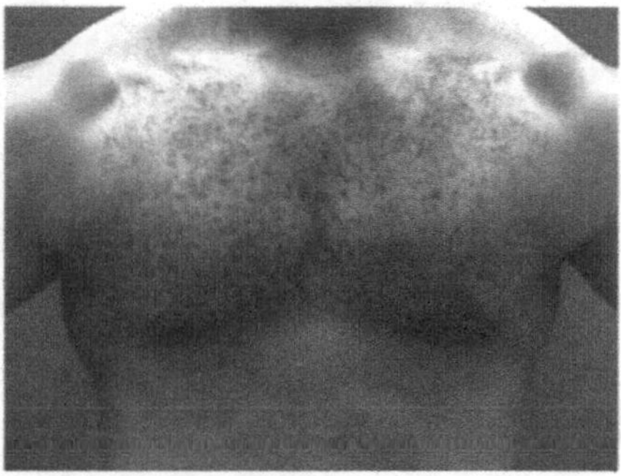

Frontal Image Arms on Hips Chest Muscles Tight

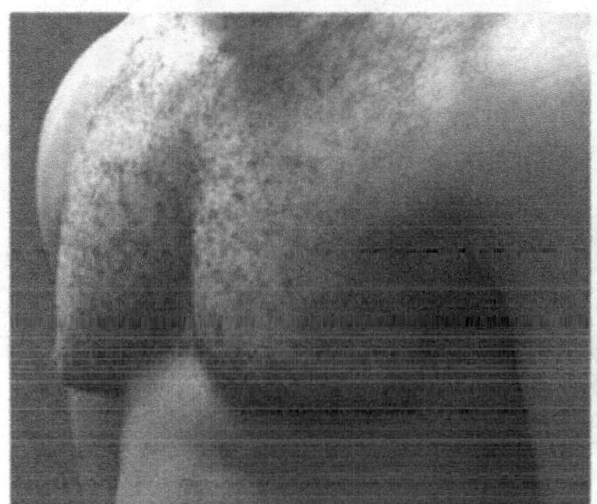

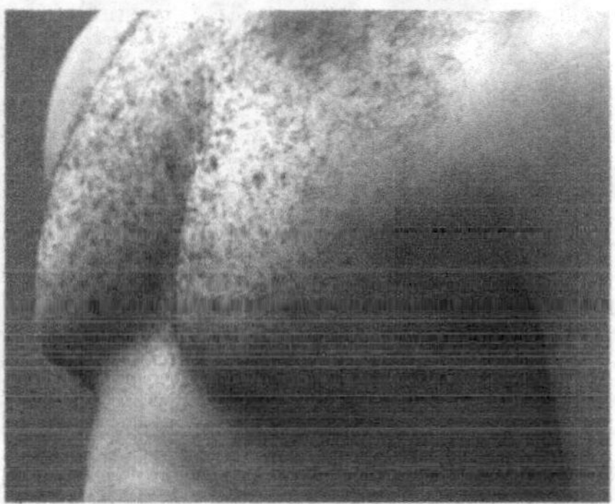

Anterior Left Oblique Image

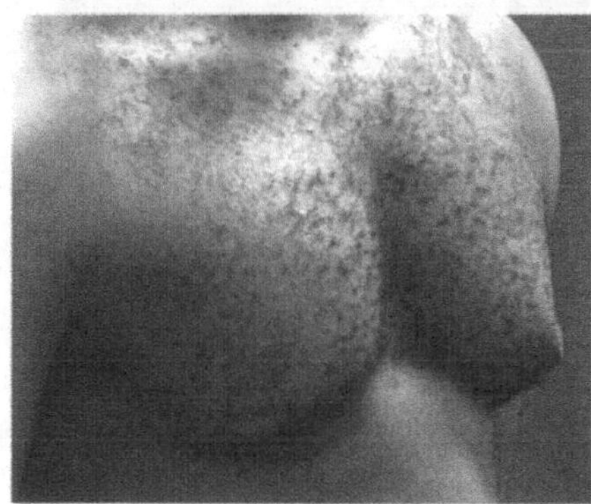

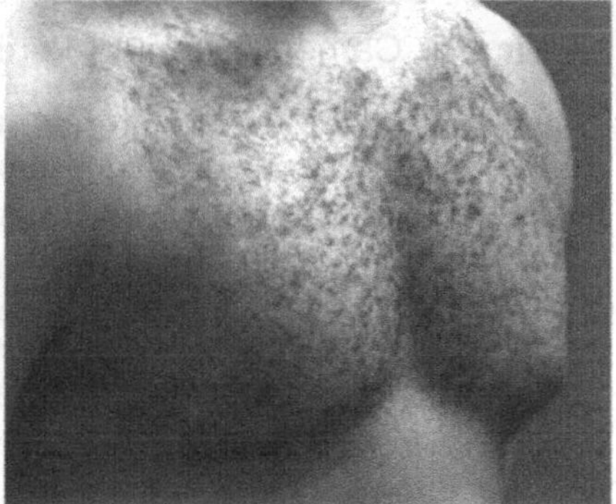

Anterior Right Oblique Image

FIGURE 2A Continued.

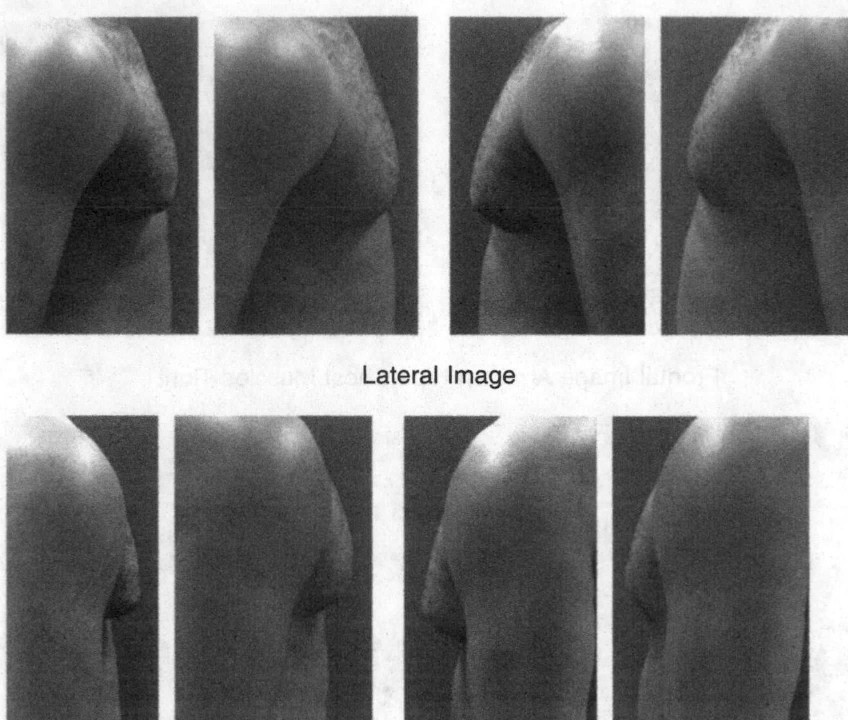

Figure 2A Continued.

Still-Image Camera Oriented Vertically

For the lateral chest position (capturing from the neck to the abdomen showing the chest abdominal relationship), the visible arm is flexed behind the back, and the following views are documented:

- left
- right

For the posterior oblique position (capturing the breast from behind just as it emerges from behind the arm), the visible arm is flexed behind the back, and the following views are documented:

- left
- right

The view with the hands straight up over the head tenses the skin revealing, some skin-movement issues. The views with the hands on the hips dem-

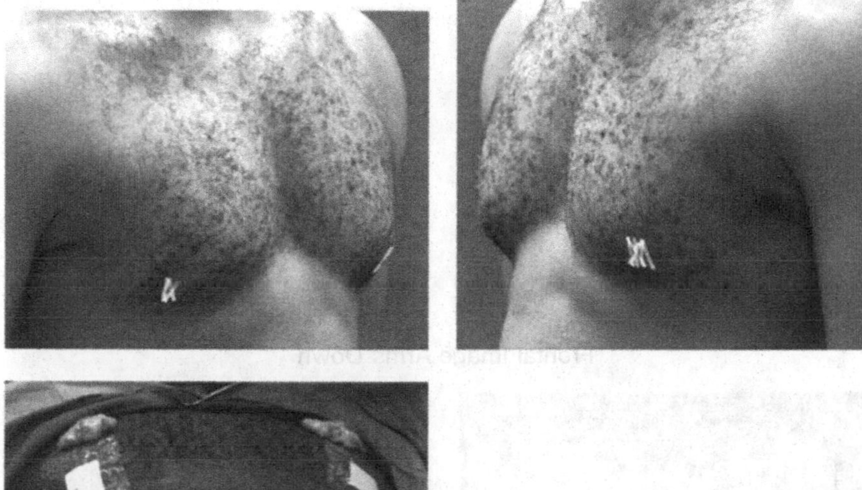

FIGURE 2B Ten days after surgery with Sertl strips in place showing minimal swelling and bruising. Excision and liposuction contouring were through a periareolar incision on each side. Each glandular mass measured 6 × 3 × 1 cm and came out through the 2-cm incision.

onstrates muscle interaction with tissues. Movies will show much more subtle issues.

Video Camera Oriented Horizontally

Chest tissue effected by arm movement, including arms starting at the side, moving straight over the head, and then back to the sides, is documented as follows:

- frontal chest
- front oblique (with the breast meridian parallel to the photograph plane)
    - left
    - right

Chest tissue affected by tightening chest muscles, including arms on the hips with pectoral muscles relaxed, then tensed, and then relaxed, is documented as follows:

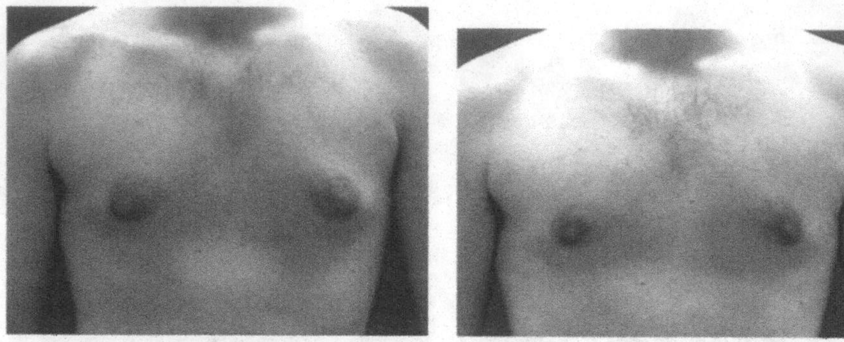

Frontal Image Arms Down

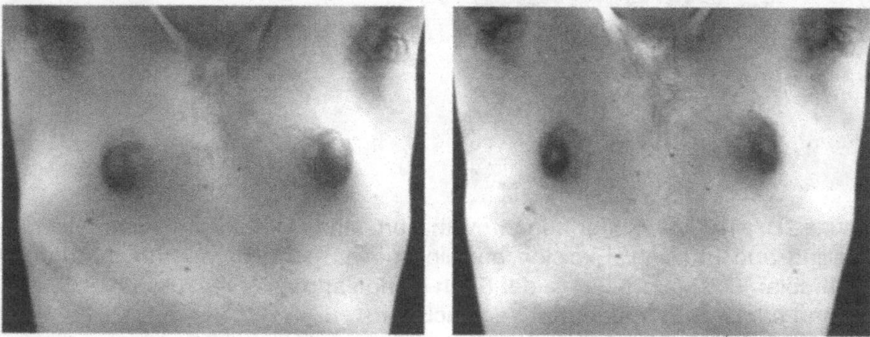

Frontal Image Arms Elevated

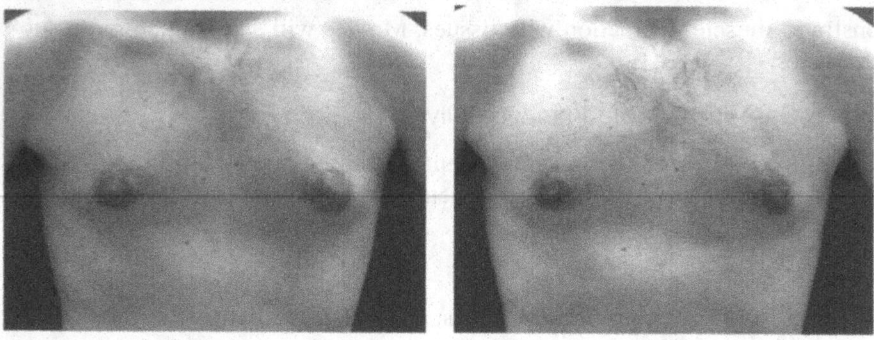

Frontal Image Arms on Hips Chest Muscles Relaxed

FIGURE 3 24-year-old male before and 9 weeks after chest surgery consisting of gland excision, fat sculpture, and liposuction. The glandular masses were 5 × 3 × 0.4 cm and 3 × 2 × 0.5 cm. Two hundred cubic centimeters of fat was removed with the liposuction. All access was through the periareolar incisions.

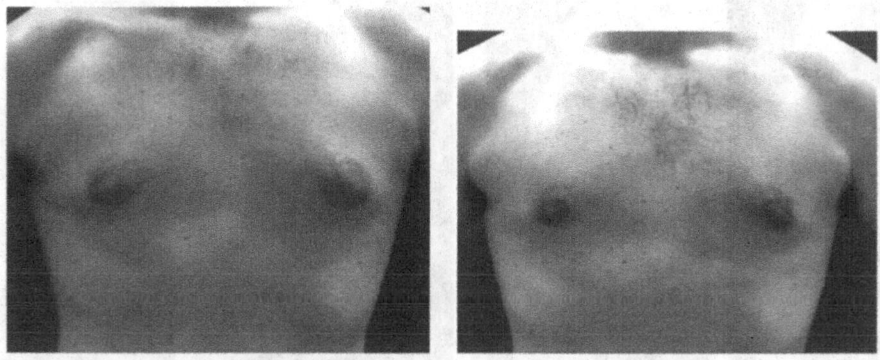

Frontal Image Arms on Hips Chest Muscles Tight

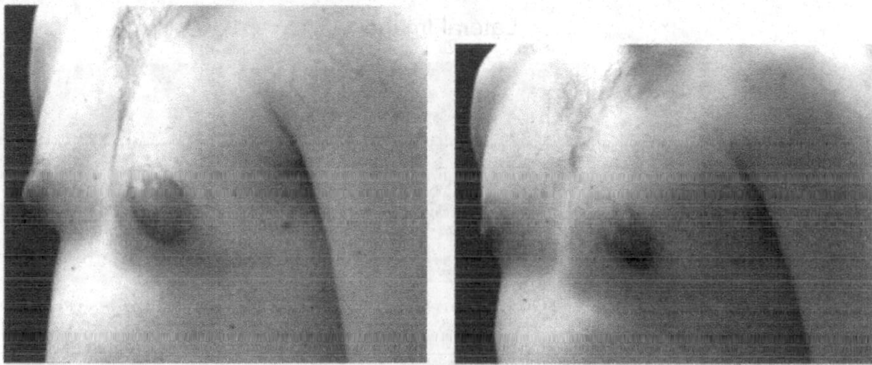

Anterior Left Oblique Image

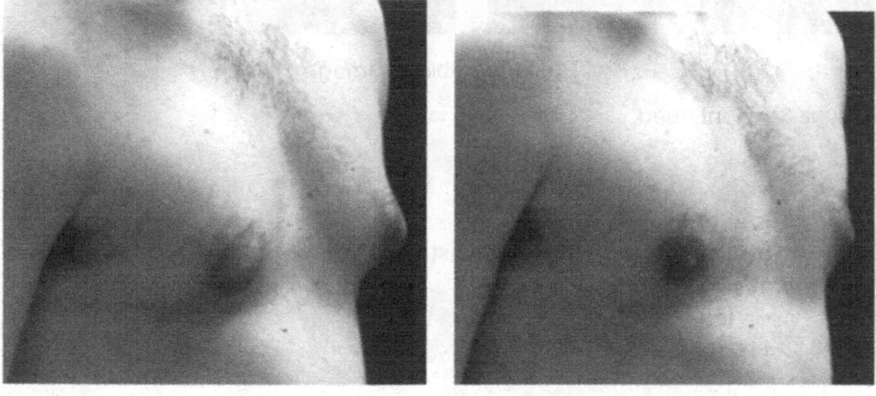

Anterior Right Oblique Image

FIGURE 3 Continued.

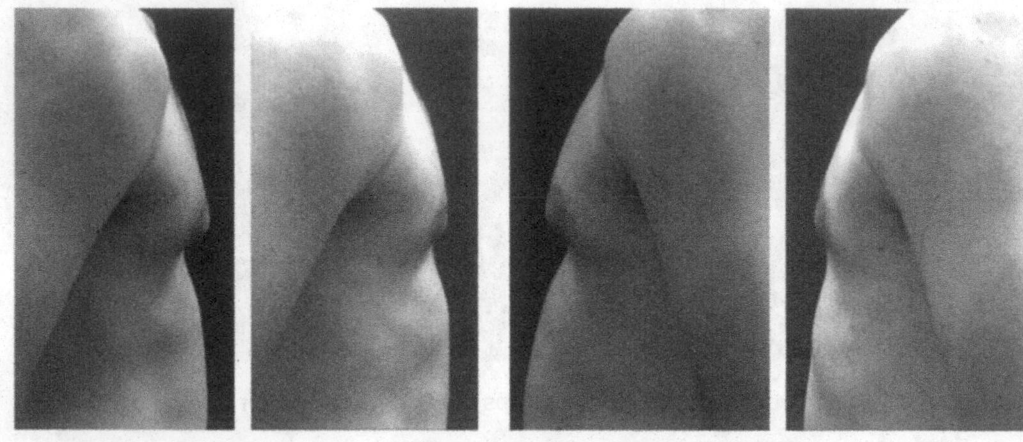

Lateral Image

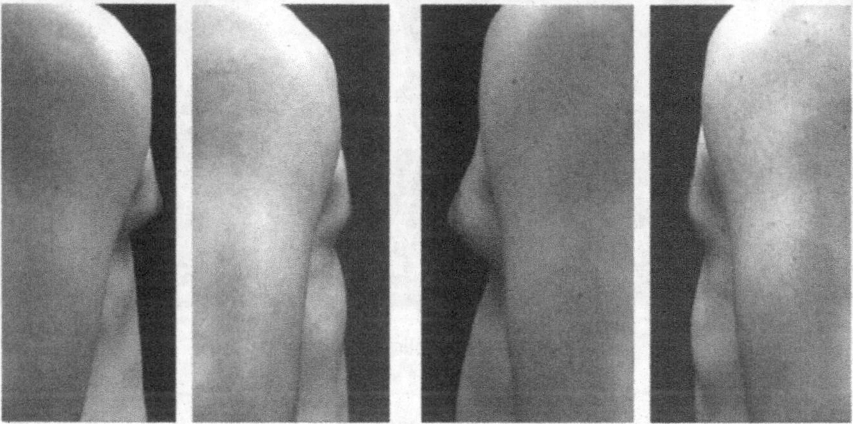

Posterior Oblique Image

FIGURE 3 Continued.

- frontal chest
- front oblique (with the breast meridian parallel to the photograph plane)
    - left
    - right

DYNAMIC MALE CHEST SCULPTURE

When skin reduction is not a factor, the surgeon must deal with an enlarged breast of an unknown combination of gland and fat. Clinical exams and mammograms are just not specific enough to determine how much gland is present [1] and what will work surgically. If there is only fat, an open technique only adds a longer scar. Liposuction alone contours fat very well. Dense gland just is not reduced with liposuction. Excision of gland alone can leave a crater and a depressed nipple and areola. Once gland is excised, the surgeon has a better idea what surrounding fat needs to be reduced or moved into the excision defect. How do you determine what is needed for any specific case? Dynamic sculpture permits the operation to be adjusted to what is found during surgery (Figs. 2A, 2B, and 3).

ANESTHESIA

Carefully placed diffuse tumescent fluid minimizes bleeding and subsequent bruising. Even with a numb chest, the forces needed for extensive chest sculpture can be stressful for patients. In such cases, I prefer to use an anesthetist to administer iv sedation. This permits me to concentrate on the three-dimensional sculpture. After appropriate sedation, local anesthesia begins with a long 27-gauge needle along the potential skin incision of the lower skin areola junction and under the potential areola dissection. A limited amount of 1% Xylocaine with epinephrine 1:100,000 buffered with NaH_2CO_3 is placed just under the skin above the gland. Dense gland is often intimately associated with the areola/nipple. Cannula penetration here is very difficult. The longer $1\frac{1}{2}$- or $1\frac{1}{4}$-in. needle permits fewer needle sticks. Typical volumes needed are 2 to 4 cc per side. After waiting enough time for the adrenaline to work, a small stab wound with a vertically oriented No. 15 blade at the caudal pole of the areola permits easy access for liposuction or tumescent cannula. Tumescent local anesthesia is placed carefully just above the pectoral fascia. This can be tough going and having a pump for the fluid flow permits concentration on technique. A low pump setting (3 on the Wells Johnson unit) is a good compromise on accuracy and speed.

Cannula placement during tumescence and liposuction is critical. You must keep parallel to the chest and above the pectoral muscles. The significant force needed to get through the tough male tissues requires precision to prevent injury to muscle or penetration through the ribs. Initial pinching of tissues with the other hand can guide to the level of this infiltration. The foot-controlled pump increases precision of fluid placement. Waiting 20 min after completing a side results in much less bleeding and better dispersal of the fluid before the surgery.

Scar tissue can increase the difficulty such that a normal blunt infiltrating cannula is just not enough. A less blunt cannula helps but requires extreme caution not to cause injury to muscle or chest penetration.

"USE THE FORCE, LUKE"

Cannula passage through fat is easy. There are some tissue attachments that are tough, but gland is a different matter. Cannula penetration of gland is very difficult. Concentrating on the feel of the infiltration with a cannula can give a good idea how much gland is present. It is easy going and you can try skipping straight to the liposuction. However, be careful. As the liposuction progresses, feel the tissues to see if there is a buildup of dense remaining gland that would be better managed by excision. Getting the gland out early means you can use the remaining fat to help with contouring. Take too much fat first, and gland excision may result in a cavity that cannot be filled easily.

GLAND EXCISION

Suspecting gland, a 2-cm incision along the caudal areola gives sufficient access for excision for most glands. The incision should be at the chest skin–areola interface. This zone can be ill defined in some men. Picking a place of maximal change of color helps hide the scar. Bipolar cautery minimizes the zone of injury and helps with the one or two 1-mm veins seen with this incision. Small scissors sharp dissection frees the gland from the nipple areola. Leave a thin layer of gland under the areola and nipple to give shape to these structures. Too much, and these structures are rigid and do not move naturally. Too little, and depression deformity can be a problem. It is difficult to compensate for lost mass under the nipple with fat. Be careful not to buttonhole, which creates unnecessary surface scars. Free the gland from the surrounding fat carefully. It is best to take only the gland, leaving as much fat for the liposuction. In most cases, the gland is centralized. When there are fingers of gland penetrating the fat, remove the firmest sections. The surgeon's finger introduced in the incision should only feel soft fat remaining.

LIPOSUCTION

The male chest, even with the tumescent infiltration, can be difficult tissue to liposuction. Skin attachments to fascia are often difficult to penetrate. Short 3-mm and smaller cannula are easier to manipulate. An aggressive tip, such as the Cobra K+, permits easier liposuction here than a blunt or bullet tip. Any cannula, especially the sharper tips or the aggressive patterns, presents a risk of injury to muscle or penetration beyond the ribs. This operation requires precision and concentration to avoid complications. I prefer straight cannula and to know at all times the location of the tip of my cannula. Long cannula are difficult to maneuver in the central chest and tend to bend. In the very large male chest, longer cannula may be necessary to reach the tail of fat in the lateral chest. Be careful not to injure the incision site skin edge during the sometimes-forceful cannula manipulations. For fine control, the 14- and 16-gauge Capistrano microcannula work well on the male chest. In most cases, a 2-cm incision at the lower skin areola interface gives satisfactory access. Rarely a second smaller axillary incision can help central contouring. Avoiding the additional axillary and lower chest incisions can look much better on the male chest.

A contour map drawn on the chest before surgery helps show the extra tissue after tumescent anesthesia. Draw the map before surgery with the patient standing, asking him to tense and loosen his pectoral muscles. This muscle movement along with rolling the tissues under your fingers helps define the redundant tissues. Liposuction is best started at the deeper fat levels just above the fascia. Be careful while getting the cannula to this deep plane. A cannula perpendicular to the chest can cause damage. Try as much as possible to keep the work strokes parallel to the chest. Pretunneling with the machine off in the deep plane is a good way to start. Then work around the entire chest systemically working each few degrees. Concentrate on the thicker fat regions, trying to leave a consistent layer of fat compared to the remaining chest. Consider any defect from gland excision while contouring the fat. As long as the surgery is not rushed, the tumescent fluid pressure dissipates permitting surface tissue manipulation. Pinching and rolling the chest tissues can help in establishing how much fat is still between the muscle and skin. Frequent checking guides the sculpting. The goal should be a fat thickness more consistent with surrounding regions. Be careful. Removing too much fat can leave skin scarred to underlying muscle. Such scars just do not move naturally and deficiencies are not easily replaced.

FAT SCULPTURE

Fat with a blood supply has a much better chance of surviving than as a graft. Fat moved in from the crater wall can fill in a glandular defect. 5-0 Vicryl suture can be used to sculpt the fat. This tissue does not hold suture very well. Using the fibrous septa for the sutures helps. Sometimes several stitches will distribute the workload. Fat moved may tug and deform the overlying surface skin. If still attached, gentle dissection from just under the skin surface can minimize such deformation. However, try to maintain the blood supply to this layer. A circular defect can close with a "dog ear"-like distortion that may need trimming or microcannula liposuction adjustment. Sometimes a second layer of fat sculpture is needed to produce a natural shape to the areola and nipple. Test the appearance by approximating the skin with your forceps and gently pulling on the surface to check the dynamic result before finishing this step.

In cases with massive glandular defects, fat layer sculpture may be needed before liposuction and removal of too much tissue (Fig. 4). Mobilize the fat, approximate the walls of the defect, and then perform the liposuction contouring. Some of the fat layer sutures may need replacing after the liposuction.

CLOSURE

Assess the quality of the skin before closure. Consider if friction has injured the skin edge. Removing a small zone of injury can be important to minimize scars. Some asymmetrical areola problems can be managed by a small ellipse skin excision along the edge of the incision. Initial placement of the gland excision is important if considering this option. At other times, very conical areola can have redundant tissues that just do not lie with an adequate contour. A small skin excision can be the difference in treating this redundancy. Be careful with areolar tissue excision unbalancing the central nipple location. Closing the subcutaneous tissue of the areola relaxes tension on the skin closure. Meticulous closure of the areola skin is essential to minimize scars. SteriStrips secured with Mastisol finish the repair.

DRESSING

Adequate tumescent technique and hemostasis during the operation often results in such minimal bruising, drains usually are not necessary. Most of the fluid has already dissipated such that a tight skin closure and dressing can be used. Mastisol, Telfa, and Tegaderm plastic sheet dressings offer a sealed minimal care design. Prominent nipples need protection under this dressing. Major skin reduction and clinical judgment may dictate different methods.

Compression Vest

A compression vest can help increase comfort, minimize bruising, and decrease swelling. This garment is available from several manufacturers and comes in many adjustable sizes. Designs with a hook and eye (instead of a zipper) offer a closure that can be adjusted for a better fit. Velcro shoulder straps permit adjustment to the many possible sizes of a male chest. Some shoulders need protection under exposed Velcro to minimize skin contact with that rough surface. Try to prevent the garment from riding too high in the axilla, which can irritate tissues.

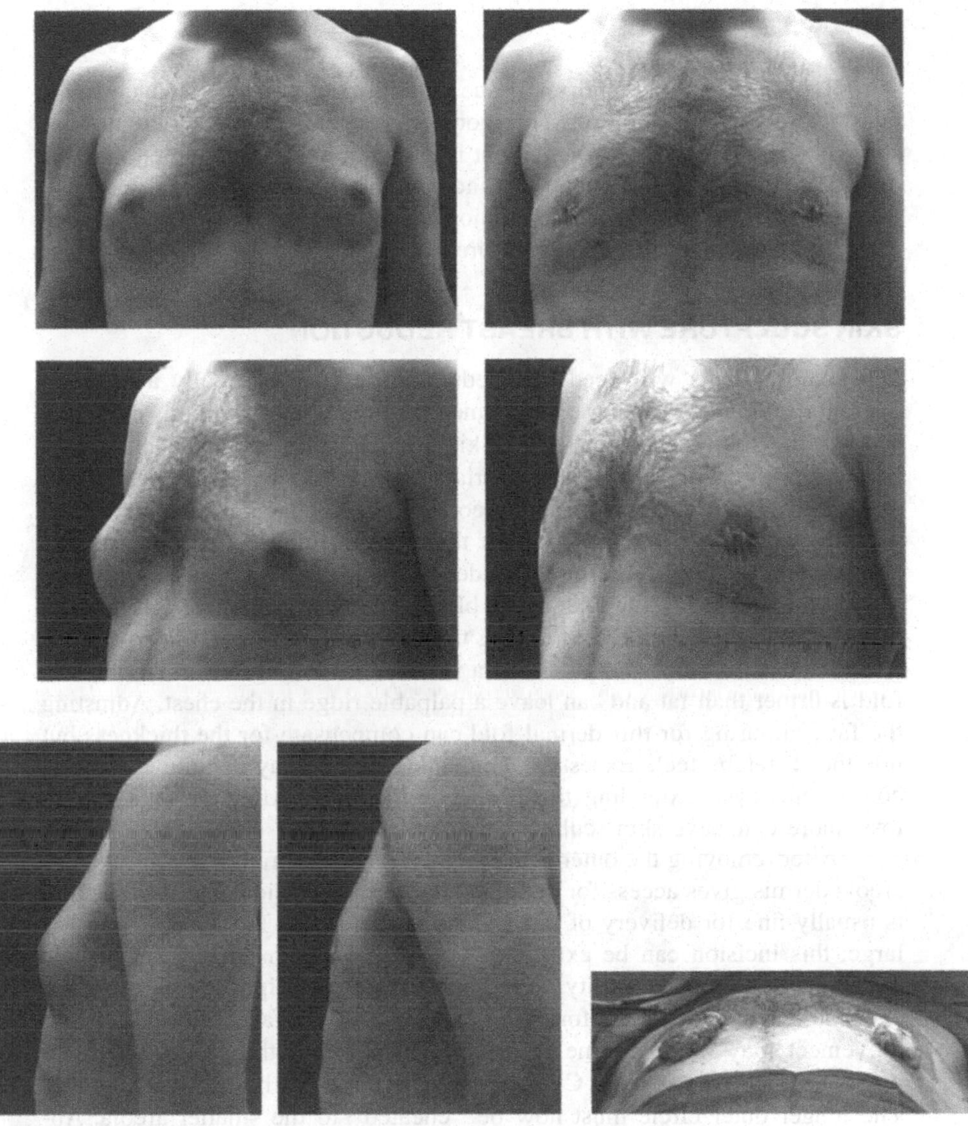

FIGURE 4 A 37-year-old male for a secondary chest sculpture. Original surgery by another doctor consisted of liposuction alone of about 500 cc fat removed through the and included the low anterior chest access. Liposuction alone in a patient with significant gland can result in such a failure. Secondary surgery removed 8 × 5 × 3 cm and 6 × 6 × 2.2 cm glandular masses through 2 cm periareolar incisions. This was followed by fat flap reconstruction and liposuction contouring. Two hundred fifty cubic centimeters of additional fat was removed during liposuction. No other incisions were needed. Images are only 11 days after his secondary surgery and show bruising and early tissue evolution of this more extensive operation.

The elastic cloth stabilizes tissues minimizing bouncing, which translates into increased comfort. This compression can impair blood flow to surgical tissues and surgical judgment is essential before recommending this device. A fold in the garment can increase pressure. Pulling the garment down from the bottom with each major position change can eliminate such folds and the danger of added pressure.

SKIN SCULPTURE WITH BREAST REDUCTION

Few male patients will need skin reduction, and this is really a different operation. When addressing a large amount of redundant skin, this reduction follows the tumescent anesthesia. Skin reduction on the male chest is a complex topic with solutions as variable as female breast reduction and mastopexy. Leaving the nipple and areola with a blood supply is complicated with the need for a thinner solution than in the fuller female breast. The doughnut mastopexy technique denudes the epidermis in a circular pattern around the areola. The nipple areola blood supply remains through the dermis, which must be protected during the surgery. The dermal layer is then folded under the skin when the areola is sewn to the larger skin circle. This fold is firmer than fat and can leave a palpable ridge in the chest. Adjusting the fat contouring for this dermal fold can compensate for the thickness but not the different feel. Excessive amounts of skin may require a vertical component, even extending to an anchor like scar. After massive weight loss, more extensive skin sculpture may be needed.

After removing the outer skin layer, an incision through the lower most areola dermis gives access for the glandular tissue excision. The 2-cm length is usually fine for delivery of most gland tissue. When the gland is just too large, this incision can be extended. Try to leave as much dermal pedicle for areola and nipple viability. Removing the fat with liposuction instead of excision leaves more septa for blood supply to the surface. However, tissue movement may require some adjustment of some of these attachments to prevent surface distortions. Close the dermal layer with absorbable suture. The longer outer circle must now be "cheated" to the smaller areola. Absorbable subcutaneous suture will take the tension off from the skin closure. Areola size can change over time as tension tends to distort. A buried permanent suture as in the female mastopexy can help. The patient needs to be warned that this stitch and buried dermal layer may be palpable and show during chest muscle movement. There is much more to a female chest that better hides such structures. Cinching the suture can result in an irregular shape. Redesigning the skin to a circle with a scalpel before closing the areola to chest skin can be important. The top-level closure must equilibrate the tissues. Any wrinkles must be well distributed and minimized. Large distortions will persist. If it does not look good on the operating table, it probably never will postprocedure.

Dressings for more extensive flap surgery depend on many factors. There is frequently more drainage. Absorbent gauze helps keep clothing clean. I rarely use a compression vest in major skin sculpture cases to protect the vascular supply.

Male skin reduction can look unnatural. The fine gradation around the areola is lost. Hair pattern around the areola is different with the migration of tissue to the areola. Bras, which can hide scars, are not worn. Any scar component away from the areola just is obvious. A little loose skin can be a much better solution than a skin sculpture scar.

Ultrasonic and Power Assisted Liposuction in the Breast

Histology studies of breast tissue after ultrasonic assisted liposuction demonstrated no destruction of glandular tissue [2]. Legal concerns can be a major issue with the use of ultrasonic liposuction of the breast [3]. Ultrasonic liposuction can make the surgeon's physical effort easier in dealing with fibrous male chest tissues [4]. Power assisted liposuction also can decrease the surgeon's workload. The surgical tools used for this procedure have a different "feel" and there is an added risk of skin injury. Your choice of instrument is determined by what is most comfortable in producing the best result.

Aftercare

Care after surgery depends on many factors and should be individualized for each patient and surgical sculpture technique. Most patients are sore. Extra Strength Tylenol seems to take care of the discomfort. Some are uncomfortable enough for pain medication such as Hydrocodone (5 mg). A compression vest helps. Teach the patient to minimize irritations from this garment.

Restriction of activities will depend on the extent of surgery. Limited activities can start the next day for a small gland excision, fat sculpture, and liposuction contouring. Helping the patient understand his limitations increases the chance of an uneventful recovery.

Sealed plastic film dressing can permit gentle showering by the second day after surgery. Alternate wound care instructions are necessary if the plastic no longer seals the wound.

Follow-up office visits depend on technique, the patient, and physician comfort. An office visit at about 1 week postprocedure permits removal of the dressing, evaluating the wounds, possible suture removal, and scar care instructions. Other visits at 1 and 6 months after surgery can help with scar and tissue evolution assessment.

REFERENCES

1. 1 Klein JA. Tumescent Technique Tumescent Anesthesia & Microcannular Liposuction. St. Louis: Mosby, 2000:404–412.
2. Walgenbach KJ, Riabikhin AW, Galla TJ, Bannasch H, Voigt M, Andree C, Horch RE, Stark GB. Effect of ultrasonic assisted lipectomy (UAL) on breast tissue: histological findings. Aesthet Plast Surg 2001; 25(2):85–88.
3. Gorney M. Caveat against using ultrasonically assisted lipectomy in aesthetic breast surgery. Plast Reconstr Surg 1998 May; 101(6):1741.
4. Rohrich RJ, Beran SJ, Kenkel JM, Adams WP Jr, DiSpaltro F. Extending the role of liposuction in body contouring with ultrasound-assisted liposuction. Plast Reconstr Surg 1998; 101(4):1090–1102; discussion 1117–1119.

14

Weekend Alternative to the Facelift

William R. Cook, Jr. and Kim K. Cook
Coronado Skin Medical Center, Inc.
Coronado, California, U.S.A

INTRODUCTION

Patients approach a cosmetic surgeon for many reasons, but perhaps the most common complaint is dissatisfaction with the appearance of the face and neck. For most people, the face they present to the world is the most important aspect of their appearance and is closely tied to their own self-image. Changes in the face and neck are often the first visible signs of aging, which may be particularly distressing to a patient who is otherwise fit and healthy (Fig. 1).

Until recently, the primary recourse for such a patient was a traditional surgical rhytidectomy or "face-lift." Thanks to the notable surgical advances of recent decades, the cosmetic surgeon now has many more tools to help patients improve their appearance. The new tools which have made new approaches possible include laser surgical instruments, improved skin peeling techniques [1], the development of tumescent liposculpture [2], and the development of laser dermal resurfacing.

We have devoted our practice for many years to improving the cosmetic treatment of the face and neck. The result is a combined procedure which we call the Cook Weekend Alternative to the Facelift™ [3]. It combines liposculpture of the face and neck with laser surgery to the neck. For

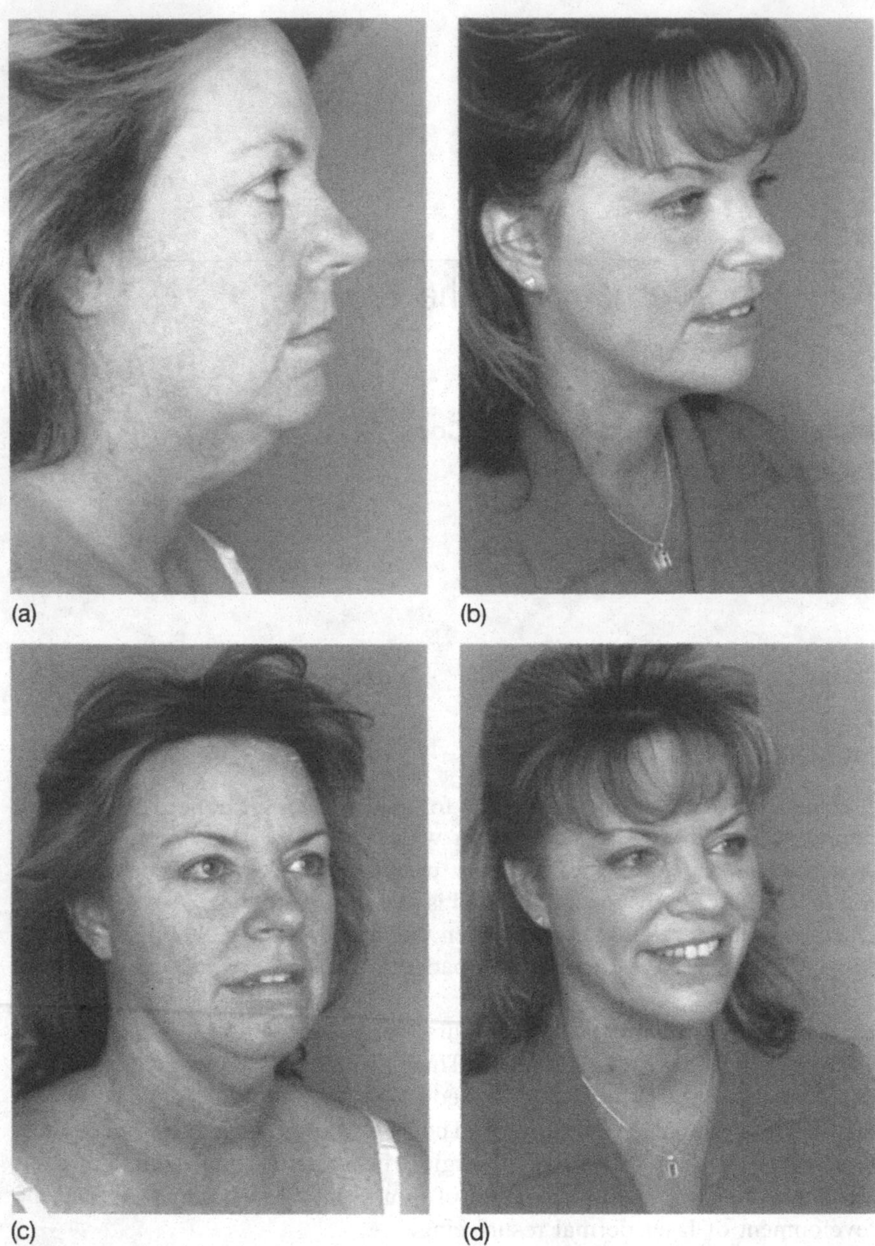

(a) (b) (c) (d)

FIGURE 1 Patient (a and c) before and (b and d) 3 weeks after the Cook Weekend Alternative to the Facelift.

some patients, a laser or chemical peel of the face and neck is also performed to further improve their appearance (Fig. 2).

We have found that this technique almost always produces a much better cosmetic result than liposculpture alone. In some patients the improvement in appearance may be striking (Fig. 3). In many cases the result may be comparable to that achieved by a traditional neck-lift, without the prolonged healing period which rhytidectomy requires and without the significant surgical scars and "tight" appearance that may result from rhytidectomy (Fig. 4).

Patient safety is enhanced by using local tumescent anesthesia; carefully observing sterile technique; controlling the blood pressure; using blunt dissection with a cannula; using a Xenon headlamp for good visibility; using a surgical drain; using a suction cautery, monitoring equipment, and a saline lock; and treating the tissues gently to minimize trauma (Fig. 5). The incidence of complications and unpleasant sequelae from this procedure has been extremely low in our experience, and scarring is minimal. The average patient can undergo the Weekend Alternative to the Facelift literally "over the weekend," with surgery on Thursday or Friday and a return to work and social activities the following week. (If the patient also undergoes a skin peel, the recovery period will be longer.)

This procedure utilizes tumescent liposculpture to remove excess fat from the face, jowls, and neck. With the tumescent technique, the operative area is infiltrated with a large volume of very dilute lidocaine solution which also contains epinephrine. The large volume of solution causes the operative area to swell, or tumesce, which greatly improves the safety of the procedure as well as enhancing the surgeon's ability to contour the area. The neck and face are sculpted precisely, and for this reason we refer to the tumescent procedure as liposculpture rather than liposuction.

In addition to liposculpture of the face, neck, and jowls, the Cook Weekend Alternative to the Facelift also includes resurfacing of the dermis from the underside to promote tightening of the skin, plication of the platysma muscle and removal of prominent platysma bands to reduce neck banding, and transection of the septae of the anterior and lateral neck so that complete redraping of the skin will occur. Where indicated, a chin implant is also inserted. Using laser technology, these surgical procedures can be performed under tumescent local anesthesia at the same time as the liposculpture.

Indications

A typical candidate for the Cook Weekend Alternative to the Facelift is a patient with lipodystrophic changes of the lower face and neck, including

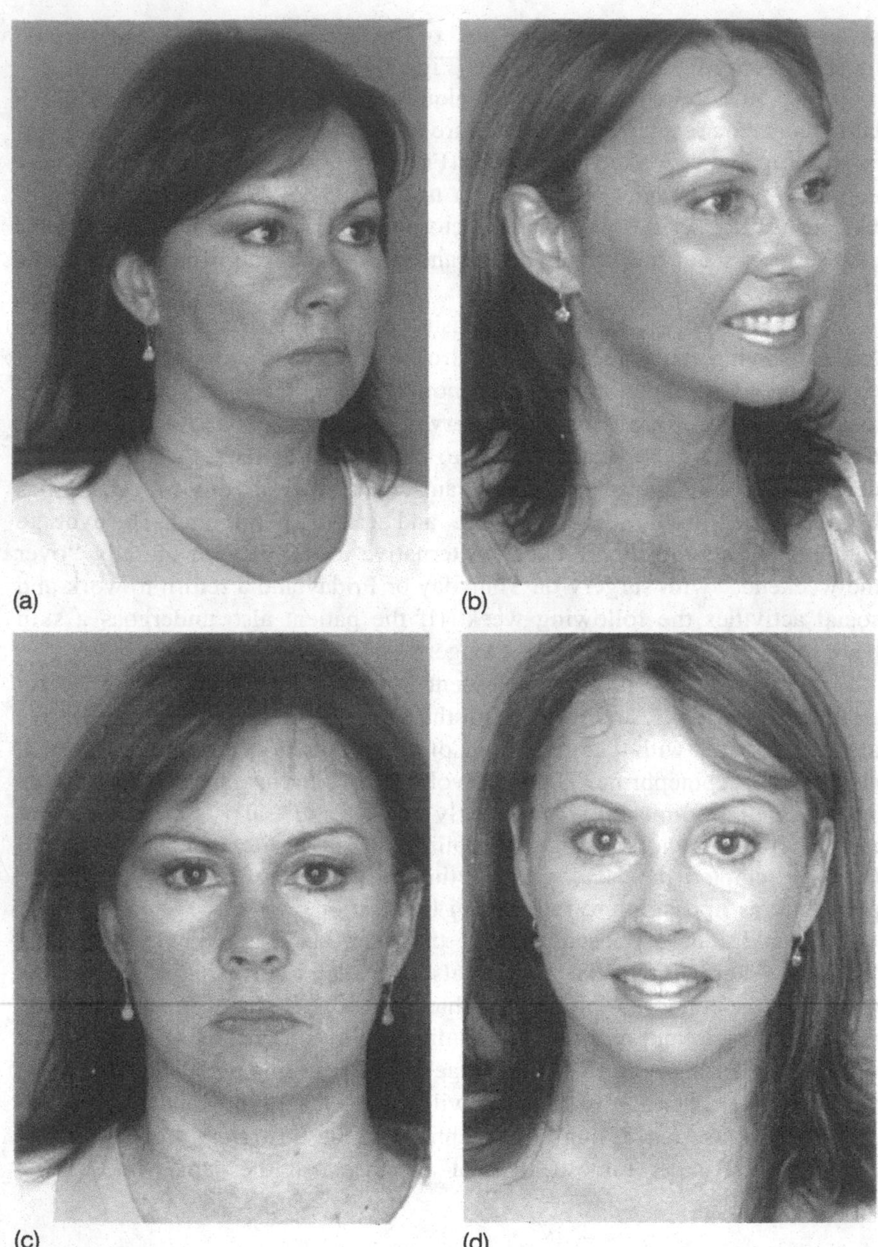

FIGURE 2 Patient (a and c) before and (b and d) after the Cook Weekend Alternative to the Facelift, facial laser peel, and Cook Total Body Peel to the neck, chest, and hands.

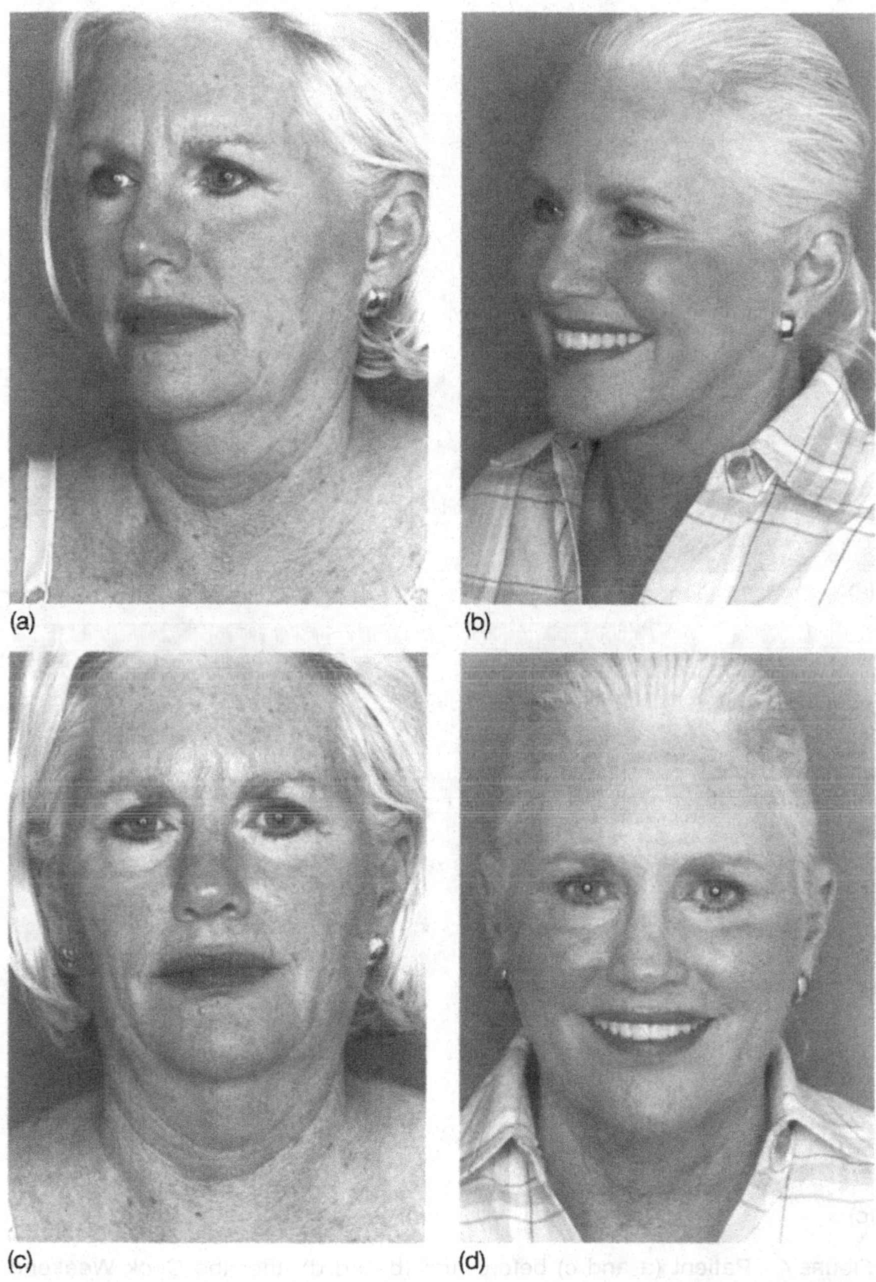

FIGURE 3 Patient (a and c) before and (b and d) after the Cook Weekend Alternative to the Facelift, facial laser peel, and Cook Total Body Peel to the neck, chest, and hands.

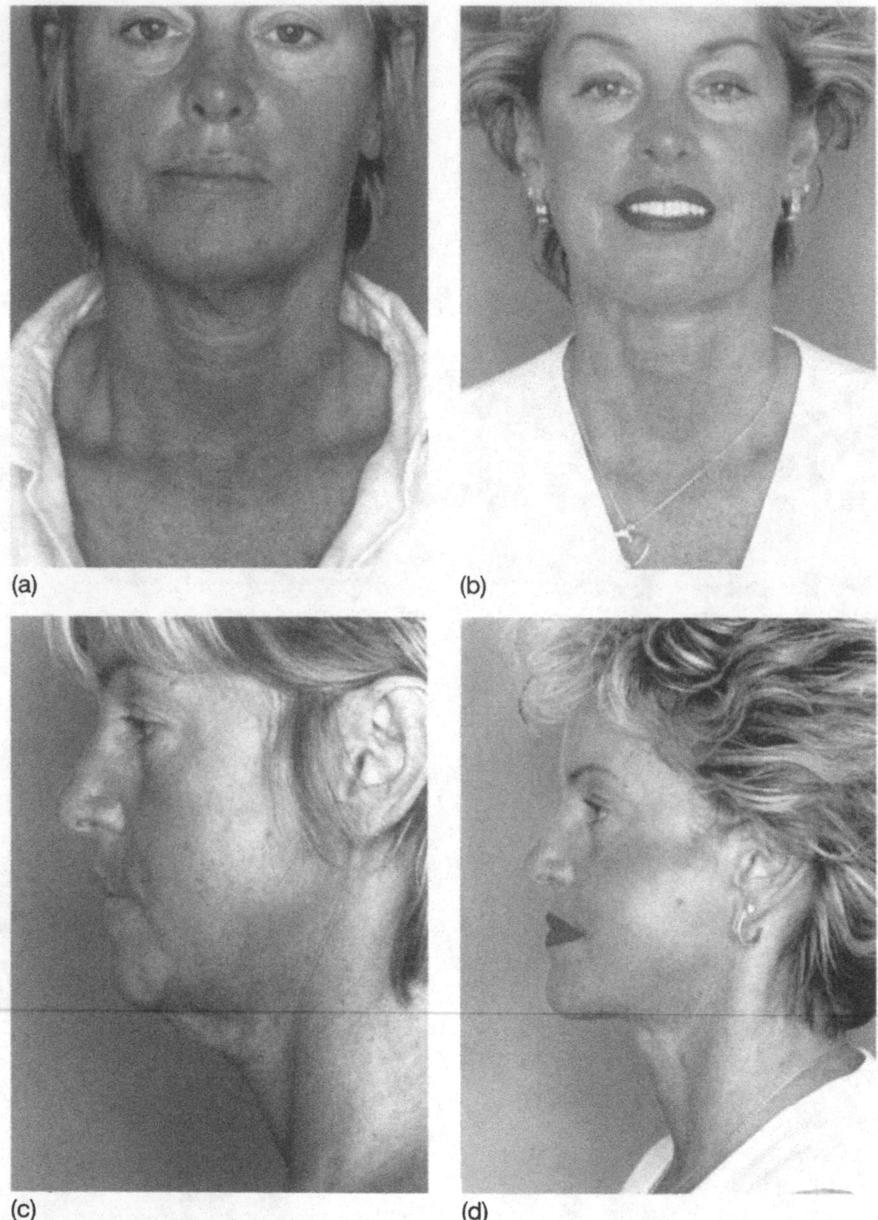

FIGURE 4 Patient (a and c) before and (b and d) after the Cook Weekend Alternative to the Facelift.

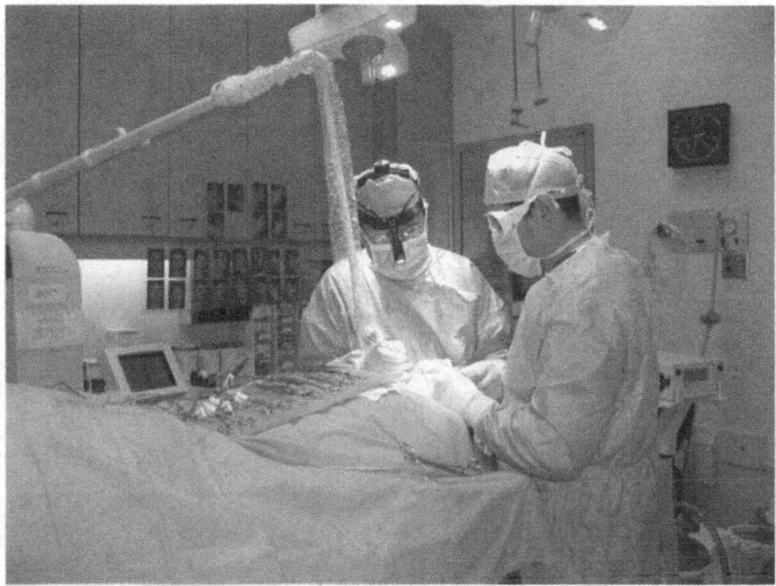

Figure 5 Cook Weekend Alternative to the Facelift procedure in progress.

"turkey neck" and "double chin" (Fig. 6). This procedure is especially useful for patients who display poor cervicomental angles, lax platysma, and mildly to moderately lax skin. Since the technique relies on the natural elasticity of the skin, it will not help a person whose skin is severely inelastic beyond repair. In some cases, individuals with poor elasticity in the skin of the face and neck may be helped by first treating the skin with a laser or chemical peel, after which they can be reevaluated for the Weekend Alternative to the Facelift [4].

Changes in the face, neck, and jowls can occur at any age but generally become more pronounced with aging. We have performed this procedure on patients ranging in age from 18 to 75.

Patients at the younger end of the spectrum generally desire correction of a genetic appearance which they find undesirable, such as a pattern of fullness of the neck and face or a recessive chin (Fig. 7). In many cases the history will reveal that these features were also present in the grandparents and parents. Liposculpture can often relieve the excessive fullness of the face and neck, and a chin implant can be inserted as part of the same procedure.

Older patients usually seek treatment for changes in the appearance of their face and neck that develop with maturity. The submental fat pad may

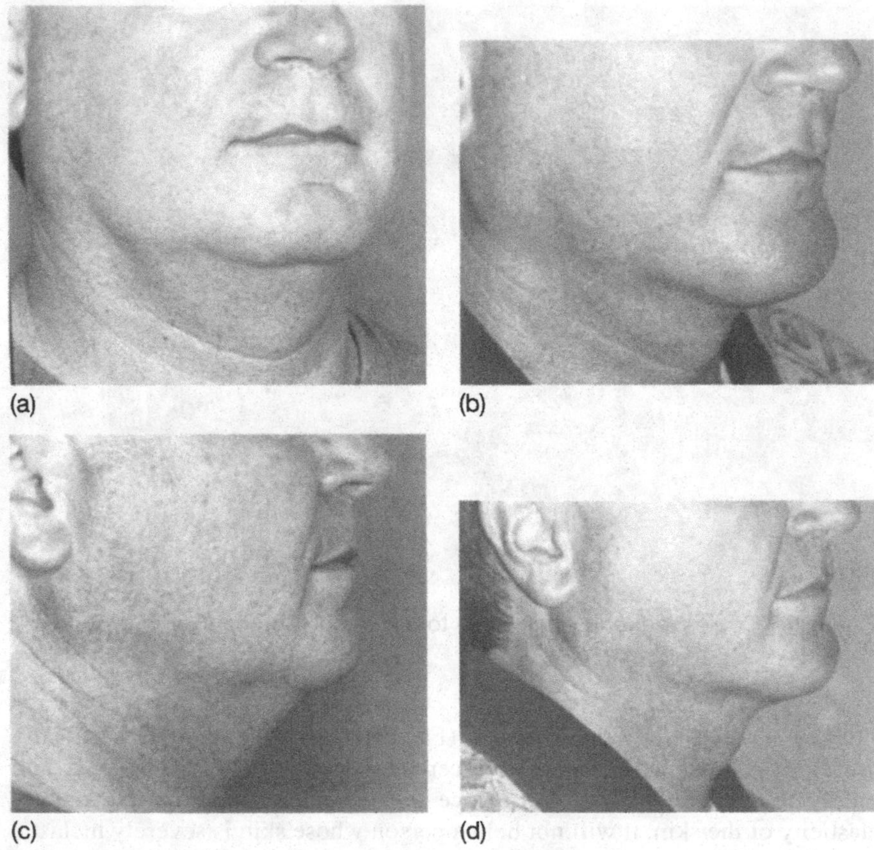

FIGURE 6 Patient (a and c) before and (b and d) after the Cook Weekend Alternative to the Facelift.

become more prominent, the platysma muscle may become weaker, and the skin may begin to lose its elasticity. A "double chin" may develop, with horizontal platysmal insertions forming a ringlike configuration around the neck in several folds. The jowls may become thickened and begin to sag. The Weekend Alternative to the Facelift may be indicated to treat these effects of time, gravity, and heredity (Fig. 8).

As with any liposculpture procedure, careful evaluation of the patient and discussion of the procedure are necessary. It is important that both the patient and the surgeon understand the clinical findings, agree on the goals of the procedure, and have realistic expectations. Patients need to understand which aspects of their appearance will be changed by the procedure and

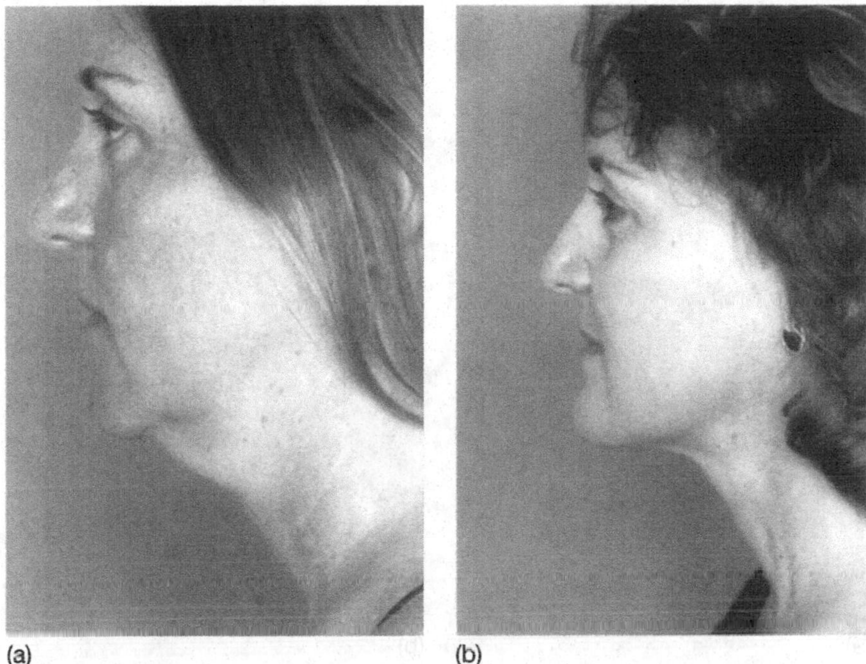

(a) (b)

FIGURE 7 Patient (a) before and (b) after the Cook Weekend Alternative to the Facelift with chin implant.

which will not. They also need to understand the timing of the results. Although significant improvement is usually seen within days, the final results will not be achieved until 2–3 months postoperatively (Fig. 9). In some cases the patient's appearance will continue to improve gradually for 6 to 12 months or even more.

Preoperative Evaluation

In planning this procedure, the distribution of the patient's facial adipose layer must be carefully evaluated. It is important to consider the general facial characteristics and underlying bone structure of that individual and also to evaluate the family history. In some cases the principal problem is bulging of excessive fat; in other cases the problems are mostly caused by lax skin and muscles. In particular, the "turkey neck" deformity needs to be evaluated as to its fat content versus the effect of the platysma muscle versus lax skin. Sagging jowls may be caused by excess fat or a hypertrophic masseter muscle. The position of the larynx and hyoid should also be con-

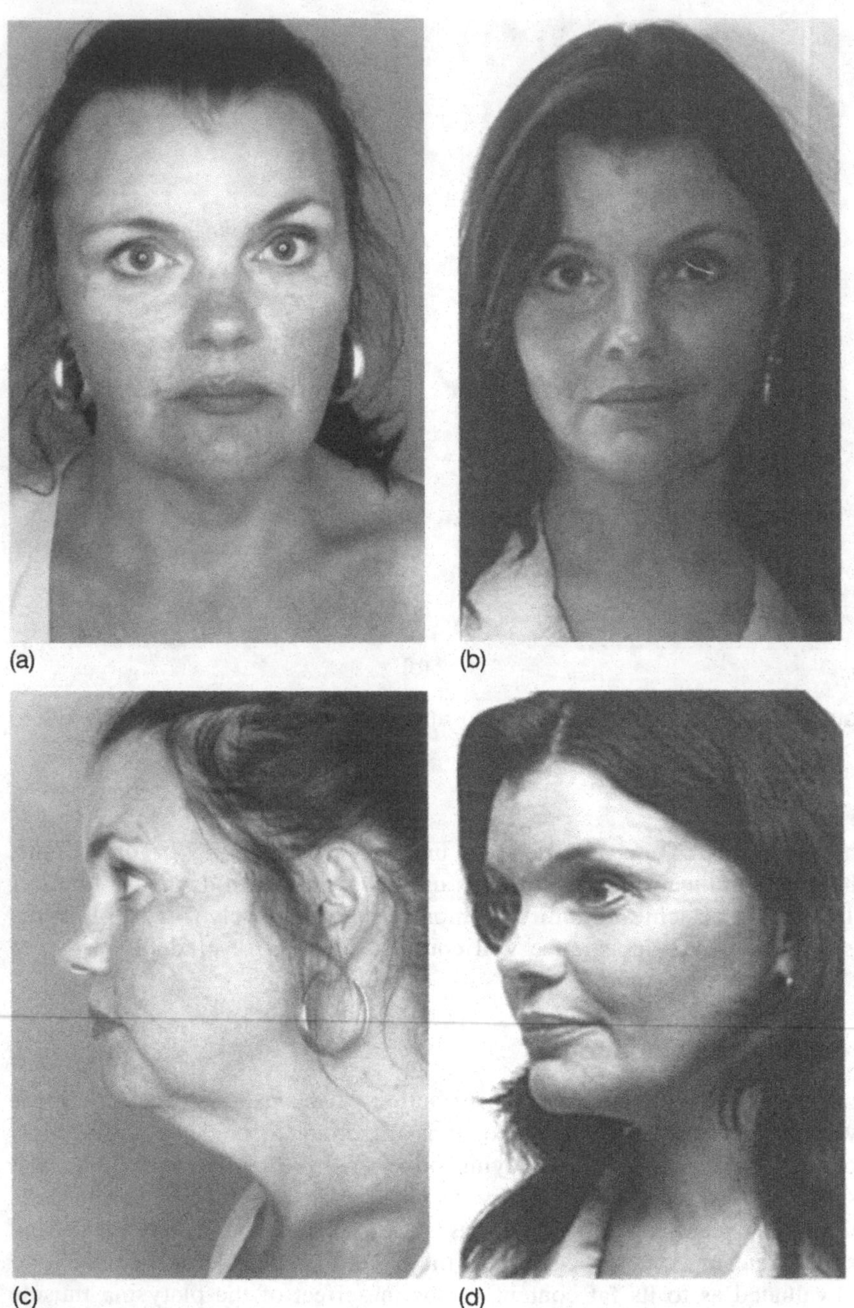

Figure 8 Patient (a and c) before and (b and d) 3 weeks after the Cook Weekend Alternative to the Facelift and upper blepharoplasty.

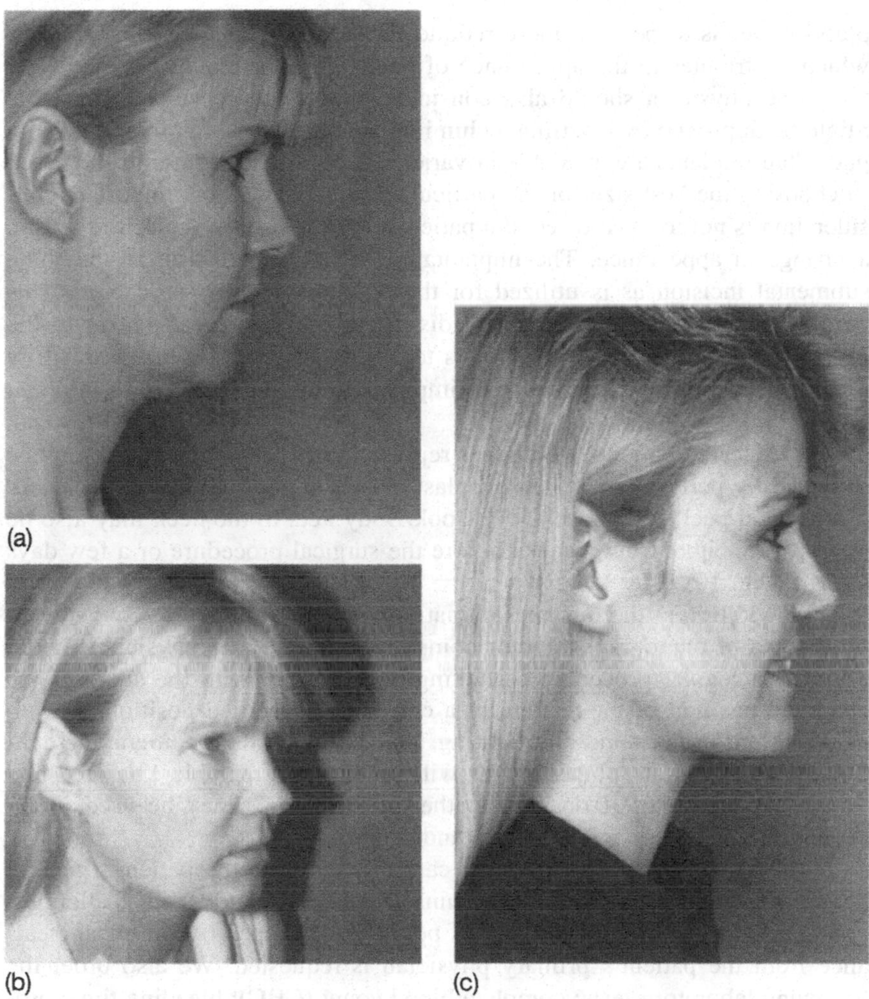

Figure 9 Patient (a) before and (b) 36 hr after, and (c) 3 months after the Cook Weekend Alternative to the Facelift with chin implant.

sidered. Patients with relatively short necks and a high position of the hyoid may need a chin implant to create a "shelf"; otherwise the results may not be as dramatic. Enlarged submandibular glands should be noted and pointed out to the patient, as these glands will remain after surgery. We have found that the platysma tuck procedure will help this condition.

The role of the platysma muscle is of particular importance in addressing any changes that have occurred in the appearance of the neck. The platysma tends to become more redundant and lax with the aging process, which contributes to the appearance of bands in the submental area.

The physician should also consider whether the cervicomental angle might be improved by inserting a chin implant and suctioning the ptotic chin pad. Chin implants are available in various sizes, and thought must be given to choosing the best size for the particular patient. The most important consideration is not to overcorrect the patient's chin so as to produce too drastic a change in appearance. The implantation is performed through the same submental incision as is utilized for the remainder of the procedure. This permits the physician to accurately dissect the subperiosteal pocket to the proper height for the prosthesis. This technique also preserves the integrity of the buccal sulcus and allows the implants to be positioned with minimal risk of injury to the mental nerve.

In selected patients, additional rejuvenation of the appearance may be achieved by performing a blepharoplasty at the same time [3]. A laser and/or chemical peel to the face and a Cook Body Peel to the neck may also be appropriate, either a few weeks before the surgical procedure or a few days after it (Fig. 10) [1].

In addition to the direct examination, clinical evaluation may be aided by the use of photographs and/or computer imaging. The physician should establish a regular procedure for taking photographs, with the angle of the head and position of the camera in a consistent, specified position, as well as consistent background and lighting. Standardizing the photographic conditions will facilitate planning and will produce comparable "before" and "after" photographs. If desired, mathematical models may be used in assessing the patient's facial features and profile [5].

Of course, the physician must carefully evaluate the patient's general health; medications, including vitamins and herbal supplements; allergies; and fitness for undergoing surgery. If possible, a preoperative surgical clearance from the patient's primary physician is requested. We also order the following laboratory tests: complete blood count (CBC); bleeding time; protime (PT); partial thromboplastin time (PTT); chemistry panel; urinalysis; HIV; and hepatitis A, B, and C.

The patient signs an operative consent form and is given written preoperative and postoperative instructions (Appendices 1–3).

SURGICAL PROCEDURE

Precautions

It is important that the surgeon be adequately trained before undertaking this procedure. It is of particular importance that the surgeon and all other op-

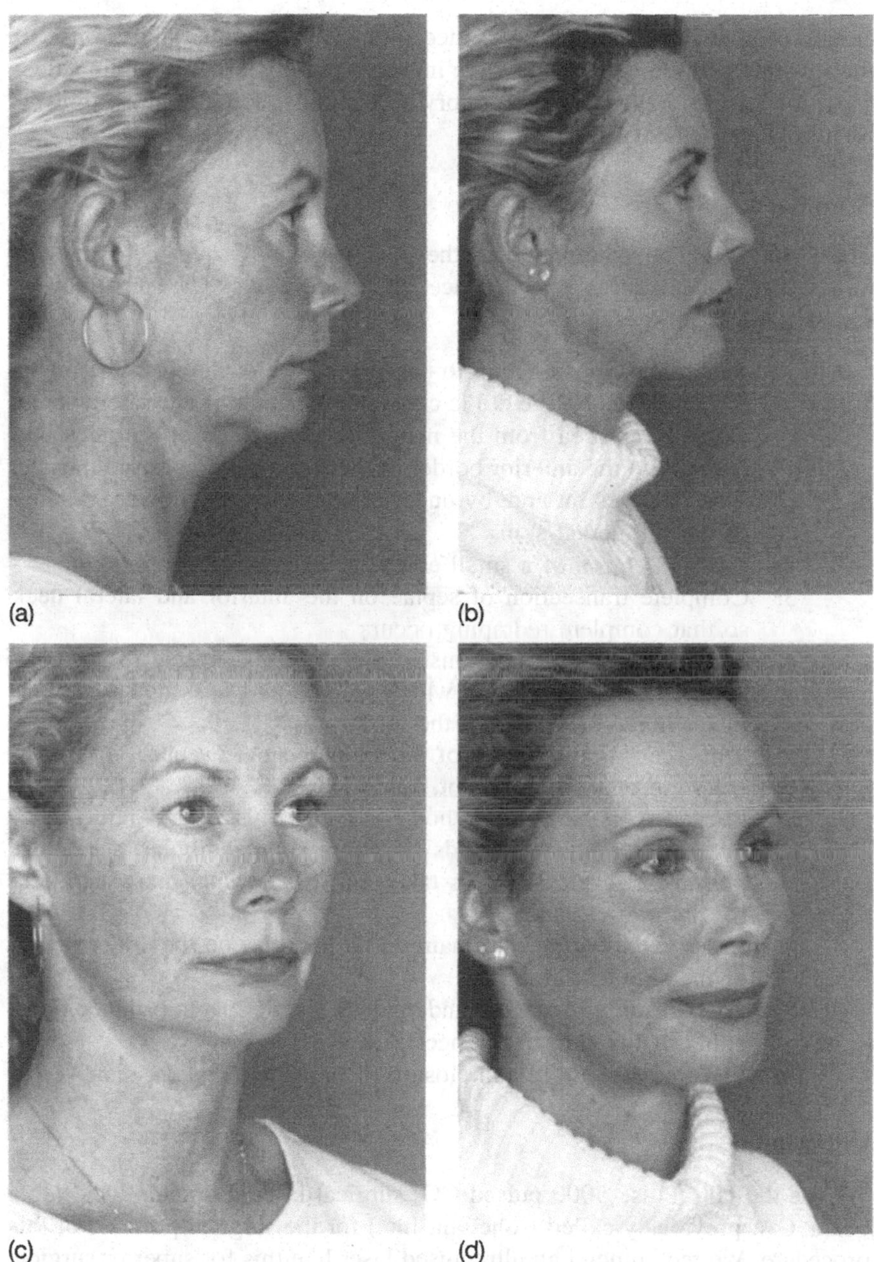

(a) (b) (c) (d)

FIGURE 10 Patient (a and c) before and (b and d) after the Cook Weekend Alternative to the Facelift, upper blepharoplasty, facial laser peel, and Cook Total Body Peel to the neck, chest, and hands.

erative personnel be thoroughly trained in sterile technique and the use of the surgical laser, since lasers involve important safety issues including electrical safety, fire prevention, respiratory precautions, and eye protection for both staff and patient [6].

Summary

The Cook Weekend Alternative to the Facelift is a 10-step technique for tumescent cosmetic surgery to the face, neck, and jowls. The steps may be summarized as follows:

1. Tumescent liposculpture to the lower third of the face, the jowls, any excess fat in the ptotic chin, and the anterior and lateral neck, covering an area from the mandible to the base of the neck and laterally to the anterior border of the sternocleidomastoid muscle. This removes fat and, by undermining the skin, allows redraping of the submental skin.
2. Laser resection of a small ellipse of excess submental skin.
3. Complete transection of septae on the anterior and lateral neck so that complete redraping occurs.
4. Separation of the insertions of the platysma muscle to the horizontal bands of the neck, which reduces and in some cases eliminates horizontal rings of the neck.
5. Tumescent liposculpture of the subplatysmal fat pad.
6. Insertion of a chin implant, when indicated.
7. Plication of the anterior body of the platysma and removal of prominent platysmal bands. If ptotic submandibular glands are present, a surgical tuck is taken in the platysma muscle to help lift the ptotic glands.
8. Laser vaporization of remaining fat globules on the undersurface of the skin of the neck.
9. Laser resurfacing of the underside of the dermis to produce tightening of the skin of the neck and jowls.
10. Placement of drain and closure of the submental incision.

Equipment

We use the UltraPulse 5000 pulsed CO_2 surgical laser (Lumenis Inc., Santa Clara, CA; previously called Coherent, Inc.) for the surgical portions of this procedure. We recommend an ultrapulsed laser like this for superior surgical results. Ultrapulsed lasers produce less heat, less coagulation necrosis, less injury to tissues, less bruising, and a greatly shortened recovery time compared to unpulsed surgical lasers or traditional metal scalpels.

For infiltrating the tumescent solution, we use a Klein infiltration pump (Wells Johnson, Tucson, AZ). For performing tumescent liposculpture, we use a mechanical vacuum pump (Wells Johnson) and a variety of Klein and Capistrano cannulas (HK Surgical, Inc., San Juan Capistrano, CA).

When a chin implant is indicated, we generally use the extended anatomical chin implants from Implantech (Implantech Associates, Inc., Ventura, CA). These implants are available in various sizes and are well tolerated by the patient.

Prior to beginning the procedure, the scrub technician prepares the instrument tray in a sterile fashion (Fig. 11, Table 1).

Marking

The lower face, jowls, chin, and neck are marked with a gentian violet pen with the patient in a sitting position (Fig. 12). Markings should clearly show the extent of the planned suctioning, any elevations or depressions, the midline of the chin, and the location of underlying bony structures such as the mandible.

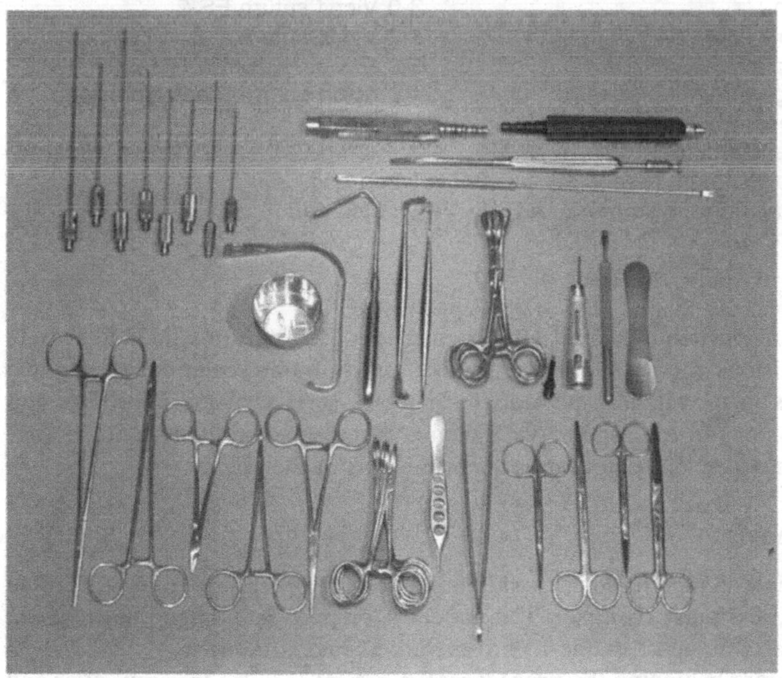

FIGURE 11 Instrument tray for the Cook Weekend Alternative to the Facelift.

TABLE 1 Instruments and Supplies Used for the Cook Weekend Alternative to the Facelift

Klein cannula handles	Six curved hemostats (sponge sticks)
4-in., 16-gauge Capistrano cannula	One "holy" pick up
6-in., 16-gauge Capistrano cannula	One laser-coated pick up
4-in., 16-gauge Klein cannula	Small gold tenotomy scissors
4-in., 14-gauge Klein cannula	Large Metzenbaum scissors
4-in., 12-gauge Klein cannula	Curved Iris scissors
6-in., 16-gauge Klein cannula	Mayo suture scissors
6-in., 14-gauge Klein cannula	Nokor 16-gauge needle
6-in., 12-gauge Klein cannula	10 French JP round drain
Rich periosteal elevator	JP reservoir, 100 ml
Toledo tissue dissector	Xenon 300 headlamp
Stainless steel bowl for lidocaine	Joystick for Xenon headlamp
Large three-hole retractor (Sweetheart)	Bovie pencil
Medium retractor	6-in. insulated Bovie tip
Two three-prong Senn rake retractors	White suction tip
Towel clips	Suction cautery
Laser tip	Stylet from suction cautery
Pineapple stick	3-0 Vicryl suture FS-2
Jaeger plate	4-0 Vicryl suture P-3
One large straight hemostat	5-0 Monocryl suture P-3
Long needle holder	4-0 nylon suture Black Sharpoint DS18
Short needle holder	2 × 2 and 3 × 3 NuGauze squares
One short straight hemostat	Trash bag
One small right-angle hemostat	Scratch pad

Incision points should also be marked. The incisions include two 1-mm incisions in the submental crease, two infra-auricular incisions, two incisions in the lateral aspect of the mucosal surface of the upper lip, and two incisions in the supraclavicular area just medial to the anterior border of the sternocleidomastoid muscle at the base of the neck.

Anesthesia

The patient is monitored with an automatic blood pressure monitor, cardiac monitor, and pulse oximeter. The patient is prepped and draped in the usual sterile fashion, and a saline-lock intravenous line is inserted.

Before beginning the procedure, the patient is given intramuscular and sublingual sedation. The intramuscular sedation generally consists of mid-

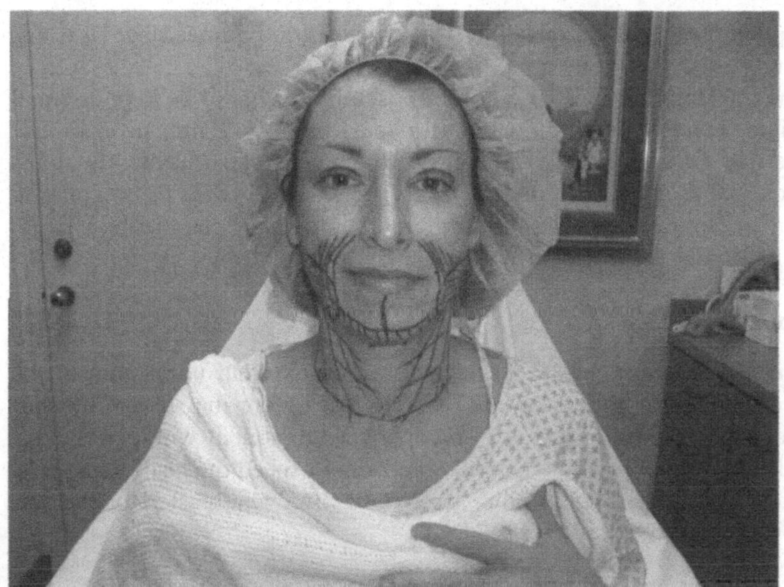

Figure 12 Patient marked for the Cook Weekend Alternative to the Facelift.

azolam (Versed), 2.5 mg if the patient is over 60 years of age or 5 mg if younger than 60; meperidine (Demerol), 50–100 mg; and hydroxyzine (Vistaril), 25–50 mg. In addition, diazepam (Valium) 5 mg is administered sublingually. In most cases this initial dose of sedation is all that is required. However, additional Versed, Demerol, or Valium can be given during surgery if necessary for patient comfort. We use no intravenous or inhalational general anesthesia.

During the initial sedation the patient is given 2 liters/min of nasal oxygen. It is important to discontinue use of the oxygen before using the laser or electrocautery.

Throughout the procedure we monitor the patient's blood pressure and control any hypertension. When indicated we use clonidine and nifedipine (Procardia) to control the blood pressure.

We use standard tumescent solution which contains 0.1% lidocaine, 1:1,000,000 epinephrine, 10 mEq/liter $NaHCO_3$, and 10 mg/liter triamcinolone acetonide (Kenalog). The tumescent solution is made up fresh on the day it will be used. Before infiltration, it is warmed to approximately 39°–40°C.

The solution is infiltrated through the small incisions in the submental and infra-auricular areas. The entire anterior and lateral neck, jowls, and lower one-third of the face should be infiltrated. The average face and neck will require 500–800 ml of fluid to achieve good tumescence for this procedure.

The incisions for infiltration and liposculpture should be kept as small as possible, ideally just 1 mm, up to a maximum of 2 mm in size. The incisions can be kept small by using a 16-gauge Nokor needle (Becton–Dickinson and Company, Franklin Lakes, NY). This needle has a constant diameter, in contrast to a No. 11 surgical blade, which can create a larger incision if it is inserted deeper.

Ultrasound

In patients with heavy necks, we usually apply external ultrasound to the tumesced areas after infiltration is complete and before the start of the surgical procedure. In our experience, preoperative treatment with external ultrasound may help to promote patient comfort and speed the healing process. It may also make the liposculpture procedure somewhat easier for the surgeon to perform [7].

Step 1

After waiting at least 20 min to allow good vasoconstriction, tumescent liposculpture is begun through the submental incision sites, using two small incisions approximately 1 cm lateral to the midline on each side in the submental fold or the area which will be utilized for the submental incision. (In some patients who require a chin implant, the submental incision will be placed inferior to the submental fold. When the chin implant insertion elevates the submental fold, the incision will still be hidden in the submental area.) Having two incisions approximately 2 cm apart permits good criss-crossing during the liposculpture of the neck. It also guarantees the exact line for incision will be maintained, since in many cases the markings may be erased during the suction process, and the skin fold that one would normally choose for the incision may disappear due to tumescent expansion of tissues. Using first a 16-gauge and then a 14-gauge Klein spatula cannula, liposculpture is performed in the submental region and jowl areas, criss-crossing the areas and forming a honeycomb pattern in the sites of involvement.

After this initial submental suctioning is completed, the infra-auricular incision is used to suction the lower one-third of the face, the jowl area, and the adjacent area of the lateral neck. Usually 16-gauge Klein and Capistrano cannulas are used, making precise passes carefully spaced. This is done in the middle or deeper plane to avoid ridging of the cheeks.

The next area of suctioning is through an incision approximately 1 mm in size in the mucosal surface of the lateral aspect of the upper lip, approximately 1.5 cm medial to the lateral commissure. A 16-gauge Klein spatula cannula and a 16-gauge Capistrano cannula, either 4 or 6 in. in length, are used to suction the mound portion lateral to the nasolabial fold, if indicated, and the jowl area. We never use larger than a 16-gauge cannula in this area so that the incision site will close nicely without suturing and leave no apparent cosmetic defect.

After the initial liposculpture is completed, an additional 50–100 ml of tumescent solution is infiltrated into the neck region. This reinfiltration helps to expand the working space and provides additional vasoconstriction. The neck region is now sculpted using first 14-gauge Klein spatula cannulas, 4 in. and then 6 in. in length, and finally 12-gauge Klein spatula cannulas, first 4 in. and then 6 in. During this final sculpting, one should thoroughly cover the areas from the mandibular ridge down to the base of the neck so that all apparent excess fatty tissue is removed. Sculpting of the entire neck is important to gain balance to this anatomical unit and to aid in the later redraping process.

Some patients develop a ptotic chin pad, sometimes called a "witch's chin." This is treated by suctioning the bottom half of the chin below the area of maximum projection of the chin. Using an 18-gauge Capistrano cannula, the left lower quarter of the chin is suctioned from the right submental incision site and vice versa.

If the patient has too narrow a space between the chin and lower lip, the upper part of the chin and the bound-down crease above the chin can also be suctioned. An 18-gauge Capistrano cannula is slipped into a pore on either side of the chin, just above and lateral to the area of maximum projection of the chin. This avoids making a visible incision on the chin.

Step 2

The submental incisions are now connected with a gentian violet marking pen to outline a 2.5-cm submental ellipse approximately 2–3 mm in width. The primary goal of this excision is to provide a working window to allow the surgeon to perform the remaining steps in the procedure, not to remove a significant amount of excessive skin. Removal of excess amounts of skin may lead to "dog ears" or poor wound healing at the incision site, due to increased stress on the wound edges. What may appear to be redundant skin in the area will be reduced by skin contraction from the dermal laser resurfacing, described below.

We use the UltraPulse 5000 laser, with initial settings of 15 mJ and 4 W, to make the initial skin incision of the ellipse. This "pulsed" mode produces a small, usually bloodless, incision with minimal tissue damage. The 7-W setting is then used to complete the excision of the elliptical piece of skin.

Step 3

A Toledo tissue dissector (Byron Medical Inc., Tucson, AZ) is inserted into the submental incision and is utilized to break all visible septae in the entire anterior and lateral neck. It is important to keep the plane of dissection relatively superficial. Hemostasis is achieved with both standard cautery and suction cautery, using a Valley electrosurgical unit (ValleyLab, Boulder, CO).

Step 4

The Toledo tissue dissector is then utilized to separate the insertion of the platysma muscle into the horizontal rings of the neck. Hemostasis is achieved with a Valley electrosurgical unit equipped with a special suction cautery tip.

Step 5

The midportion of the platysma muscle is now infiltrated with a solution of 2% lidocaine and 1:100,000 epinephrine, approximately 1.5–2.0 ml injected directly into the muscle. This will provide anesthesia and vasoconstriction for the subplatysmal suctioning described below.

A small incision is made in the midline of the superior aspect of the platysma muscle. The subplatysmal fat pad is carefully visualized through this small opening and is gently aspirated using a 12-gauge Klein spatula cannula. The fat in this area is very soft, and extreme caution and very slow movements of the cannula are needed so as not to traumatize any of the adjacent structures. Following suctioning, the area must be carefully monitored for good hemostasis.

After the excess subplatysmal pad is removed, direct visualization is made of the jowl areas. Any residual globules of fat in this area are carefully removed, using the same 12-gauge Klein spatula cannula with the openings toward the skin surface.

Step 6 (Optional)

In patients with slight to moderate microgenia, the mandible may be augmented to maximize the cervicomental angle. The implant procedure is begun by using the UltraPulse 5000 laser on the 7-W continuous setting to carefully separate the platysma muscle in a horizontal line just beneath the submental skin incision. The laser is then used to elevate the muscle off the periosteum of the lower half of the chin, corresponding to the desired position for the implant. The periosteum is then incised with the UltraPulse 5000 laser. A Rich periosteal elevator (Byron Medical Inc., Tucson, AZ) is utilized to create a pocket subperiosteally along the border of the mandible.

The pocket for the implant should be located so that the implant will seat comfortably and squarely over the chin prominence and will not extend higher than the natural labiomental groove. The pocket must accommodate the prosthesis comfortably; otherwise the implant will slide inferiorly over the symphysis and rock back and forth. Most patients respond best with the "wrap-around" or anatomical type of implant. These give a very natural appearance.

Once the pocket is freed and hemostasis is achieved, the implant is positioned and is secured to the periosteum with 4–0 clear nylon sutures. The fibers of the platysma muscle are then reapproximated with 3–0 Vicryl sutures (Ethicon, Inc., Somerville, NJ).

Step 7

Platysmal tightening is then performed to further improve the cervicomental angle and to reduce neck banding. After liposculpture, severing of the septae, and removal of the platysmal insertions into the skin of the neck, the pattern of the particular individual's platysma muscle can clearly be noted. Because of the support given by the platysma and its role in the creation of the cervicomental angle, there is no substitute for a very thorough plication of the medial platysma to create the best results in the neck. The exact amount of tightening and the linear extent of the plication will vary from patient to patient.

The medial borders of the platysma muscle are carefully sutured together using a vertical mattress plication stitch of 3 0 Vicryl suture. By the time this suture is absorbed, there will be good firm support of the muscular filaments and the overlying fascia. The number of sutures and their placement will vary considerably, depending on the anatomy of the underlying platysma muscle.

After plication, any platysmal bands can be trimmed away using Metzenbaum scissors (Miltex Inc., Bethpage, NY). With the resulting change in the position of the platysma muscle after plication and the removal of existing bands, postoperative banding has been minimal.

Below the point of plication, a small horizontal wedge of muscle is resected from each of the anterior platysmal borders to break the continuity of the band and allow the creation of a sharp cervicomental angle. Alternatively, a small cross cut can be made into the platysma muscle to help demarcate the crease at the cervicomental angle. This allows the muscle to conform to the cervicomental angle rather than forming a "bowstring" across it.

If the patient has ptotic submandibular glands, the glands can be elevated by taking a tuck in the platysma muscle overlying the glands with 3-0 Vicryl suture.

Step 8

Persistent excess fat lobules on the undersurface of the skin are spot vaporized with the laser. It is important to use the most defocused handle position with a 7-W continuous wave setting and the minimum time necessary to vaporize the globules. Try not to remove all of the fat.

Step 9

To tighten the skin, the undersurface of the dermis of the neck and jowls is carefully resurfaced in a crisscrossing randomized fashion, using the UltraPulse 5000 laser on a 7-W defocused setting. Care must be taken to keep the laser beam moving continuously. The amount of resurfacing done on the undersurface of the skin will depend upon the skin laxity, the skin thickness, and the amount of tightening desired. Resurfacing should only be done on no more than 20% of the skin undersurface. It helps to evert the skin and hold the nondominant "smart" hand behind the area being resurfaced to stabilize the skin and to guard against any areas of heat, which would indicate the need to adjust the laser concentration for the thickness of the skin in that particular area. Lase evenly over all areas of the exposed dermal surface, extending into the lateral neck to obtain even contraction. Avoid excessive lasing, which can lead to excesssive contraction of the skin. Miminum lasing has been shown to produce excellent contraction. In fact, in our clinical experience the skin shrinkage continues for almost an hour after the lasing is complete.

Step 10

With good hemostasis achieved in all areas, a Jackson-Pratt 10 French drain with an attached Jackson-Pratt 100-ml sterile reservoir (Allegiance Healthcare Corporation, McGaw Park, IL) is placed in the base of the neck. The drain is inserted through the previous suction site opening generally at the right base of the neck. The drain is sutured in place with 4-0 Nylon suture. The insertion site is covered with Tegaderm dressing (3M Company, St. Paul, MN) to retard any contamination of the drain exit site by surface bacteria. The drain is usually removed in 2 days.

The submental incision is then closed, using 4-0 Vicryl interrupted sutures in the subcutaneous layer and 5-0 clear Monocryl absorbable running subcuticular sutures (Ethicon, Inc., Somerville, NJ) in the skin surface. Steri-Strips (3M Company) are also applied. The small incisions in the infra-auricular, lip, and lower neck areas are left open to promote drainage. These sites usually close in the first 24 hr postoperatively.

If a blepharoplasty is to be performed in connection with the Weekend Alternative to the Facelift, the lower eyelids are infiltrated with local anesthetic (2% xylocaine with 1:100,000 epinephrine) just before suturing the submental incision. By the time the drain is placed and the neck incision sutured, the lower eyelids will be anesthetized and blepharoplasty may be commenced immediately using the Ultrapulse 5000 laser. The upper eyelids are done after the lower eyelids. A detailed description of the blepharoplasty procedure has been published elsewhere [3].

POSTOPERATIVE CONSIDERATIONS

Postoperative Care

Stretch foam tape is applied to the neck and lower facial areas (Fig. 13). The stretch foam tape must be positioned very carefully so as not to induce any folds in the skin. The tape is then covered by an elastic neck strap to hold the tissues in the appropriate position (Fig. 14).

Patients must leave the office after surgery with a responsible adult who will drive them home and remain with them for the remainder of the day and night. Upon returning home, the patient is advised to rest for the remainder of the day, with the head elevated and ice packs in position over the lower face and neck, 15 min "on" and 15 min "off." This will help to reduce tissue swelling and help to prevent ecchymosis of the areas. Good hydration should be maintained through adequate water intake.

The first full postoperative day is spent in quiet activities, with periodic rest and head elevation. Patients are instructed to leave the stretch foam tape in place and keep it dry until it is removed in the office and to wear the elastic neck strap for 1 day. Excessive activity immediately after surgery is not recommended.

The day after surgery, patients may return to the physician's office for inspection or changing of the tape. If the tapes are well positioned, not loose, and giving good support, they are left in place for 2 days. In cases where there has been a large amount of tissue contraction after the procedure, it is best to replace the tapes on the first postoperative day.

On the second postoperative day the patient returns to the office again for removal of the tape and the surgical drain. Rarely, in patients with large necks who still show significant drainage on the second postoperative day, the drain is left in until the third postoperative day. After removal of the drain patients can return to work and normal activities; however, they should avoid vigorous exercise for a week or more, depending on the activity. Immersion in water such as a swimming pool, hot tub, or tub bath is prohibited until all the incisions have closed and the sutures have dissolved (approximately 3 weeks).

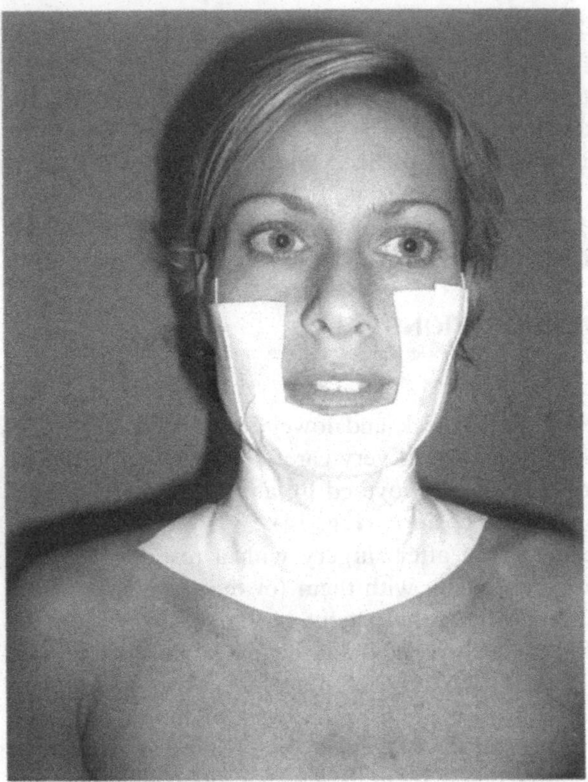

Figure 13 Stretch foam tape in place following the Cook Weekend Alternative to the Facelift.

Complications and Sequelae

Patients undergoing this procedure generally experience no to minimal postoperative ecchymosis or discomfort. Occasionally the chin implant site may be tender for 1–2 days postoperatively. Patients are usually able to return to work and social activities on about the 3rd postoperative day. Exercise of any strenuous type should be avoided for the first 2 to 3 weeks postoperatively, particularly in patients who have received a chin implant.

Although patients will show significant cosmetic improvement as soon as the tape is removed, the final result of the surgical procedure may not be apparent for 2–3 months postoperatively or even longer. This must be emphasized before the operation so that the patient's expectations will be in line with the natural healing processes which will take place.

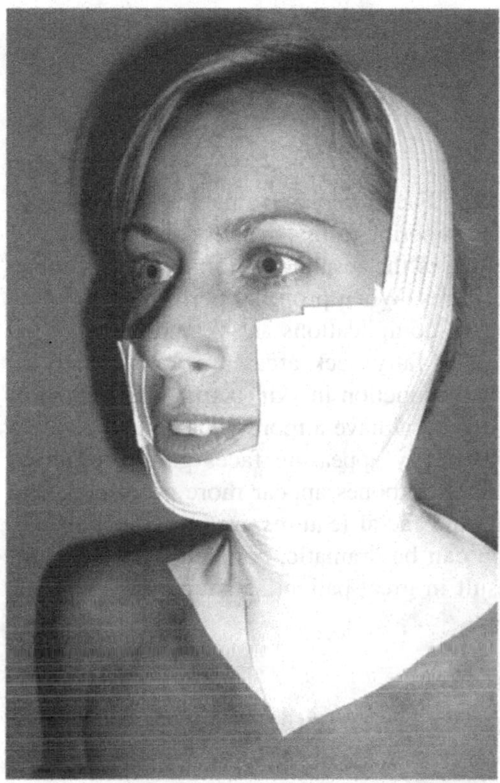

FIGURE 14 Elastic neck strap in place following the Cook Weekend Alternative to the Facelift.

We have had no serious complications to date. Some individuals will recover more rapidly than others, depending on the amount of skin retraction which must occur. Rarely a small seroma may develop during the postoperative period. Placement of the surgical drain at the base of the neck almost eliminates the incidence of postoperative seromas. If one develops after the drain is removed, it may be easily drained with an 18-gauge needle and a 10-cc syringe, and recovery will then proceed uneventfully with generally excellent clinical results.

Individuals with a history of hypertrophic scarring or keloid formation need to be monitored carefully. Seromas can also heal with excess fibrosis. If excess scarring appears it can be treated with intralesional Kenalog. This treatment should be started postoperatively as soon as any excess scar tissue is noted and continued weekly as needed. The concentration of the Kenalog solution should be low initially (2–5 mg/cc) and increased as indicated. Also, silicone sheeting may be helpful in reducing any scarring.

RESULTS

The Cook Weekend Alternative to the Facelift creates a natural-looking cosmetic improvement that can be far superior to that which can be achieved with liposculpture alone. In many cases the results are comparable to those achieved from rhytidectomy procedures. When properly performed the procedure is very safe and postoperative complications are very rare.

After this procedure, sagging or fatty neck areas are transformed by good tightening of the neck, marked reduction in skin laxity, and reduction of the platysmal bands. Patients in general have a more youthful appearance (Fig. 15). Patients with round and heavy appearing faces gain a slimmer, more attractive look (Fig. 16). The cheekbones appear more prominent, the mandible is more sharply defined, and facial features are in better balance. The cosmetic improvement, which can be dramatic, coupled with the rapid recovery period will generally result in great patient satisfaction.

APPENDIX 1

PATIENT'S OPERATIVE CONSENT FOR FACIAL SURGERY

Patient name: ______________________

Patient states: I am aware that the Cook Weekend Alternative to the Facelift™ (including but not limited to liposculpture, platysma muscle revision, laser dermal resurfacing, etc.) is a contouring process. Dr. Cook and assistants have carefully explained to me the nature, goals, limitations, and possible complications of this procedure and alternative forms of treatment. I have had the opportunity to ask questions about the procedure, its limitations, and possible complications.

All items contained herein apply to these procedure(s):

1. Cook Weekend Alternative to the Facelift™
2. ______________
3. ______________

I clearly understand and accept the following:

1. The potential benefits of the proposed procedure(s).
2. The possible alternate medical procedure(s).

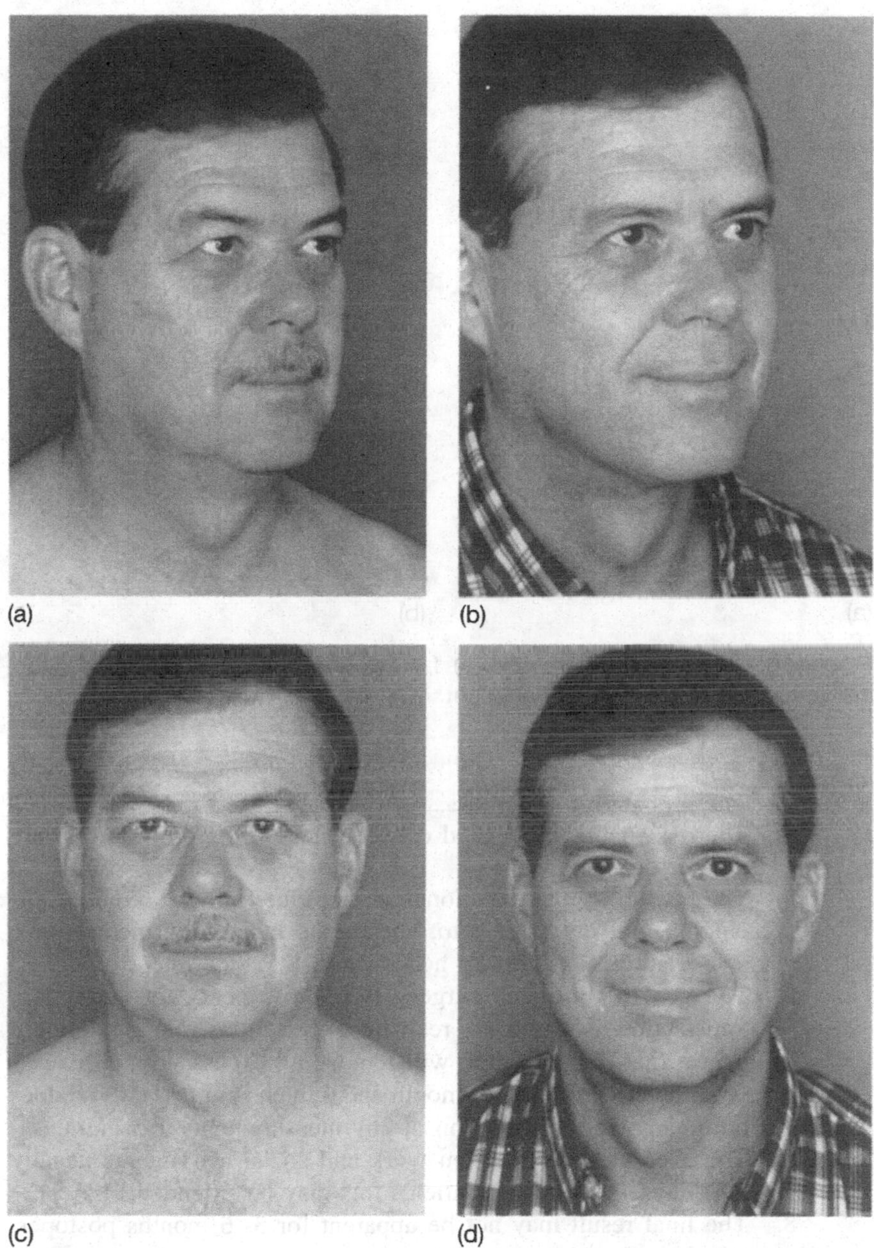

(a) (b) (c) (d)

FIGURE 15 Patient (a and c) before and (b and d) 6 months after the Cook Weekend Alternative to the Facelift with chin implant and upper blepharoplasty.

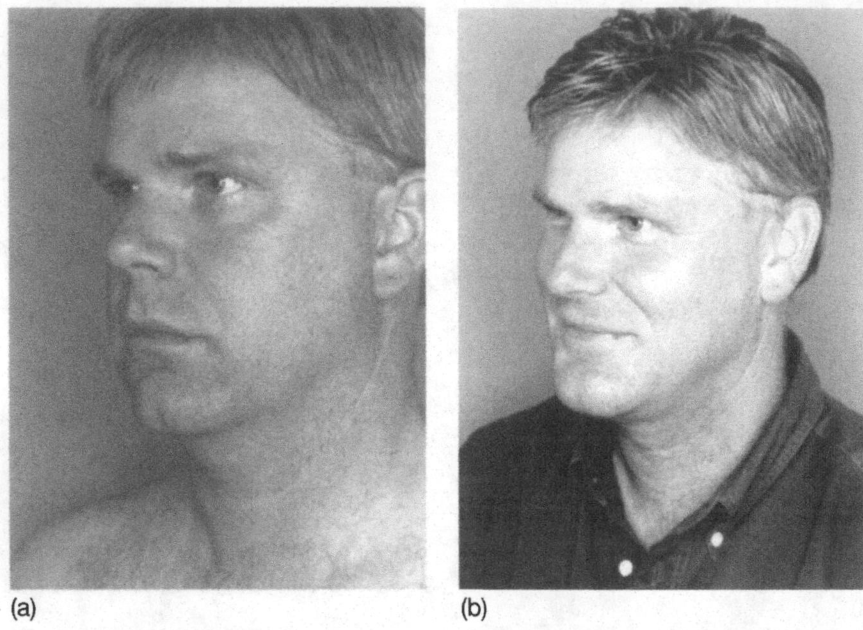

(a) (b)

FIGURE 16 Patient (a) before and (b) 1 week after the Cook Weekend Alternative to the Facelift with chin implant.

3. The probability of success.
4. The reasonable anticipated consequences if the procedure(s) are not performed.
5. The possibility that additional services/fees may be required, including, but not limited to, anesthesia, laboratory, medications, and/or surgical facility or hospital use.
6. The goal of cosmetic surgery is improvement, not perfection. Satisfaction is based on realistic expectations. No one should expect that the procedure will remove all excess skin, all excess fat, or every wrinkle, or smooth and tighten skin perfectly. It does not guarantee the reduction of any measurements or weight.
7. The average time off from work and social activities is usually 2–3 days, but in some patients this may be extended.
8. The final result may not be apparent for 3–6 months postoperatively or longer.
9. Occasionally, to achieve the best possible result, additional procedures may be required. There will be a charge for any additional operation performed.

10. Strict adherence to postoperative instructions is necessary in order to achieve the best possible results.
11. The surgical fee is paid for the operation itself and subsequent postoperative visits.
12. I will not drive for 24 hours after the procedure.
13. I give my permission for the administration of anesthesia, as deemed appropriate by the physician.
14. Protective eye covering will be provided to protect my eyes from accidental laser exposure. Accidental exposure to laser is extremely rare but possible.

Although complications following surgery are infrequent, I understand that the following may occur:

1. Bruising, bleeding, thrombophlebitis (inflammation of the veins), and blood clots are rare, and in rare instances could require hospitalization and blood transfusion. It is possible that blood clots or fluid may form under the skin, requiring surgical drainage.
2. Swelling, crusting, skin irregularities, lumpiness, hardness, and dimpling may occur postoperatively. Most of these problems will disappear with time and massage, but they may persist permanently.
3. If loose skin is present in the treated areas, it may or may not shrink to conform to the new contour. In rare cases wrinkling may persist.
4. Infection is rare, but should it occur, treatment with antibiotics and/or surgical drainage may be required.
5. Possible numbness or increased sensitivity of the skin over treated areas may persist for months, and in rare cases may be permanent.
6. Objectionable bruising and scarring is rare but possible, and may result in discoloration or texture changes of the skin. This is usually temporary but may rarely be permanent. To minimize the chances of this, I understand that it is important for me to follow all preoperative and after-care instructions carefully.
7. Dizziness may occur following surgery, particularly upon rising from a lying or sitting position. If dizziness occurs, exercise caution while walking and do not attempt to drive a car.
8. As the dermal resurfacing heals and the skin redrapes itself, in rare instances the skin may appear more wrinkled and the neck may feel tighter. In almost all cases this resolves, but in rare instances it may persist.

9. Allergic or toxic responses to anesthesia are extremely rare, but possible.
10. In addition to these possible complications, I am aware of the general risks inherent in all surgical procedures and administration of anesthetic.
11. (For chin implant procedures only) Rare but possible complications include: extrusion (pushing out of the implant), malposition (abnormal location of the implant), bone absorption, hypesthesia of the lip (full or partial loss of sensation), and allergies. These complications may require removal of the implant.

My signature certifies that I have discussed the above material thoroughly with Dr. Cook and assistants. I understand the goals, limitations, and possible complications of the above procedure(s). I wish to proceed with the operation. I authorize and direct Dr. Cook and/or associates or assistants of his choice to perform these procedures on me and/or to do any other additional therapeutic procedure that his judgment may dictate to be advisable, reasonable, or necessary for my well-being.

Patient signature: ______________________ Date: __________

Witness signature: ______________________ Date: __________

Physician signature: ______________________ Date: __________

APPENDIX 2

PREOPERATIVE INSTRUCTIONS FOR PATIENTS

1. Please inform our staff of any health problems, previous surgeries, allergies, and any medications that you are taking
2. DO NOT TAKE ASPIRIN OR IBUPROFEN PRODUCTS OR VITAMIN E PRIOR TO SURGERY AND FOR 1 WEEK AFTER SURGERY. These products can cause bleeding. These include aspirin, Advil, Aleve, Empirin, Anaprox, Nuprin, Motrin, Naprosyn, Feldene, vitamin E, any other anti-inflammatory medicine, arthritis medicines, vitamins, and cold/flu medications. Call our nurse if you have any questions. The only pain medication allowed prior to your surgery is Tylenol.
3. Be sure that you take all medications as directed.
4. Please advise our staff of any removable dental appliances or contact lenses. Please do not wear contact lenses the day of surgery.

5. Please do not wear any jewelry or bring any valuables such as purse, wallet or watch on the day of your surgery. We cannot be responsible for any lost items.
6. DO NOT CONSUME ANY ALCOHOLIC BEVERAGES FOR SEVERAL DAYS PRIOR TO SURGERY AND 1 WEEK AFTER SURGERY. Alcohol may cause bleeding and may interfere with the other medications you are taking.
7. Arrange for a responsible adult to bring you to and from the office, NOT A TAXI DRIVER OR YOURSELF. DO NOT PLAN TO DRIVE A VEHICLE FOR 24 HOURS.
8. Arrange for a friend to stay with you for the first night after your surgery.
9. Take 2 showers, one the night before surgery and one before surgery. Wash your hair and face with Hibiclens cleanser (may be purchased at the drug store). DO NOT GET THIS IN YOUR EYES. You may apply conditioner to your hair, but do not use hair spray or mousse.
10. Eat a light meal the morning of surgery. NO CAFFEINE OR ALCOHOL. Limit your fluid intake on the morning of surgery to 1 glass.

YOUR SURGERY HAS BEEN SCHEDULED FOR (date): ____________

PLEASE REPORT TO THE OFFICE AT (time): ____________

APPENDIX 3

POSTOPERATIVE INSTRUCTIONS FOLLOWING FACIAL SURGERY

Swelling may be present following facial surgery. This is usually minimal and temporary, but varies from person to person. Careful attention to these postoperative instructions will help to minimize any swelling, discoloration, and discomfort after surgery.

You must have an adult friend drive you to and from the office on the day of surgery and stay with you for the first night. You may not leave the office in a taxi.

Plan to rest in bed the remainder of the day of surgery to help prevent bruising and swelling.

Elevate your head at all times. Sleep on 2 pillows for 1 week. This will help to prevent swelling.

Apply cold packs to your face for the first 8 hours after surgery until bedtime, alternating 15 minutes "on" and 15 minutes "off." This will reduce bruising and swelling. Bags of frozen peas or soft ice packs are excellent for this purpose. Purchase four such packs so you can keep two in the freezer while using the other two. Do not put ice cubes directly on your skin; just gently lay the cold packs on your face. Remember to keep the operative area and tapes dry.

For the first 48 hours after surgery, confine your activities to resting and gentle activities which do not elevate your heart rate or blood pressure. If you are receiving a chin implant, avoid contact sports for 2–3 weeks.

Be gentle to your face and neck, and avoid trauma to the area.

Tapes will be applied to your face and neck postoperatively. Do not remove these tapes. They will be removed at your follow-up office appointment. Keep them dry.

Sutures under your chin will absorb on their own.

You will be given a chin strap to wear after surgery for approximately 2 days. Wearing this strap helps to prevent bruising, decreases swelling, and gives your neck a better shape.

You may shower in lukewarm water, but keep your neck tapes dry. After we remove the tapes, you should wash your neck incision sites twice a day for 1 week. Wash with soap and water, then hydrogen peroxide. Do not use Band-Aids in this area.

You will be given various medications to take. Keep a written record of the times medications are taken. Take all medications as prescribed; do not skip or double up on medication. Do not take aspirin or other nonsteroidal anti-inflammatory medications for 1 week after surgery. See the separate medication sheet for a list of medicines to take and to avoid.

Do not drive on the day of surgery.

If at any point in your recovery you experience swelling, resume the application of cold packs to the area.

Avoid sun burning of your face and neck. Wear a hat and protect yourself from the sun. The incision sites may darken if they receive too much sun.

Do not use self-tanning creams for 1 month following surgery.

Feel free to call our office at any time, day or night, if you have questions or problems.

REFERENCES

1. Cook KK, Cook WF Jr. Chemical peel of nonfacial skin using glycolic acid gel augmented with TCA and neutralized based on visual staging. Dermatol Surg 2000; 26:994–999.

2. Klein JA. The tumescent technique for liposuction surgery. Am J Cosmet Surg 1987; 4:263–267.
3. Cook WR Jr, Cook KK. Manual of Tumescent Liposculpture and Laser Cosmetic Surgery. Philadelphia: Lippincott/Williams & Wilkins, 1999.
4. Koch RJ, Cheng ET. Quantification of skin elasticity changes associated with pulsed carbon dioxide laser skin resurfacing. Arch Facial Plast Surg 1999; 1: 272–275.
5. Farkas LG, Sohm P, Kolar JC, Katic MJ, Munro IR. Inclinations of the facial profile: art versus reality. Plast Reconstr Surg 1985; 75:509–519.
6. Alster TS. Manual of Cutaneous Laser Techniques. Philadelphia: Lippincott-Raven, 1997.
7. Cook WR Jr. Utilizing external ultrasonic energy to improve the results of tumescent liposculpture. Dermatol Surg 1997; 23:1207–1211.

15

Ultrasonic Liposuction

Rhoda S. Narins
Dermatology Surgery and Laser Center
New York and White Plains, and
New York University Medical School
New York, New York, U.S.A.

Ultrasonic liposuction employs the use of ultrasonic energy to disrupt the adipocytes and liquefy the fat, making it easier for the surgeon to remove. I find it helpful in some patients as an adjunct to liposuction.

Michele Zocchi first presented the technique in 1988 and promoted it throughout the world in 1992 [1]. It was used as far back as the early 1980s by Zocchi and Yves Illouz [2,3]. Zocchi believed that ultrasonic energy had a direct micromechanical effect on fat as well as a cavitational effect resulting from prolonged energy delivery to the fat cells and thermal effects that he found insignificant but that others would soon find a problem. Zocchi felt the heat was distributed through the infiltrated tissue [3]. (I have measured the temperature of the tissue and of water after using the ultrasound machine and found no elevation of temperature, but patients report feeling heat if I use the machine for more than a minute or so in one area.) In addition, it was felt that the use of ultrasonic liposuction selectively targeted the low-density fat tissue and spared the intervening higher density connective and neurovascular tissue.

In the 1990s, ultrasonic liposuction became very popular in South America and Europe. Five U.S. plastic surgery societies formed a task force to study ultrasonic liposuction in 1995 [4]. It was then used extensively in the United States because many surgeons mistakenly thought that the benefits of markedly decreased bleeding and pain were due to the ultrasonic procedure rather than to the tumescent solution which was necessary for the technique to work. Imagine the amazement of a surgeon exposed to the tumescent anesthetic technique for the first time! Unfortunately, all of the benefits of the true tumescent technique of local anesthesia alone were not seen because the tumescent solution that was necessary for ultrasound to work was used along with general anesthesia (Chap. 1; Table 1). The use of general anesthesia allowed the removal of more fat at one time. In fact, the problems due to ultrasonic liposuction as well as to the large volumes of fat sometimes removed with this procedure were often mistakenly blamed on "tumescent liposuction" [5,6]. This, however, is not the "tumescent technique." The true "tumescent technique" using local anesthesia alone is extremely safe and general anesthesia is not used at all [7].

Ultrasonic liposuction was widely acclaimed throughout the plastic surgery world until complications such as seroma, burns, and sloughing were reported and many surgeons no longer use the technique (Table 2) [3,8]. It has been reported that although there is less blood seen in the canister as compared to regular liposuction without tumescent fluid, with ultrasound liposuction there is marked decrease in blood volume, which is still diminished 20% 1 week post surgery [8]. It was also feared that the use of ultrasound might affect the hearing of the patient or the surgeon as although ultrasound is outside the range of human hearing an audible sound can be

TABLE 1 Benefits of Tumescent "Safe" Liposuction

1. Minimal blood loss	No transfusions necessary
2. Anesthesia long lasting	Minimal pain
3. General anesthesia not needed; patient awake	Quicker recovery Patient move into position needed Less thrombophlebitis/pulmonary embolism None of general anesthesia's risks Less risk of perforation of body cavities Patients feel better post-op
4. Surgery limited by safe amount of lidocaine	Fewer ancillary procedures (e.g., face-lifts) Quicker recovery Shorter procedures
5. Tumescent solution antibacterial	Fewer infections
6. High volume of solution	Provides fluid replacement
7. Infiltration of fluid into fat maximizes tissue	Smaller cannulas and smaller incisions

TABLE 2 Ultrasonic Liposuction

Pros	Cons
Good for fibrous areas	Burns
Good for secondary procedures	Seromas
Good for gynecomastia	Skin sloughs
Good for male flanks	Learning curve
Good for female backs	Patient feels heat
Skin retraction	Cannulas limited shapes/size
Good for large fat deposits	Expensive equipment

heard during surgery. In a study done by Kenkel et al. it was reported that the sound intensity fell within the acceptable limits set by the Occupational Safety and Health Administration and was deemed to be safe [9].

Some surgeons use a hollow cannula to remove the fat with aspiration done at the same time while others, such as Zocchi, use a solid probe to liquefy the fat and then manually express it or use regular liposuction to remove it. The aspiration machine is used on low power, about .5 atm, and a hollow titanium cannula is used to remove the fat. The cannula is moved slowly to selectively target the fat. The probe is also titanium. The problem with using a probe is that there is no feedback to the surgeon about what is going on under the skin plus the procedure is very time consuming, necessitating two steps. The first step after injecting the tumescent fluid into the subcutaneous tissue is the emulsifying with the probe and the second is the evacuation of the fat [2,7]. Most of the cannulas are at least 5 mm in diameter. When I use ultrasonic liposuction, I use a shorter cannula only 4 mm in diameter. The shorter cannula gives me better control and the smaller diameter allows me to make smaller incisions that are still larger than the ones I make using regular liposuction. I use a No. 11 blade or a 16-gauge NoKor needle in order to make the smallest incision possible and then I spread it using a Gradle scissor. I use a Lysonics 2000 machine set on 4 or 5, which is 40–50% of available power. I do not use sutures or drains. I do use the crisscross cannula technique moving in a deep plane to avoid thermal injury and I stop as soon as I feel decreased resistance (Table 3). I have not needed to use a skin protector to avoid burns although they are available. The skin protectors do necessitate a larger incision.

Some surgeons use ultrasonic liposuction for the entire surgery. I have always thought it safer to use ultrasonic liposuction for only a short time to get through fibrous or scar tissue or to treat areas that need more destruction like male gynecomastia and then immediately go to conventional liposuction

TABLE 3 Tips to Decrease Ultrasonic Liposuction Complications

1. Use for short time only in any one area—stop when no resistance
2. Suction thoroughly postultrasonic liposuction using conventional liposuction
3. Use wet towel near incision to protect skin
4. Keep cannula 1 cm under skin
5. Use true tumescent local anesthesia so patient can tell you when they feel heat
6. Use compression garment post-op
7. Use shorter smaller (4-mm) cannula

to thoroughly evacuate the remaining as well as the liquefied fat. I have not seen a seroma develop. I believe this is because of the limited amount of ultrasonic liposuction I do in any one area, the adequate evacuation with conventional liposuction of all areas, and the postoperative use of French tape to provide support and get rid of any dead space. Others, including Rod Rohrich, agree with the increased safety of this limited use of ultrasonic liposuction (H. Brody, personal communication, 1997). However, many surgeons who do not use ultrasonic liposuction for the entire procedure still will use up to 10 min in an area where I might use 30 sec to 1 min [4].

One of the reported benefits of ultrasonic liposuction is the ease with which the surgeon can get through fibrous tissue when doing a repeat liposuction in an area where it was previously done or in scar tissue or in areas that are inherently more fibrous such as male gynecomastia, male flanks, and female backs. It is also useful in areas with large deposits of fat. Many surgeons feel that other benefits have never been adequately documented such as the elimination of cellulite, the retraction of skin, and the lack of harm to septae that carry nerves, blood vessels, and lymphatics. However, Mateo and Perez reported a "profound" retraction of skin in 2000 [10].

For the future, Illouz is working on a water-cooled ultrasonic machine that will be safer and easier to control and not have a problem with heat [3]. Ultrasonic liposuction has a definite learning curve and if you get good results with conventional liposuction, you may not need or want this technology. However, if you do repair (secondary) liposuction on patients who have had problems with previous surgery then ultrasonic liposuction may be a procedure you want to have available. When used carefully in a limited fashion, ultrasonic liposuction is a useful adjunct to conventional liposuction in the right patient.

REFERENCES

1. Zocchi M. Ultrasonic liposculpturing. Aesth Plast Surg 1992; 16:287–298.
2. Zocchi M. Clinical aspects of ultrasonic liposculpture. Perspect Plast Surg 1993; 7(2):153–174.
3. Illouz YG. History and current concepts of lipoplasty. Clin Plast Surg 1996; 23(4):721–730.
4. Baker JL Jr. A practical Guide to ultrasound-assisted lipoplasty. Clin Plast Surg 1999; 26(3):363–368.
5. Grazer FM, Meister FL. Complications of the tumescent formula for liposuction. Plast Reconstr Surg 1997; 100:1893–1896.
6. Coleman WP III. The history of liposuction and fat transplantation in America. Dermatol Clin 1999; 17(4):723–727.
7. Klein JA. The two standards of care for tumescent liposuction. Dermatol Surg 1997; 23:1194–1195.
8. Troilius C. Ultrasound-assisted lipoplasty: is it really safe? Aesth Plast Surg 23:307–311.
9. Kenkel JM, Donnell FJ, Rohrich RJ, Adams WP Jr, Roeser RJ. Hearing and Ultrasound-assisted liposuction: the effect on surgeon and patient. Plast Reconstr Surg 2000; 105:150–153.
10. Mateo JM, Vanquero Perez MM. Systematic procedure for ultrasonically assisted Lipoplasty. Aesth Plast Surg 2000; 24:259–269.

16

New Techniques: Powered Liposuction

Bruce E. Katz
Columbia University and Juva Skin and Laser Center
New York, New York, U.S.A.

William P. Coleman III
Tulane University Health Sciences Center
New Orleans, Louisiana, U.S.A.

EVOLUTION OF POWERED LIPOSUCTION DEVICES

Liposuction was originally developed by Giorgio and Arpad Fischer in Italy in 1975 [1]. When the Fischers first began to develop tools for this new technique, they assumed that some sort of cutting instrument would be required to efficiently remove subcutaneous tissue. Up to this date, all attempts at removing fat had been based on curettage. Eventually, however, the Fischers settled on blunt tipped cannulas for tunneling through the fat [2]. To assist, however, in this effort, they designed blunt instruments with sharp blades contained within the shafts. This so called cellusuciatome was a cannula with a removable blunt tip and internal blades to break up aspirated fat. Some of the Fischers' designs incorporated a motorized system to move the blades within the shaft of the cannula.

Subsequently, the Fischers as well as a second generation of liposuction pioneers, including Fournier and Illouz, recognized that liposuction could be performed just as well using only blunt-tipped cannulas without any sort of internal blade or powered function. When liposuction was introduced into the United States the standard method utilized large-diameter (8- to 10-mm) blunt cannulas containing one or two apertures. It was assumed that fat removal was primarily accomplished by the negative pressure generated within subcutaneous tissue by the suction device.

As liposuction became more widely used throughout the world, surgeons and manufacturers experimented with a variety of different cannula designs to reduce surgical effort. Areas of firm fat or those which had been operated on previously were resistant to the penetration of cannulas and required great physical effort to tunnel through. More aggressive cannulas with the apertures near the tip became popular. These sharper instruments allowed the surgeon to more easily penetrate through firm fat, but also increased bleeding.

Meanwhile, other surgeons began using smaller cannulas. Although originally designed to provide greater finesse, it soon became apparent that smaller (2-mm) diameter cannulas penetrated through fat more easily. The concept of using smaller cannulas to make numerous smaller tunnels instead of a few larger ones also resulted in smoother contours.

In the late 1980s, experimental work with ultrasound led to the development of ultrasonic liposuction cannulas [3]. These rapidly vibrating instruments were designed to penetrate fat more easily by liquefying adipocytes and creating cavitation in the subcutaneous tissue. Although these ultrasonic cannulas decreased surgical effort, complications such as thermal burns and skin necrosis were reported [4]. Many surgeons also complained of a lack of control because these instruments penetrated subcutaneous tissue so easily (much like a hot knife through butter). Manufacturers also produced ultrasonic cannulas only in larger diameters (4–6 mm) and many designs required skin protectors to avoid burns. The larger incisions restricted the ability of the surgeon to make multiple tiny incisions to approach the fat from multiple angles as had become commonplace using 2-mm cannulas.

In an attempt to obtain the benefits of decreased surgical effort provided by ultrasonic liposuction, but at the same time eliminate many of the negatives of this technology, a number of manufacturers began to experiment with power-assisted liposuction instruments in the mid-1990s. The first designs incorporated a blade within a cannula [5]. These were derived from orthopedic and head and neck instruments which incorporated burrs and various blade designs within a cannulalike sheath. Blades were exposed to tissue only through small apertures in the cannulas. The first instruments designed somewhat resembled the blade-within-a-cannula designs of the Fischers' 20 years before. They were intended for use in submental lipectomy through an open incision. Early researchers were enthusiastic about the potential of these devices to remove submental fat more efficiently than with closed blunt liposuction.

Eventually more sophisticated blade-within-a-cannula instruments were designed to be used for whole-body liposuction in a closed environment [6]. These instruments were quite successful in tunneling through more fibrous fat in certain anatomic locations such as the male breasts and flank. They were also useful in penetrating subcutaneous tissue which had undergone previous liposuction. However, because these instruments were more aggressive there was some concern about the potential for increased bleeding and they were never widely used.

In the late 1990s a number of U.S. manufacturers began to experiment with vibrating cannulas which moved several millimeters in a to-and-fro motion. These instruments were designed to vibrate at a rate of between 800 and 10,000 movements per minute. Because these devices did not create the thermal energy generated by ultrasonic instruments they were shown to have a similar safety profile to manual liposuction. However, the vibration allowed easy penetration of fat and more rapid removal of subcutaneous tissue. Powered liposuction instruments were designed to be used with a wide variety of cannula shapes and sizes, including those with very small diameters. Consequently, many of the same surgical techniques employed with manual liposuction, including multiple small crisscross tunneling, could be employed.

POWERED LIPOSUCTION EQUIPMENT

The first powered liposuction devices developed were driven by compressed gas. The advantage of these systems was that they could generate significant torque, but the chief disadvantage was that they were quite noisy. They also required the extra expense and inconvenience of maintaining compressed gas to drive the devices. Subsequently, several electric powered liposuction devices came onto the market. These were much quieter than the gas-driven devices and simply required normal 110-V electrical current.

One manufacturer (Byron Surgical) developed a disposable powered liposuction handle which was driven by the air discharged by a liposuction aspirator. This arrangement allowed the aspirator to perform two different functions. The chief disadvantages of this design, however, were the increased noise, comparable to that of gas-driven instruments, and the recurring cost of the disposable handles.

Recently the following powered liposuction instruments available in the United States were tested by an independent laboratory (Accelerated Reliability Test Centers, Winterpark, Florida) [7].

1. The Medtronic/Xomed PowerSculpt is an electric system driven by a 140-W brushless motor. It has a back-and-forth stroke of 2.8 mm. It has the lowest noise and vibration of the available units.
2. The Numed unit is electric and driven by a 90-W brush motor. It has a stroke of 2.5 mm. This unit displays higher noise levels than many of the other units.
3. The Wells–Johnson unit is electric and driven by a 40-W brush motor. It has a stroke of 2.0 mm. This unit has low vibration and is moderately noisy.
4. The Micro-Air PAL 100 is a pneumatic system driven by gas. It has a stroke of 2.0 mm. This unit has low vibration, but is quite noisy compared to the other units.
5. The Byron ARC unit is pneumatic, driven by the Byron PSITEC aspirator exhaust. It is available in 12-mm and 6-mm throw lengths. Testing revealed low vibration, but high noise, with this unit.

This demonstration of increased efficacy of powered over manual liposuction was apparent in all of the studied devices. However, some of the instruments appeared to be more effective than others. This may be due to differences in the rate of vibration. It is currently unclear whether slower or faster vibration provides optimal efficiency for removing fat. This is further complicated by the variations in the length of the to-and-fro movement generated by each instrument. The Byron device, for instance, is available in two different lengths of throw with the longest set at 1 cm. Many of the other devices have throws between 2 and 3 mm.

Radial movement intrinsic to vibrating cannulas is another potential variable. Some of the instruments appear to have more side-to-side vibration than others. This potentially increases the diameter of the tunnel in subcutaneous tissue and may lead to increased problems. There have been anecdotal reports of increased seromas from some surgeons who have begun to use powered liposuction. These appear to be more common with certain devices and with the use of larger diameter and longer cannulas.

Clearly powered liposuction is a more advanced way to remove fat which also reduces surgical effort. Patients also prefer the pleasant vibratory sensation associated with powered liposuction over the sensation felt during manual liposuction. This is much more critical as increased numbers of liposuctions are being performed under local anesthesia with minimal or no sedation. In one study, over 53% of patients preferred powered liposuction over manual liposuction while no patients preferred manual over powered liposuction [8]. (The remaining patients had no preference.)

Most surgeons prefer the decreased physical effort of powered over manual liposuction. Although powered liposuction still provides much of the "feel" of manual liposuction (as opposed to ultrasonic techniques). It enables the surgeon to more easily penetrate more fibrous fat. It also allows more finesse in sculpting more difficult areas such as the periumbilical region. The surgeon can literally hold the cannula still and allow the back and forth micromovement of the cannula to gently sculpt away fat.

The decision to choose among these various units should be based on the manufacturer's reputation and warranties, preference of electrical or pneumatic, the vibration of the unit, and the noise produced by the unit. All of these devices are capable of increasing fat removal per minute although studies have demonstrated that the Byron and Medtronic/Xomed units provided the largest increase in fat extraction.

THE POWERED LIPOSUCTION PROCEDURE

As with traditional liposuction, preoperative photos and informed consent are obtained. The patient is marked in the standing position and incision sites are placed asymmetrically to minimize any future stigmata of liposuction. Surgical prepping is performed in the normal fashion and an intravenous access line is started. Since the most commonly treated areas are the hiproll and outer thigh, the patient assumes either the prone or lateral decubitus position. The incision sites are injected and stab incisions are made.

Using a variflow pump, local tumescent anesthesia is infiltrated (0.05–0.075%) lidocaine according to the Klein formula with a maximum total dose of 50 mg/kg. Up to four sites are injected at one time. After 15 min. liposuction commences.

The powered cannula is assembled and connected to the aspiration hose. The number of strokes per minute (spm) are preset on the power console (depending on the brand of cannula) and range from 800 to 10000 spm. It is important to know the recommended spm setting for the particular power cannula being used as each type of cannula is most efficient at particular settings (Fig. 1).

The reciprocating powered cannula, at the tissue level, parallels in an extreme microcosm the manual movements that are performed using the traditional nonpowered cannula. It differs significantly in that the powered cannula stroke distance measures in millimeters, the distance traveled is always constant, and lateral movement is minimized thus reducing trauma to adjacent adipose tissue. The key to maximizing the benefits of powered liposuction is to introduce as few of the variables produced by vigorous manual movements. Thus moving the powered cannula as slowly as possible maximizes fat extraction and allows for more precise sculpting [8]. This is what has been described as the "learning curve" involved in power liposuction. The tendency to move the powered cannula quickly to and fro as

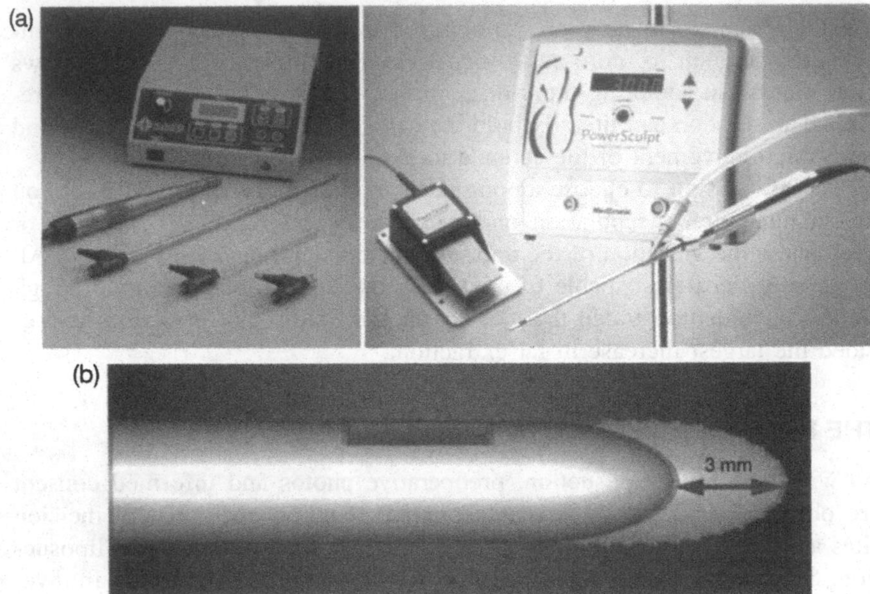

FIGURE 1 (a) Two types of reciprocating powered cannulas. (b) Reciprocating power cannula with 3-mm stroke distance.

with a traditional cannula minimizes the benefits of the powered device. This overly vigorous technique also creates similar trauma to adipose tissue and reverses the benefits of less edema and ecchymoses seen with the powered approach.

Once the customary aesthetic endpoint is reached, the patient is asked to stand for final contouring. Multiple digital images of the patient from various angles may be taken in the standing position so she or he can view her- or himself on the operating room television monitor to be sure he or she is satisfied with the results. Incision sites may be closed with sutures if gaping and the patient is placed in a compressive surgical garment, which is worn 24 hr a day for the first week and 12 hr a day for the second week. Follow-up visits occur at 4 to 6 days, 1 month, 3 months, 6 months, and 1 year postoperatively.

Power Liposuction and the Standing Technique

Performing liposuction with the patient in the standing position has obvious advantages over doing so in the supine position. It is not as precise to perform the procedure on fat contours that have changed position once the patient becomes supine. This is clearly why, preoperatively, surgeons mark the areas to be suctioned with the patient in the standing position. A better view of the areas to be contoured and how they blend with adjacent anatomic sites is also achieved with the patient standing. The tumescence from local anesthesia infiltration distorts the adiposities to some degree and must be taken into consideration.

A variety of devices and techniques have been described in order to perform liposuction in the standing position though they have had their limitations. An orthostatic liposuction operating table has been developed [9] which, during the procedure, moves the patient from the horizontal to vertical position. It incorporates a safety sling and footrest to hold the patient in place. In the event of sudden hypotension, the table quickly allows for the return to the supine position. Aside from the considerable expense of the table, the compression of tissues against the table even while in the vertical position limits accurate viewing of all the suctioned sites.

A technique of "standing epidural liposuction" has been proposed [10] due to the difficulty of assessing the patient while lying flat on an operating table. An epidural catheter instilling a combination of anesthetics is placed between T10 and L2 vertebrae. As this removes most sensory innervation while leaving motor tone intact, patients are able to stand during the liposuction procedure. The improved visualization of fatty contours when in the standing position led to improved results and more satisfied patients. Problems encountered with this approach included relaxation of the abdominal muscles leading to distortion of fatty contours. This prevented the use of the standing position for this anatomic site. Frequent transient hypotension necessitated fluid loading with 2 liters of Ringer's lactate preoperatively. The risks from the sudden movement of an in-dwelling epidural catheter while a patient is in the standing position are obvious.

When powered liposuction is performed in the standing position, only tumescent local anesthesia can be used and the patient is allowed to have a light breakfast. We have found that this virtually eliminates the occurrence of postural hypotension. If the patient has not eaten and begins to become light-headed upon standing, a 500-cc bolus of Ringers lactate or 0.3–0.5 mg of iv atropine may be given to correct this problem. Two operating-room nurses assist with supporting the patient and monitoring for vasovagal signs. "Fine-tuning" of fatty contours is performed with 2.5- and 2.0-mm powered cannulas. Because powered cannulas move very precisely and with short strokes, the "to and fro" movement is not "rough" on the patient as would be the case with a manual liposuction cannula.

Power liposuction performed with the patient in the standing position allows for precision of contouring and aesthetic results that we have found to be far superior to the traditional approach. The ability of patients to view themselves on a television monitor while standing and be satisfied with the results before leaving the operating room create a greater sense that their aesthetic goals have been fulfilled.

ADVANTAGES OF POWERED LIPOSUCTION

When any new medical technology comes along, its efficacy and risk/benefit ratio have to be carefully evaluated by controlled studies. If the results are positive, clinicians will wish to incorporate this technology into their practices. Ultrasonic-assisted liposuction is an example of a technology that was initially positively received. It was thought to improve the ease of fat removal and possibly increase skin retraction [11–13]. However, the greater incidence of complications with this technque, including burns, seromas, and skin necrosis, has led to a waning of its popularity among surgeons [4].

The results of two multicenter studies have shown that the use of motor-driven reciprocating powered cannulas when performing liposuction has significant advantages over traditional hollow manual cannulas [8,14]. When four different brands of power cannulas were compared to traditional cannulas in the first study, the powered devices were found to have a mean increase in fat extraction ranging from 21 to 45% [8]. In the second study, powered liposuction was performed on one side of the body and traditional liposuction was performed on the matching contralateral side. The amount of time taken to perform powered liposuction was 35% less, intraoperative pain was 45% less, and surgeons' strain was rated as 49% less than for traditional liposuction [14]. Postoperative pain, ecchymoses, and edema ranged from 32 to 38% less for the side of the body undergoing powered liposuction (Fig. 2). At 5 days and 2 weeks postoperatively, patient satisfaction with the powered liposuction side was greater but there was no difference in surgeons' satisfaction.

This data suggest that powered cannulas improve the safety profile of the procedure as patients are in surgery for shorter time periods (particularly when having intravenous sedation) and can return to normal activities more quickly (usually by the second or third postoperative day). The significantly faster recovery times achieved with this technology are also a major advantage. From the patients' perspective, the vibration of the power cannulas was found to be gentler and more relaxing than the shearing sensation of the traditional cannulas. The fact that surgeons' strain was significantly reduced with powered cannulas transforms this often physically strenuous procedure into a "no-sweat" technique. Reduced surgeon strain will be particularly appreciated in larger volume cases. A less fatigued surgeon can perform longer at a higher level of precision.

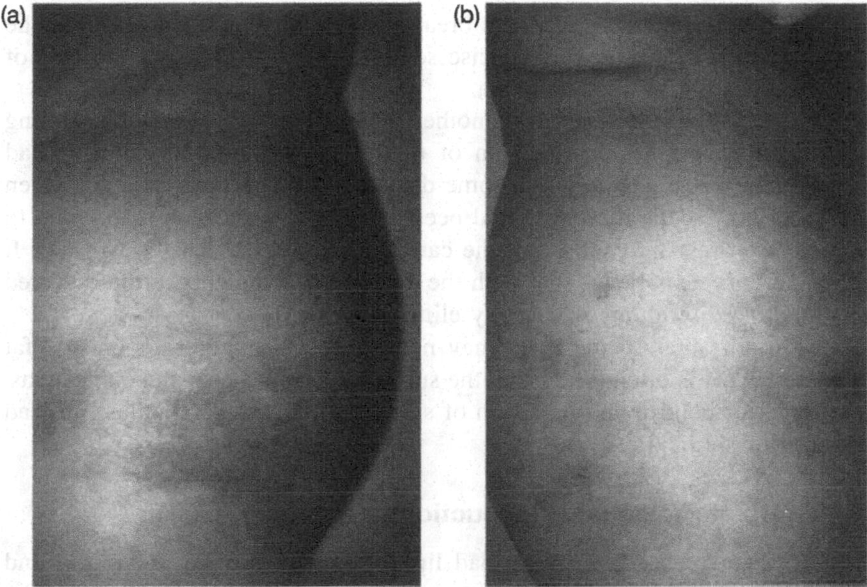

FIGURE 2 (a) Ecchymoses from manual liposuction cannula at 5 days post-operation. (b) Minimal ecchymoses from powered cannula at 5 days post-operation.

With any new procedure or technique some time and effort is required in order to master it (the "learning curve"). To an experienced liposuction surgeon who chooses to integrate powered liposuction into his or her armamentarium, the learning curve may not be apparent at first. The authors initially thought there was a minimal learning curve involved. However, review of the study data showed that there does appear to be a significant learning curve involved in powered liposuction in order to achieve its specific advantages. However, the advantages of faster healing and recovery for patients, shorter procedure times and greater fat aspirated per minute all make learning this procedure well worthwhile. Furthermore, surgeons have found the procedure significantly less fatiguing, resulting in safer and more precise surgery.

Special Considerations for Certain Anatomic Sites

Powered liposuction offers particular advantages when the procedure is performed in certain anatomic locations. It enhances surgical results by its increased precision and the reduced surgeon strain. The latter benefit is particularly appreciated in larger volume cases. However, fibrous areas like the hiproll, upper abdomen, and male breast require less physical effort by the surgeon while affording very precise sculpting with the fine movements of the reciprocating powered cannula.

The periumbilical area is another site where this superior sculpting ability is appreciated. Liposuction of this area with manual cannulas had been found in the past to cause some discomfort for the patient, even when adequate tumescent anesthesia had been infused. This was probably due to the gross jerking movements of the cannula against the sensitive tissues. It is the authors' experience that with the exacting movements of the powered cannula this discomfort is virtually eliminated.

Certain areas of the body may need only very small amounts of fat aspirated. This is often the case in the submental, arm, knee, and ankle areas. The superior control and precision of small reciprocating cannulas can lead to superior surgical results.

Touch-Up of Previously Liposuctioned Areas

Patients may present who have had liposuction of an area previously and either wish to have more adipose tissue removed or are unhappy with the results. If excess fatty tissue is still present, a repeat procedure may be performed. However, when liposuction is carried out in a previously suctioned area, the adipose tissue is often found to be more fibrous and the procedure becomes more difficult. The powered cannula offers advantages in such a case for reasons discussed above.

If the patient is unhappy with the previous liposuction surgery, it is often due to waviness and irregular contours of the subcutaneous tissues. This problem was seen more frequently when liposuction was performed under general anesthesia and the patient could not stand at the end of the procedure in order to be evaluated for contour irregularities. However, this complication can occur with any approach. To correct these contour defects requires careful marking of areas requiring more fat removal and areas that need to be avoided. Sometimes even autologous fat transfer may be necessary to fill in depressions. The reciprocating powered cannula has been a great aid in these cases where meticulous sculpting of often extremely small amounts of fat is required to even out these irregular contours. We have found this new technology very helpful in correcting problem cases which could not have been dealt with as well by manual cannulas.

COMPLICATIONS OF POWERED LIPOSUCTION

Multiple complications of traditional liposuction have been described, including ecchymoses, edema, skin irregularities, asymmetry, skin necrosis, drug interactions, seromas, infection, pulmonary embolism, and death [15]. This includes cases where liposuction was performed under general anesthesia and when ultrasonic-assisted liposuction was employed. Traditional liposuction carried out with only local tumescent anesthesia has had much fewer complications [16–17].

In over 161 powered liposuction cases performed at one of the authors' (BEK) center, complications included three seromas (2%) which resolved with aspiration and compression. Three cases of skin irregularities and asymmetry required touch-up procedures several months later (touch-up rate of 2%). Touch-up rates for traditional liposuction reported in the literature range from 10 to 12% [18]. The lower rate of complications and subsequent touch-up procedures seen with powered liposuction is probably due to the greater precision and control afforded by reciprocating cannulas and reduced trauma to surrounding tissues. Further studies are needed to confirm these findings.

SUMMARY

Powered liposuction offers significant benefits for both the patient and surgeon, resulting in safer and more precise surgical outcomes. Although long-term benefits have not been clearly delineated, there does appear to be a lower incidence of complications and touch-up procedures when the powered reciprocating cannula is utilized. A significant learning curve appears to be involved with this new technology. Powered liposuction appears to be a significant advance for the liposuction procedure.

REFERENCES

1. Fischer A, Fischer G. First surgical treatment for molding body's cellulite with three 5mm incisions. Bull Int Acad Cosmet Surg 1976; 3:35.
2. Fischer G. Liposculpture: the correct history of liposuction. Part I. J Dermatol Surg Oncol 1990; 16:1087–1089.
3. Zocchi ML. Utrasonic-assisted lipectomy. Adv Plast Reconstr Surg 1995; 11: 197–221.
4. Gingrass M, Kenkel J. Comparing ultrasound-assisted lipoplasty with suction-assisted lipoplasty. Plast Reconstr Surg 1999; 26:283–287.
5. Gross CW, Becker DG, Lindsey WH, Park SS, Marshall DD. The soft tissue shaving procedure for removal of adipose tissue. Arch Otolaryngol Head Neck Surg 1995; 121:1117–1120.
6. Coleman WP. Powered Liposuction. Dermatol Surg 2000; 26:315–318.
7. Flynn TC. An evaluation of current instrumentation available for powered liposuction. Dermatol Surg 2001. In press.

8. Coleman WP, Katz B, Bruck MC, Narins R, Lawrence N, Flynn TC, Coleman WP, Coleman KM. The efficacy of powered liposuction. Dermatol Surg 2001; 27:735–738.
9. Fischer G. Orthostatic liposculpture. Am J Cosmet Surg 1995; 12:211–218.
10. Shuter D, Drourr NR. Liposuction with standing technique: the true lipo "sculpture." Plast Reconst Surg 1999; 104:1546–1550.
11. Scuderi N, DeVita R, D'Andrea F, Vonella M. Nuove prospettive nella liposuzione: la lipoemulsificazone. Giorn Ital Chir Plast Ricostr Estet 1987; 2:1.
12. Zocchi M. Ultrasonic liposculpturing. Aesth Plast Surg 1992; 16:287–291.
13. Zocchi M. Clinical aspects of ultrasonic liposculpture. Perspect Plast Surg 1993; 7:153–158.
14. Katz B, Bruck MC, Coleman WP. The benefits of power liposuction versus traditional liposuction: a paired comparison analysis. Dermatol Surg. In press.
15. Klein JA. Tumescent Technique: Tumescent Anesthesia and Microcannular Liposuction. St. Louis: Mosby, 2000.
16. Klein JA. Tumescent technique for local anesthesia improves safety in large-volume liposuction. Plast Reconstr Surg 1993; 92:1085–1098.
17. Hanke CW, Coleman WP. Morbidity and mortality related to liposuction. Dermatol Clin 1999; 17:899–902.
18. Teimourian B, Adham MN. A national survey of complications associated with suction lipectomy: what we did then and what we do now. Plast Reconst Surg 2000; 105:1881–1884.

17

Assessing the Results and Liposuction Tips

Patrick J. Lillis
New York University Medical Center
New York, New York, U.S.A.

Rhoda S. Narins
Dermatology Surgery and Laser Center
New York and White Plains, and
New York University Medical Center
New York, New York, U.S.A.

There are a number of situations and body sites in which the results of liposuction may be inconsistent and/or the approach to treatment may present unusual challenges or controversy.

MALE NECK

In general, the skin of the male neck is very thick and heavy, with much more fibrous tissue. This is even more of a problem in older men where the skin is not only heavy, but loose. Neck lifts are difficult because the heavy skin tends to fall again. It is quite resistant to trauma. More aggressive instruments have to be used during liposuction. A more aggressive approach, including special maneuvers with the "smart" hand, is used to increase the amount of fat removed. A more thorough fat removal with more unloading of the compartment leads to better skin retraction. Most male necks benefit from this more thorough liposuction. Female neck skin, as well as some male's neck skin, is much thinner and lighter and contracts much more easily. Less aggressive liposuction is needed in these cases.

No matter what you do the amount of contraction in males with heavy skin is not as dramatic as in females. In addition, jowls do not contract and lift as well in men. Postoperative fibrosis can make touch-ups quite difficult. Dr. Narins uses ultrasonic liposuction for the first few passes in these difficult cases as well as in early cases of loose skin. This helps to get through the fibrous tissue as well as causing more skin contraction. A round and full neck with significant lateral fat also presents a problem. The skin directly underneath the chin retracts far better than the skin on the anterolateral neck underneath the angle of the mandibles. This becomes more of a problem with advancing age as the skin becomes less elastic and more loose.

Men with an anterior hyoid will not get as good a result because there is not much room between the chin and the neck mass.

Men in their mid-40s sometimes have the firmer skin of a younger man and sometimes the looser skin of an older man. In these latter patients and in most men over 55, skin elasticity is poor. In these cases liposuction may not be sufficient. Platysmaplasty and skin excision should be used along with liposuction to get the best results. Patients must be realistic about what they can expect to achieve. The physician should be very confident that the patient would accept a less than ideal result. Dr. Lillis uses the snap test, as one would in a lower lid blepharoplasty, to assess the

TABLE 1 Summary of Procedure for the Male Neck

Problems
- Round necks with significant lateral fat may not do well.
- Retraction is often better centrally than laterally.
- Men with an anterior hyoid do not get dramatic results.
- Jowls contract better in women.
- Heavier male skin does not retract well.
- Over age 45, skin laxity may be poor and the skin may not retract well.
- Do a snap test for skin elasticity.
- Make sure the patient will accept a less than ideal result.

Treatment
- More aggressive liposuction should be done in the male neck.
- Have patients wear the postoperative garment for a longer period of time.
- Consider ultrasonic liposuction for a short period of time.
- Consider skin excision and/or platysmaplasty.
- Consider the "Lilax" procedure with liposuction, laser resurfacing on the undersurface of the skin and excision with or without platysmaplasty.

laxity of the skin. Dr. Narins will often use a "Lilax" procedure, originally described by Dr. William Cook, that combines liposuction of the neck and subplatysmal fat, resurfacing using the CO_2 laser on the undersurface of the dermis, platysmaplasty, and excision of a small amount of skin in the submental crease. Many men do not want a face or neck lift and are usually satisfied with more subtle results if this is well discussed at consultation (Table 1).

MALE CHEST

None of the authors have seen a single case of skin damage from aggressive liposuction in this area. The skin in this area retracts consistently well in young men. The fat, however, is very fibrous and difficult to remove. Aggressive liposuction must be done with the use of the "smart" hand. This is another area where more thorough fat removal leads to a better result. Younger men also have significant glandular tissue. Removal of this tissue is necessary to obtain an ideal result. Some physicians make an incision around one-third of the way along the breast areola junction and remove the fat that way. After thorough liposuction, the authors use the liposuction incision sites and advance toward the glandular site that is under the nipple. Dr. Narins also uses ultrasonic liposuction for a short time in this area to get through the fibrosis and for skin retraction. Using a forceps or hemostat the glandular tissue is pulled out through the incision sites with visible retraction of the areola and nipple as this is done. Some of the glandular tissue is removed and the rest allowed to fall back into the subcutaneous space. When enough glandular tissue has been removed, the procedure is finished. The surgeon can palpitate the glandular tissue under the areola to determine when enough tissue has been removed. Subcutaneous fibrosis may be quite significant for several months postoperatively. This does not affect the final result.

In older men the area is more easily treated, as there is less glandular tissue and less fibrosis. Thorough fat removal is easily achieved in this age group. It is important to make sure that the tail of fat that runs from the lateral breast under the arm is removed. This can be quite significant in the older man or the younger man who is overweight. The skin will retract to a considerable degree in the older patient but not as completely as in the younger individual. Patients should be counseled preoperatively as to the result they might be likely to achieve. Revisions for fine-tuning are rarely necessary in younger men and older men usually want nothing further done (Table 2).

Table 2 Summary of Procedure for the Male Chest

Problems
Young men have very fibrous breast with a lot of glandular tissue.
Young men may have prolonged postoperative fibrosis.
Young men usually achieve excellent results.
Older men get very good results without as complete skin retraction.
Older men have less glandular tissue.
Treatment
Aggressive and thorough liposuction is necessary in this area.
Aggressive cannulas must be used in this area.
Excision of glandular tissue is necessary especially in the younger individual.
The tail of fat from the lateral breast under the arm must be removed for the best results.
Revisions are seldom necessary in the younger person but may give 10–20% improvement in the older patient who is generally not interested in having anything further done. Dr. Narins uses ultrasonic liposuction for 1–2 min before regular liposuction just to get through the fibrosis and retract the skin.

MALE ABDOMEN

The male abdomen should be divided into two age groups (young and old) and the upper and lower abdomen should be discussed separately. The skin of the abdomen in men is quite thick and resistant to trauma. Neither author has observed cases of ulcerations or erosions in the abdominal skin in hundreds of male patients despite very thorough liposuction. This is another area where better results are seen with aggressive liposuction. A thin layer of fat should be left under the skin for the smoothest results but it can be thinner than that left in women because of the thickness of the male dermis.

Dr. Lillis has had difficulty achieving total anesthesia consistently in this area while Dr. Narins has not had this problem. The upper abdominal fat can be quite fibrous in both younger and older men and retracts better than upper abdominal skin in women. In many older men with "beer bellies" it is hard to achieve any result in this area because the skin is right on the muscle and the fat is around the organs behind the muscle. This is the so-called beer belly. This type of fat deposit only responds to diet, although the lower abdomen is usually amenable to surgery. This problem with visceral fat that does not respond to liposuction surgery leads to a high rejection rate of 25–30% of men consulting for liposuction in both author's offices.

Table 3 Summary of Procedure for the Male Abdomen

Problems

- Thick skin with fibrous tissue, especially in the upper abdomen.
- Skin contracts well.
- Some physicians find it difficult to get total anesthesia using local anesthetic solution. (Dr. Narins feels that using 5–10 cc of 1% lidocaine around the umbilicus and 0.1% lidocaine tumescent solution rather than 0.05% solution helps in achieving total anesthesia in this area.)
- Seromas can be seen if liposuction very thorough. (Dr. Narins believes that wrapping the area with French Tape prevents the formation of seromas.)
- Periumbilical area may require touch-ups. (Dr. Narins sometimes uses ultrasonic liposuction for a few seconds around the umbilicus to decrease the number of touch-ups required.)
- Men tend to have more bleeding in this area than in women.
- Older men may have a lot of visceral fat in the upper abdomen, which is not amenable to liposuction.
- In older men, skin retraction is less in the upper abdomen and suprapubic areas.

Additionally, in older men, the heaviness of the dermis as well as the loss of elasticity with age can produce significant laxity. This also occurs in the suprapubic area, which does not contract as well as the suprapubic area in women. Dr. Lillis feels that the aspirate in men is usually bloodier than in women.

It is important to remove all of the periumbilical fat as in women so that the need for touch-ups is diminished or eliminated. Dr. Lillis has had three men who developed seromas 1–2 weeks after surgery due to vigorous physical activity. He warns his patients to curtail explosive physical activities for 3–4 weeks postoperation. Dr. Narins has her patients avoid contact or jarring activity for 3–4 weeks as well. She also wraps the area for 1–2 days postop with French Tape and has them wear an abdominal binder for 3 weeks (Table 3).

LOVE HANDLES

Liposuction of the flanks, or love handles, in young men is a consistently rewarding procedure. Skin contraction is usually complete and a more youthful contour can easily be achieved. The skin is much thicker and more fibrous than that of the female waist. Dr. Lillis has seen one case of "erythema ab igne" by another physician, who may have been overly aggressive

TABLE 4 Summary of Procedure for Love Handles in Males

Problems
Consistently good results in younger men.
Skin is usually thick and area often fibrous.
Significant improvement in older men but some skin laxity usually is present.
Treatment
Consider doing the lower back in selected individuals due to the collapse of lower back fat after the flank fat is removed.
Vigorous liposuction can be done in this area but leave a thin layer of fat just under the skin.

with liposuction as well as coming too close to the underside of the dermis and leaving no fat at all.

In older men, a significant improvement is the rule, but it is common to have some skin laxity. These fat pads tend to go right around the back almost to the spine. Dr. Lillis believes that removal of the flank fat sometimes exposes lower back fat in older men, which then tends to fall without support from the flank fat. This underscores the importance of preoperative evaluation. This can occur in older men as well as younger men who are overweight (Table 4).

FEMALE UPPER ABDOMEN

Skin contraction of the upper abdomen in women is rarely complete and this is discussed with all patients at consultation. It is common in both younger and older women to have some degree of laxity as compared with the impressive contraction and tightening of the skin seen in the lower abdomen. When the patient bends her head forward to look at the upper abdomen, this accentuates the wrinkling in this area even when there is no apparent laxity when the patient is in the erect standing position. Dr. Narins feels that small touch-ups in this area, when required, improve results.

Fat is usually more fibrous in the upper abdomen and more difficult to remove. It may be more difficult to anesthetize and usually requires 0.1% lidocaine tumescent solution rather than 0.05%. It is not uncommon to leave a strip of fat underneath the submammary line, which may have to be removed at a later date. Careful marking can obviate this problem. This same phenomenon can occur of the wrapping does not go all the way up to this line leaving some swelling and persistent fullness behind.

TABLE 5 Summary of Procedure for the Female Upper Abdomen

Problems
Skin contraction not as good as that of the lower abdomen.
When the patient leans forward to look at the upper abdominal fat, this increases the folding and irregularity. This is what the patient sees.
The fat in this area is more fibrous than that of the lower abdomen.
Skin retraction is worse in the area just above the umbilicus where "hooding" can be seen.
Treatment
Liposuction should continue all the way up to the submammary line if significant fat is present in this area.
Liposuction of the upper abdomen should usually be done when operating on the lower abdomen even if it appears to be unnecessary.
Touch-ups in this area may provide enhanced results.

Skin retraction is often poor in the area just above the umbilicus. If the rest of the skin of the abdomen contracts well but this are does not then this may lead to "hooding" or a "frownlike" appearance, with a little extra skin pouching over the umbilicus. Excision of the skin in this area leaves a noticeable surgical scar and both authors rarely do this.

Both authors treat the upper abdomen 90% of the time when doing the lower abdomen even if it appears to be unnecessary. If this is not done, a touch-up in this area will often be needed after liposuction of the lower abdomen alone. After liposuction of the lower abdomen with the excellent skin retraction in this area, the upper abdominal fat becomes more apparent. It is also possible that in a patient who stays the same weight or gains weight after liposuction the fat accumulates in other areas, including the upper abdomen, which then becomes more prominent (Table 5).

FEMALE LOWER ABDOMEN

Uniformly good skin retraction occurs with liposuction of the lower abdomen, especially if the patient is young with good skin turgor. Even in the older, overweight woman there is significant retraction of the skin, even when a panniculus is present. Thorough liposuction, always leaving a small smooth layer immediately under the skin, gives excellent results. The thicker the skin, the thinner the layer of fat that should be left behind. The deep and midabdominal fat should be removed. If the patient has very thin skin with multiple striae, their expectations should be much lower and a thicker layer of subdermal fat should be left behind to keep the area smooth.

The abdominal musculature must be taken into account. A patient with a rounded abdominal muscular wall will not achieve a totally flat abdomen without a muscle repair. Most women past 35 with children will have some muscular rounding even if it is minute. Some patients who are markedly overweight have a protrusion similar to a "beer belly" with the fat around the organs and these people are not candidates for liposuction.

Some patients, especially if they are very young, may just need liposuction of the lower abdomen alone. Most need liposuction of the lower and upper abdomen. If the patient is a little overweight, they may need a procedure called the Hourglass Abdomen with liposuction of the upper and lower abdomen as well as the waist, hips, posterior waist and lower back for the best result.

When a shelf of fat hangs over a suprapubic (Pfannensteil) incision, this can be easily removed with thorough liposuction and undermining of the bound-down incision with a Toledo undermining instrument. Significant improvement occurs.

Stretch marks do not affect the procedure but they do not disappear. Remember to treat the pubic area in most patients. It can also become more noticeable postoperatively unless it is treated.

Do not sweep the cannula in a windshield washer fashion and remove all the fibrous septa in the area. This will create large open spaces that will increase the rate of seroma formation. Dr. Lillis feels that when the fat is thoroughly removed in very large abdomens, seromas may develop and are easy to treat with two to three simple evacuations of the serosanguinous fluid. Dr. Narins has not seen a seroma in this area and she feels it is because she wraps the area with French Tape postoperatively and this closes the dead space.

Dr. Lillis uses punch openings of 1.5–2 mm in diameter as per Dr. Jeffrey Klein's recommendation. He uses these primarily in the lower abdomen and in the suprapubic area, where the most drainage occurs. Dr. Klein and Dr. Lillis feel that these round holes stay open and drain better than slits. Drainage is necessary for the best results. Dr. Narins sees no difference between slits or punch holes and in fact has more ecchymoses on the lateral thigh with punch holes than with slits.

Dr. Lillis uses Reston Foam to wrap the abdomen postoperatively underneath a compression garment. This is left on for 48 hr. He feels this improves drainage and enhances his results. Both Dr. Narins and Dr. Klein are opposed to Reston Foam as they have both seen the skin ripped off when the tape is removed, causing pain and scabbing of the area. Dr. Lillis has seen skin erosion on two occasions. He has not seen it in 3000 other patients on whom he has used it. Dr. Klein knows of a case where presumably the Reston Foam Wrap caused sloughing of the skin. Dr. Lillis uses Reston

TABLE 6 Summary of Procedure for the Female Lower Abdomen

Problems

- Most women have excellent contraction of this area even if they have a panniculus.
- Make sure to treat the area around a Pfannensteil or other incision.
- Point out rounded muscle wall to patient at consultation.
- Evaluate patient for Hourglass Abdomen.
- The suprapubic area may need to be treated if liposuction is not done at the same time as liposuction of the lower abdomen.
- Seromas can be seen postoperatively.
- Fat pocket may be seen postoperatively around the umbilicus.
- The most sensitive area for pain is around the umbilicus.

Treatment

- Wrap the area with tape postoperatively to avoid seromas.
- Do not use windshield wiper movements with the cannula, which increase the chance of seromas.
- Do liposuction of the suprapubic area at the same time.
- Make sure the area around the umbilicus is treated thoroughly. Dr. Narins feels that ultrasonic liposuction for a few seconds is often helpful in this area.
- Dr. Narins uses 10 cc of 1% lidocaine around the umbilicus for greater anesthesia of this area.
- Drainage incisions are important for this area.
- Thorough liposuction around incisions, including the Pfannensteil, and undermining of the bound-down fibrous scar with a Toledo underminer.

Foam on the abdomen and on large lateral thighs and occasionally on the waist. There is also a risk of allergy to the adhesive in the foam (Table 6).

FEMALE WAIST

The female waist responds beautifully to liposuction and the entire female form is enhanced. Even a small amount of liposuction in this area produces a pleasing curvature. It is often necessary to treat the hips and sometimes the back for the best results. This area contracts well in virtually every women and is a major "patient pleaser" (Table 7).

FEMALE HIPS

The female hips are another great area for liposuction. Results are consistently good. This is a wonderful area for beginners to do for their first cases.

Table 7 Summary of Procedure for the Female Waist

Problems

- Consistently great results in everyone.
- This is a major "patient pleaser."
- May need to be blended into other areas for best results.

Treatment

- Do liposuction of the hips in most patients and the back where necessary for the best results.
- This is part of the Hourglass Abdomen.

Table 8 Summary of Procedure for Female Hips

Problems

- Consistently great results.
- Usually cannot remove too much fat in this area. Can occasionally do too much in thin-skinned individuals.
- Great area for beginners.
- May need to do other areas for best results and blending.

Treatment

- Do not remove too much superficial fat in thin-skinned people.
- Make sure top get the deep fat pad.
- Liposuction may need to be done at the same time on the waist and the back for the best results.

Small cannulas can be used. Dr. Narins uses two incision sites and Dr. Lillis uses three to four. It is difficult to have a problem in this area. As mentioned previously, the back and waist may need to be done at the same time for the best results (Table 8).

BACK

The back is rarely done in men except to blend in the flanks in older men. The back has by far the thickest skin in the body with the most fibrous tissue. Skin damage does not occur in this area from regular liposuction even when it is extremely aggressive. More aggressive instruments can be used in this area. It is not necessary to worry about removing too much fat in the back. The more you remove, the better the skin contraction (Table 9).

TABLE 9 Summary of Procedure for the Back

Problems
Fat is usually quite difficult to remove as skin is thick and the area has a lot of fibrous tissue.
The greater the fat removed, the better the contraction of skin.
Warn the patient that a bulge may still be present when the bra is on and a roll may still be present postoperatively.
Treatment
Use aggressive cannulas and take out as much fat as possible. Make significant use of the smart hand.
In selected patients, consider doing the upper back for blending.

ANTERIOR AXILLA (ANTERIOR "BRA FAT") AND POSTERIOR AXILLA (POSTERIOR "BRA FAT")

Female patients are very bothered by bulges of the anterior or posterior axillae, anterior or posterior "bra fat," because they cannot wear strapless dresses or other revealing clothing. Wearing a bra actually accentuates these fatty lumps. Significant improvement is seen with liposuction, especially of the anterior axillae. Thorough liposuction gives the best results. Again, the more thorough the liposuction, the better the skin contraction. Aggressive or nonaggressive cannulas are used for the anterior pockets and aggressive cannulas are used for the posterior pockets. The fat comes out easily in these areas. It is important to treat infra-axillary fat at the same time if excess fat is present. If this fat is not treated the area will bulge and hang over the bra (Table 10).

TABLE 10 Summary of Procedure for the Anterior and Posterior Axillae

Problems
There will still be some redundant skin postoperatively when the arms are at the side.
Patients are asymmetric preoperatively and may be postoperatively as well.
Treatment
Thorough liposuction with small and aggressive cannulas gives the best results.
Consider doing the infra-axillary fat if a significant amount is present.

UPPER ARMS

In the past, the upper arms had the reputation of being very difficult areas to do. Patients are often told they need skin removal, which requires a long and unsightly vertical scar. Liposuction of the arms is limited strictly to females. Thorough deep liposuction leaving pinchable subdermal fat produces the best skin contraction and the best postoperative appearance. The usual area treated is the posterior compartment but the biceps area should be treated if there is excess fat. It also can take longer than the usually stated 6 months to get maximal results from contraction.

Patients with thick skin can have very thorough liposuction and achieve excellent results. The more thin-skinned patient needs more subdermal fat left in place. The wrinkled skin of older patients will contract well but occasionally the wrinkles become more accentuated. The patient should be made aware of this at consultation. These wrinkles are still superior to the brachioplasty scar. Take into account that the skin over the biceps is thinner when doing the procedure.

There are usually fat pads, which the patient is often not aware of, present just distal to the medial condyle. If any fat is present in this are it

TABLE 11 Summary of Procedure for the Upper Arms

Problems
- Impressive contraction is usual.
- Be careful of irregularities in thin-skinned people.
- Thin skin with fine wrinkles will contract well but the wrinkles may become accentuated. Make the patient aware of this.
- Circumferential liposuction is never done in this area but biceps fat should be treated if present. The biceps skin is thinner so be careful here.
- Postoperative fat lumps can occur over the medial condyle, in the more fibrous skin above the posterior elbow and in the most proximal area to the axillae if they are not treated thoroughly at the time of the initial surgery.

Treatment
- Thorough fat removable leaving some subcutaneous fat gives the best results.
- Leave more subcutaneous fat in the more thin-skinned individual.
- Treat the fat pads over the medial condyle, over the posterior elbow and the area most proximal to the axillae with extra attention to prevent the need for touch-ups.

must be removed. If this is not done, it will become very evident postoperatively and a touch-up will be required. All experienced liposuction surgeons routinely do this area initially. Fat is very soft in the arms and is easily removed except in the area immediately above the posterior elbow where it is more fibrous and the smart hand must be used to immobilize the fat and suction it more aggressively.

The areas that commonly require touch-ups by the inexperienced operator include the area just proximal to the elbow and the most proximal arm fat near the axillae. Make sure to concentrate on these in the initial procedure (Table 11).

OUTER THIGH

Beginners often assume that this area, "saddlebags," is the easiest to treat and would be a good choice for their first case. The upper outer thighs can, however, be problematic. If the patient has poor skin tone, even with a perfect technique, cellulite, irregularities, and some skin laxity may persist. This should be discussed at consultation. Perhaps the biggest mistake is to take too much fat out over the trochanteric area leaving a depression that is often impossible to totally correct. Proper positioning of the patient and experience are necessary to avoid this pitfall. In addition, always leave a small subdermal fat layer for the best results.

The lower outer part of the buttock is involved in the saddlebag deformity and is always done with the outer thighs by Drs. Lillis and Narins. Dr. Narins almost always does some liposuction of the buttock and hip areas as well when a violin deformity is present for the best results. A moderate amount of deep and midlevel liposuction is done in this area and in patients with good skin tone actual lifting and rounding of the lower outer buttock will be seen. Patients that have "banana" deformities should be warned that these may never be totally corrected [see Upper Posterior Thigh (Banana Roll) below].

Drs. Lillis and Klein use 2-mm punch holes at the most dependent area of the upper outer thigh to enhance drainage while Dr. Narins uses an incision with a Nokor needle or a No. 11 blade. Dr. Lillis uses Reston foam postoperatively over large saddlebags for 48 hr while Dr. Narins uses French Tape for 24 hr. Dr. Lillis has occasionally seen a patient at 48 hr where one side has drained more thoroughly than the other, which at times may leave a persistent irregularity requiring touch-up at a later date. Dr. Narins has not seen this complication. Occasionally Dr. Narins will have a patient with large outer thighs stand toward the end of the procedure to better evaluate the endpoint. Dr. Lillis feels that he does the most touch-ups on the outer thighs and abdomen (Table 12).

Table 12 Summary of Procedure for the Outer Thigh

Problems

- The lower outer part of the buttock is usually involved in the saddlebag deformity.
- The hips and buttocks are involved with a violin deformity.
- Drainage can be a problem in this area.
- Small touch-ups of the outer thighs are not uncommon in patients with very large volume and if skin tone is poor.
- Trochanteric depressions may occur that can be severe when too much fat is removed from the area over the joint.

Treatment

- Proper positioning of the patient can prevent trochanteric depressions in susceptible individuals.
- Drainage incision or punch hole at most inferior point.
- Do liposuction on the lower outer buttock as well as the outer thigh for all saddlebag deformities and the hips and buttocks, especially the lower outer buttock, for a violin deformity.
- Tell patients with extremely large fat volumes in the outer thigh that they will probably need a touch-up.
- Dr. Narins has patients stand occasionally towards the end of the procedure to better evaluate the results.
- Always leave a small subdermal fat layer for the best results.

CIRCUMFERENTIAL THIGH

Some liposuction surgeons routinely do circumferential liposuction of the thighs. Dr. Lillis rarely does the lower two-thirds of the anterior thigh or the posterior thigh. He feels that in patients with average or poor skin, skin retraction is often poor in these areas. He avoids these areas unless the problem is significant enough to warrant the risk of laxity. There rarely is fat in the posterior thigh except in the unusual patient or in the banana roll. Dr. Narins agrees that it is usually the upper third of the anterior thigh that is the problem. She will, however, do circumferential liposuction of the thighs in the patient with very heavy legs and a large amount of anterior thigh fat evaluated with the patient standing on their toes. Otherwise she would prefer to sculpt the outer thighs, inner thighs, and knees. Results after circumferential liposuction take many months to be realized, sometimes up to a year postoperatively for total contraction.

Be careful not to remove all of the superficial fat so that patients do not get erythema ab igne from disruption of the vascular system. Also, do not perform circumferential liposuction of the thighs at the same time as

TABLE 13 Summary of Procedure for the Circumferential Thigh

Problems
- Dr. Lillis feels that people with poor skin may have poor skin retraction in the lower two-thirds of the thigh.
- Circumferential liposuction takes a longer time to recover from.
- Severe swelling may occur when circumferential liposuction is done at the same time as the calves and ankles. Do not do both of these areas at once.
- Patients can get erythema ab igne from disruption of the superficial vascular system in this area.

Treatment
- Do circumferential liposuction only if the patient really needs it; otherwise sculpt the outer thighs, inner thighs, and knees.
- Do not do circumferential liposuction at the same time as the calves and ankles.
- Stay away from the superficial fat so that patients do not get erythema ab igne.

circumferential liposuction of the calves and ankles as you can overwhelm the lymphatic circulation and get severe swelling (Table 13).

INNER THIGH

Skin tone of the inner thigh is usually poorer than that of other areas. This is discussed with the patient preoperatively to make sure that patients with poor skin turgor have realistic expectations. A thicker layer of subdermal fat should be left in this area as compared to other areas such as the hips and waist. This gives a smoother result and allows the deep fat to be suctioned more thoroughly, giving more skin contraction and a better result.

It is important to have the garment fit correctly going all the way up to the inguinal crease, otherwise a touch-up procedure may be necessary. If a garment comes a few centimeters below the crease, it will create a proximal bulge, which may not go away. If this bulge is observed in the first 24 hr, proper instruction on how to wear the garment may correct the problem.

For the beginner, failure to suction the anterior fat thoroughly is another reason a touch-up might be required. It is often difficult to blend the inferior part of the inner thigh with the midthigh if there is no good demarcation. Blending is necessary in this area. If the medial knee and the inner thigh need to be done, then the bridge between them should also be

TABLE 14 Summary of Procedure for the Inner Thigh

Problems
Many patients have poor skin tone in this area. Expectations must be realistic as laxity and/or some irregularity can occur.
Beginning liposuction surgeons often leave fat bulges in the anterior as well as the proximal posterior inner thigh.
Thin-skinned individuals may have more laxity and/or irregularities postoperatively.
If the garment is not pulled up to the inguinal crease a persistent bulge may appear.
Treatment
Counsel the patient preoperatively as to poor skin turgor and postoperative laxity and/or irregularities.
Be sure to remove the fat in the anterior inner thigh and proximal posterior inner thigh.
Leave adequate subdermal fat, especially in the more thin-skinned patient.
The entire medial knee, inner thigh, and the area in between should be blended to give optimal results.
Positioning is important for beginners.

done for blending. In addition, the posterior inner thigh needs to be blended into the banana roll if it is present.

Patients, even those with poor skin turgor, are usually happy to have these uncomfortable protuberances removed (Table 14).

UPPER POSTERIOR THIGH (BANANA ROLL)

Liposuction of the banana roll can be very problematic; never tell the patient that you can totally improve this area. If thorough liposuction of this area is done, there may be ptosis of the buttock. When the patient bends forward, a significant concavity may be seen. A double or triple skin roll may occur postoperatively that can be treated only surgically, and then not very well. This roll occurs where the posterior thigh fascia thins out and the deep fat bulges through. If too aggressive liposuction is done to get at this fat destroying some of the fascia, that is when buttock ptosis can appear. The deep fat in this area should be avoided for this reason. Both Drs. Narins and Lillis stay away from this area in patients with very poor skin turgor and use small nonaggressive instruments superficially to try to flatten the convexity in patients with better skin tone (Table 15).

TABLE 15 Summary of Procedure for the Upper Posterior Thigh

Problems

Overaggressive suctioning can lead to ptosis of the buttock as well as double and triple rolls that are usually not amenable to treatment.

A deep depression may appear in this area when the patient bends forward if too much fat is suctioned from this area.

In patients with poor skin tone and overaggressive suctioning, the area may appear worse postoperatively.

Treatment

Do not suction the deep fat in this area.

Use nonaggressive cannulas and suction superficially.

Do not suction this area in a patient with very poor skin tone.

In a patient with good skin turgor, suction the upper half of the superficial fat for the best results, which will not be perfect.

Counsel the patient preoperatively that the results in this area are never perfect.

KNEES

The knee can be divided into four compartments. The most commonly done and most gratifying is the area over the medial condyle. There is usually a tail extending inferomedially under the patella and this should be addressed at the same time to give a nice curve to the calf. Dr. Narins does some liposuction on the entire medial upper calf to really enhance the shape of the leg. Skin contraction is virtually complete over the medial condyle. As mentioned previously, consideration of blending the midthigh should be given if the upper inner thighs are to be done.

The second compartment is the area over the lateral condyle that is present in 5–10% of people. Fat should also be removed from this area if it is present to obtain the best results. This area has consistently good results with good skin contraction.

The third compartment is the suprapatellar area that patients often complain about. Skin retraction is poor here and the weight of the anterior thigh presses down on it. Often this is only loose skin and suctioning may result in little visible improvement. In addition, overzealous suctioning can lead to a depression in this area with a noticeable "shelf" above it. It is hard to blend it in to the thigh above it. Dr. Narins may do a little liposuction in this area using small nonaggressive cannulas, and Dr. Lillis avoids doing it.

The fourth compartment is present in a small percentage of people who have three to four fibrous pockets of fat over the patella. Short, small,

TABLE 16 Summary of Procedure for Knees

Problems

Fat deposits are common in the medial knees and great results are the norm.

The tail of fat under the inferomedial patella should be addressed.

Suprapatellar fat does not respond well to liposuction and carries the risk of leaving a depression with a shelf above it. This skin does not retract well.

In 5–10% of people, the fat pad over the lateral condyle can be prominent.

Treatment

The fat over the medial condyle responds easily to liposuction.

Always remove the ail of fat inferomedial to the patella if it is present. Dr. Narins also removes some of the fat from the upper medial calf to get the shapeliest legs.

Suprapatellar fat removal should be done lightly or not at all because of the many problems in this area, including postoperative depression with an overhanging shelf, as well as the difficulty in blending this into the thigh above this area.

Always remove the fat over the lateral condyle if it is present.

Small fibrous pads over the patella can be suctioned aggressively using the smart hand to pinch and immobilize the fat and these may or may not improve in appearance.

and aggressive cannulas should be used in these areas and the surgeon must make use of the smart hand to pinch and immobilize the fat. The area is quite fibrous and gristly and the fat can be very difficult to remove. These fat deposits really bother the patient and they are very grateful to have them treated. Results are not uniformly good (Table 16).

CALVES AND ANKLES

Calves and ankles have the reputation of being problematic. In our experience, liposuction of the ankles and calves gives consistently good results. The patient is often evaluated with the patient standing, sometimes on their toes and occasionally there seems to be no fat over the calves, just skin and muscle. These latter patients should be reevaluated with a pinch test with the leg raised and the muscle relaxed to more accurately decide how much fat is present. For the beginner, it is sometimes difficult to differentiate relaxed muscle from overlying fat.

Liposuction of the ankles and calves should be done using multiple small incisions and multiple small nonaggressive cannulas. The tight circumference and shape of the leg and ankle may make positioning difficult initially. Thorough deep fat removal is desirable. A variable layer of subdermal fat should be left to give a smooth result. As in other areas, more subdermal fat should be left in the more thin-skinned patient. The patient turns during the procedure 360 degrees so that all areas can be done around the entire leg and ankle.

The patient needs to walk to the kitchen and bathroom to prevent deep venous thrombosis but also needs to elevate the legs above the heart for the first 3–4 days when they are not walking to prevent swelling. This will decrease recovery time. A medical-grade support stocking should be worn for 2 weeks and longer if swelling persists. Debulking of the thighs should not be done at the same time as that of the calves and ankles as this puts too much stress on the lymphatic drainage system.

Liposuction of the calves and ankles is one of the most gratifying areas to treat, as the fat in this area is quite diet and exercise resistant. Most patients with thick ankles and calves have had problems with this area since their early adolescent years and are thrilled to have the fat gone (Table 17).

Table 17 Summary of Procedure for Calves and Ankles

Problems

- More difficult to do because of the tight circumference of area, the need to turn 360 degrees during the surgery, and the need for good positioning to get to the fat, especially that around the ankle.
- Thorough deep removal of fat leaving some subdermal fat gives the best results.
- Swelling can be severe and may persist for several days to weeks.
- Uniformly good results can be expected.

Treatment

- Because of positioning problems and the tight circumference, multiple small incisions must be made.
- Leave some subdermal fat, especially in the thin-skinned patient, for the best results.
- Use small nonaggressive cannulas.
- Elevate the legs for much of the first 3–4 days to speed up recovery. Swelling can last 2–8 weeks and it is important to wear medical grade support hose for the first 2 weeks and longer if swelling persists.
- Do not overwhelm the lymphatic system by debulking the thighs at the same time as liposuction of the calves and ankles.

18

Megaliposculpture and Therapeutic Megaliposculpture

Pierre F. Fournier
Private Practice
Paris, France

INTRODUCTION

Ten years ago, we proposed the name megaliposculpture to all liposculpture procedures during which is extracted 10 liters or more of a mixture composed of adipose tissue, the normal saline from the subcutaneous infiltration, and the patient's blood. The proportions of each of these elements vary according to the case, and only the quantity of adipose tissue is taken into consideration. The evaluation at the same time of the hemoextraction, the visible fraction of the blood loss that conditions the pursuit or the abandonment of the intervention, is of such importance that it is necessary to closely watch over this parameter. Its qualitative and quantitative importance determine the volume of pure lipoextraction.

At the time of his initial demonstration in Paris in March 1977 at the Muette Clinic, Giorgio Fischer, father of this technique, declared before the observing surgeons that lipoextraction (the name given to this operation at the time) was not a treatment of obesity and that he had conceived this technique, as a cosmetic surgeon, solely to be part of the cosmetic surgeon's armamentarium to treat localized adipose parts of the body. He offered to his colleagues, cosmetic surgeons, a closed operation that eliminated the dermolipectomies (proposed by Ivo Pitanguy) in many cases, thus making it a preferred procedure.

This closed technique of lipoextraction avoided the long scars and, at the same time, transformed dermolipectomy (a procedure also designed to modify the shape of the body and not excess weight) into a procedure of lesser importance. Nevertheless, the idea of using this procedure to treat obesity and to extract large quantities of adipose tissue readily occurred to everyone, both surgeons and patients, even if this concept only corresponded to the treatment of the consequence, being overweight, and not to the cause itself of obesity.

This affirmation of Giorgio Fischer, creator of the technique and the conditions in which the procedure took place at the time [hospitalization, frequently the use of general anesthesia, the use of large cannulas and of the machine, absence of infiltration ("dry technique" or infiltration without adrenaline), a large number of blood transfusions, problems with fluid and electrolyte balance, hypovolemic shock, long convalescence, lack of practice by surgeons, complications or unsatisfactory results, and lack of updating the procedure] made surgeons fear that a lipoextraction of more than 2 liters was the cause of the difficulties of resuscitation and of more frequent and more serious problems. The taboo of 2 or 2.5 liters was created from this fact and so respected that from time to time, those extractions of 5–6 liters were considered exceptional performances.

Little by little, the quantity of adipose tissue extracted increased once it became certain that large extractions would pose no additional risk to patients who were candidates for such operations. With Nestor Asurey, my assistant, we first practiced megaliposculptures in two stages at 6-month intervals: 8 liters was extracted from the lower extremities during the first stage and 6 months later 6–8 liters was extracted from the abdominal wall. After the cap of 8 liters, corresponding to 6 liters of pure adipose tissue, we reached the limit of 10 liters for a large number of patients, then that of 12 liters, then 14 liters, then 16 liters, then 18 liters, then 20 liters and so on, until we reached a maximum of 23 liters, corresponding to about 17 liters of pure adipose tissue.

This quantitative work was spread out over 10 years and it was found to be greatly stimulated by an identical work occurring almost simultaneously by our colleagues M. Eed in Saudi Arabia and A. Fikioris and G. Ioannidis in Greece, who treated cases similar to ours and used the same technique. In this way, little by little, the taboo of 2.5 liters was destroyed and was replaced by confidence in megaliposculpture. This procedure must only be performed by a surgeon trained in megaliposculpture; selection of patients must be careful, and the anesthesiologist must be trained for operations on obese persons and must work in coordination with the surgeon and his team. Both the anesthesiologist and the surgeon must each know when to stop before going too far and never induce greater risks to the patient than would be possible during the course of a standard liposculpture.

To this day more than 800 cases have been performed with no mortality by the following surgeons, who currently practice this operation: Dr. Eed, world leader in this kind of surgery; Drs. Fikioris and Ioannidis; Dr. Carson Lewis in California; Dr. Giorgio Fischer in Rome; Dr. Furio Ferrari in Torino; Dr. Yelda Felicio in Brazil; Dr. Louis Madgdi Fanous in Abu Dhabi; Dr. Cesar Morillas in Peru; Dr. Hernandez Perez in El Salvador; Dr. Eduardo Krulig in Venezuela; and Dr. Louis Benelli in Paris. This permits us to be optimistic, even if, one day or another, as in any surgical operation, a serious complication should arise.

WHY PERFORM MEGALIPOSCULPTURE?

Failures in current medical or surgical therapies for the obese justify megaliposculpture. Athough the cause itself of the obesity is not treated by this megalipoextraction of adipose cells, the target is reached, but only in part, since lipectomy is concerned only with superficial excess and not the deeper excess of adipose tissue.

A certain part of hypertrophied or hyperplaised adipose cells are definitively removed from the catastrophic influence of the cause of the obesity. In this way, one can expect an improvement in the physical condition of the patient while provoking disturbances in the generative process of the obesity. One could compare this disease, obesity, to a war in which there is one enemy and several victims. If a counterstroke leading to victory is not possible, the first thing to do is to protect the victims or at least, in the case of obesity, to shield them from the catastrophic action of this cause. In this way, one can expect that the lesser the quantity of vulnerable tissue subjected to the disastrous cause, the better the body can fight against this biologic and metabolic anomaly. This attempt to reduce the vulnerable tissue territory can attenuate the potential life-threatening consequences of obesity.

It is well known that obesity can cause or aggravate the following pathologies: cardiac diseases, high blood pressure and stroke, pulmonary diseases, diabetes, gall bladder disease, gout, certain cancers, osteoarthritis of weight-bearing joints, an abnormal level of lipids and plasma lipoproteins, and irregularity of the menstrual cycle. Moreover, obesity is often an enormous psychological burden. When all the conventional treatments have failed, megalipoextraction is the last course of action. It should be regarded as a major life-saving operation and not just as an esthetic procedure.

The goals of megaliposculture or therapeutic megalipoextraction are (1) to extract in a single operation the greatest possible quantity of subcutaneous adipose tissue for the patient without running a greater risk than that in the course of a normal liposculture and without needing to perform any type of blood transfusion (autologous or not): The result of this operation is a numerical reduction of the subcutaneous adipose cells; and (2) to provoke biological metabolic or psychological modifications in the patient, following a diet, exercise, or medical treatment, which will result in decreasing the intraabdominal and intramuscular adipose tissue and residual components of the excess adipose tissue. The result of these postoperative biological modifications is a reduction in the volume of the adipose cells in these two areas, where a mechanical reduction is impossible to perform.

INDICATIONS

Megaliposculpture is a major operation that can produce serious complications and is selected only after thorough reflection by both patient and surgeon. Another criterion is that other medical or surgical treatments have failed to reduce obesity. The patient must be informed of the risks and is asked to reflect for a period of time.

In the beginning, we operated on patients weighing between 100 and 150 kg presenting with no comorbidities, e.g., high blood pressure, cardiac or pulmonary problems, and diabetes. Eventually we operated on patients over 150 kg, the heaviest patient weighing 210 kg. It was only on his insistence that we decided to operate. The ideal patient does not exceed 100 kg; it is with these patients that one achieves the best results. At the present time, we accept, with the agreement of our anesthesiologist, certain obese patients who also have high blood pressure, cardiac, pulmonary, or diabetic problems only if the risk does not appear to be too great.

Our results indicate that megaliposculture does not solve obesity, but rather additionally treats people with obesity, high blood pressure, certain cardiac or pulmonary problems, and other problems associated with obesity. In certain cases of ambulatory difficulties, e.g., vertebral osteoarthritis of the hip, an abdominal megaliposculture can reduce chronic vertebral pain or chronic pain in the hips or knees or, as orthopedic surgeons have suggested, it might prolong the life of hip prostheses by removing the excess weight.

Having obtained positive results, we became more and more adventurous in our applications. We are convinced megaliposculture has a place in the treatment of obesities, whether general or regional.

MATERIAL AND METHODS

Anesthesia

Therapeutic megaextractions are done under general or epidural anesthesia. We prefer epidural, which is the least toxic for the obese patients and permits them to be moved without risk, if necessary (Fig. 1). However, general anesthesia is often requested by the patients, even if they are informed that it is slightly more risky and that there will be more bleeding. The anesthesiologist must be accustomed to operations on obese people and be trained for this type of operation, which is completely different from the current cosmetic liposculture. The anesthesiologist and the surgeon work in close collaboration with each other [2].

Once the actual operation has been completed, the surgeon must monitor the operated regions and must take part in the follow-up. Our anesthesiologist has the major responsibility for the patient's fluid and electrolyte balance and the monitoring of the vital functions. His role during a mega-extraction is of utmost importance in the selection of the patient, the resuscitation, the follow-up of the operation, and the convalescence.

Surgical Technique

This is obviously preceded by the physical and psychological selection done by the surgeon and anesthesiologist. Megalipoextraction is possible due to

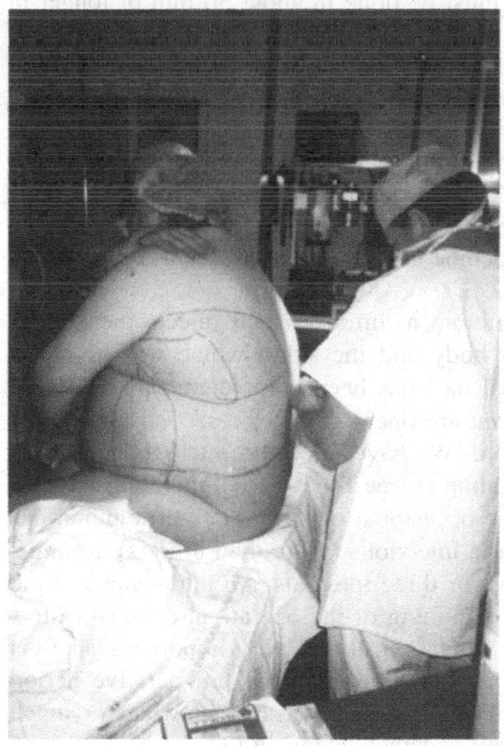

FIGURE 1 Epidural anesthesia is preferred to general anesthesia.

use of a large amount of normal saline. We have learned that it is possible to inject into the subcutaneous area 10, 15, or even 20 liters of a normal saline which is cold at 2°C, and each liter can contain 1 mg of adrenaline (1 ml if 1:1000). This amount of normal saline allows us to avoid postoperative hypovolemia and considerably limits pre- and postoperative bleeding.

Subcutaneous Infiltration Technique

The operation begins as soon as the epidural anesthetic has taken effect or immediately after induction of general anesthesia. The surgeon will do this by her- or himself or, as is more often the case, with the assistance of an operating assistant, who must be equally competent.

The only syringes used are the 60-cc syringes with a Luer-Lock tip fitted with a cannula of 2.5 mm external diameter and 28 cm length. A second assistant fills them in a basin that contains several liters and hands them over to the operating surgeons. The infiltration is made in the thick part of the subcutaneous tissue and is a retrograde injection, each operating surgeon making injections in symmetrical locations drawn in advance. Quick infiltration should be avoided. It must be done in about 30 min or longer if the area to be operated is very extensive. The infiltration is done at one time or, if the area is extensive, at three sequential separate times, allowing $\frac{1}{2}$ hr between infiltration and lipoextraction. The first infiltration is in the abdomen, then the sides, the thorax, the gynecomastia, then last the hips, outer and inner thighs, the front of the thighs, and the knees. The head of the operating table is elevated 15°. The four-handed operation begins as soon as the abdomen is ready to be operated on, i.e., 20–30 min after the end of the infiltration. An infiltration machine could also be used but we prefer to infiltrate with syringes.

During the abdominal operation, a third assistant injects the second region to be operated, the upper body and the sides, which will be ready for operation when the abdominal part has been completed. Finally, while the surgeon and his or her assistant are operating on the second region, the third and the last region is injected. We have injected up to 10 or 12 liters of cold normal saline with adrenaline at one time before operating with no major complications. Even so, the occasional occurrence of arrhythmia has made us prefer, in the case of large injections (more than 8 liters), to inject the areas to be operated on in two or three intervals. An intravenous of the normal saline is instituted at the beginning of the operation; only 1–2 liters is given during the course of the operation, this is very important. There is no reason to start this intravenous rehydration in the preoperative period even though certain surgeons do. Fatal complications happen when too much fluid is given intravenously as well as subcutaneously [3].

Operative Technique

The operation is done exclusively with the aid of 60-cc plastic Toomey syringes. The vacuum machine is not used and could be even harmful in the cases of esthetic liposculpture and even more so during a therapeutic megalipoextraction. We use 60-cc syringes mounted with cannulas of 4 or 5 mm in external diameter. The French model of the cannula, passing through the barrel of the syringe, is preferred over the American Tulips, which is fixed externally on the end of the syringe. In order to lock the plunger of the syringe during an extraction, a groove in the form of a hook is made on one of the wings of the plunger of the syringe. This system of locking the plunger allows us to avoid the use of metallic, heavy, cumbersome, and useless locks. This instrument is therefore light and thus does not "scrape" the adipose tissue, as did the cumbersome and heavy instruments when the machine was used (an operation during which there was significant pre- and postoperative bleeding, as confirmed by Vladimir Sidor, our anesthesiologist, in a hematological study) [2].

A light instrument is more enjoyable, more efficient, better controlled, and less fatiguing for the surgeon. In order not to lose time, one will have at his or her disposal four systems of cannula–syringes with intrinsic lockage, and one will commence the operation after having waited 30 min once the injection has been made. Once the syringe is filled, each surgeon exchanges it for another cannula–syringe unit prefilled with 5 cc of normal saline, which is given to him or her by a third assistant. The role of this assistant is solely to empty and fill in advance the syringes that he or she takes from or returns to the two operating surgeons. It takes about 10 s to fill a 60-cc syringe.

This method, with two operating surgeons and one assistant (Fig. 2), allows a considerable amount of time to be gained and is much more rapid than the machine technique and overall does not have one of the disadvantages of pre- and postoperative bleeding, which becomes more important without the buffering action of the 5 cc of normal saline which is present in the syringe at the moment of the extraction.

An average operating surgeon will extract about 5 liters/hr. Thus 2 hr are necessary to extract 20 liters (Fig. 3). The injection itself and the time waiting for it to take effect takes 1 hr. The preparation of the patient and the epidural anesthesia takes another hour. The preoperative drawing, which determines the operating regions in exactly symmetrical zones, permits each operating surgeon to do his or her job efficiently, rapidly, and of identical quality. The work of the first assistant must replicate that done by the principal operating surgeon.

Throughout the entire operation, the anesthesiologist informs the surgeon of all possible variations in vital functions and assures fluid and elec-

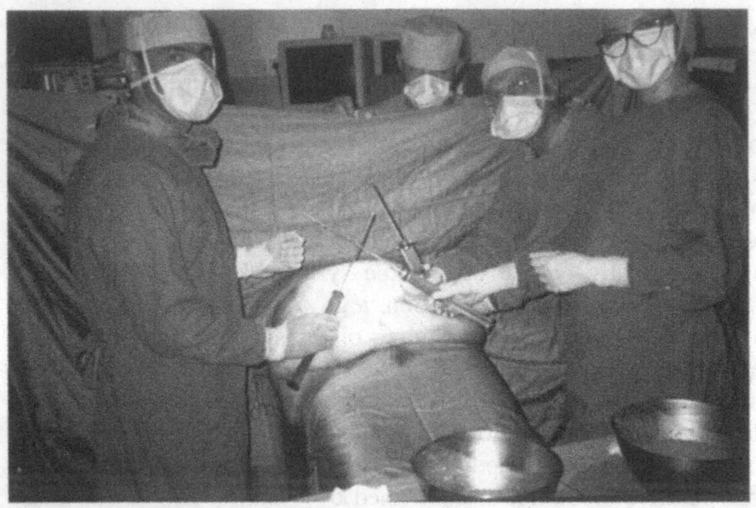

FIGURE 2 Two surgeons extract and another exchanges full syringes.

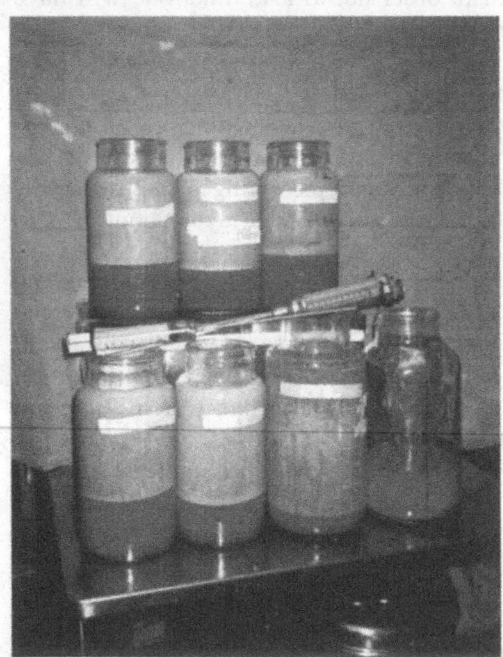

FIGURE 3 Extraction of 20 liters of adipose tissue: use of 14 liters of cold normal saline (1 mg of adrenaline per liter).

trolyte balance of the patient. The operation must also be as minimally hemorrhagic as possible. A prolonged extraction that is too bloody will force the procedure to be stopped. Sometimes it will be necessary to turn the patient over, which is done with the usual precautions. The operating table is head-up at 15° during the entire operation. The extraction will be done according to the usual criss-cross technique. Once the operation has been terminated, the cutaneous penetration points are sutured, and the elastoplast bandage (10-cm-wide-strips) is used unless one uses the elastic garment right away. The patient then remains in the recovery room under strict observation for 2 hr before being taken back to his or her room.

During the majority of large lipoextractions, megaliposculpture is interrupted when there is no more subcutaneous adipose tissue to be extracted. In the regions that are completely treated, the residual excess of the patient's adipose tissue is represented only by the intraabdominal or intramuscular adipose tissue. Even for a patient weighing 210 kg, once 21 liters have been removed, the operation has to be interrupted since almost the entire subcutaneous tissue has been extracted. This demonstrates the importance of a postoperative dietary regime, as the problem is not entirely solved by a single surgical operation.

Follow-up and Postoperative Care

In his or her room, the patient is kept in a semirecumbent position in order to facilitate easy breathing and to avoid compression of the diaphragm muscle. The same evening the patient will sit up and, as soon as he or she is able, recommended to move his or her legs several times per hour and to breathe deeply.

The postoperative monitoring (electrocardiogram, pulse, blood pressure) is maintained for 24 hr. The epidural catheter is maintained for 24–48 hr, and only the anesthesiologist decides when the analgesic solution should be injected. The urinary Foley catheter is maintained for 24–48 hr. Temperature and urine output are monitored, as well as hemoglobin, serum proteins, and electrolytes. The anesthesiologist must be accustomed to such operations because hemodilution can persist for several days. Antibiotics are routinely administered (vibramycin 100 mg b.i.d. for 5 days), as well as anti-inflammatories (Reparil or Extranase, 2 pills t.i.d.). In our patients, fluid and electrolyte balance is done by the anesthesiologist. In general, one gives either 1 liter of normal saline or Ringers solution every 6 hr for 2–3 days.

The surgeon observes the dressing, which sometimes needs to be changed due to light bloody saline discharge. The importance of this discharge should be explained before the patient's operation in order to avoid useless worries. It is psychologically beneficial to tell the patient that the greater the discharge, the better the postoperative result and the less residual edema. Thus the patient views this unavoidable discharge favorably.

RESULTS

In the days following the operation, an inflammatory reaction occurs that lasts 6–8 weeks. The operated tissues will harden and become sensitive, which is completely different from the immediate postoperative period, when they were soft. When the bandages are changed after 24 hr, the modification of the silhouette is impressive (Fig. 4). Then, over a few days the inflammatory reaction begins and the patient finds her- or himself with the same configuration as in the preoperative period. It is this inflammatory reaction that explains why the patient's weight is not modified in the first few weeks. It is not until 2, 3, or sometimes 4 weeks that the weight loss begins. It is more or less rapid right away, but it varies from one patient to

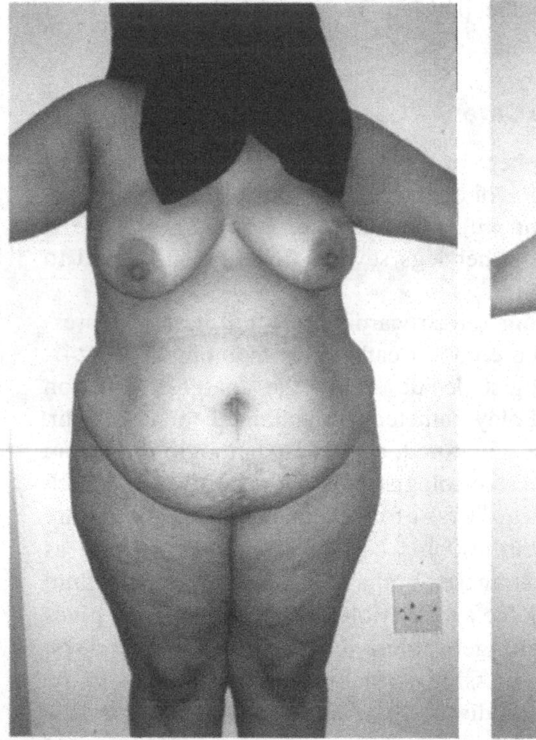

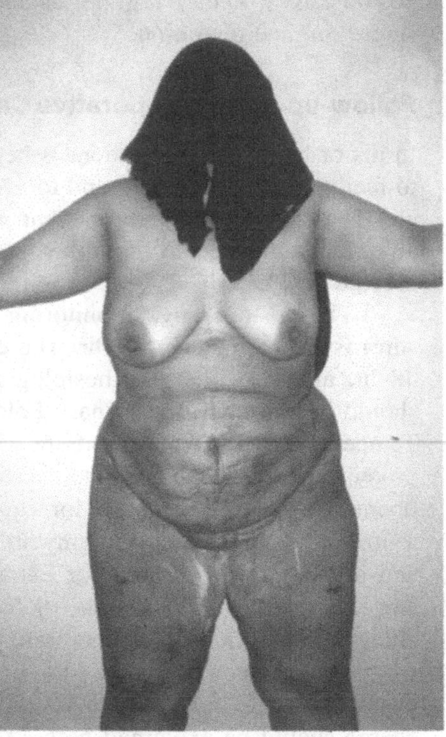

FIGURE 4 Before (left) and after (right) (result after 24 hr) a 12-liter extraction.

the next. It is also associated with a softening of the operated tissues, which become less tender, allowing the patient to move more easily. The urine output also increases considerably. This weight loss will be approximately equivalent to the weight of the quantity of adipose tissue that was extracted. It is after this weight loss begins that it is determined whether the patient should follow a diet. In about 20% of patients, the weight loss in the months following the operation is less than the quantity of adipose tissue extracted.

The majority of patients notice a sudden loss of appetite that lasts several months. Whatever its origin, whether psychological or due to metabolic modifications, it is very frequent. Fatigue is variable from one patient to another and is not necessarily linked to volume of blood loss. The drop in hemoglobin is not as important as one would think. Megaliposculptures of 15 liters do not vary the hemoglobin level by more than 1 g. The drop can sometimes be greater than 1–3 g, but one must take into account hemodilution, which makes the appreciation of the true blood loss difficult. Strict iron therapy is, however, routine for several weeks.

The hospital stay varies from 2–5 days according to the patient. Following discharge from the hospital, convalescence of 1 week is necessary. Normal activities may be resumed 10–15 days after the operation. Aided by a nutritionist, the patient commences dieting after 8–10 days. Iron supplements, vitamin C in normal doses, and a high-protein diet is recommended. The patient will see the surgeon at frequent intervals (Figs. 5–10, patients before and after 1 year).

Complications

Moderate anemia, fatigue, and a loss of appetite may occur postoperatively. It is unavoidable for a large extraction of adipose tissue to cause localized as well as generalized reactions, and a patient who cannot understand this should not be operated on. The psychological motivation of the patient is indispensable for a favorable outcome. It is more a matter of therapeutics rather than aesthetics even if aesthetics play a role (Fig. 11). The goal is to obtain an almost certain weight loss due to lipoextraction that is followed in most patients by a second weight loss which is related to dieting, exercise, and to therapeutic medication administered postoperatively (Figs. 12–14).

Local Complications

A moderate cutaneous necrosis of a few square centimeters occurred on the abdomens of three patients, attributed to a liposculpture that was too superficial. This healed in a few weeks. A larger one on the thighs took 2 months to heal, as the patient refused a skin graft (Fig. 15). After 6 months surface irregularities, excess of skin, and depression of the adipose tissue are treated

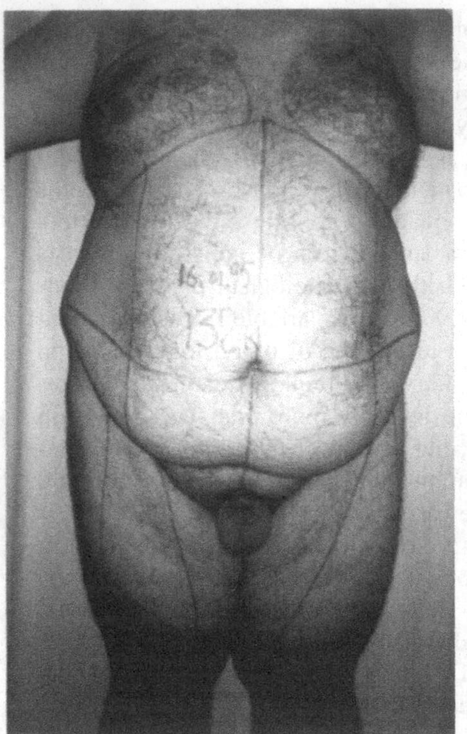

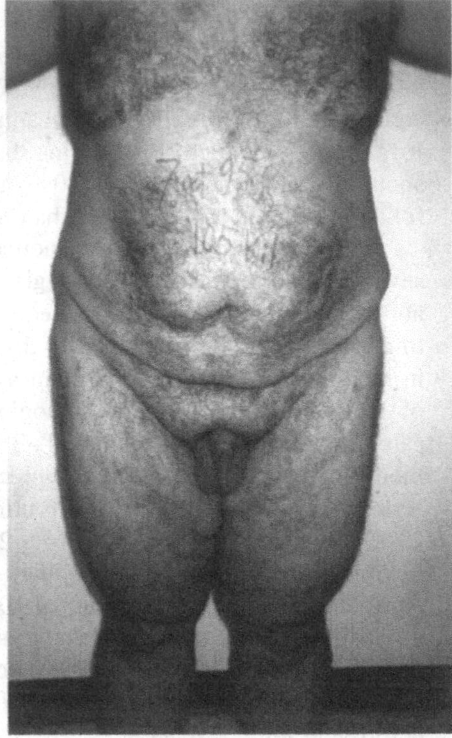

FIGURE 5 Before (left) and after (right) (9 months) 27 kilos lost. The result was maintained for 6 years.

by dermolipectomy if the patient wishes, but few patients ask for it since cutaneous retraction is good or the patients simply does not wish to be treated. A normal appearance is often noted spontaneously because of the thinning process postoperatively. Before the operation the patient is duly informed of the possible local aesthetic discrepancies and the possibility of eventual surgical operations.

When working on the abdominal region, we have had several lymphatic effusions. They are frequent when the megaliposculpture reaches 15, 17, or 20 liters. One can notice them on the third postoperative day. They disappear after 5–6 weeks and can be tapped two to three times. The quantity extracted varies from 1 to 3 liters. We have not had an infection in between the punctures. Patients receive moderate compression postoperatively from the elastic garment and also antibiotics.

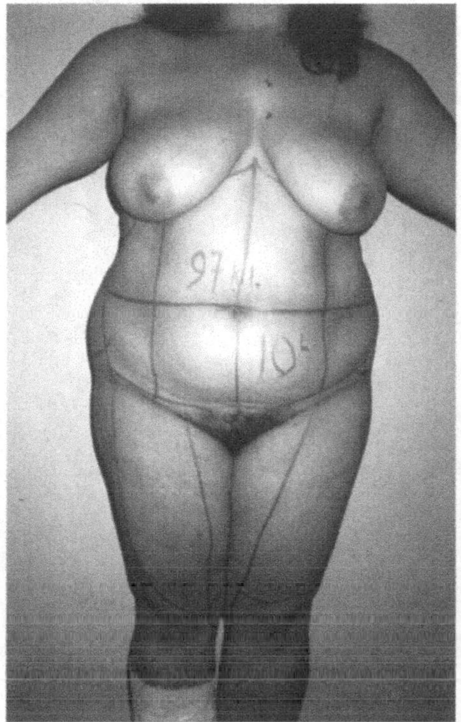

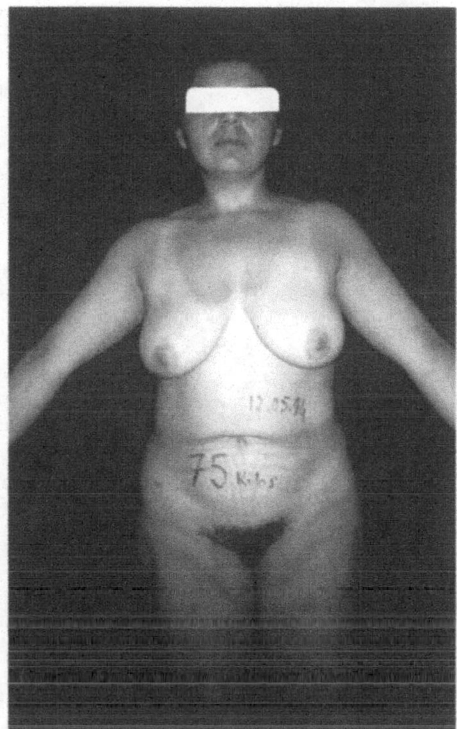

FIGURE 6 Before (left) and after (right) (1 year) 22 kilos lost.

General Complications

We have not had hypovolemic shock due to the pre- and postoperative fluid and electrolyte balance. Aside from the cold saline injections, the intravenous therapy is left entirely to the anesthesiologist. This intravenous treatment is discontinued 24–48 hr after the operation. In one patient, acute pulmonary edema occurred the night following the operation. Blood letting of 1 liter rapidly improved the condition of this 150-kg patient, from whom 15 liters of adipose tissue had been extracted without difficulty. The 15-liter lipoextraction corresponded to the essential excess of subcutaneous adipose tissue from the abdomen and thorax, the remaining excess being mostly intra-abdominal. The patient left the hospital on the fourth day, and when he returned 6 weeks later, he had lost 26 kg.

The analysis of this unusual and dramatic complication was a learning experience. The obese patient was breathing mostly with his diaphragm and little with his ribs, which were laden with adipose tissue. The cause of this

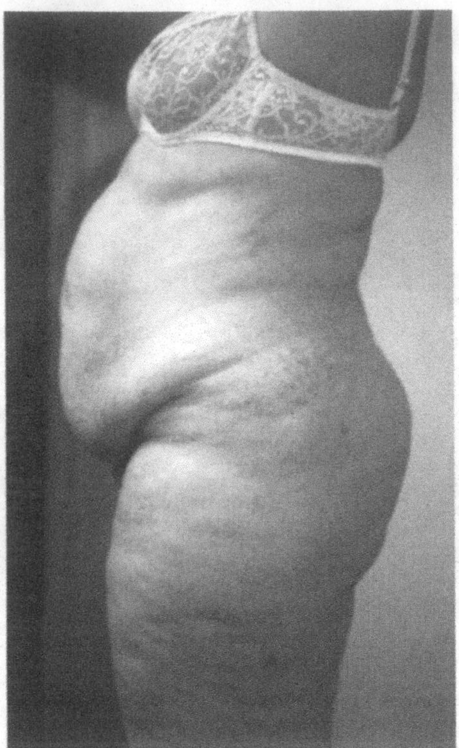
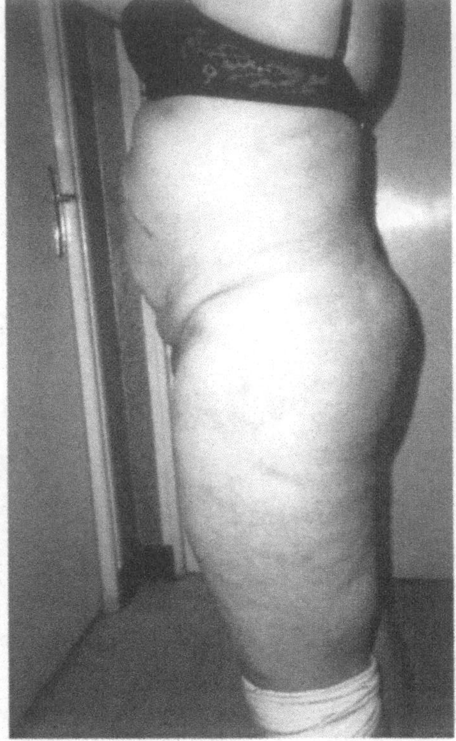

Figure 7 Before (left) and after (right) (1 year) photos showing excellent skin retraction.

acute edema appeared to be due to the abdominal bandage made of elastoplast strips that were unintentionally too compressive and also due to the strictly horizontal position of the patient in his bed. This excessive compression and the vertical pressure due to the weight of the intra-abdominal internal organs (where excess blood had accumulated) considerably hindered the movements of the diaphragm, further accentuated by the strict horizontal position of the patient on the operating table and then in his bed. The 15° head-up position of the operating table has subsequently been adopted as a matter of routine. This semirecumbent position is maintained long after the operation while the patient recovers in his or her hospital bed. The bandaging should be occlusive but not compressive. One could think that the acute edema in this case was due to a fluid excess, due to the 8 liters of normal saline that were injected subcutaneously. However, we have injected in all

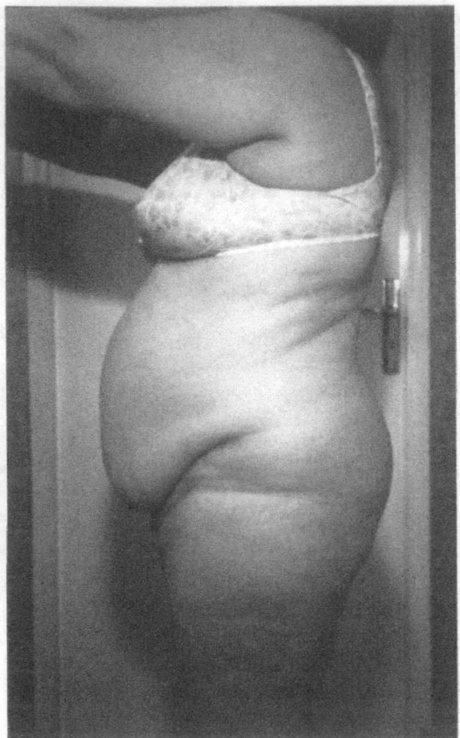
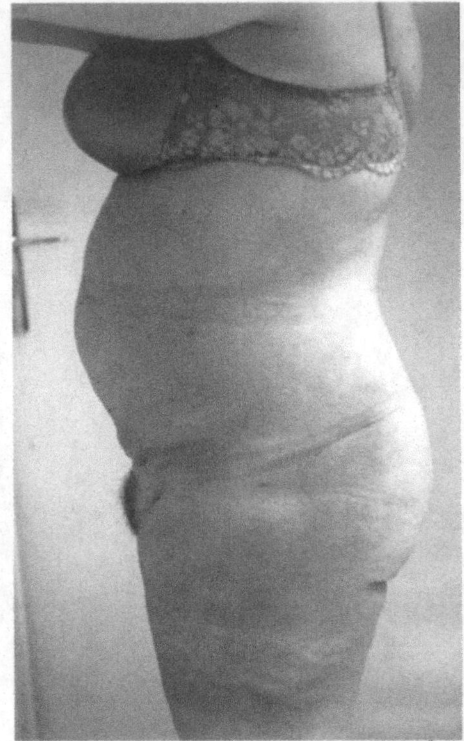

Figure 8 Before (left) and after (right) (1 year) photos showing excellent skin retraction.

patients large quantities of normal saline at 2°C (with 1 mg of adrenaline per liter) and sometimes up to 21 liters with no problems.

We have never experienced complications due to the utilization of normal saline at 2°C. Sometimes we register a moderate decrease in the central temperature of 0.5°C in the postoperative period, but with no serious consequences. The 2°C cold saline injection produces a better quality anesthetic than a pure local anesthesia, either classical or Klein's formula, and above all a more important local vasoconstriction. The work of Nestor Asurey in Buenos Aires on the white rat demonstrated this. One side of the femoral pedicle of a white rat was dissected and moistened with an adrenaline xylocaïne solution at 2°C while the other femoral pedicle was equally dissected and moistened with an identical adrenaline xylocaïne solution, but at room temperature (22–23°C). The examination of the pedicles under a microscope demonstrated that in the side that was moistered with the solu-

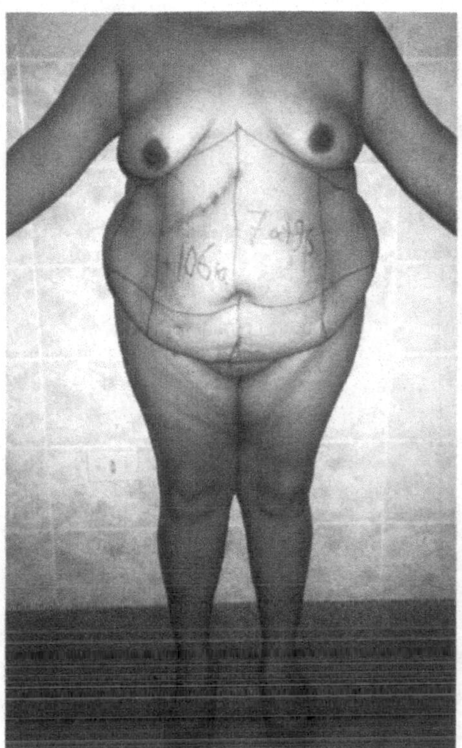

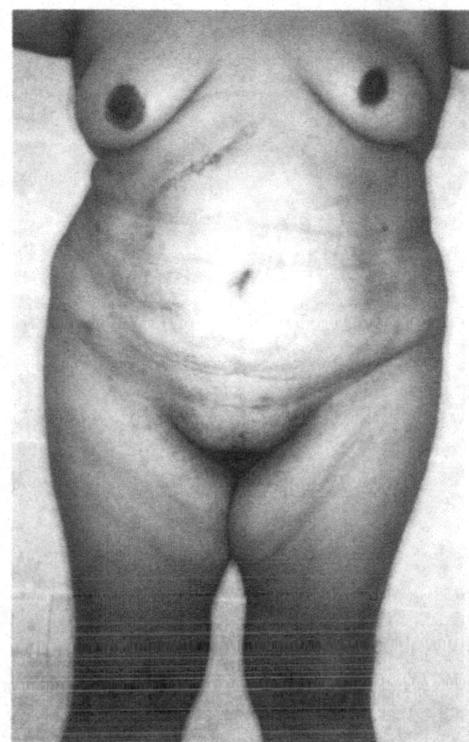

FIGURE 9 Before (left) and after (right) (after 6 months) 26 kilos lost.

tion at 2°C, the arterial vasoconstriction was more rapid, intense, and prolonged than on the opposing side, where the solution was at room temperature.

DISCUSSION

In 1974 in Rome Giorgio Fischer used a specially built suction machine and blunt cannulas of different diameters for the extraction of adipose tissue from localized fat deposits on the body. The equipment used was simplified in 1977. Karmann's abortion cannulas and suction machine allowed the surgeon to perform a procedure identical to Fischer's. In 1985, 60-ml plastic syringes were used, and a special cannula was passed through the syringe mounted on the tip of the barrel. For many surgeons, the syringe replaced the suction machine. Lipoextraction is simple, efficient, and more rapid.

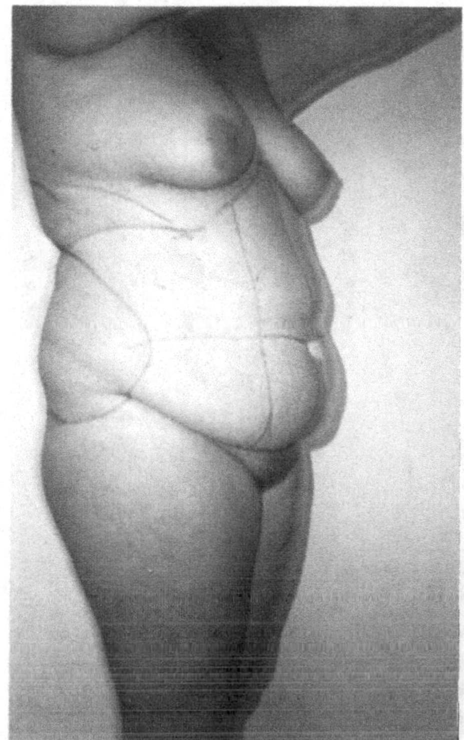
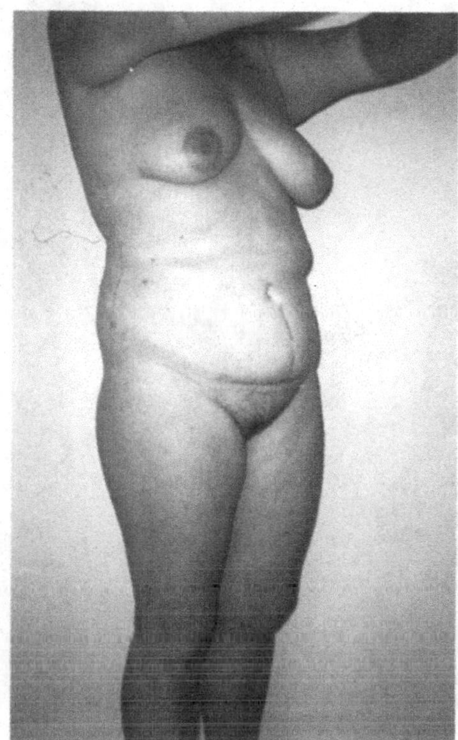

Figure 10 Before (left) and after (right) (1 year) 18 kilos lost.

Liposculpture is indicated for patients who have excess fat in some part of the body. For a long time extraction of greater than 2 or 3 liters was considered too risky. However, over the past 10 years, we have increased the amount of adipose tissue extracted. To achieve this, the surgeon has to inject large amounts of normal saline at 2°C with epinephrine (1 mg/liter). The lipoextraction is performed with 60-ml syringes by one or two surgeons to decrease the duration of anesthesia. Up to 20 liters of adipose tissue mixed with normal saline and some blood can be extracted in one session with no blood transfusion. In most patients, we inject only between 5 and 10 liters, and in only a few patients have we injected 15–20 liters. It appears that adrenaline is quickly metabolized after the injection. In many cases we inject in two or three stages during the operation to avoid major modifications in blood pressure.

Our specific indications are patients between 100 to 130 kg with no major diabetes, high blood pressure, or heart or pulmonary disease who have

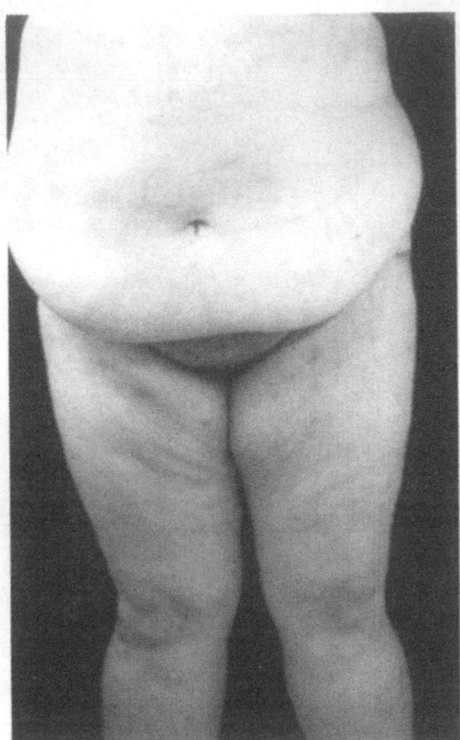

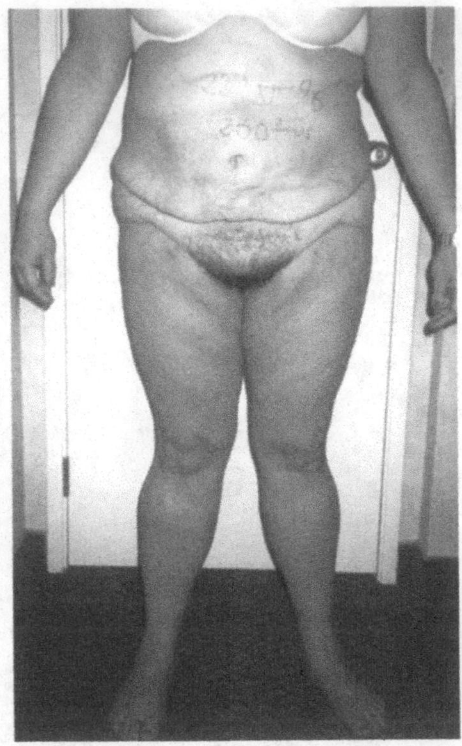

FIGURE 11 Before (left) and after (right; 1 year later) photos of a depressed patient who lost 42 pounds. A normal life was attained and the result was maintained for 6 years.

tried diets and medical and surgical treatment without success. Patients should understand that this is not intended as an aesthetic procedure, that complications may occur, and that "touch-up" may be necessary as well as other operations to get rid of skin excess, should it occur. Lipoextraction can be performed in patients with a maximum weight of 160 kg, but these patients should understand that the risks of the operation are slightly increased. Contraindications are (1) patients who have never tried dieting, exercise, or medical treatment; (2) patients who do not understand that this is a major procedure, that there are some risks, and that a "touch-up" or a future skin resection may be necessary; and (3) patients who have serious disease secondary to their obesity.

I and my colleagues have lost contact with many patients, as they live abroad or do not return for follow-up. Our main goal has been to prove that

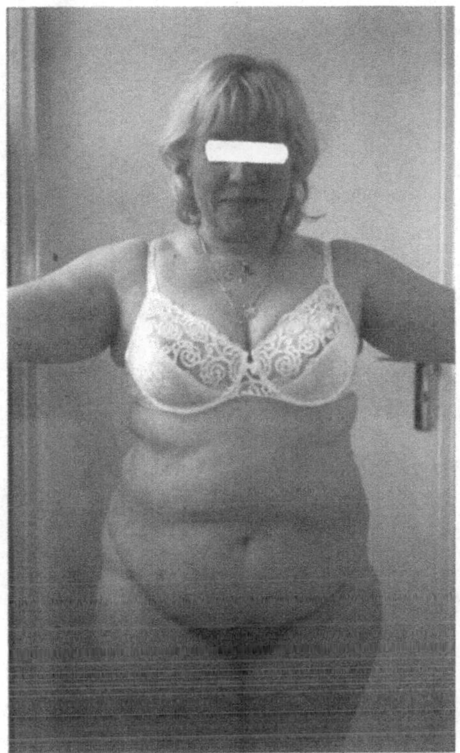
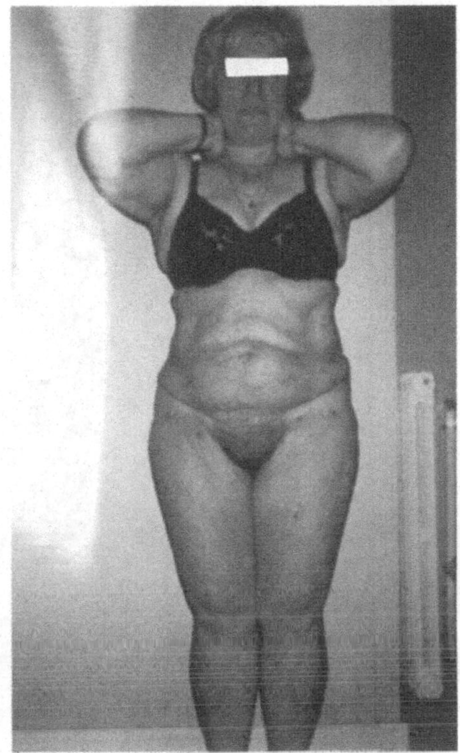

FIGURE 12 Before (left) and after (right; 7 months) photos of a diabetic patient who also had moderately high blood pressure. At 7 months postoperation, normal blood sugar was maintained with diet only (no insulin). Normal blood pressure and the result were maintained for 6 years.

major amounts or subcutaneous fat can be removed with minimum risk and without blood transfusion. The complications that we had have been accepted by our patients who understood that it was a life-saving operation and not a cosmetic procedure.

Gastrointestinal operations for massive obesity have significant morbidity. In the long-term, regain of weight may occur. All bariatric abdominal operations leave the fat cells in place that can once again hypertrophy if the cause of the obesity has not been suppressed at the same time. Only large dermolipectomies which are major operations reduce the number of adipose cells. They are burdened with a significant morbidity in the obese patient. On the contrary, a closed megaliposculpture reduces greatly the number of adipose cells. This treatment is minor compared to large dermolipectomies.

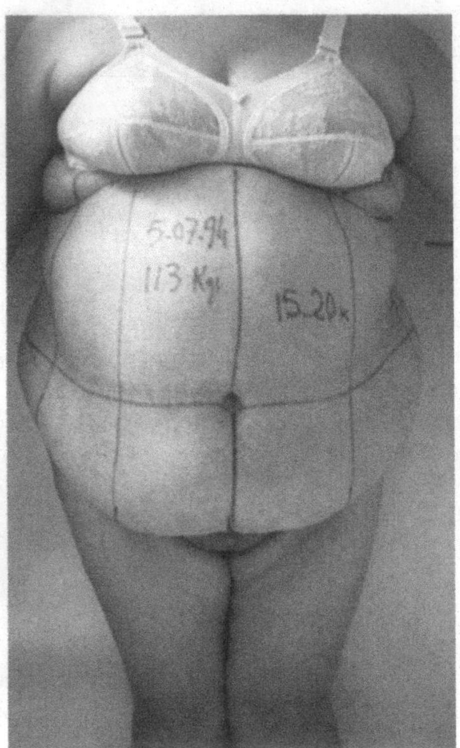

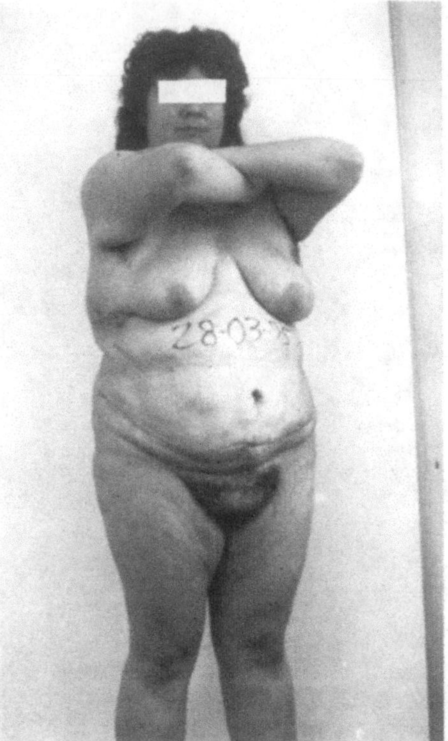

FIGURE 13 Before (left) and after (right) photos of a patient presenting with high cholesterol, mild diabetes, and mild high blood pressure. After a year 22 kilos were lost, blood sugar was normal, cholesterol was normal, blood pressure was normal; and the result was maintained for 7 years.

If a large quantity of adipose cells remain and can once again hypertrophy, megaliposculpturing is the only moderately aggressive treatment compared to other techniques. Although it does not treat the cause of the obesity, it considerably diminishes the quantity of the patient's adipose cells. Megaliposculpture has shown that large quantities of adipose tissue can be extracted without minimal risk and that large, localized obesities provoking a functional hinderance can be definitively improved or eliminated. It opens new horizons in the treatment of osteoarthritis of the lower extremities and possibly of the comorbidities. This operation can be used to treat residual adiposities following gastroplasties or bypass procedures and may be used for patients who have insufficient weight loss from dieting.

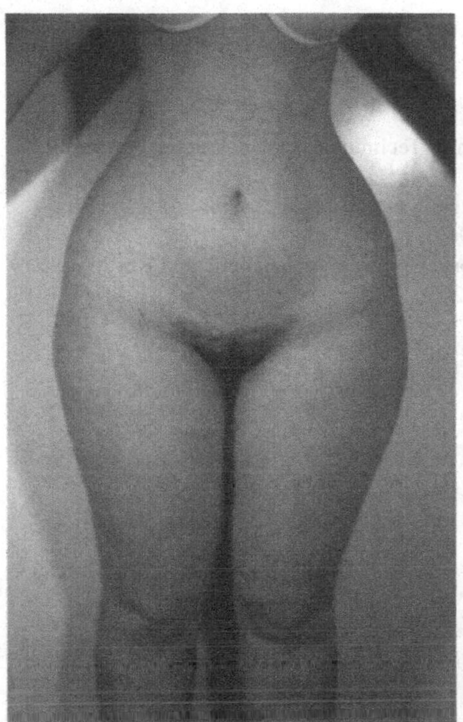

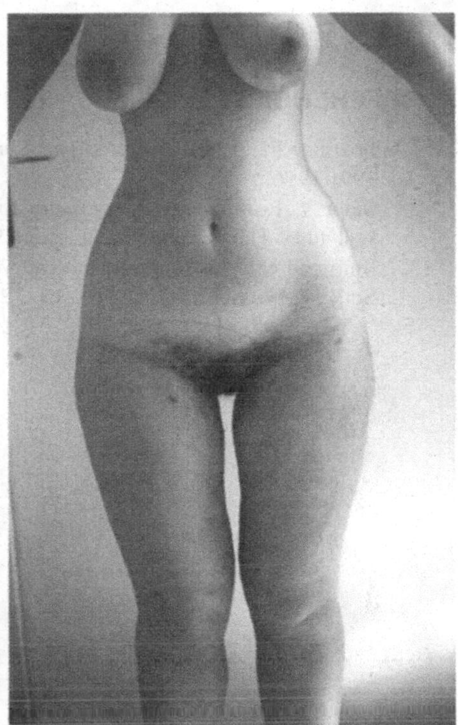

Figure 14 Before (left) and after (right) photos of a patient treated for infertility for 10 years. The patient became pregnant 6 months after the megaliposuction and now has two children. The weight loss was maintained for 8 years.

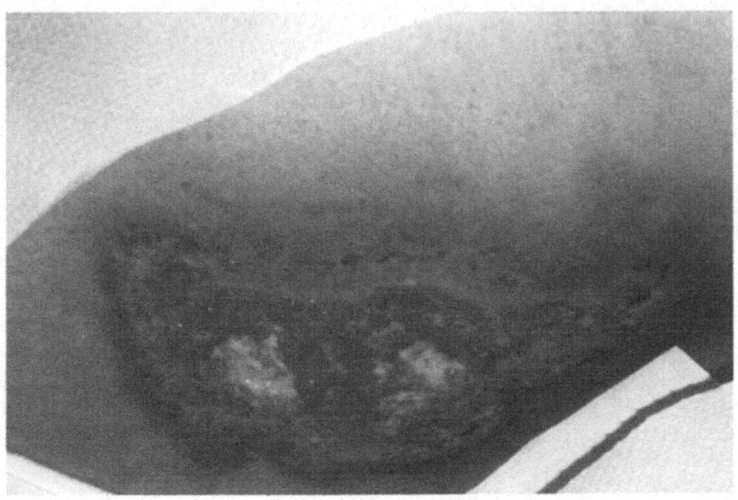

Figure 15 Skin necrosis on the thigh, healing in 2 months (patient refused a skin graft).

REFERENCES

1. Fournier PF. Liposculpture: The Syringe Technique. Paris: Arnette Blackwell, 1991/1996.
2. Sidor V. From megaliposculpture to therapeutic megalipoaspiration. In: Liposculpture: The Syringe Technique. 1996.
3. Shiffman M. Liposuction disasters. World Congress of Aesthetic and Restorative Surgery, Mumbai, India, Feb. 10–12, 2001.

19

Immediate and Long-Term Postoperative Care and Touch-Ups

Naomi Lawrence
Cooper Health System
Marlton, New Jersey, U.S.A.

Kimberly J. Butterwick
Dermatology Associates
La Jolla, California, U.S.A.

INTRODUCTION

Liposuction with tumescent anesthesia has a relatively low maintenance and an uncomplicated postoperative course when compared to other cosmetic procedures such as skin resurfacing. The postoperative course differs greatly from that of traditional dry or wet technique liposuction, which can cause blood loss significant enough to require transfusions, extensive bruising, hematomas, and seromas. The postoperative course is best divided into three phases: immediate, short term, and long term.

IMMEDIATE: FIRST TWENTY-FOUR HOURS

Immediately after the liposuction it is beneficial to have the patient shower. This allows them to clean off the blood-tinged anesthetic solution and warm up. It is best if the shower has a built-in seat as the patient is more subject to orthostatic hypotension by taking a standing shower. In addition the patient can use a small towel to compress over the treated areas and help drain excess tumescent fluid. Gauze pads or sanitary napkins are taped over cannula entrance sites to absorb drainage. If the patient is sensitive to tape, a tubular elastic retainer (Surgilast Glenwood Inc., Tenafly NJ) can be used to hold the pads in place. The staff usually needs to help the patient put on the compression garment. It is best to order two compression girdles: one the patient wears the day of surgery and is true to the measurements taken preoperatively and one a size smaller.

Postoperative edema is thought to be caused by increased interstitial fluid secondary to capillary injury. Application of ice is recommended in the first 24 hr after liposuction [1]. Crushed ice or a bag of frozen peas or corn are wrapped in a thin towel and held in place over the girdle. Cryotherapy has a vasoconstrictor effect on blood vessels which minimizes bleeding into injured area [1a,2]. As a result cryotherapy reduces accumulation of inflammatory cells and exudate into injured tissue [1a,3]. Cooling lowers the local metabolic rate, decreasing the injured cell requirement for oxygen, which makes the tissue more resistant to further damage through hypoxia [4,5]. Lowering tissue temperature may block the release of histamine, thereby blocking further vasodilatation and increase of tissue edema [1a,6]. Tissue cooling also has an important analgesic effect. Application of cold decreases the excitability of free nerve endings and depresses nerve impulse conduction [1a,7]. It may do this by bombarding the pain receptors with cold impulses, effectively blocking pain impulses [1a,8]. (The optimal tissue temperature to achieve therapeutic effects is thought to be 25°–35°C.)

Most of the literature on tissue cooling is from the physical therapy and orthopedic specialties, in which the main goal is to cool muscle. In this literature ice is cited as more effective in reducing muscle temperature than frozen gel, chemical ice pack, or refrigerated injected splint [1a,9]. The duration of ice application may vary with the depth of injury. Skin will begin to cool within 5 min of application. Muscle temperature is not reduced until the area has been iced for at least 10 min [1a,10,11]. The thicker the adipose layer, the more prolonged the application should be (up to 20 min) [1,12]. There have been cases reported in which nerve injury has occurred with prolonged use application [13,14]. Ice chips should be put in a bag or wrapped in a towel so as not to directly injure the skin.

The optimal cycle for ice application after injury is still under some dispute. Karunakara et al. studied forearm blood flow during single 20-min cold application in comparison with a 20- to 30-min cold application followed by cycles of 10 min on/10 min off for 1 hr. They found a significant advantage by maintaining the decrease in tissue temperature with intermittent ice application without reactive vasodilatation [13].

Compression

With tissue injury there is transudation of fluid across healing capillary membranes resulting in edema. Fluid moves from intravascular to extravascular responding to the gradient of hydrostatic and oncotic pressures between the two compartments [1a]. Compression increases interstitial hydrostatic pressure and equalizes the gradient between the two components. In addition the increase in tissue pressure may create a better environment for hemostasis of injured vessels (see Figs. 1–5).

Klein details the postliposuction environment that leads to postliposuction edema [15]. The liposuction cannula movement disrupts the lymphatic capillaries in the adipose tissue. Leakage of large protein molecules results in decreased plasma colloid osmotic pressure and an increased interstitial osmotic and hydrostatic pressure. Klein also describes the preoperative and postoperative circumstances that can worsen postliposuction edema [15]. General anesthesia with secondary limb immobilization and loss of sympathetic vascular tone increases capillary hydrostatic pressure. Trapping excess tumescent anesthetic solution by suturing the incisions exacerbates the fluid load to be reabsorbed by the capillaries. Klein also believes that prolonged high-grade compression collapses the lymphatic capillaries and cre-

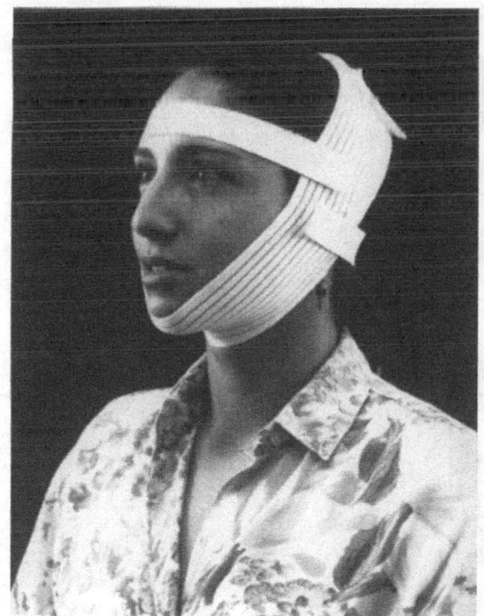

FIGURE 1 Compression garment for submandibular area and jowl.

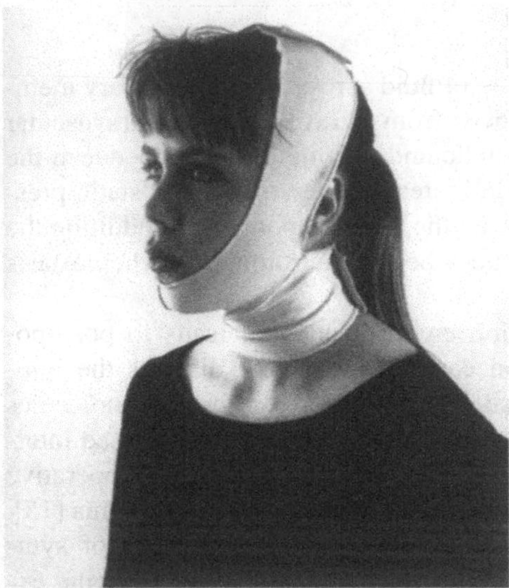

FIGURE 2 Compression garment for neck and jowl.

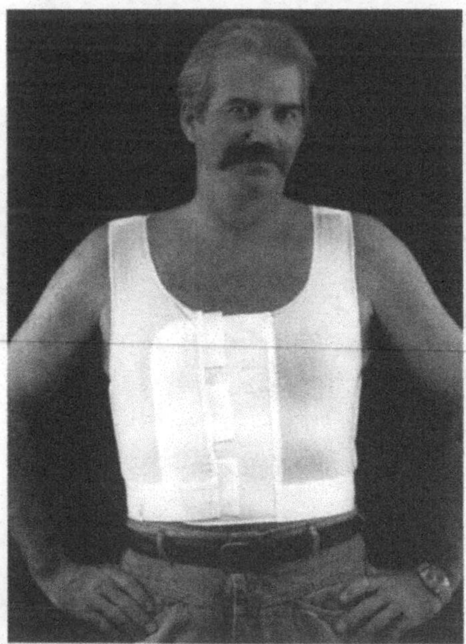

FIGURE 3 Compression garment for the male chest.

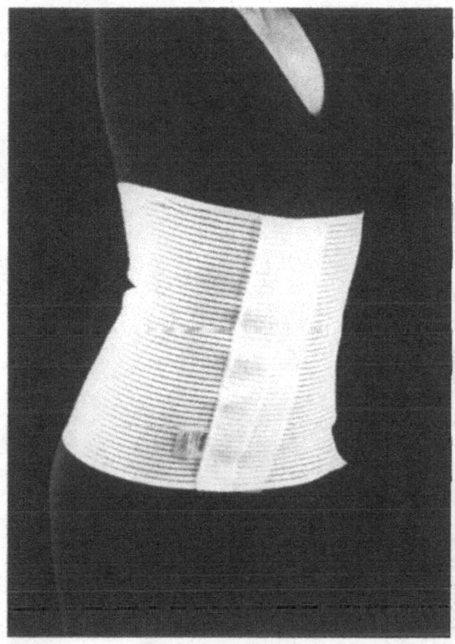

FIGURE 4 Compression garment for abdomen, hips, and back.

ates worse postliposuction edema [15]. Klein advocates bimodal compression: (1) high-grade compression in the first 24 hr postsurgery to facilitate drainage through open incisions and (2) mild compression after the first 24 hr [15a]. Most liposuction surgeons recommend that their patients wear a liposuction garment that adequately compresses the entire area treated for 2–4 weeks.

There are some area specific differences in the postoperative course of liposuction edema and the requirement for compression [15a]. The breasts require extra compression because this is a higher risk area for postoperative bleeding and hematoma. Circumferential thighs or calves and ankles have a greater risk for excessive or prolonged edema. Compression hose and leg elevation (above the level of the pelvis) during the first 3 days postoperatively will minimize edema in the legs. The abdomen is also an area where edema may be more persistent.

Klein describes a clinical scenario which he terms "*amplified liposuction edema syndrome*" [15]. The combination of excessive liposuction, iatrogenic hemodilution by giving excessive iv fluids intraoperatively, closure of cannula insertion sites (preventing open drainage of tumescent fluid), and high-grade compression can lead to progressive generalized edema. Extreme

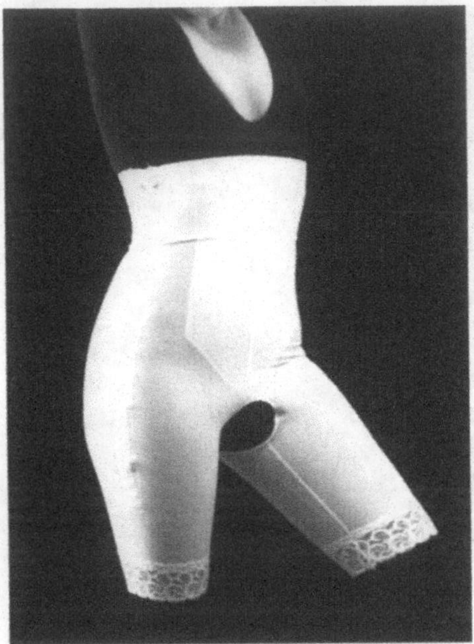

Figure 5 Compression garment for hips, abdomen, and outer and inner thighs.

cases of this syndrome can result in pulmonary edema, effusions, acute renal failure, and death [15].

Compression not only can reduce the risk of postoperative hematoma and decrease edema but also decreases discomfort during the postoperative period. Patients often maintain that the compression garment splints or supports the area that has been treated, making it less painful.

Some liposuction surgeons advocate the use of Reston foam under the compression garment [16]. Reston foam (3M, St. Paul, MN) is an adhesive-backed porous dressing. The most common areas to use it are the abdomen and neck. Advocates of Reston use feel that it decreases postoperative waviness; cushions the compression of the overlying garment, making it more comfortable; and stabilizes the skin's capillary network, leading to less bruising. Although these effects sound beneficial, none are supported by scientific research. In addition, there are reports of the foam causing an irritant or allergic contact dermatitis with bullae and postinflammatory hyperpigmentation [15]. The company no longer recommends their foam postliposuction (due to infections and sloughing blamed on Reston). As an alternative

TopiFoam (LySonix Inc., Carpinteria, CA), a nonadherent foam could be used.

SHORT-TERM POSTOPERATIVE PERIOD

Incision Sites

The majority of surgeons who perform tumescent liposuction leave the incision sites open for optimal drainage of the anesthetic solution. Most incision sites have a small amount of surrounding echymosis. The skin surrounding the sites can be erythematous as is typical for an actively healing second intention wound. It is important that these are treated with moist occlusion to encourage more rapid healing and a better cosmetic result. A spot Band-Aid is a better choice than a strip Band-Aid as it seals on all four edges. To avoid allergic contact dermatitis a plain ointment such as Vaseline (Sherwood Medical, St. Louis, MO) or Aquaphor (Beiersdorf Inc., Wilton, CT) is preferable to a topical antibiotic ointment. It is important to explain to the patient that allowing scab formation on the incision sites will delay healing and may result in a more noticeable scar. When appropriate postoperative care is implemented the 2- to 3-mm incision heals very well with a scar that is often difficult to identify in a year. Once the incision site has reepithelized but while it is still pink, patients should be instructed to cover the healing site with sunscreen to prevent postinflammatory hyperpigmentation. This is particularly critical in patients with skin types IV and VI.

Surgical Site

During the immediate postoperative period the patients experience soreness of the surgical area, bruising, and swelling. There can also be areas that are indurated. Most patients tolerate the postoperative course of tumescent liposuction with no adjunctive care. They are easily able to perform their normal activities after a day or two and often only refrain from heavy exercise for a week. The postoperative morbidity for tumescent liposuction is drastically improved over that of traditional dry technique or wet technique liposuction. The old dry technique of liposuction was extremely traumatic to the soft tissues and the patients had extensive bruising and soreness that took 4–6 weeks to improve.

Several adjunctive therapies have been investigated to evaluate their effect on the postoperative course. External ultrasound has been used as a therapeutic modality for over 40 years [17,18]. Most of the literature attribute the therapeutic effects of ultrasound to heat production. Dyson reports that tissue temperatures must be elevated to 40°–45°C and maintained for 5 min to achieve a useful therapeutic effect [19]. The physiologic effects of tissue heating include increased blood flow, increased extensibility of collagenous tissues, decreased pain, and decreased muscle spasm. According to Dyson there are also some useful nonthermal effects of ultrasound which produce stimulation of tissue regeneration, soft tissue repair, blood flow of clinically ischemic tissues, decreased sensitivity of neural elements, protein synthesis, and bone repair [19]. This nonthermal effect can be useful in the immediate postoperative period.

Butterwick et al. looked at the application of external ultrasound (EUS) to relieve postoperative discomfort and swelling after tumescent liposuction [20]. In Butterwick's study 25 patients had tumescent liposuction of the abdomen or hips. The patients were treated biweekly for 8 treatments in 22 patients and 6 treatments in 3 patients. In the first 2 weeks the patients were treated with 1 MHz U/S at 20% duty cycle .3–.75 W/cm^2 on the treatment side and 10% 0–5 W/cm^2 on the control (placebo) side. After 2 weeks the treatment side dose was increased to 1–2 W/cm^2 continuous-wave ultrasound (for the thermal effects) and the control side with pulsed EUS at placebo settings. Application ranged from 5 to 10 min. The study was double blinded. The results showed no advantage to the application of ultrasound. Of the 25 patients 17 reported no difference between the two sides. Three patients reported improved symptoms and 5 reported worse symptoms on the EUS-treated side.

Draper et al. looked at the effects of pulsed short-wave diathermy (PSWD) on postoperative course [21]. Pulsed short-wave diathermy, like ultrasound, heats the tissue. The application of PSWD has three advantages over ultrasound. Pulsed short-wave diathermy treats a large area—an average diathermy drum is 200 cm^2 compared to the average U/S soundhead of 5 cm. The treatment application is static and therefore requires no ancillary personnel time in comparison to U/S, which requires constant movement of the soundhead. In addition the temperature retention in the tissue is better. When evaluation tissue temperature changes from a 10-min application of 3 MHz U/S, Draper et al. found an increase in fat temperature from 33° to 40.5°C (7.5°C) and a subsequent drop by 4.0°C at 5 min after application and a 5.5°C decrease at 10 min [22]. When this same study was done with PSWD the increase in temperature was 7.5°C and the decrease less precipitous: 2.6°C at 5 min and 3.7°C at 10 min [23]. They postulate that better heat retention from PSWD is due to the larger area heated and less diffusion of heat [21].

In their study on the effect of PSWD on the postoperative course for liposuction, Draper et al. applied PSWD with the Megapulse (Accelerated Care Plus-LLC., Topeka, KS) at 27.12 MHz for 20 min preoperatively and at 1 and 5 days postoperatively. Liposuction to the thighs was performed on 10 patients with a treatment side and a "no treatment" control side. The doctor was blinded to the application of PSWD. Two objective measures were used: girth measurements of the thigh and measurement of bruises. They found a significant difference between the treatment and control sides at both 1 and 5 days. Bruising showed a significant difference at day 1 but not at day 5. Even though the bruising difference was statistically significantly different, a 3-cm difference in bruising (15.31 cm^2 vs. 18.92 cm^2) is probably not clinically significant. They found no difference in postoperative pain by patient subjective assessment.

The use of magnetic field therapy during the liposuction postoperative period was evaluated by Men et al. [24]. Externally applied magnetic fields are theoretically thought to stimulate biologic homeostatic feedback and trigger tissue repair [24]. They are thought to enhance blood flow and oxygen delivery to an injured site [24]. In this double-blinded study 10 patients had a magnetic patch placed in their treatment area and 10 had a sham patch placed. Evaluations of discoloration (bruising) and edema were made by a blinded observer on postoperative days 1–4, 7, and 14. They found a difference in discoloration they felt to be both clinically and statistically significant on days 1 (43%), 2, and 3 (28%). No significant difference in discoloration was seen on days 4, 7, and 14. Edema measurements were also clinically and statistically different on days 1 through 4 (40–53%) but not on day 7 and Pain scores were significantly decreased on days 1–4 and 7 but not on day 14. In this study they split their patients population rather than using a split site (treatment vs. control in same patient) design. The problem with their design is that there is a great individual variability between patients in bruising, swelling, and subjective pain assessment. In such a small cohort the impact of a few patients who simply have a greater tendency toward any one of these variables could be great.

Another concern is that the photos shown in this article all show the treatment patch applied to superior aspect of the surgical site. Bruising and edema typically settle down to the most dependant area of a region so the apparent "clearing" of these areas may be due to gravity rather than magnetic fields.

LONG-TERM POSTOPERATIVE COURSE

Patient Expectations

The final result of any cosmetic procedure is evaluated by both objective and subjective standards. To best handle the patient's subjective evaluation it is important to set appropriate patient expectations, before the procedure is done. The patient should be prepared for a reasonable percentage reduction of an area. This is particularly important in areas where other anatomic structures contribute to the protuberance in the treatment area. In the abdomen a lax rectus or fat in the omentum contribute to outward rounding. In the hip and thigh area pelvic bony structure size and configuration contribute to outward contour. Pre- and postoperative pictures and measurements can help show the patient that significant improvement (but not perfection) has been achieved. It is also important to get a preoperative weight. Some patients will come back 6 months to a year after liposuction dissatisfied with their result. On reweighing these patients many have gained a significant amount of weight. These patients need to be encouraged to find a diet-and-exercise program that can stabilize their weight. On the contrary, it is not infrequent that patients are so inspired by their new contour that they lose weight after liposuction.

Touch-Ups

A touch-up procedure is by definition retreatment of a subunit of the original area treated to remove a residual pocket of fat. Because remodeling of scar tissue takes a full year, it is best to encourage the patient to wait to evaluate any irregularity until the scar has matured. The need for touch-up should be determined by the physician. Sometimes there is an obvious irregularity in fat removal. This could be due to positioning during fat removal. Alternately it can be due to incomplete fat removal because the patient was hypersensitive to the entire procedure or "touchy" in a certain area because fat was more fibrous (i.e., periumbilical area). Finally it may be that the physician incorrectly assessed the endpoint in all areas suctioned such as in patients who have lax skin. An obvious irregularity is often easily corrected by reinfusion and suctioning. The area is usually limited as to make sedative and pain medications unnecessary. More difficult is the situation in which the patient perceives the need for a touch-up for an irregularity that is not appreciable by clinical assessment. This type of patient is often a perfectionist and may have unrealistic expectations of what can be achieved by liposuction in this area. This can lead to a chain of touch-ups with no clear endpoint.

Butterwick et al. did a retrospective review of their touch-up procedures over a 2-year time period (1998–2000) [25]. Of the 954 liposuction procedures done during this period, 118 patients had touch-up procedures, giving a rate of 12.3%. Males and females had an equal incidence of touch-up procedures. The touch-up rate per area was 9% of 1613 areas treated. The most common areas for touch-up, the neck and abdomen, were also the most common areas to be treated. The areas with the highest incidence of touch-ups were fibrous areas of the back, chest, and ankles. Over 80% of patients had their touch up procedure 6 months or longer after the original procedure. In comparing weight at time of touch-up to baseline weight 36%

of the patients had decreased weight, 47% increased weight, and 17% had no weight change. The amount of supernatant fat removed during the touch-up procedure was usually small; less than 100 ml in 38% and 300 ml or less in 66%. Touch-up site per physician did not necessarily correlate with experience. Patients appeared to have continued confidence in the physician after the touch-up and undergo more liposuction (over 33%) or other cosmetic procedures (over 50%).

Serial Suctioning

Patients who are 20% over their ideal body weight may benefit from serial liposuction procedures. In this circumstance the second procedure is not done because of an irregularity in contour, but rather to achieve greater reduction. It is best that the physician make this possibility clear at the initial evaluation. A patient will usually understand that because of the thickness of their layer of adipose and the limitation of maximum safe dose with lidocaine limits, you may not be able to remove all of the excess fat in one session.

CONCLUSION

Tumescent liposuction is a safe procedure with high patient satisfaction. The postoperative period requires simple supportive care. Although there have been trials on adjunctive therapies, the results of these trials have not shown a clear indication for any of these. Touch-up procedures should be used when there is an irregularity to correct. Touch-up procedures should probably be avoided when there is no clear endpoint.

REFERENCES

1. Coleman WP. Liposuction In: Coleman WP, Hank CS, Alt TH, Asken S, eds. Cosmetic Surgery of the Skin: Principles and Techniques. Philadelphia: BC Decker, 1991:213–238.

1a. Landry GL, Gomez JE. Management of soft tissue injuries. Adolesc Med 1991; 2(1):125–140.

2. Knight KL. Cryotherapy: Theory, Technique, and Physiology. Chattanooga: Chattanooga Corp., 1985: Chapts. 7 and 10.

3. Farry PJ, Prentice NG, Hunter AC et al. Ice treatment of injured ligaments: an experimental model. NZ J Med 1980; 91:12–14.

4. El Hawary R, Stanish WD, Curwin SL. Rehabilitation of tendon injuries in sport. Sports Med 1997; 24(5):347–358.

5. Knight ATC. Cold as a modifier of sports-induced inflammation. In: Leadbetter WB, Buckwalter JA, Gordon SL, eds. Sports-Induced Inflammation: Clinical and Basic Science Concepts. Park Ridge: American Academy of Orthopaedic Surgeons, 1990:463–478.
6. Adamson C, Cymet T. Ankle sprains: evaluation, treatment, rehabilitation. Md Med J 1997; 46(10):530–537.
7. Kellett J. Acute soft tissue injuries—a review of the literature. Med Sci Sports Exerc 1986; 18:489–500.
8. Olson JE, Stravino VD. A review of cryotherapy. Phys Ther 1972; 52:840–853.
9. McMaster WC. A literary review on ice therapy in injuries. Am J Sports Med 1997; 5:124–126.
10. McMaster WC, Liddle S, Waugh TR. Laboratory evaluation of various cold therapy modalities. Am J Sports Med 1978; 6:291–294.
11. Thorsson O, Lilja B, Ahigren L. The effect of local cold application on intramuscular blood flow at rest and after running. Med Sci Sports Exerc 1985; 17:710–713.
12. Lehman JF, de Lateur BJ. Cryotherapy. In: Lehman JF, ed. Therapeutic Heat and Cold. Baltimore: Williams & Wilkins, 1990:605–607.
13. Karunakara RG, Lephart SM, Pincivero DM. Changes in forearm blood flow during single and intermittent cold application. J Orthop Sports Phys Ther 1999; 29(3):177–180.
14. Drez D, Faust DC, Evan JP. Cryotherapy and nerve palsy. Am J Sports Med 1981; 9:256–257.
15. Klein JA. In: Klein JA, ed. Tumescent Technique: Post Liposuction Edema. St. Louis MO: Mosby, 2000:79–87.
15a. Klein JA. In: Klein JA, ed. Tumescent Technique: Open Drainage and Bimodal Compression. St. Louis, MO: Mosby, 2000:281–293.
16. Schlesinger SL, Kaczynski AJ. Use of Restontm foam in liposuction. Aesth Plast Surg 1993; 17:49–51.
17. Dyson M. Therapeutic applications of ultrasound In: Nuborg WI, Siskin MC, eds. Biological Effects of Ultrasound: Clinics in Diagnostic Ultrasound. New York: Churchill-Livingstone, 1985:121–131.
18. Kitchen SS, Partridge CJ. A review of therapeutic ultrasound, part 1: background and physiological effects. Physiotherapy 1990; 76(10):593–600.
19. Dyson M. Mechanisms involved in therapeutic ultrasound. Physiotherapy 1987; 73:116–120.
20. Butterwick KJ, Tse Y, Goldman MP. Effect of external ultrasound postliposuction: a side-to-side comparison study. Dermatol Surg 2000; 26(5):433–435.
21. Draper DO, Abergel RP, Castel JC, Schlaak C. Pulsed short-wave diathermy restricts swelling and bruising of liposuction pations. Am J Cosm Surg 2000; 17(1):17–20.
22. Draper DO, Abergel RP, Castel JC. Rate of temperature change in human fat during external ultrasound: implications for liposuction. Am J Cosmet Surg 1998; 15(4):361–365.

23. Draper DO, Castel JC, Abergel RP. The effect of pulsed short wave diathermy on temperature elevation in adipose tissue. J Athl Train 1998; 33(2):S70.
24. Man D, Man B, Plosker H. The influence of permanent magnetic field therapy on wound healing in suction lipectomy patients: a double-blind study. Plast Recon Surg 1999; 104(7):2261–2268.
25. Butterwick KJ, Amiry S, Goldman MP. Touch-up procedures following tumescent liposuction: a two-year retrospective study of 954 cases. In press.

20

Liposuction Complications

Jean-Francois Tremblay
University of Montreal Hospital Centre
Montreal, Quebec, Canada

David A. Wrone
Northwestern University
Chicago, Illinois, U.S.A.

Ronald L. Moy
David Geffen School of Medicine at UCLA, Los Angeles, and West Los Angeles Veterans Administration Hospital, Los Angeles, California, U.S.A.

Brian Shafa
Los Angeles, California, U.S.A.

Liposuction was first introduced as a fat-removal procedure in 1979 and since then has evolved dramatically, resulting in better outcomes and fewer complications. In the early days of liposuction, general anesthesia as well as aggressive fluid and blood loss replacement were often necessary and patients undergoing liposuction faced the risks of a major surgical procedure. Tumescent liposuction, which is today's standard of care, is performed on an ambulatory basis and requires neither heavy surgical anesthesia nor volume replacement. Tumescent liposuction is performed by definition under local anesthesia, specifically excluding additional anesthesia medications at dosages that may impair the protective airway reflexes and respiratory drive. Expected and common complications of liposuction such as bruising, edema, and contour irregularities are for the most part self-resolving or easily treatable. No significant morbidity or mortality has been reported in association with tumescent liposuction alone under local anesthesia with or without oral sedation. Cases of severe complications and deaths have only been described when liposuction was performed under general anesthesia, conscious sedation or with concomitant additional procedures such as surgical lipectomy. These isolated events have led to the development of conservative guidelines of care and recommendations by the different medical specialties involved in liposuction. Tumescent liposuction is considered as a safe and effective procedure when performed in medically fit patients by qualified physicians. In this chapter the common sequelae as well as the uncommon and rare complications of tumescent liposuction are discussed (Table 1).

SCARRING

At least two forms of scarring can occur after liposuction. Skin entrance points for liposuction cannulas inevitably leave scars. Those are almost never bothersome to patients as they are usually less than 3 mm in size and strategically placed in covered areas or skin folds. Cases of keloids and hypertrophic scars have nevertheless been reported and predisposed individuals should probably be informed of that risk.

A second form of scarring results from the expected dermal healing response stimulated by superficial liposuction. Liposuction near the subcutaneous-dermal plane is believed to stimulate collagen formation which usually results in a desirable retraction of redundant skin. Some patients may develop an exaggerated fibroblastic response resulting in significant subcutaneous induration (Fig. 1). In most cases, this firmness resolves spontaneously within 6 months or less but rarely some of it may be permanent. External ultrasound has been reported as helpful in accelerating the softening of indurated areas [1,2,3]. Prudent liposuction of the immediate subdermal plane may also help to prevent excessive fibrosis.

SKIN WRINKLING AND LAXITY

Some skin wrinkling or laxity is expected to appear shortly after liposuction especially when large volumes are removed. Normal skin retraction may take up to 6 months to occur. The skin of the neck, back, buttocks, and thighs tends to redrape invariably well, whereas that of the proximal arms and the periumbilical area may not do as well. Patients with poor skin tone preoperatively generally obtain less skin contraction after liposuction. In some patients, better long-term results may be obtained in areas showing poor skin tone by avoiding removal of immediate subdermal fat.

CONTOUR ABNORMALITIES

Undesirable minor contour abnormalities and "skin lumpiness" are not uncommon during the first few weeks to months after liposuction although most of it usually subsides spontaneously. The use of smaller 3- to 6-mm

TABLE 1 Sequelae and Complications of Liposuction

Common sequelae	Uncommon complications	Rare complications
Minor scars at cannula entry sites	Keloids and hypertrophic scars	
Bruising	Minor hematomas/seromas	Large hematomas or seromas
Localized and gravitational edema (including scrotal, labial, and lower limb edema)	Persistent edema (>6 months)	Important blood loss[a] Skin burns and necrosis[b]
Transient induration	Persistent induration (>6 months)	Lidocaine toxicity due to dose error or drug interaction
Transient dysesthesia/ hypoesthesia	Persistent dysesthesia (>4 months)	Mycobacterial infections, necrotizing fasciitis[a] and toxic shock syndrome[a]
Minor contour irregularities	Significant contour abnormalities and body asymmetry	Hypovolemic shock due large volume liposuction[a]
Fluid and blood drainage	Fluid drainage (>7 days)	Pulmonary edema[a]
Minor postoperative pain and discomfort	Persistent postoperative pain (>3 weeks)	Deep vein thrombosis and pulmonary embolism[a]
Postoperative fatigue	Postoperative fatigue (>2–3 weeks)	Fat embolism[c]
Skin laxity	Noninfectious panniculitis	Abdominal peritoneal wall perforation[a]
	Minor infections	Cardiopulmonary complications of sedatives and general anesthesia[a]
	Permanent hyper- or hypopigmentation	Deaths from above-mentioned complications[a]
	Minor adverse drug reactions	
	Vasovagal episode	

[a]No cases reported in association with tumescent liposuction alone.
[b]Reported cases in association with ultrasonic liposuction.
[c]One case in association with tumescent liposuction and concomitant surgical lipectomy.

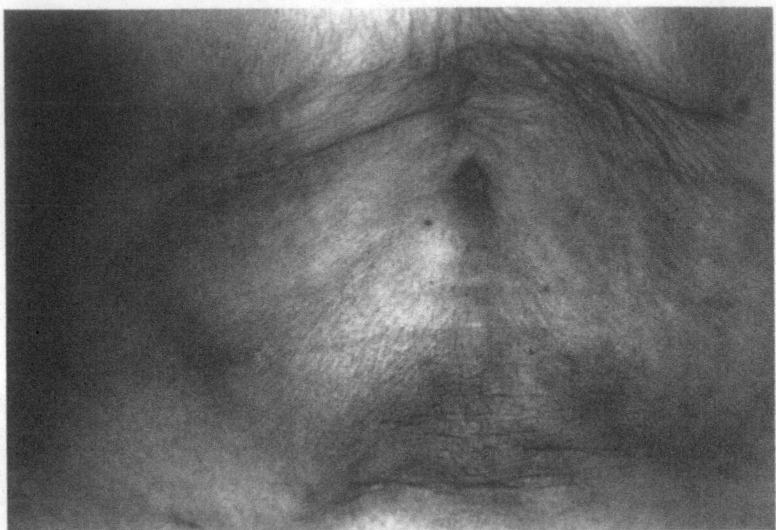

FIGURE 1 This patient developed permanent skin induration and hyperpigmentation in the area surrounding the incisional site of a previous abdominal surgery.

cannulas following a crisscross pattern allows for more precise and uniform liposculpturing. Compressive garments worn during the first 2–3 weeks after liposuction may also promote more even remolding of the subcutaneous compartment.

Contour revision should not be performed within less than 4 to 6 months after the initial procedure while subcutaneous tissue remodeling and edema resorption may be still ongoing. A revision liposuction can be used to correct body asymmetry, remove residual lumps, or liposculpture areas surrounding focal depressions. Alternatively, contour depressions can be corrected by autologous lipoinjections harvested from local or distant donor areas. However, fat injections do not take well in areas of high mobility and may be of limited value in filling hollows on upper and lower extremities.

BLEEDING PROBLEMS

Excessive blood loss is no longer considered a major threat as long as tumescent liposuction is used. In the past, patients who underwent the dry (or nontumescent) procedure routinely needed intravenous volume replacement and autologous blood transfusions for liposuction volumes exceeding 1500–2000 ml [8].

The tumescent liposuction technique using Klein's solution with 0.05–0.1% lidocaine and 0.5–1.0:1,000,000 epinephrine in buffered normal saline results in a profound decrease in blood loss, which is mainly attributable to the vasoconstrictive effect of epinephrine. The use of smaller blunt-tipped cannulas in modern-day liposuction may also be less traumatic to the neurovascular bundles and consequently reduce the amount of bleeding. In the largest survey ever published, on 15,336 tumescent liposuction patients, none required blood transfusions [4]. Blood loss using the tumescent technique was shown to represent approximately 1% of the aspirate total volume [5,6], which favorably compares to 20–45% using the dry technique [7–10] and 15–30% using the wet technique [11,12].

The tumescent technique is standard of care nowadays and the dry technique is contraindicated as per the *Liposuction Guidelines of the American Society for Dermatologic Surgery*, the American Academy of Cosmetic Surgery, and the American Academy of Dermatology. Although hemorrhages are rare, patients should be advised to avoid anticoagulants such as aspirin, alcohol, and vitamin E before and early after surgery. A personal and family history probing for bleeding disorders should be systematically performed preoperatively. The bleeding risk should be further evaluated with a baseline complete blood count, partial prothrombin time/international normalized ratio tests, and liver function tests.

HEMATOMA AND SEROMA

Well-fitted compressive garments are critical in the immediate postoperative period to promote subcutaneous hemostasis and effective open drainage of blood and interstitial fluid through cannula insertion sites. Some degree of bruising is expected following liposuction but significant hematoma formation rarely occurs. Patients who develop a hematoma may complain of increased pain associated with reactive localized warmth and erythema (see Fig. 2) which may be difficult to differentiate from early cellulitis. When in doubt, a soft-tissue ultrasound examination may help demonstrate the presence of a blood collection. Early hematomas that have not yet coagulated can be immediately syringe-drained with a large-bore needle. Most hematomas start liquefying 1 week after formation, at which point they can be evacuated more easily.

Seromas are rare in tumescent liposuction unless the patient is very active immediately after surgery. Compressive garments help minimizing third spacing and are thought to further decrease that risk. However, seromas appear to be more frequent with ultrasonic liposuction. Maxwell and Gingrass [13] reported a 13.6% complication rate in 250 patients treated with ultrasound-assisted liposuction and seromas accounted for 83% of those

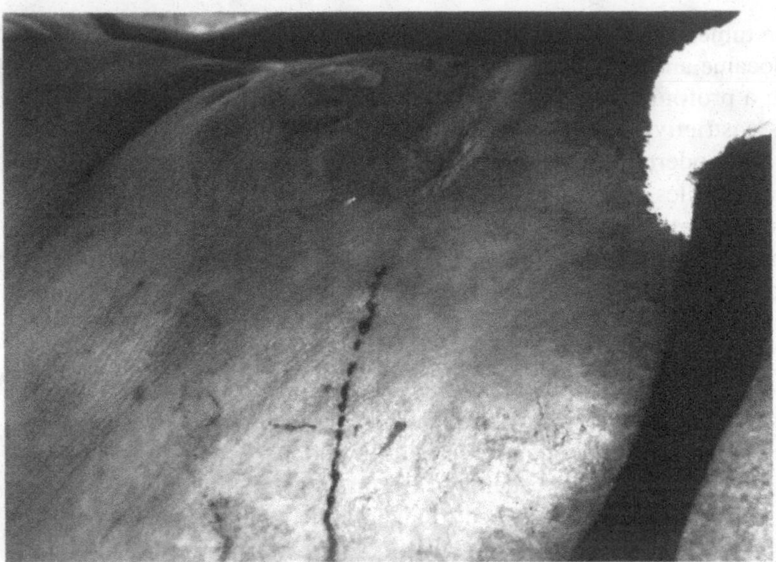

FIGURE 2 This patient developed postoperatively a small-sized hematoma on the right lower abdomen associated with some reactive erythema and edema. Over 100 cc of liquefied coagulated blood were drained 10 days later and the patient recovered with no permanent sequelae.

complications. Seromas are filled with a clear yellowish fluid that can be easily aspirated with a large-bore needle although repeated drainage may be necessary until the condition resolves. Seromas are not usually associated with significant pain and inflammation. These symptoms are suggestive of a secondary bacterial infections and warrant fluid analysis for bacterial culture and sensitivity and antibiotic treatment based on clinical evidences.

INFECTION

Infectious complications after tumescent liposuction are extremely rare, with a reported incidence of less than 0.5% [4]. This may be explained by the fact that many surgeons provide prophylactic gram-positive antibiotic coverage to their patients perioperatively. Dilute lidocaine also has weak bacteriostatic properties which may account for this low infection rate [14,15] although the significance of this effect has been called into question [16]. The use of the open-drainage technique may also further contribute to the elimination of microbial contaminants introduced subcutaneously during the procedure.

Over 99% of infectious complications are caused by bacterial pathogens. The great majority of those are minor superficial infections limited to the incisional sites and respond in due course to antibiotics. Two cases of mycobacterial infections have also been reported [17,18]. We reported a case caused by *Mycobacterium fortuitum* following neck liposuction in which the infection did not become apparent for a full 2 months after an otherwise uneventful procedure (Fig. 3). Isolated cases of serious infections have also been reported, including necrotizing fasciitis [19] and toxic shock syndrome [20], but fortunately those are extremely rare.

NONINFECTIOUS POSTLIPOSUCTION PANNICULITIS

Postliposuction panniculitis is an uncommon complication of tumescent liposuction that may occur focally in 2–4% of patients [21]. Patients present with localized tender mildly erythematous subcutaneous nodules which fail to respond to antibiotics These respond within a few days to a short course of oral prednisone or can be treated with nonsteroidal anti-inflammatory

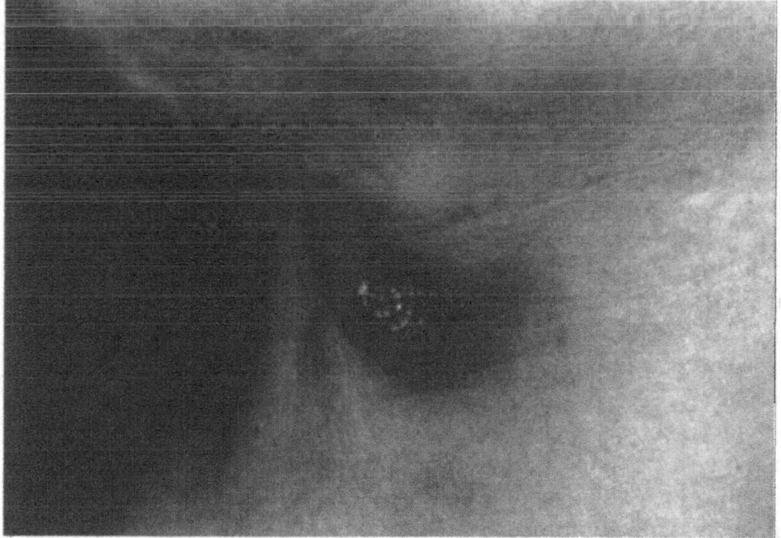

FIGURE 3 This patient presented 2 months after uneventful neck liposuction recovery with an erythematous, slightly tender, fluctuant subcutaneous mass in the submental area caused by *M. fortuitum*. The patient was treated with a combination of clarithromycin, ciprofloxacin, and minocycline. The lesions resolved completely after 6 weeks and did not recur.

drugs. Some authors sustain that this complication may be prevented by adding triamcinolone (10 mg/liter) to the tumescence solution.

LIDOCAINE TOXICITY

The safe maximal dose of lidocaine in tumescence liposuction recommended is 55 mg/kg [22]. Nevertheless, some authors have reported in the past using up to 75 mg/kg without complications. Lidocaine is exclusively eliminated by hepatic cytochrome P450 3A4 (CYP3A4) enzymatic metabolism. Normal metabolism and elimination of lidocaine may be compromised by conditions decreasing hepatic blood flow, including poor cardiac function, hypotension, and the use of beta-blockers. Numerous commonly prescribed medications are known to specifically inhibit CYP3A4 metabolism, including benzodiazepines, macrolide antibiotics, selective serotinin reuptake inhibitor antidepressants, azole systemic antifungals, and carbamazepine [23]. Although lidocaine toxicity is extremely rare, one should probably consider reducing the total dosage of lidocaine or when possible discontinuing certain medications preoperatively when there is a potential risk of drug interaction.

CAUSES OF DEATH

Death from tumescent liposuction alone performed under local anesthesia with or without oral sedation has never been reported. Cases of severe morbidities and fatalities have been reported when liposuction was performed under general anesthesia or conscious sedation with the use of intravenous anesthetics or when other cosmetic procedures were performed concomitantly. The benefits and safety of using local anesthesia only is also evidenced in a large review of liposuction malpractice cases in which virtually all claims occurred in patients who underwent the procedure under general anesthesia [24]. Additionally, 71% of those liposuction malpractice cases were performed in a hospital-based setting, further supporting the safety of liposuction as an office procedure conducted under local anesthesia.

The plastic surgery literature suggests that the risk of death from liposuction is 1 in 5000 procedures [25]. Intraabdominal penetration is a feared complication of liposuction that has only been reported with general anesthesia and is unlikely to occur in a conscious patients [4,26]. Other rare severe complications that have been reported include fat embolism, deep vein thrombosis and pulmonary embolism, cerebrovascular accident and transient ischaemic attack, anesthesia complications, transfusion complications, pulmonary edema, acute respiratory distress syndrome, and cardiogenic shock [4,7,27,28].

CONCLUSION

Tumescent liposuction is a safe and effective procedure providing excellent patient satisfaction when performed in suitable surgical candidates by qualified physicians. To further minimize complications of liposuction, the guidelines of care of the American Society for Dermatologic Surgery recommend: (1) limiting the total aspirate volume to 5000 cc or less, (2) using a maximal dose of lidocaine of 55 mg/kg or less, (3) using as little systemic anesthesia as possible, (4) monitoring vital signs perioperatively, and (5) minimizing the number of procedures and operating time per surgical session. In addition, physicians and medical personnel involved in liposuction surgery should be capable of managing acute cardiopulmonary emergencies.

REFERENCES

1. Bernstein G. Advanced seminar of ultrasonic liposuction. Annual Scientific Meeting of the American Academy of Cosmetic Surgery, New Orleans, LA, Feb 1, 1998.
2. Dyson M. Therapeutic applications of ultrasound. In: Nyborg WL, Siskin MC, eds. Biological Effects of Ultrasound (Clinics in Diagnostic Ultrasound). Edinburgh: Churchill-Livingstone, 1985:121–133.
3. Bernstein G. Liposuction of the thigh. Dermatol Clin 1999; 17(4):849–863.
4. Hanke CW, Bernstein G, Bullock S. Safety of tumescent liposuction in 15,336 patients: national survey results. Dermatol Surg 1995; 21:459–462.
5. Klein JA. Tumescent liposuction for local anesthesia improves safety in large-volume liposuction. Plast Reconstr Surg 1993; 92:1085–1098.
6. Lillis PJ. Liposuction surgery under local anesthesia: Limited blood loss and minimal lidocaine absorption. J Dermatol Surg Oncol 1988; 14:1145–1148.
7. Dillerud E. Suction lipoplasty: a report on complications, undesired results, and patient satisfaction based on 3511 procedures. Plast Reconstr Surg 1991; 88:239–46; discussion 247–249.
8. Courtiss EH, Choucair RJ, Donelan MB. Large-volume suction lipectomy: an analysis of 108 patients. Plast Reconstr Surg 1992; 89:1068–1082.
9. Pitman GH, Holzer J. Safe suction: Fluid replacement and blood loss parameters. Perspect Plast Surg 1991; 5(1):79–89.
10. Chrisman B, Coleman WP. Determining the maximum volume of liposuction before transfusion is required. J Dermatol Surg Oncol 1988; 14:1095–1102.
11. Goodpasture JC, Burkis J. Quantitative analysis of blood and fat in suction lipectomy aspirates. Plast Reconstr Surg 1978; 78:765–772.
12. Dolsky RL. Blood loss during liposuction. Dermatol Clin 1990; 8(3):463–468.
13. Maxwell GP, Gingrass MK. Ultrasound-assisted lipoplasty: a clinical study of 250 consecutive patients. Plast Reconst Surg 1998; 101(1):189–194.
14. Miller MA, Shelley WB. Antibacterial properties of lidocaine on bacteria isolated from dermal lesions. Arch Dermatol 1985; 121:1157–1159.

15. Thompson KD, Welykyj S, Massa MC. Antibacterial activity of lidocaine in combination with bicarbonate buffer. J Dermatol Surg Oncol 1993; 19:216–220.
16. Craig SB, Concannon MJ, McDonald GA, Puckett CL. The antibacterial effects of tumescent liposuction fluid. Plast Reconstr Surg 1999; 103:666–670
17. Behroozan DS, Christian MM, Moy RL. Mycobacterium fortuitum infection following neck liposuction: a case report. Dermatol Surg 2000; 26:588–590.
18. Murillo J, Torres J, Bofill L et al. Skin and wound infection by rapidly growing mycobacteria: an unexpected complication of liposuction and liposculputure: The Venezuelan Collaborative Infectious and Tropical Diseases Study Group. Arch Dermatol 2000; 136:1347–1352.
19. Heitmann C, Czermak C, Germann G. Rapidly fatal necrotizing fasciitis after aesthetic liposuction. Aesthetic Plast Surg 2000; 24:344–347.
20. Umeda T, Ohara H, Hayashi O, Ueki M, Hata Y. Toxic shock syndrome after suction lipectomy. Plast Reconstr Surg 2000; 106:204–207; discussion 208–209.
21. Klein JA. Anesthetic formulation of tumescent solutions. Dermatol Clin 1999; 17(4):751–759.
22. Ostad A, Kageyama N, Moy RL. Tumescent liposuction with a dose of lidocaine of 55 mg/kg is safe for liposuction. Dermatol Surg 1996; 22(11):921–927.
23. Klein JA, Kassarjdian N. Lidocaine toxicity with tumescent liposuction: a case report of probable drug interactions. Dermatol Surg 1997; 23:1169–1174.
24. Coleman IW, Hanke CW, Lillis P, Bernstein G, Narins R. Does the location of the surgery or the specialty of the physician affect malpractice claims in liposuction? Dermatol Surg 1999; 25:343–347.
25. Grazer FM, de Jong RH. Fatal outcomes from liposuction: census survey of cosmetic surgeons. Plast Reconstr Surg 2000; 105:436–446; discussion 447–448.
26. Talmor M, Hoffman LA, Lieberman M. Intestinal perforation after suction lipoplasty: a case report and review of the literature. Ann Plast Surg 1997; 38:169–172.
27. Rao RB, Ely SF, Hoffman RS. Deaths related to liposuction. N Engl J Med 1999; 340:1471–1475.
28. Boezaart AP, Clinton CW, Braun S, Oettle C, Lee NP. Fulminant adult respiratory distress syndrome after suction lipectomy: a case report. S Afr Med J 1990; 78:693–695.

21

Safety of Liposuction

C. William Hanke
Laser and Skin Surgery Center of Indiana, Carmel, and
Indiana University School of Medicine, Indianapolis, Indiana, U.S.A.

INTRODUCTION

High profile tragedies involving office surgical procedures have prompted regulation and oversight of office surgical facilities. Tumescent liposuction (liposuction using tumescent local anesthesia), despite an exemplary safety record, has attracted the attention of regulators. The first two sections of the chapter review multiple studies and guidelines that relate to the current status of liposuction. The final section discusses accreditation. Current and future regulation of office surgery will involve accreditation organizations, such as the Accreditation Association for Ambulatory Health Care (AAAHC), to insure that patient safety standards have been satisfied.

LIPOSUCTION SAFETY AND COMPLICATION STUDIES

Teimourian and Rogers [1] reported survey data on 112,756 liposuction procedures performed by 935 plastic surgeons. The survey divided the 112,756 procedures into three categories: (1) major liposuction (75,591), (2) dermatolipectomy (10,603), and (3) abdominoplasty (26,562). All procedures were performed between January 1984 and January 1988. The mortality rates were 2.6/100,000 for major liposuction, 18.0/100,000 for dermatolipectomy, and 41.4/100,000 for abdominoplasty. A total of 15 fatalities were reported. The largest number of nonfatal complications reported for liposuction were listed under deep venous thrombosis, anesthesia complications, transfusion complications, and pulmonary thromboembolism (Table 1). Bernstein and Hanke [2] reviewed survey data on 9478 patients who received liposuction on 24,643 body areas. Seventy-one percent of the cases were performed using local anesthesia and 29% had liposuction under general anesthesia. There were no significant complications or fatalities. There were three hospital admissions. All three patients made a complete recovery. The first patient was admitted for 24 hr for observation following profound muscle weakness which resulted from succinylcholine. The second patient was admitted for observation for 24 hr following development of a left bundle branch block intraoperatively. The block resolved during observation. The third patient had bleeding from a left flank incision postoperatively. The bleeding resolved spontaneously during a 48-hr hospitalization. No transfusions were required. Complete recovery occurred.

Survey data from the American Society for Dermatologic Surgery revealed no fatalities in 15,336 patients who underwent liposuction using tumescent local anesthesia [3]. Forty-four thousand fourteen body areas were treated in 15,336 patients. Serious complications such as emboli (pulmonary or fat), hypovolemic shock, perforation of peritoneum or thorax, thrombophlebitis, seizures, toxic reaction to drugs, and fatalities did not occur in any of the patients. Only one medical liability action was reported. No patients required blood transfusions or were admitted to the hospital for treatment of complications. Complications were minor and infrequent. Two patients developed cardiac arrhythmias requiring treatment. Two patients developed tachycardia necessitating delay in discharge.

Jackson and Dolsky [4] reported liposuction safety results from American Academy of Cosmetic Surgery survey data. The study reported results on nearly 200,000 liposuction patients operated on between 1995 and 1998. One fatality was reported during the 3-year study period. This was equivalent to a fatality rate of 2.4/100,000.

Grazer and de Jong [5] studied liposuction fatalities reported in a survey of 917 plastic surgeons. The time frame of the study was 1994–1998. Ninety-five fatalities were reported which corresponded to a fatality rate of 19.1/100,000 cases. A similar fatality rate (20.6/100,000 cases) was reported by the ASPRS Task Force on Lipoplasty in 1998. The authors attributed the upward trend in fatalities to the use of large volumes of wetting solution, trivialization of the procedure, poorly trained physicians, and possibly lidocaine/epinephrine toxicity. However, there were no cases of lidocaine/epinephrine toxicity reported in the study. The authors found no association between fat volume removed and fatal outcomes. They noted a trend for

TABLE 1 Liposuction Safety Studies

Study/author	Reference	Year	Number of procedures	Specialty	Number of fatalities	Fatality rate
Newman, Dolsky	4	1984	5458	Cosmetic surgeons (Derm, ENT, etc.)	0	1/38,426
Bernstein, Hanke	2	1988	9478	Dermatologic surgeons	0	0
Temourian, Rogers	1	1989	112,756	Plastic surgeons	15	12.7/100,000
Dillerud	16	1991	3511	Plastic surgeons		
Hanke et al.	3	1995	15,336	Dermatologic surgeons	0	0
ASPRS Task Force on Liposuction	17	1998	24,295	Plastic surgeons	5	20.6/100,000
Jackson, Dolsky	13	1999	200,000	Cosmetic surgeons (Derm, ENT, etc.)	1	2.4/100,000
Grazer, de Jong	5	2000	496,245	Plastic surgeons	95	19.1/100,000
Hughes	6	2001	94,159	Plastic surgeons	Not stated	1/47,415 (lipo only); 1,7314 (lipo & other procedures); 1/3281 (lipo & abdominoplasty)

death to occur on the first postoperative night and advocated overnight medical supervision, home nurse, or pulse oximeter use by home care-givers. Of the fatalities 77.7% originated in an office surgical facility or free-standing ambulatory surgery center. The most common causes of death were thromboembolism (23.1%), abdomen/viscus perforation (14.6%), anesthesia/sedation/medication (10%), fat embolism (8.5%), cardiorespiratory failure (5.4%), massive infection (5.4%), and hemorrhage (4.6%) (Table 2). The authors concluded that the high fatality rate was reason to reconsider patient safety issues such as procedural limitations and postoperative discharge guidelines. The authors reported that a number of changes in liposuction technique were responsible for the reduced fatality rates compared to earlier studies. The changes included proper patient selection, the use of lower levels of fluids and local anesthetics, elimination of high-volume fat removal, and elimination of lengthy combination procedures.

Hughes [6] analyzed complication/fatality survey data on 94,159 liposuction procedures performed by 754 plastic surgeons between September 1, 1998 and August 31, 2000. The purpose of the study was to determine whether plastic surgeons had modified their practice patterns in recent years in order to reduce complications and fatalities reported in earlier plastic surgery surveys. The survey included queries regarding liposuction complications and fatalities, combined procedures, patient selection, facility accreditation, and changes in anesthesia and liposuction technique.

The results of the survey revealed that in 66% of the procedures, liposuction was performed alone. In 20% of the liposuction procedures, additional surgical procedures (excluding abdominoplasty) were performed during the same operative session. In 14% of the liposuction procedures,

TABLE 2 Liposuction Causes of Death

Cause of death	*N*	Percentage
Thromboembolism	30	23.1
Abdomen/viscus perforation	19	14.6
Anesthesia/sedation/medication	13	10.0
Fat embolism	11	8.5
Cardiorespiratory failure	7	5.4
Massive infection	7	5.4
Hemorrhage	6	4.6
Unknown	37	28.5
Total	130	100.1

Source: Ref. 5.

abdominoplasty and other procedures were all performed during the same operative session. The fatality rate for liposuction as a single procedure was 1 in 47,415. The fatality rate increased to 1 in 7311 when liposuction was performed in conjunction with other procedures (excluding abdominoplasty). The fatality rate was 1 in 3251 when liposuction was performed in conjunction with abdominoplasty with or without other procedures.

Three additional articles have been abstracted in order to provide complete coverage of the subject. The publication by Rao et al. [7] reported on five liposuction fatalities in New York. Studies by Coleman et al. [8] and Bruner and de Jong [9] analyzed insurance malpractice claims data for liposuction.

Rao and co-workers [7] from New York University, mistakenly attributed five liposuction fatalities to lidocaine toxicity from tumescent anesthesia. Four of the liposuction procedures were performed by plastic surgeons and one by a general surgeon. All five patients were given general anesthesia or intravenous sedation by an anesthesiologist. All patients underwent autopsy and there was no evidence of lidocaine toxicity. Intravenous fluids were given intraoperatively to three of the patients in the following volumes: 7.3, 3.0, and 1.7 L (Table 3). Two of the patients had a surgical procedure time of 4.5–7 hr and had liposuction of multiple body areas. These two patients developed pulmonary emboli. One of the patients also had breast implants performed during the same operative session as the liposuction.

Coleman and co-workers [8] analyzed Physicians Insurance Association of America (PIAA) malpractice data for liposuction for the years 1995–1997. The PIAA includes approximately 60% of physician-owned insurance companies. Of 253 claims 226 involved plastic surgeons. Only two claims

TABLE 3 Current Specialty Society Guidelines for Liposuction

Specialty society	Reference	Total lidocaine dose (in mg/kg)	Extraction volume (in liters)
American Academy of Dermatology	11	55	4.5 (supranatant fat)
American Society for Dermatologic Surgery	12	45–55	5 (supranatant fat)
American Academy of Cosmetic Surgery	13	55	5 (supranatant fat)
American Society of Plastic Surgery	—	35	5 (total aspirate)

were against dermatologists. Seventy-one percent of the 253 liability claims resulted from liposuction in the hospital operating room. Twenty-one percent of claims resulted from office-based liposuction. Practice data from the American Society for Dermatologic Surgery and the American Society of Plastic Surgery indicated that more plastic surgeons than dermatologists perform liposuction procedures (3:1 ratio). However, the vast majority of the liability claims were against plastic surgeons. Overall losses for claims against plastic surgeons were nearly $9 million compared to less than $4000 against dermatologists.

Bruner and de Jong [9] reported on PIAA medical liability claims for liposuction for the years 1995–1998. The report involved essentially the same data that were analyzed by Coleman and co-workers [8] in a previous publication. Although 255 of 292 liposuction claims (86.3%) were brought against plastic surgeons, it was pointed out that 67% of claims involved informed consent on breach-of-contract issues. Seven fatalities were reported. The authors felt that more complex, longer duration liposuction procedures were performed in the hospital as opposed to the outpatient setting. It was further stated that serious liposuction complications occur less commonly in the hospital than office-based surgery because hospital surgeons are board certified in a surgical specialty and are subject to peer review. The discussion of the article by Gorney reported that the plastic surgeon's problems with serious complications and fatalities had "vanished from the radar" by October 1, 2000.

LIPOSUCTION GUIDELINES

Liposuction surgery is performed by multiple specialties. Consequently all of the specialities have developed guidelines. The first liposuction guidelines to be published by any specialty were written in 1991 by the American Academy of Dermatology [10]. The most recent AAD Guidelines of Care for Liposuction were published in 2001 [11]. Similarly, the most recent American Society for Dermatologic Surgery Guidelines of Care for Liposuction were published in 2000 [12]. The American Academy of Cosmetic Surgery published its most recent Guidelines for Liposuction Surgery in 2000 [13]. Clinical Practice Guidelines for Lipoplasty have also been published by plastic surgery societies.

The various speciality society liposuction guidelines are summarized in Table 3. In general, all specialty society guidelines subscribe to total lidocaine doses of less than 55 mg/kg, and total supranatant fat extraction values of less than 5 L. The plastic surgery guidelines recommend a lower total lidocaine dose (35 mg/kg) presumably because they utilize general anesthesia or intravenous sedation as the primary method of anesthesia. In addition, plastic surgeons are generally unfamiliar with liposuction using tumescent local anesthesia as performed by dermatologists [14–15].

ACCREDITATION OF OFFICE SURGICAL FACILITIES

When a physician elects to offer office liposuction services, increased scrutiny by regulators and/or hospital credentialing committees usually follows. At least 31 states have imposed regulations on office surgery or are considering them. With ambulatory surgery on the rise, regulatory oversight is likely to escalate. Accreditation is one way to provide the oversight that will satisfy state regulators and the public interest.

Although several accreditation organizations exist, this chapter will discuss only the programs of the largest accreditor of ambulatory health care organizations, the AAAHC.

Accreditation is an indicator of health care quality and demonstrates a commitment to patient safety. Currently more than 1400 ambulatory health care organizations are accredited by AAAHC. Eight core standards apply to all ambulatory health care organizations seeking AAAHC accreditation. The eight core standards are listed in Table 4. Additional adjunct standards such as Anesthesia Services, Surgical Services, Pharmaceutical Services, and Pathology and Laboratory Services may apply to many office surgical facilities (Table 5). In 2001, the AAAHC introduced a new, streamlined accreditation program for office-based surgical facilities. This Office-Based Surgery Accreditation Program involves a single surveyor who performs a 1-day survey (Table 6).

Considerable preparation is required for an AAAHC Survey. AAAHC educational courses are offered each year for staff members from organizations that are preparing for accreditation surveys. Alternatively, organizations can hire an AAAHC consultant who will provide varying levels of on-site consultation and staff training. The OBS Guidebook and self-help materials are an excellent starting point for organizations seeking accreditation. Most often the surveyor who performs the AAAHC survey is from the same specialty as the organization being surveyed. Thus, the surveyor can provide useful consultative guidance to the organization during the survey.

An organization must be operational for at least 6 months before an AAAHC Survey can be done. The organization submits a Pre-Survey Questionnaire to the AAAHC to request a survey (Table 7). The PSQ allows AAAHC staff and the designated surveyor to become familiar with the organization in advance of the survey.

TABLE 4 AAAHC Core Standards

Rights of Patients
Governance
Administration
Quality of Care
Quality Management and Improvement
Clinical Records and Health Information
Professional Improvement
Facilities and Environment

TABLE 5 AAAHC Adjunct Standards[a]

Anesthesia Services
Surgical Services
Pharmaceutical Services
Pathology and Medical Laboratory Services
Teaching and Publication Activities
Research Activities

[a] Selected for office-based surgical facilities.

TABLE 6 AAAHC Office-Based Surgery Accreditation Program

Newly developed in 2001
Designed for practices with fewer than four surgeons and fewer than two operating suites
One-day, single-surveyor survey
Special Guidebook identifies specific standards for office-based surgery
Self-help materials available including templated forms and policies/procedures
Survey fee reduced to an affordable $2990

TABLE 7 AAAHC Contact Information

Accreditation Association for Ambulatory Health Care
3201 Old Glenview Road, Suite 300
Wilmette, IL 60091
Phone: 847-853-6060
Fax: 847-853-9028
Web: www.aaahc.org
Email: info@aaahc.org

Each on-site survey begins with a surveyor-led orientation meeting and concludes with a summation conference. Following the survey, the surveyor files a report with the AAAHC. An accreditation decision is granted within a matter of weeks. The AAAHC awards full accreditation for 3 years if the organization is in compliance with AAAHC standards. Organizations who demonstrate lessor compliance with standards may be granted a 1-year accreditation. Uncommonly, the accreditation decision is deferred or provisional accreditation is given. Occasionally an organization is denied accreditation.

The focus and emphasis of the AAAHC Accreditation process is always quality improvement. AAAHC views accreditation as a method for organizations to improve the patient care they deliver. A written, operational quality management and improvement program is required. Organizations who are new to accreditation may be somewhat familiar with quality improvement activities. However, they often require consultative assistance in designing and formatting studies and documenting that they have been done. Organizations who achieve accreditation generally feel more prepared and better organized after going through the process.

SUMMARY

Tumescent liposuction, performed totally under tumescent local anesthesia by dermatologic surgeons, has a superior safety record compared to more aggressive forms of liposuction. There have been no reported fatalities from liposuction using tumescent local anesthesia. A number of factors are responsible for the increased fatality risk from liposuction under general anesthesia or intravenous sedation: (1) multiple surgeries performed during the same operative session, (2) prolonged surgeries lasting many hours, (3) removal of excessive amounts of fat (i.e., "megaliposuction") during a single operative session, (4) intravenous fluid overload, and (5) administration of toxic doses of lidocaine used in conjunction with general anesthesia.

Tumescent liposuction utilizes tumescent local anesthesia as the primary method of anesthesia and postoperative pain control. Patients treated in this manner are extremely comfortable following the procedure. They recover in a matter of several days and the aesthetic results are superior.

Modern tumescent liposuction surgeons are committed to maximizing patient safety. Tumescent liposuction has contributed greatly to patient safety by allowing liposuction to be performed with minimal complications and excellent results. Accreditation of office surgical facilities, whether voluntary or mandated by the states, will further assure patient safety.

REFERENCES

1. Teimourian B, Rogers WB. A national survey of complications associated with suction lipectomy: A comparative study. Plast Reconstr Surg 1989; 84:628–631.
2. Bernstein G, Hanke CW. Safety of liposuction: a review of 9478 cases performed by dermatologists. J Dermatol Surg Oncol 1988; 14:1112–1114.
3. Hanke CW, Bernstein, Bullock S. Safety of tumescent liposuction in 15,336 patients: national survey results. Dermatol Surg 1995; 21:459–462.
4. Newman J, Dolsky RL. Evaluation of 5,458 cases of liposuction surgery. Am J Cosmet Surg 1984; 1(4):25–80.
5. Grazer FM, de Jong RH. Fatal outcomes from liposuction: census survey of cosmetic surgeons. Plast Reconstr Surg 2000; 105:436–446.
6. Hughes CE. Reduction of lipoplasty risks and mortality: an ASAPS survey. Aesthet Surg J 2001; 21:120–125.
7. Rao RB, Ely SF, Hoffman RS. Deaths related to liposuction. N Engl J Med 1999; 340:1471–1475.
8. Coleman WP, Hanke CW, Lillis P, Bernstein G, Narins R. Does the location of the surgery or the speciality of the physician affect malpractice claims in liposuction? Dermatol Surg 1999; 25:343–347.
9. Bruner JG, de Jong RH. Lipoplasty claims experience of U.S. insurance companies. Plast Reconstr Surg 2001; 107:1285–1291.
10. Drake LA, Ceilley RI, Cornelison RL et al. Guidelines of care for liposuction: Committee on Guidelines of Care. J Am Acad Dermatol 1991; 24:489–494.
11. Coleman WP, Glogau RG, Klein JK et al. Guidelines of care for liposuction. J Am Acad Dermatol 2001; 45:438–447.
12. Laurence N, Clark RE, Flynn TC, Coleman WP. American Society for Dermatologic Surgery Guidelines of Care for Liposuction. Dermatol Surg 2000; 26:265–269.
13. Jackson RF, Dolsky RL. Liposuction and patient safety. Am J Cosmet Surg 1999; 16:21–23.
14. Klein JA. The tumescent technique for liposuction. Am J Cosmet Surg 1987; 4:263–267.
15. Klein JA. Tumescent technique for regional anesthesia permits lidocaine doses of 35 mg/kg for liposuction. J Dermatol Surg Oncol 1990; 16:248–263.
16. Dillerud E. Suction lipoplasty: a report on complications, undesired results, and patient satisfaction based on 3511 procedures. Plast Reconstr Surg 1991; 88:239:246.
17. ASPRS Task Force on Lipoplasty. 1997 Survey Summary Report. Arlington Heights (IL): American Society of Plastic and Reconstructive Surgeons, 1998.

22

Managing Adverse Events: A Medicolegal Perspective

Abel Torres
Loma Linda University School of Medicine
Loma Linda, California, U.S.A.

DEFINING AN ADVERSE EVENT AND A MEDICOLEGAL PERSPECTIVE

The *Macmillan Dictionary* defines an adverse event as "not helpful to what is wanted" [1]. Professional liability companies tend to define an adverse event as "occurrences which could result in claims or suits" [2]. As defined above, a clinical/surgical adverse event has a component which requires medical decision making in that it is an event which can impede a desired clinical/surgical outcome. It is also an event or occurrence that may activate the legal process and precipitate litigation. As a result the management of a clinical/surgical adverse event related to liposuction surgery requires that the clinician approach the situation with a perspective that minimizes the impedance to the desired clinical outcome and minimizes the activation of the legal process. Thus, the reason for the title of this chapter being "Managing Adverse Events: A Medicolegal Perspective."

CONSEQUENCE OF AN ADVERSE EVENT

As defined above, an adverse event is undesirable in that it may not be helpful to the wanted clinical outcome and could result in a claim or suit.

When the latter occurs, it usually signals that the trust between the patient and doctor has eroded to a point of no return [3]. Thus, a key component of the medicolegal perspective needed in dealing with adverse clinical/surgical events is one that emphasizes maintaining and strengthening the trust between the clinician and the patient.

HONESTY IS THE CORNERSTONE OF TRUST

Few would dispute the statement that honesty is the cornerstone of trust. In 1996 the results of a survey of patients attitudes toward doctors' mistakes was published in the *Archives of Internal Medicine.* The survey interviewed 149 responders, 400 of whom were randomly chosen from among 10,000 patients seen in the general internal medicine outpatient clinics at the Loma Linda University Medical Center located in Loma Linda, California. The latter is a health sciences university medical center which includes a medical school. Patients were presented with three hypothetical scenarios, including a minor, moderate, and severe mistake made by a doctor. An identical set of questions geared toward determining patient responses to physician error followed each scenario. Not surprisingly, the results revealed that patients want physicians to acknowledge their mistakes no matter how minor. In addition, although the survey revealed that patients would lose some measure of trust with a disclosure by the physician, it was even more damaging to the physician–patient trust if the physician failed to disclose a mistake and it was later discovered by the patient. In fact the latter circumstance was more likely to lead the patient to sue or report the doctor [4]. Yet, not every mistake leads to an adverse event either because it is intercepted before it can cause harm or it is insufficient in and of itself to significantly affect the desired outcome. Is not disclosing this type of mistake dishonesty? Some physicians recommend that if the mistake is intercepted and does not harm the patient, it should be disclosed internally to correct a system weakness but not disclosed to the patient and risk needless damage to patient trust [2]. An extension to this position is that medical care and medical decision making can be simple or complex [5]. Human beings are also complex creatures and the end result of a medical intervention is unpredictable. What may be considered the correct approach for one person may in fact be the wrong approach for another. Thus, it can be debated that whether a given act or omission by a clinician is in fact a mistake may be better judged by the final outcome rather than intervening outcomes during medical interventions. Do these intervening acts or omissions need disclosure or do they also needlessly erode patient trust and ultimately patient care? Finally, not all adverse events are the results of mistakes but rather truly unexpected outcomes. Although few would argue with honesty being the cornerstone of trust, what constitutes dishonesty is not always so clear and it is up to each individual to decipher which of their morals and professional ethics they construe as honesty. Regardless, it is clear that patients value honesty in their interactions with doctors and physicians would do well to keep honesty foremost as the guide to their actions when dealing with adverse events. What is critical in dealing with adverse events is that the physician needs to honestly communicate with and manage the patient and as part of this process needs to assure that the events which transpire are accurately assessed to assure honest communication. What should not occur is a premature rush to honesty without a full reconciliation of the facts since this may in fact be dishonest communication and lead to needless erosion of patient trust, patient angst, the impediment of corrective action, or premature litigation.

REMEDYING AN ADVERSE EVENT

It goes without saying that when an adverse event occurs, the clinician needs to take steps to minimize the impact of that adverse event on the desired clinical outcome. The chapters in this book, especially the one on complications by Dr. Ronald Moy, can provide much useful guidance as to the clinical direction to follow in that regard. The purpose of this chapter is to provide education as to useful steps that can be followed to ease the process of helping the patient maintain and strengthen his or her trust in the clinician, thereby facilitating any necessary clinical intervention. As always, when dealing with issues that can precipitate litigation, the clinician should not rely on this or other written material as a substitute for legal counseling from their attorney.

The approach to an adverse event will be influenced by whether the physician is the treating or consulting physician or whether the physician has been asked to serve as an expert witness. Honesty is the key to success in all these settings but the approach by necessity varies according to the role of the physician and is discussed in each context.

TREATING PHYSICIAN

When dealing with an adverse event, the treating physician should take positive and not negative measures. They should be honest with the patient and the family as appropriate. All facts should be reconciled with the health care team (office staff). Assessments and interventions should be well documented in the medical record with special care not to alter or give the appearance of altering the medical record. Any type of evidence involved in the occurrence should be preserved. Contacting the physician's liability carrier, risk management service, or attorney should also be foremost in the mindset of the physician since risk of litigation is part of the definition of an adverse event.

Positive Measures

Positive measures refers to dealing with the situation in a manner that is productive as opposed to counterproductive. It may be appropriate to empathize or sympathize with the patient's distress. This would be productive since it communicates that you are concerned about his or her well-being. On the other hand expressing remorse when the facts have not been fully sorted may be premature and lead to distrust that hinders patient care. Likewise, expressing self-criticism or thinking out loud may stimulate the physician to be creative in remedying the situation and perhaps preventing future problems. However, the same actions can be misconstrued by nonmedically savvy individuals as admissions of wrongdoing or negligence when in fact the physician is attempting to sort out the problem. Physicians are trained to consider differential diagnoses no matter how unlikely and ultimately discard those that are not plausible. A nonmedically trained individual can misconstrue a differential diagnosis of what went wrong as a list of mistakes or omissions that occurred or incompetence by the physician. Hence, physicians can certainly approach the occurrence as a differential diagnosis type of evaluation but should not do so by thinking out loud in the presence of the patient. To do so would be akin to a pilot turning on the loudspeaker and discussing his options when the airplane is having difficulties. The latter would not inspire confidence or be appreciated by the passengers.

Another productive positive measure is to acknowledge any complaint by a patient as an opportunity to gather more data and investigate a situation more fully. It is counterproductive and a negative to dismiss a patients complaint no matter how trivial. Of all the productive positive measures that can be taken, one of the most important is to make sure that the patient's medical needs are appropriately addressed, including referral for consultations when needed. Timely consultations can help and reassure the patient. They may also prevent needless litigation by assuring that the patients needs are adequately addressed by competent individuals familiar with the circumstances of the adverse events. On the other hand procrastinating a referral is a negative measure that forces the patient to shop around for help and risk treatment by clinicians that may not be properly trained for the problem or who may make comments to hide their own inadequacies. Such comments have been documented to be a frequent source for inflaming the situation and initiating litigation (oral communication, Southern California Physicians Insurance Exchange, 1998).

Communication

It is important to recognize that people are social beings who seek comfort from others such as family and friends. As physicians we are well aware of the importance of the latter in the care of the patient. When performing cosmetic procedures we should be cognizant of the folly of not including family and friends as part of the presurgical consultation process, since when an adverse event occurs it is those same family and friends that the patient will look to for comfort and advice. Thus, it is important that we include them in our discussions with the patient as soon as possible. If family and friends understand what is happening they can assist the patient as needed; provide reassurance; and, almost as important, avoid making inflammatory remarks. Studies have shown that aside from the inflammatory remarks of other health care practitioners being a leading cause of precipitating litigation so too are the remarks of friends and family (oral communication, Southern California Physicians Insurance Exchange, 1998). Dealing with an angry patient and their support group can be uncomfortable for a physician but if the physician puts him- or herself in their shoes it is easier to understand the anxiety involved and avoid becoming defensive. During the communication the physician should empathize, accept responsibility for the care of the patient, and find a solution to the problem but not accept blame prematurely. The discussion should center around factual issues and clearing up misperceptions as well as clarifying the course of action that will be taken. Premature opinions and theories by the physician should be avoided and those of the patient and support group politely acknowledged with the clarification that data will be gathered and all possibilities explored. Finger pointing at anyone, including another health care practitioner, should be avoided. The latter is important because without all the facts, finger pointing may be premature and human nature is such that it only makes others defensive and want to point back, initiating an endless cycle of blame. Communication requires access and however uncomfortable for the physician, access must be present at all times. Avoiding the patient and the support group will not make the problem go away but it will inflame the situation. If the physician is not available to the patient to discuss his or her concerns he or she will look for someone who will listen. That is what attorneys do well, often with a bias toward promoting their business as evidenced by the fact that they see "clients" not patients. Thus, physicians should make sure that they or a designated member of their staff are readily reachable and available to the patient to answer any and all questions and assist as needed. As always, in our haste to communicate honestly with the patient and his or her support group we must not forget that patients are autonomous individuals with a right to privacy [6]. The new Health Insurance Privacy and

Portability Act (HIPPA) rules further underscore the need to protect confidentiality [7]. Thus, prior to initiating any communication with a patient's family or friends a physician should procure the patients consent for this action, preferably with documentation in writing. In fact depending on the jurisdiction, the new HIPPA regulations or local laws may mandate the process to be followed and physicians would be wise to know these.

Facts versus Assumptions

In dealing with an adverse event it is important never to assume anything. Embarrassment and misunderstandings are more likely to be the result of assumptions. This is well understood in legal circles and in depositions a deposed person is cautioned against guessing. When an adverse event occurs, the situation should be fully investigated. The facts as understood by the patient and the health care team need to be reconciled. This reconciliation is not to conjure up a defense as one plaintiff's attorney once assumed and tried to chastise me for. Rather it is part of the process of a thorough investigation and as an attorney I support such a thorough exploration of the facts just as I support depositions to sift for an reconcile valid facts and not to conjure up frivolous causes of action. Reconciliation of the facts assures that the physician is aware of all the facts pertaining to the patients care. As physicians we know that it is not uncommon for a patient or staff member to be aware of a fact that the physician has not been made privy to. Often, this is because it may be embarrassing to the patient. Also, it is common knowledge that if you whisper a comment in a person's ear and wait to hear the comment as it travels around a circle of people, the comment you hear at the end will often be very different than what you initially said. Likewise, when an adverse event occurs, the whispers that take place in and out of the office as well as the staff, patient, and physician perceptions of the facts can vary widely. Knowing all the facts allows us to clear up misperceptions by the patient, physician, and/or the staff. Furthermore, it can be very confusing for a patient to hear different versions of instructions or explanations to their questions. It is only natural for each staff member to communicate in a manner customary for them but unfortunately any differences can be interpreted by the patient as inconsistencies or hint at subterfuge. Thus, even before the facts are reconciled and certainly afterward, the physician should either handle all inquiries from the patient and support group him- or herself or designate one staff member for that task. The latter assures consistency for the patient and accuracy of communications and eases anxieties.

Just as it is important to reconcile the facts before making any conclusions and treatment decisions, so also is it important to avoid voicing premature opinions without weighing all the facts. As medical students physicians are often trained to discuss differential diagnoses with the health care team. This is part of the education process for all the health care personnel. The sharing of opinions helps to stimulate discussion, learning, and quality assurance. Therefore, it is only natural that physicians would carry on these same type of exercises in their offices and discuss opinions with their staff as to what occurred during an adverse event. Unfortunately, the legal process takes a different view of this kind of activity and can misinterpret any comment or opinion by a physician or staff member as an admission of guilt [8]. The logic is that in the ordinary course of business or in the heat of the moment people will be candid and say the truth [8]. Regardless of the scientific soundness of this assumption, it is not uncommon for a physician or staff member to be asked during a deposition about what comments or opinions have been voiced out of the courtroom in an effort to ferret out these so-called admissions. Thus, until our legal system can be reformed to recognize the value of this activity for patients, it is wiser for the physician to only discuss facts with his or her staff or others until they have sufficient facts to arrive at a valid opinion and conclusion. Nevertheless, the need to speak out loud or express an opinion is often a way for a physician to release anxiety since after all we are social creatures who seek comfort from others as well. Fortunately, the legal process has recognized this innately human need and allows us the privilege of communicating with our spouse, attorney, and sometimes clergy to express our frustrations and opinions without fear of repercussion. Such communications are privileged and can be used by physicians as an outlet instead of having to carry the world on their shoulders. Yet such communications are only privileged if not shared with others and physicians should remember the old adage of "loose lips sink ships."

Documentation

Patient care is best served by good documentation. A well-documented patient chart will assure that the information needed to take care of that patient is available as the physician ponders a course of action or should another health care provider need to be consulted. The written communication (patient record) should reflect the oral communications. Hence, the physician should factually record the adverse event and response. Unless it adds to the care of the patient, premature opinions and conclusions should be avoided as this may confuse future caregivers or be legally misinterpreted as an admission. Risk management comments, or comments about any individuals, including the patients, usually add little if anything to the patients care and should be avoided in the records. The key consideration should be how any entry will help the patient's care. With this in the forefront, the value of any addenda should be appraised before adding it to the record.

Although the record reflects hearsay, it is a business record and the presumption is that in the ordinary course of business it is accurate and truthful and accepted as a legal hearsay exemption [9]. Thus, the patient record serves a dual importance for patient care as well as evidence for any future litigation. For this reason it is important that the record not be altered in any way that gives the appearance of impropriety. If the latter happens, the credibility of the record and consequently the physician will be called into doubt during legal proceedings. Thus, the record should only be altered when essential for patient care. Attorneys, often advise that any alteration should reflect by whom and when it was made (a simple line to cross out an error with a date and initials or signature) to reflect that there is no attempt at subterfuge (oral communication, Southern California Physicians Insurance Exchange, 1998). The latter also helps assure a subsequent caregiver reading the chart that the correction or addition was appropriately made for patient care.

Preserving the Medical Record and Evidence

Since the patients medical record is important for patient care as well as evidence, it must be carefully guarded to preserve its accuracy and confidentiality [7]. As such the original records should never be released although copies can be made if authorized by a patient via written consent or through other legal proceedings [7]. This protects the accuracy of the records for patient care, the privacy of the patient and for the physicians defense if necessary. Often, a medical device will be used in providing patient care. It may ultimately turn out that an adverse event was the result of a defective device. Therefore, medical devices used in a patient care should be preserved for later inspection whenever feasible. Advise from a manufacturer or vendor regarding the device should be sought when needed but if the device was used in association with the adverse event it should not be returned until its defect or lack of defect has been properly documented. A premature return of the device could lead to loss of or tampering of crucial information regarding the adverse event both from a patient care as well as a legal evidence perspective. Often, a manufacturer will be subject to strict product liability for their devices, which can ease the litigation burden for the physician [10].

Legal Advice

It cannot be overemphasized that if a physician receives a request for patient records, a summons or legal complaint, or a threat or demand for compensation he or she should immediately advise his or her attorney and or medical malpractice carrier. Failure to do so can have significant consequences among which is noncoverage by the carrier if not notified in a timely manner as required by the malpractice contract. Whether all adverse events need to be reported to the latter is a judgment call by the physician more likely to be prudent when patient injury occurs. Certainly, the advisability of writing off a bill should be discussed with and coordinated with an attorney or malpractice carrier. Some patients will see this as a gesture of goodwill while others will see it as an admission of guilt and sue regardless of the adjustment [2]. The courts and the National Practitioner Data Bank have not considered writing off a bill as either an admission of guilt or a reportable incident [2]. This could change but for now, this should make writing off a bill a more attractive option for physicians. Patients, especially cosmetic surgery patients, may have paid for a service with specific expectations. Just as we would not want to pay in full for a service that was only partially performed, a patient may not want to pay in full for a cosmetic procedure that only partially met their expectations. It is my belief and experience that these type of patients may be satisfied by a complete or partial waiver of a debt. It behooves the physician to understand the motives behind his or her patient's request for cosmetic surgery as well as later complaints to accurately assess whether writing off a bill can help defuse a potentially inflammatory situation after an adverse event. I would be wary of naysayers who insist writing off a bill is never an option.

CONSULTANTS

The principles that a subsequent treating physician or consultant should follow in evaluating a patient after an adverse event are the same as those for an initial treating physician. However, consultants or subsequent treating physicians need to be wary of the fact that these patients may now be distrustful of health care providers. They may also be introducing their own perception bias into any history provided and have preconceived notions of what constitutes appropriate care. Thus, the consultant or subsequent treating physician needs to be vigilant for misperceptions and document carefully, especially with photographs if possible. He or she should refrain from pointing fingers or assigning blame and should strive to keep discussions on a factual level. When asked for an opinion by the patient the physician should be mindful that it is unlikely that he will be able to accurately form an opinion until all facts have been ascertained and this may sometimes require the patient's permission to contact the prior treating doctor. Of particular concern is the fact that the patient may have had a long-standing relationship with the prior treating doctor and may be mad at that physician but still have mixed feelings about suing him or her. This is much like one may be mad at a friend or family member but think twice before suing. On the other hand, the relationship with the consultant is only beginning and if the patient needs someone to blame, the consultant or subsequent treating physician would be a logical outlet for the patient's frustrations. That this phenomenon does occur has been well documented in psychiatry as the process of transference [11]. It is not hard to imagine that the patient can perceive any adverse effects to be the result of inadequate follow-up care rather than poor original care. This can justify preserving a long-standing relationship with the original treating doctor while seeking redress. So while it may seem that the consultant or subsequent treating physician should have a less arduous task than the original treating physician, it is wise to guard against complacency.

EXPERT WITNESSING AND ADVERSE EVENTS

Unlike the original treating physician and the subsequent treating physicians or consultants, the physician who is called to act as an expert witness, be it for the plaintiff or defendant, does not have to worry about providing patient care or maintaining the patient's trust. Nevertheless, the effectiveness of that physician as an expert witness will depend on whether he or she is perceived to be honest and unbiased. Therefore it behooves the expert witness to assure that he or she has thoroughly reviewed all of the facts before rendering an opinion. An attorney who is sizing up the effectiveness of the expert witness testimony will look at the thoroughness of the experts preparation as one guide in deciding whether to proceed further, settle, or dismiss the case. A hallmark of an expert is that he or she is being called upon to render an opinion. Thus, a factual review will not be sufficient but will be critical in assuring that the opinion is based on a solid foundation. The opinion will also bear more weight if it is perceived to be honest and unbiased. Thus, an expert witness must concede the obvious and if the facts do not clearly support the position that the expert was asked to support the better part of valor should be to make this clear to the requesting party early on rather than walking the line of honesty versus dishonesty.

CONCLUSION

In summary, maintaining the patient's trust is essential when an adverse medical event occurs. Key to that goal will be honesty in communication and actions. Physicians should take positive measures and be honest with the patient and the family yet reconcile facts with the health care team before arriving at premature conclusions. Assessments and interventions should be well documented in the medical record with special care not to alter or give the appearance of altering the medical record and preserve any type of evidence involved in the occurrence. Contacting the physicians liability carrier, risk management service, or attorney should also be foremost in the mind set of the physician since risk of litigation is part of the definition of an adverse event and unfortunately the current social climate gravitates to this way of solving problems. Yet at the forefront of a physician's thoughts should be how to care for the patient's needs.

REFERENCES

1. Levey JS. Macmillan Dictionary for Children. 2nd ed. New York: Simon and Schuster, 1989, p 12.
2. Keyes C. Responding to adverse events, forum: Risk Management Foundation of the Harvard Medical Institutions Inc., Keyes C, ed. 18(1):2–3, 1997.
3. Localio AR, et al. Relationship between malpractice claims and adverse events due to negligence. N Engl J Med 325(4):245–251, 1991.
4. Witman A, Park D, Hardin S. How do patients want physicians to handle mistakes? Arch Int Med 156:2565–2569, 1996.
5. Anderson CA, et al. Evaluation and management services guidelines: current procedural terminology. Chicago: AMA Press, 2001, pp 1–7.
6. National Commission for the Protection of Human Subjects of Biomedical and Behavioral Research. The Belmont report: ethical principles and guidelines for the protection of human subjects in research. DHEW Pub No. (05) 78-0012, Washington D.C.: U.S. Government Printing Office, 1979.
7. Health Insurance Portability and Accountability Act of 1996, Pub. L No. 104-191, Codified at 42 USC Sec. 1320d, 1996.
8. California Jury Instructions 2.25: Extrajudicial admissions, cautionary instructions. BAJI 9th ed. 1:27, 2000.
9. People v Brust, 1957, 47 Cal 2d 776–785.
10. California Jury Instructions 9.003: Products liability—strict liability in tort-defect in manufacture. BAJI 9th ed. 5:324, 2000.
11. Nicholi A. The therapist-patient relationship. In: Nicholi A, ed., The Harvard Guide to Psychiatry. 3rd ed. Cambridge: Belknap Press, pp 1–25, 1999.

23

Handling the Dissatisfied or Difficult Patient

Paul Jarrod Frank
New York University Medical Center
New York, New York, U.S.A.

A cosmetic surgeon's familiarity with the difficult and dissatisfied patient is a popular topic of discussion both professionally and medically/legally. Long problem lists, unrealistic expectations, and incessant dissatisfaction despite satisfactory results persevere as the common thread among this population that is, at the least, demanding of special treatment. As much as these individuals serve as a source of simple frustration among professionals they can also provide significant anxiety in regard to medical/legal and ethical issues pertaining to the proper treatment of patients. In order to maintain a healthy doctor–patient relationship and avoid unnecessary stress it is important to recognize the "red flags" of the difficult patient and to practice problem-avoiding techniques in order to minimize the sometimes stressful kinetics between patient and doctor.

THE IDEAL VERSUS THE PROBLEM PATIENT

Recognizing patients at high risk for both medical and psychological complications is of utmost priority in our profession. It is not as easy as "good patient/bad patient" as there are often shades of gray. Each patient and doctor may, under different circumstances, present with characteristics that threaten a healthy professional relationship. Often the surgeon's personality and his or her transference of emotions toward patients can play a significant role as well. Physicians, typically under significant amounts of stress, must be aware that their personal and professional issues can potentially affect the interaction that they have with patients. A rule of constant self-monitoring and objectivity is always an advantage for doctors as they too are not perfect.

So who is a good cosmetic patient? An individual with realistic desires and expectations for aesthetic improvement is best. One who seeks improvement without the need for perfection and is aware that magical transformation is never an accomplishment of cosmetic procedures. Patients who have or are willing to educate themselves in the potential options for treatment and seek the advice and expertise of a physician that they have chosen on their own volition. Specific concerns that are realistic, limited, and perceivable by the doctor clearly relieve some of the pressure to satisfy the patient upon consultation. The ability to understand, weigh, and respond to the risks and benefits that are described to them without hastiness in decision making allows the doctor to understand the willingness and tolerability of a patient to a given treatment option. Confident and proactive in their health and well-being, ideal patients seek improvement for themselves rather than from outside pressures [1]. As for the problem patient, we can all make a long list of characteristics to watch out for, most of which are dichotomous to the traits mentioned earlier. Because patients from a wide variety of ethnic, cultural, and socioeconomic groups present for cosmetic consultation, we must acknowledge that the desires of each patient fall upon a wide spectrum of characteristics. The red flags, though, tend to be universal among the high-risk patients and strict avoidance in performing unnecessary procedures on this population should be practiced. Often enthusiastic to hone skills and to achieve pleasant results, cosmetic surgeons young and old are, way too often, eager to perform procedures on anyone who wants them. This is often the Achilles heel of the cosmetic surgeon that, in the end, provides more frustration and anxiety than satisfaction for both the doctor and patient.

Of primary concern, again, is the proper perception of the patient. The presurgical expectation of the end result is the most reliable predictor of the degree of procedural satisfaction [2]. Even when the results are excellent, patients may be severely disappointed if their image of themselves postoperatively is different from the preconceived notion they had prior to the procedure. Unfortunately, we live in a world of "media hype" where "before" and "after" pictures, advertising promotions, and procedural promises falsely educate patients on the proper expectations. Lack of monitoring and control of the media has been a doubled-edged sword for dermatologic surgeons. As the number of individuals seeking cosmetic procedures has risen dramatically, so has the percentage of difficult patients. For example, a 45-year-old woman who is 40 lbs overweight and has had three children is unhappy after tumescent liposuction. Although she has dropped a few clothing sizes and has excellent results, her figure and skin tone are not what they were before having her children. "Before" and "after" pictures she had seen on the Internet gave her this drastically unrealistic expectation of what liposuction could do for her. To avoid this, the initial consultation should clearly state the objective of the procedure, which is to contour, not recreate skin tone. If the patient as perceived by the physician does not acquire an understanding of the risks and benefits, then it is an obvious sign that the patient is a poor surgical candidate [3,4]. A patient's reasoning for getting a cosmetic procedure does not always imply reason, as many people have motives with secondary gain [2]. Wanting a husband to stop cheating, avoiding having to exercise and eat well to control weight, or trying to emulate an idol are not uncommon incentives for the difficult or dissatisfied patient. Such motives are frequently encountered when patients come in requesting a specific procedure, signifying some level of education and thought on the matter. It is always imperative to determine the motivation of one's patients. Approaching the topic with open-ended questions often reveals the patient's motivation on consultation. "What do you expect from liposuction" should be answered with "help in removing my trouble spots that I can't achieve with diet and exercise." "So I can have the body I did when I was 20" in a 55-year-old is clearly a red flag for a potentially dissatisfied patient. In addition, avoidance of those individuals who are going through life's stressful events is generally a good rule as their perceptions of themselves change frequently through difficult times [2]. If and when the physician and patient can agree upon a realistic outcome with good intentions, further workup can successfully commence.

Caution should always be maintained with individuals with extreme vanity and concern for their appearance. Given, cosmetic surgeons are in a field of medicine where external appearance is of primary concern; but nonetheless, a clear delineation can be made between those who want to improve their appearance and those who are obsessed with their physicality. These patients can clearly be the most difficult as their self-esteem is dependent only on others. A dysmorphic body image often pervades their daily behaviors with unrealistic demands and/or exaggerated perceptions of their appearance [5]. The obsession with real or imagined defects brings them to your office when they have frequently seen many doctors before you. You are first perceived as the one that will be able to see their flaws and help them. Regardless of what you can do, they will almost universally be disappointed and/or begin to focus on other aspects of themselves. Often with mirror in hand, they are pointing out blemishes and marks that are barely perceivable to nonexistent. The inability to accept one's asymmetries, minor flaws, or aging is a hallmark of patients with this problem. The syndrome is a much bigger problem that often requires professional help other than cosmetic surgery [1].

Individuals with body dysmorphism are often susceptible to surgical addiction [6–9]. Constantly in search for the fountain of youth, these patients have no tolerance for imperfection and are always on the hunt for the newest procedures with better results. Using cosmetic surgery to obtain acceptance provides a false perception of happiness that takes them from one procedure to the next [6].

One of the most important skills expected of a doctor is that of communication. The ability to educate, console, and guide a patient through treatments and procedures is necessary in all aspects of medicine. One of the more frustrating and potentially deleterious situations is when the patient clearly lacks the ability to communicate and correspond with his or her doctor. A telltale sign of more significant emotional difficulties, the inability of a patient to communicate makes them undesirable cosmetic candidates. Those who look but do not listen fall into this category [6]. Often unable to understand the risks or goals of a procedure, these individuals, rather than demanding a clearer understanding, often appear disinterested when the risks of procedures are discussed. Quick glancing and signing of consent forms are frequent maneuvers to avoid the potential consequences. Pressured speech, total silence, or erratic behaviors are additional traits to be wary of. The potential for patients to lie and become aggressive and impulsive is great in these circumstances. Spending the time to talk and share information with the patient, either by yourself or with your staff, often reveals the potential for such problems.

Given the inundation of information on cosmetic surgery in the media and on the Internet, it is recommended to ask the patient what he or she may know already about a given procedure. With his or her patient's preconceived notions in mind, the doctor can build upon and/or augment what the patient needs to understand in order to have a satisfactory outcome. When it is evident that a patient either cannot comprehend or that he or she is unwilling to deal with the risks and expected outcomes of a procedure, the doctor should make clear that the procedure is not for them. And finally, doctor–patient relations with those who are verbally manipulative, overdemanding, and/or threatening should immediately be dissolved in a calm and cautious manner.

Given the elective, cosmetic nature in much of dermatologic surgeon's practice, it is important to first do no harm. Differentiating a good and poor candidate for a procedure and guiding treatment based on that perception is often the best way to achieve the best results and maintain a healthy relationship with one's patients.

COSMETIC PATIENTS WITH PSYCHIATRIC CONDITIONS

It is evident to all cosmetic surgeons that consultations almost always involve the use of psychology. Because patients judge themselves based on their appearance, it is not uncommon for those with psychiatric conditions to come for consultation [10–13]. These patients, because of their illnesses, are at the highest risk for dissatisfaction. It is imperative for doctors to recognize when these problems exist and to learn how to deal with those patients who have them. While some cases are quite obvious, others are subtle; therefore, it is essential in the initial consultation to rule out both subjectively and objectively any potential pathology. Often doctors can get a sense of a patient's disposition that guides them through the initial consultation. Objectively, doctors must include a psychiatric history in their initial questionnaire. These questions should be open ended so as to request "if ever" a situation occurred. Questions should include past therapy, psychiatric medications, hospitalization, recent changes in life (i.e., divorce, loss of a loved one, etc.). Because psychiatric illness is quite common, it is not necessary to exclude all patients who have had a psychiatric history from cosmetic procedures; but is essential to weigh the risks and benefits for that patient with all the appropriate information available. There are a great number of patients who have overcome many of life's difficulties and can be very good candidates for cosmetic procedures. Contacting a patient's psychiatrist is of great help to determine the appropriateness of a procedure for a particular patient [13].

Individuals with many types of personality disorders have an affinity for cosmetic surgery. Of these, cosmetics surgeons most frequently encounter those who have narcissistic and borderline personality disorders and obsessive compulsive disorder [1,10,11]. Narcissistic patients are often the most grandiose in speech and mannerism. Overindulgence in their beauty and the things that can enhance it are hallmark traits. Frequent glances into a nearby mirror while talking to them are not uncommon. When asked what they would like to have done they usually interject that they think very highly of themselves as is. "Arrogant," "demanding," and "pushy" are best used to describe these individuals. Because of these characteristics, they are never satisfied and are at high risk for unrealistic expectations. When complications or dissatisfaction do occur, they believe you are in practice for them only and should act accordingly.

Patients with borderline personality disorder often pose specific threats to a proper doctor–patient relationship [10]. First, these patients develop characteristic images of their physician as either an idol or an enemy. Upon consultation, these patients make you feel as if you are the only one capable of helping them. Unfortunately, this perception is very labile. When dissatisfaction sets in, you quickly become quite the opposite and can easily be a target for personal or legal harassment. They can become aggressive, angry, and inappropriate if their exceedingly high expectations are not met. Recognizing and avoiding erratic behavior is important. Second, these patients almost always have a dysmorphic body image, which can cloud their judgment in weighing the risks and benefits of procedures. They often have several complaints and feel that a total cosmetic "makeover" is essential. Once one problem is attended to there is another immediately. Concerns are usually out of proportion with reality for borderline patients and they can be quite seductive in convincing doctors of the necessity for a procedure.

The final condition worth discussing in detail is that of obsessive–compulsive disorder. These patients are true perfectionists and therefore pose specific concerns to the cosmetic surgeon [5]. They incessantly focus on their cosmetic faults and are rigid in their own perception, often unwilling to accept other's opinions. Defects that are invisible to the surgeon are outlined frequently without regard to the big picture. Often during one consultation the same concerns are repeated several times in great detail. When compulsive behavior is a part of their condition, it is not uncommon to see self-induced scars, excoriations, and picking that is uncontrollable. These activities relieve some aspect of their obsession and are very difficult for the doctor to effectively advise against. These traits can drastically alter the outcome of any cosmetic procedure given their uncontrollable nature. Patients with this problem often cannot follow pre- and postoperative instructions appropriately, therefore making them poor surgical candidates.

Several other psychiatric conditions can pose management difficulties [11]. Mood disorders, histrionic or dependent personality disorders, and psychotic diseases each have their own characteristics traits. Regardless of a psychiatric patient's specific disorder, it is essential to recognize the "red flags" of patients suffering with mental disease. Excessive anxiety, confusion, inappropriate behavior, neurosis, and anger are clear indications of underlying psychological distress. These patients, regardless of their exact diagnosis, should be deterred from getting cosmetic surgery. The ability to handle them is unique for each doctor and should be a skill that cosmetic surgeons seek to develop for their practice.

MINIMIZING DISSATISFACTION AT THE CONSULTATION

The initial consultation with a cosmetic patient can be used as an essential tool to minimize dissatisfaction [14]. With a good history and physical examination many of the high-risk patients can easily be recognized. The appropriate information should be presented to patients in order for them to educate themselves of the procedural course and their risks and benefits

[15,16]. By identifying different risk factors and providing information to the patients, physicians can then determine whether a patient is a good surgical candidate.

During the initial visit the physician should describe the reality of a procedure and its risks, being careful not to downplay any facet of it or the patient's responsibility to follow instructions before, during, and after the procedure [17,18]. Expected results cannot be exaggerated as this always leads to a dissatisfied patient. Avoiding "selling" a procedure is always good behavior. Convincing a patient that a procedure is best for them puts a tremendous responsibility on the physician to ensure significant results. Often patients feel "duped" or "swindled" if the results are not what they expected [18,19].

In order to establish a good doctor–patient relationship it is necessary to have good communication skills. Ensuing trust is an essential part of the first visit. To acquire the proper rapport, one's manner of speech as well as body language are considerable aspects in the first meeting. Seat yourself at eye level across from the patient. Avoid excessive note taking during the conversation as this dissociates your attention from the patient. Create pauses in your conversation and question the patient frequently to ensure his or her understanding of what you are trying to explain. Using open-ended questions that start with "how," what," or "why" are best suited to gaining insight into your patient's needs [1,16]. Answering their questions slowly and thoroughly with appreciation, not judgment, shows patients your concern for their well-being. Allow patients to finish their thoughts before commenting on their concerns and questions. Patients are more nervous to see you than you are to see them; be sensitive to this fact. Smiling and projecting a confident self-image often gives patients a sense a security that they are in need of when faced with the unknown.

Many factors external to the physician help to develop the proper rapport with the patient. A clean and attractive office provides a good impression for the patient. Being well groomed and friendly gives patients comfort when they discuss their concerns with you. An attentive and well-informed staff is one of the most essential aspects to any cosmetic practice. They allow the patient several opportunities to interact, ask questions, and get formal attention rather than sitting alone in the consultation room awaiting the doctor [20,21]. In addition, some patients develop bonds with specific staff members that make their experience an easier one [18]. Any aspect of a patient's experience from the moment they walk into your office could affect their impression of you either positively or negatively, so pay attention to detail.

When the consultation is nearing its close, it is helpful to ensure that the patient's concerns have been attended to. Using another open-ended question such as "is there anything else I can do for you" gives the patient a final opportunity to ask any additional questions. Let the patient know that if they should think of any additional questions that you and/or your staff are always available. Providing them with a means to contact the office gives them the satisfaction that you are working in their best interest by educating them. Sometimes a second presurgical consultation allows the patient to reflect on the information given to them and then ask more specific questions prior to a procedure.

PATIENT SELECTION

It is easy for most surgeons to recognize the "red flags" of the potentially difficult patient. In the same manner, one can recognize those candidates who are ideal. Unfortunately though, most individuals who enter our practices fall somewhere in between. What is essential for all cosmetic surgeons is to follow their instinct and avoid patients and situations that can pose problems in the future. Using objective measures as well as subjective ones are desirable. It is important to remember that much of what we do is elective and unnecessary; therefore, it is in our own best interest to make a strong effort to decipher who is and who is not a good surgical candidate. Using the opinions of your office staff often makes this decision an easier one [20,21]. If there is at all any doubt, then it is likely that the patient is a poor candidate.

Any patient who is, in your opinion, not a good surgical candidate should be declined. This should be done in a manner that is not offensive to the patient. Absolving the blame of the patient is often the best technique. In this manner, the physician can express to the patient that he or she would not benefit from a procedure relative to the desired outcome. In addition, it can be expressed to the patient that his or her concerns do not fall within your field of expertise. It is very tempting as a young cosmetic surgeon to acquire surgical experience with those patients who are eager, regardless of whether they are good candidates. It is advantageous, though, to avoid such temptation for the adverse consequences of acquiring a dissatisfied or difficult patient can often ruin the enthusiasm and expectations of the budding surgeon [2].

USING COMMUNICATION TO PREVENT DISSATISFACTION

Probably the most single important factor that leads to malpractice claims, in all fields of medicine, is poor doctor–patient relationship [22,23]. This is particularly true for cosmetic surgery. Often the relationship between the doctor and patient holds greater weight than the actual technical and clinical acumen required for each procedure. For this reason, it is necessary to guide and comfort patients every step along the way. When problems arise, they must be attended to quickly and with assertiveness. Regardless of the level of complications, the physician should never abandon the patient. If it is obvious that the patient is dissolving the relationship it should prompt the doctor to make a greater effort to strengthen the interaction. Follow-up is essential and each patient should be encouraged to keep their follow-up appointments regardless of satisfied or dissatisfied results.

Many factors contribute to a good doctor–patient relationship and therefore strongly influence the perceived outcome for a patient [6]. In a study on the communication behavior in physicians, those primary care physicians without a history of malpractice claims spent significantly more time with patients than did physicians with malpractice claims [24]. Patients seen by nonclaims doctors were informed more often of their progress and told what to expect with each visit. They were also asked questions more frequently and were able to verify their understanding of their condition. In addition, the no-claim physicians used humor more often to put their patients at ease. Although these differences between claims and nonclaims physicians were identified among the general and orthopedic surgeons evaluated, it is fair to say that these differences would hold true for dermatologic cosmetic surgeons.

A good rapport with the patients that is nurtured by the physician throughout the surgical course is a strong guard against dissatisfaction. By communicating with the patient several times throughout the treatment course it is possible for the doctor to detect any difficulties that may arise and subsequently deal with them early and effectively [17]. In order to do this, the patient must be provided with significant "hand holding." This means having an attentive and caring staff that keeps open lines of communication with the patient. Frequent phone calls to go over the details prior to the procedure plus postsurgical checkup calls are great techniques [25]. The patient can be reassured as they likely maintain some level of stress regarding the procedure. Several follow up visits, regardless of the results, also ensures a proper psychological as well as physical recovery.

HOW TO RESPOND TO THE DISSATISFIED PATIENT

When a situation with dissatisfied patient arises, it often creates significant distress in the cosmetic surgeon [26]. Most surgeons develop a high degree of regard for their skills and strive for excellence in their practice; therefore, it is a personal blow when a dissatisfied patient threatens that sense of security [23]. It is common for surgeons to remember more clearly the dissatisfied patients rather than the satisfied ones due to the actions necessary to accommodate the distress of the patient and themselves. Because of strong correlation between confidence and competence, sometimes the surgeon is unable to cope with the difficulties that arise when complications occur [23]. Feelings of incompetence, rejection, frustration, and anger are not uncommon as the physician often questions his or her capabilities. These feelings can be significant threats to patient care and can impede the physician from handling a patient's problems. By recognizing the potential for these expected psychological reactions, the surgeon can approach the dissatisfied patient in a more level-headed manner.

When surgical complications do occur, the physician must be attentive. Each individual expresses his or her dissatisfaction in a variety of ways. Some show anger while others do not even show up at all for follow-up appointments. Regardless of the manner in which they express themselves, the physician must remain calm and confident in their judgment. If patients do not express satisfaction, they should be asked if they are pleased with the results. If a patient does not show up for a follow-up appointment they should be contacted. If a patient appears confused it is essential to explain once again what the purpose and expected outcome of the procedure is. It is important to determine if there is a problem with patient satisfaction early on so it can be managed appropriately.

Whether or not the patient is dissatisfied with a favorable or unfavorable result, the doctor should respond in a similar manner. Concern, compassion, and support are vital to handling the dissatisfied patient [26]. The physician should be soft-spoken and caring without showing fragility. Confidence is essential in restoring a patient faith. Asking patients to clarify and elaborate their concerns allows them to relieve themselves of the frustrations that often make them angry toward the doctor. Again, open-ended questions such as "How do results make you feel?" are always best. The physician must listen meticulously even if the patient does not make sense. Defensive behavior is the worst way to handle a situation. Although patients can be frustrating at times it is never productive to argue or interrupt a patient. "Do you feel you were misled about the potential risks of the procedure?" is certainly more appropriate than "You did sign a consent form that informed you of that risk."

The best prescription for many patients is often reassurance. Patients often feel guilty that they endured a procedure when the results are not what they expected. By reassuring them of their decision, the physician can ease their distress [1,27]. The surgeon should focus on the healing power of time, as patients fear permanence and irreversibility. Assuring patients, when relevant, that many complications improve over time or that things can be done that may improve an outcome are useful approaches. Reinforcing the patient to continue with follow-up allows you to document their progress and allows them to diffuse much of their anxiety along the way. It is your main objective to convince the patient that your efforts are in their best interest and that your are experienced in dealing with complications if they should arise.

Depression and anxiety can occur during the postsurgical course [16]. The physician should express concern and reassure the patient that he or she is available to help them through the difficult period. Many patients in this scenario may benefit from psychiatric help but by no means should the physician push the patient away to somebody else's care. Adding another caregiver may be beneficial, as would pharmacological intervention in some cases. When patients complain of excessive pain, beware of potential narcotics abuse. Although chronic pain can be a complication of the postsurgical course, it can also be a sign of depression or chemical dependence.

No matter the level of skill of the surgeon, each and very one will experience the dissatisfied patient. Some patients are dissatisfied when technical and cosmetic results are optimum while others are dissatisfied when results are not [17,28,29]. A rare situation is when the surgical patient is satisfied with the results while the surgeon recognizes adverse effects of the procedure. It is important in these circumstances not to alarm the patient by expressing these concerns. Continuing the appropriate management of the patient as outlined above will minimize the chances of the patient becoming dissatisfied with his or her care.

FAVORABLE RESULTS AND DISSATISFIED PATIENTS

It is not uncommon to encounter patients who are dissatisfied with their results despite an appropriate outcome of a procedure. In these cases, it is misconceived expectations and goals that usually lead the patient astray. A physician must first revaluate the manner in which the procedure was presented. Were the objectives of the procedure detailed? Were the expected recovery phase and reactions of treatment discussed in depth? Did the goals of the patient match the proposed advantages of the given cosmetic procedure? In several cases, the physician may have properly informed the patient yet unrealistic goals were not recognized. Remember, it is always necessary to tell the whole truth about a procedure, both positive and negative. This way there are no surprises for the patient or physician.

When this situation arises, it is counterproductive to act defensively by reiterating what you already discussed in the past. Reassurance is the first essential step. Assure the patient that you are available to "hand-hold" them through the postoperative period. Fortunately, when the results are favorable, handling expected postoperative discomforts are not difficult. In time, most patients who are dissatisfied due to unrealistic expectations develop a more favorable impression [30].

Using several novel techniques, the physician can devise ways to relieve some of the postoperative discomfort, both physically and mentally [31]. Makeup tips, hair-styling techniques, and pain-relieving maneuvers give the patient the impression that you are trying make them more comfortable. Such is the case in post-CO_2 resurfacing, in which the patient must tolerate several weeks of waning redness. In many cases, the postoperative appearance, regardless of how good it is, can be shocking to patients despite warnings. Let your patients know that they are in good company with other patients who have had similar procedures. This shows that the physician has experience and that the patient is not alone. Showing "before" and "after" pictures at several stages postoperatively often gives the patient a better visual of what to expect from a procedure. In many cases, a verbal discussion alone leaves too much to the imagination for the patient.

UNFAVORABLE RESULTS AND DISSATISFIED PATIENTS

The most difficult situation for cosmetic surgeons is when a patient is dissatisfied when true complications arise. This is an occasional and unfortunate consequence for any surgeon who has been in practice long enough. Complications are always difficult to approach for both the patient and surgeon. In general, the surgeon takes complications personally, which can compromise his or her confidence and ability to cope with the patient who may be suffering or angered. Unfortunately, many patients act unaware of the potential complications that were pointed our during the initial consultation due to their inattentiveness when reviewing the risks and benefits of a procedure [32].

When a patient first comes for follow-up, it is not long before a sense of dissatisfaction can be recognized. The patient usually expresses a variety of emotions ranging from anger to silence. Often the doctor is aware of the complication by phone prior to the visit. This may allow time before the follow-up visit to reevaluate the course of events before, during, and after the procedure via notes, staff, and memory. If you do not have this opportunity prior to the visit, it is always best to take a moment alone before responding to the patient extensively [6]. What is most important for the physician is to confront the problem directly. There is temptation to avoid complications that may arise due to the overwhelming guilt and self-deprecation that may be involved in accepting such consequences. By doing so, larger problems are cultivated. Accepting the complication or poor outcome in a concerned and conscientious manner is always the best approach.

When suboptimal results are evident, the first step is to search for confounding or causative factors that may have led to the poor result. By reviewing the patient's initial consultation and surgical course in front of them, including medical history and medications, the physician can reevaluate the appropriateness of the procedure and detect any contributing factors that may have caused the problem. Check instrumentation, staff protocol, and medications used. In this manner, the doctor shows his or her concern to find a reason for the complication without focusing the blame on the patient. In many cases, the actual cause is due to poor patient compliance or disclosure of information. Such is the case when patients fail to include vitamins or herbs in the medication history. It is well known to physicians that megadoses of vitamins may anticoagulate a patient and cause complications. It is also common for patients to treat themselves without consulting the physician. The surgeon must document the postoperative activities of the patient and inquire about any changes in care or the use of any medications for any reason.

If there is evidence that the patient's actions contributed to the complication or poor result, do not blame them directly. You may inform them of the contributing factor without totally deferring blame to them. "Your surgical site bleeding and opening up was likely caused by several factors, including the use of aspirin after the procedure" is better than "if you hadn't taken aspirin after I recommended not to, this wouldn't have happened." Accusations make patients defensive and exacerbate their dissatisfaction. Patients are distressed enough when complications occur. Be sensitive to this fact. No matter what the blame, the physician must make efforts to rebuild rapport with the patient.

Physicians must encourage communication with their patients. Inquire about how they feel and what their concerns are. Often dissatisfied patients do not reveal all that they are thinking, both positive and negative. Availability and frequent follow-up are essential to handling these patients. Special care should be enforced by your staff, who should be informed of the patient and the nature of the problem. Private telephone numbers, after-hours appointments, and phone calls are excellent techniques to show concern for the problem at hand. While attending to the needs of the patient, it is imperative to remain confident and calm. Your attention should not appear fearful even if the patient becomes angered. You can only do your best to appease the dissatisfied patient; it is easy yet unnecessary to become emotional in their presence.

When specific complications are a well-known risk of a procedure make sure the consent clearly states this. Most complications are predictable and the patient needs to be aware of them. Underplaying them during the consultation is not advantageous for either the patient or the doctor. Many patients do not remember being informed of the risks until they are reexposed to the consent form. If an adverse reaction does occur, reassure the patient that he or she made a conscious decision to have the procedure done with consideration to both the risks and benefits. When the patient calms, he or she begins to comprehend and accept the reality of the situation. Your support and concern make it easier for them to understand the potential uncertainty of many cosmetic procedures.

Rather then dwelling on the permanence of an unfavorable result, the doctor should focus on improving the condition. Prioritizing the patient's concerns is the first step. "What specifically bothers you regarding the look of the scar" is a good start. Then approach and treat each aspect of their complaints. If the redness is most bothersome, you may want to treat it with a laser. If it is the elevation of the scar, then you may want to start with cortisone injections. Regardless of the nature of problem, the physician must show the patient that options are available and that their concerns will be dealt with one by one. Organizing the treatment of a complication helps the patient relax and feel that there is hope. Reinforcing the prescription for "tincture of time" is always advantageous. When complications occur for patients there is always a great sense of urgency. Reiterating that it takes time for healing and resolution allows the patient to reinvest his or her faith in your treatment rather than turn away immediately.

When additional procedures are performed to augment suboptimal results, they should be approached with the same enthusiasm and optimism as the first. Although promises should not be made, the surgeon should explain the purpose, the course, and the hopeful result of the procedure. In most cases the term "improvement" should be used, not "correction." Take the same precautions as any other procedure and make sure to document everything discussed or done with the patient. Be aware that the patient is now sensitized to any potential risks that a procedure may have. Hand holding, both physically and mentally, is essential.

If the patient chooses to seek a second opinion or the care of another physician, do not discourage this. It is important to try to include yourself in the care of the patient. By cooperating with the patient and other physicians in a collective effort, the patient's faith in the surgeon can be restored. In addition, the patient feels that the cooperative doctor has nothing to hide. The surgeon should offer his or her assistance in finding another physician but should give the patient total control in the final decision. Suggesting doctors who are renowned for the particular procedure may be beneficial for both parties. Contacting the consulting physician prior to evaluating the patient may also be of benefit in order to prepare the doctor on the matter at hand. The patient should be told that copies of records, photographs, and a letter explaining the nature of the complications could be forwarded to the consulting doctor. This shows your enthusiasm to be involved in their care and the appreciation for the opinion of a peer. Deterring a patient from seeking a particular physician can always appear arrogant and defensive.

After the patient consults with the other physician, do not lose contact. Keep open lines of communication between all parties in order to achieve an optimal solution.

When complications are severe, the issue of risk management needs attending to. In larger institutions there are usually departments dedicated to these scenarios. By consulting them, the physician can learn how to both cope with complications and minimize the likelihood and severity of medical/legal intervention. In smaller working environments, such as private practice, the surgeon should notify his or her lawyer. Under no circumstances should the physician alter medical records, blame another for the outcome, or be untruthful regarding the case [33].

DISSATISFACTION WITH PRIOR SURGERY

It is not uncommon for patients who are dissatisfied with prior procedures to seek consultation from another physician. These patients require certain expertise [6,16]. Because they have already had negative reinforcement for surgical procedures their threshold for dissatisfaction is very low. Often you are their choice in a desperate situation; therefore, they should be approached with greater caution and care. As with any patient, a detailed history is mandatory. The course of events, from the patient's perspective, should be documented in detail. In addition, determine how the patient heard about you. Did the original surgeon, another doctor, or a friend refer the patient? By contacting the original surgeon it is usually easier to decipher the reality of the situation as the patient may not completely understand the nature and cause of the problem. Patients can be dissatisfied for one of several reasons. Some do not like their actual result while others do not like the experience they had despite satisfactory results. Others are satisfied but require a second opinion in order to reassure themselves that everything went fine. Never slander or defend another physician when discussing a prior surgery with the patient. This is a bad practice and can only reinforce or exacerbate the patient's anger. If the patient has negative comments about the prior surgeon take a neutral stance. Reassure the patient that the doctor was likely working in their best interest and that no harm was intended.

When evaluating and managing a patient with dissatisfaction from earlier procedures the physician must proceed cautiously. If the outcome is satisfactory, in your opinion, then it is important to reassure the patient of this without ignoring his or her concerns. Reviewing the proper expectations, risks, and benefits of a procedure may clarify things for them and put them at ease. When results are suboptimal then a cooperative decision must be made between the patient, the consulting physician, and preferably the original surgeon. When the patient presents to the physician's office they may expect the consultant to assume responsibility for their care. This is up to the consulting physician to decide based on the nature of the case, the patient, and the original doctor. The consultant should never force the patient to return to the original doctor nor insist on taking total responsibility for the patient. The best scenario is when the original surgeon and consultant work together to determine the best level of care for the patient, allowing him or her to make the final decision on all interventions. Allowing time for communication between all parties should be done before deciding on any additional procedures. The original surgeon should provide all the relevant history and documentation in order to assess the best manner in which to deal with the situation.

When a second procedure is decided upon, the patient must understand the nature and purpose of the intervention. As with all procedures, details of the risks and benefits must be discussed in depth as well as the hopeful outcome. Often the patients dwell on the prior procedure. Both the patient and surgeon should focus on the future rather than on the past. This provides hope for the patient and convinces him or her of your proactive approach in patient care [6].

CONCLUSION

All cosmetic surgeons are familiar with difficult and dissatisfied patients. Several methods of screening, both subjective and objective, can be used to avoid patients who are at high risk for difficulties. Differentiating those who are good candidates for cosmetic procedures is the first step. Educated, personable, and attentive patients with clearly defined and limited cosmetic concerns are often the best candidates. Meticulous history taking and cooperative interaction with the patient is essential. Using subjective impressions, based on historical, aesthetic, and psychological factors, a surgeon and his or her staff should determine their ability to properly treat and satisfy a patient, both technically and emotionally. Taking special precautions to recognize and carefully interact with psychiatric illness is important given the prevalence of these patients within our specialty. Body dysmorphism and narcissistic, borderline personality, and obsessive–compulsive disorders are most prevalent.

Regardless of our screening capabilities and efforts to provide the best care, at times patients become disgruntled with results of a procedure and/or the surgeon. Sometimes this is the circumstance when complications and unfavorable results occur, but also when results are satisfactory. Several factors can lead to this disposition, including misdirected expectations, poor relations with the staff or surgeon, and failure to recognize the risks and benefits of a particular procedure on the part of the patient. Regardless of the cause, special care must be given to these patients. Attentiveness, availability, and empathy must be provided in order to regain rapport with patients and minimize the chance of emotional and legal interventions. Using the techniques outlined in this chapter, cosmetic surgeons should be able to minimize the sometimes-unavoidable consequences of patient dissatisfaction within the specialty of cosmetic surgery.

REFERENCES

1. Wright MR. How to recognize and control the problem patient. J Dermatol Surg Oncol 1984; 10:389–395.
2. Vuyk HD, Zijlker TD. Psychosocial aspects of patient counseling and selection: a surgeon's perspective. Fac Plast Surg 1995; 11:55–60.
3. Lewis CM. Dissatisfaction among women with "thunder thighs" undergoing closed aspirative lipoplasty. Aesth Plast Surg 1987; 11:187–191.
4. Popp JC. Complication of blepharoplasty and their management. J Dermatol Surg Oncol 1992; 18:1122–1126.
5. Sarwar D. The "obsessive" cosmetic surgery patient: a consideration of body image dissatisfaction and body dysmorphic disorder. Plast Surg Nurs 1997; 17: 193–197 and 209.
6. Wright MR. Management of patient dissatisfaction with results of cosmetic procedures. Arch Otolaryngol 1980; 106:466–471.
7. Wright MR. Surgical addiction: a complication of modern surgery. Arch Otolaryngol Head Neck Surg 1986; 112:870–872.
8. Menninger KA. Polysurgery and polysurgical addiction. Psychanal Q 1934; 3: 173–199.
9. Knorr NJ, Edgerton MT, Hoopes JE. The "insatiable" cosmetic surgery patient. Plast Reconstr Surg 1967; 40:285–289.
10. Napoleon A. The presentation of personalities in plastic surgery. Ann Plast Surg 1993; 31:193–208.
11. Wright MR, Wright WK. A psychological study of patients undergoing cosmetic surgery. Arch Otolaryngol 1975; 101:145–151.
12. Jacobson WE, Edgerton MT, Meyer E. Psychiatric evaluation of male patients seeking cosmetic surgery. Plast Reconstr Surg 1960; 20:356.
13. Edgerton MT, Jacobson WE, Meyer E. Surgical-psychiatric study of patients seeking plastic (cosmetic) surgery: ninety-eight consecutive patients with minimal deformity. Br J Plast Surg 1961; 13:136–145.
14. Flynn TC, Narins RS. Preoperative evaluation of the liposuction patient. Dermatol Clin 1999; 17:729–734.
15. Findley C, Kaye BL. Care of the office surgery patient. Clin Plast Surg 1983; 10:333–356.
16. Baker TJ. Patient selection and psychological evaluation. Clin Plast Surg 1978; 5:3–14.
17. Macgregor FC. Patient dissatisfaction with results of technically satisfactory surgery. Aesth Plast Surg 1982; 5:27–32.

18. Katez P. The dissatisfied patient. Plast Surg Nurs 1991; 11:13–16.
19. Caputy GG, Flowers RS. Computer imaging: true or false. Hawaii Med J 1993; 52:349–351.
20. Hockenberger SJ. The nurse's role and responsibilities regarding patient satisfaction. Plast Surg Nurs 1995; 15:187 and 189.
21. Dugas B. Dealing with the dissatisfied patient. Plast Surg Nurs 1983; 3:33–35.
22. Macgregor FC. Cosmetic surgery: a sociological analysis of litigation and a surgical specialty. Aesth Plast Surg 1984; 8:219–224.
23. Wright MR. Self-perception of the elective surgeon and some patient perception correlates. Arch Otolaryngol 1980; 106:460–465.
24. Levinson W, Roter DL, Mullooly JP, Dull VT, Frankel RM. Physician-patient communication: the relationship with malpractice claims among primary care physicians and surgeons. J Am Med Assoc 1997; 277:553–559.
25. Fallo PC. Developing a program to monitor patient satisfaction and outcome in the ambulatory surgery setting. J Post Anesth Nurs 1991; 6:176–180.
26. Goin JM, Goin MK. Changing the Body: Psychological Effects of Plastic Surgery. Baltimore: Williams & Wilkins, 1981.
27. Adamson PA, Kraus WM. Management of patient dissatisfaction with cosmetic surgery. Fac Plast Surg 1995; 11:99–104.
28. Leist FD, Masson JK, Erich JB. A review of 324 rhytidectomies, emphasizing complication and patient dissatisfaction. Plast Reconstr Surg 1977; 59:525–529.
29. Scheflan M, Maillard GF, de St Cyr BC, Ramirez OM. Subperiosteal facelifting: complication and the dissatisfied patient. Aesth Plast Surg 1996; 20:33–36.
30. Goldwyn RM, ed. The Unfavorable Result in Plastic Surgery: Avoidance and Treatment. 2nd ed. Boston: Little, Brown and Co, 1984.
31. Hoefflin SM. Surgical pearls in the management of the aging face from A to Z. Dermatol Clin 1997; 15:679–685.
32. Goin MK, Burgoyne RW, Goin JM. Face-lift operation: the patient's secret motivation and reactions to "informed consent." Plast Reconstr Surg 1976; 58:273–279.
33. Gorney M. Malpractice. In: Courtiss EH, ed. Aesthetic Surgery: Trouble, How to Avoid It and How to Treat It. St. Louis, MO: Mosby, 1978.

24

Fat Transfer Microliposuction and Liposuction for Advanced Repair of Liposuction Defects

Rhoda S. Narins
Dermatology Surgery and Laser Center
New York and White Plains, and
New York University Medical Center
New York, New York, U.S.A.

Liposuction has become the most commonly performed cosmetic surgery in the United States. One would expect to see some unsatisfactory results requiring secondary procedures. I have treated patients who are unhappy after liposuction and who do not want to go back to the original surgeon for obvious reasons. Some of these problems are amenable to repair, even when an entire area is uneven, using a combination of liposuction done both by hand and with an aspiration machine along with fat transfer. Fat transfer procedures have advanced over the past decade and now one can achieve long-lasting improvement, especially when the fat is harvested from an area near the recipient area.

It is important to counsel patients so that they are realistic in their expectations. All depressions as well as fat accumulations must be pointed out. Preoperative photos must be taken, including those of the marking. It is very important to mark the areas of fat that will be harvested or undergo liposuction in a different color from the depressed areas requiring fat transfer (Fig. 1 and Table 1).

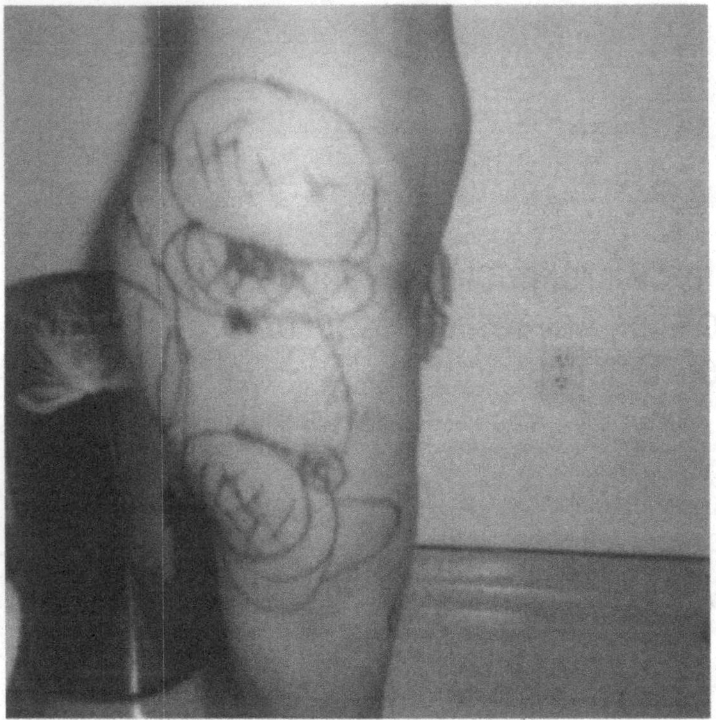

Figure 1 Marking the patient.

Surgery begins in the usual way with infiltration of local tumescent anesthesia into the entire area using shower-head infiltrators and a Klein electric pump. Multiple tiny incisions are made where necessary using a 16-gauge NoKor needle. For the small fat accumulations I remove the fat by hand using a Coleman extractor attached to a 10-cc syringe. I collect the fat I intend to save using minimal backward pressure on the plunger so as not to injure the fat cells. When removing fat I do not intend to keep, I am not concerned with the amount of pressure I exert on the plunger. For large accumulations of fat that do not need to be saved, I use a liposuction aspirator and regular liposuction cannulas (Table 2). The fat that is saved is then prepared for reinjection. First the fat is centrifuged for 1–2 min. Then the supranate consisting of broken fat cells and oil and the infranate consisting of anesthetic fluid and blood are discarded. Any remaining supranatant oil is then wicked off with sterile gauze pads. A female-to-female adaptor is used to push the fat into 1-cc syringes. Any extra fat is frozen (Table 3).

TABLE 1 Advanced Liposuction Repair—Pre-Op Procedure

1. Consultation and discussion
2. Preoperative photos
3. Mark areas of liposuction and fat transfer with different-colored markers

TABLE 2 Advanced Liposuction Repair—Surgery

1. Infiltration of tumescent anesthetic
2. Multiply tiny incisions made with NoKor needle
3. Harvest fat by hand using a 10-cc syringe and Coleman extractor
4. Prepare fat for reinjection (see Table 3)
5. Inject fat into recipient sites (see Table 4)

TABLE 3 Preparing the Fat

1. Centrifuge 1–2 min
2. Discard supranate and infranate
3. Wick off remaining supranate
4. Inject fat into 1-cc syringes through female-to-female adaptor
5. Freeze extra fat

TABLE 4 Fat Transfer

1. Use 1-cc syringes with Coleman injection cannulas
2. Incisions made with 16-gauge NoKor needle
3. Toledo underminer used to detach skin if bound down
4. Injection of small aliquots of fat at multiple levels from various directions

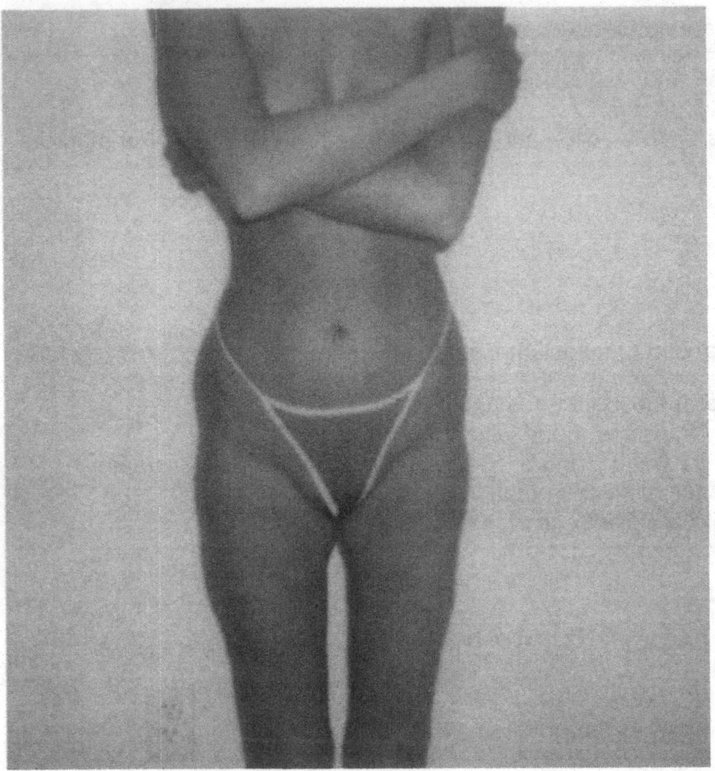

FIGURE 2 Preoperative photo of patient.

NoKor needles are used to make incisions for the fat transfer. One-cc syringes are attached to a Coleman injector and tiny aliquots of fat are injected at multiple levels in the tissue defect from multiple directions. If the skin is really bound down to the underlying tissue, a Toledo underminer is used prior to injection of fat to detach the skin and allow the infiltration of the necessary amount of fat (Table 4). The incisions are left open for drainage. Postoperatively support garments are worn that are tight enough to prevent dead space but loose enough to let the fat grafts take.

Results have been gratifying even when not totally perfect (Figs. 2 and 3). The fat is long lasting and often permanent. We do have extra fat saved if needed. Complications have not been a problem and I have seen no infections, seromas, or hematomas.

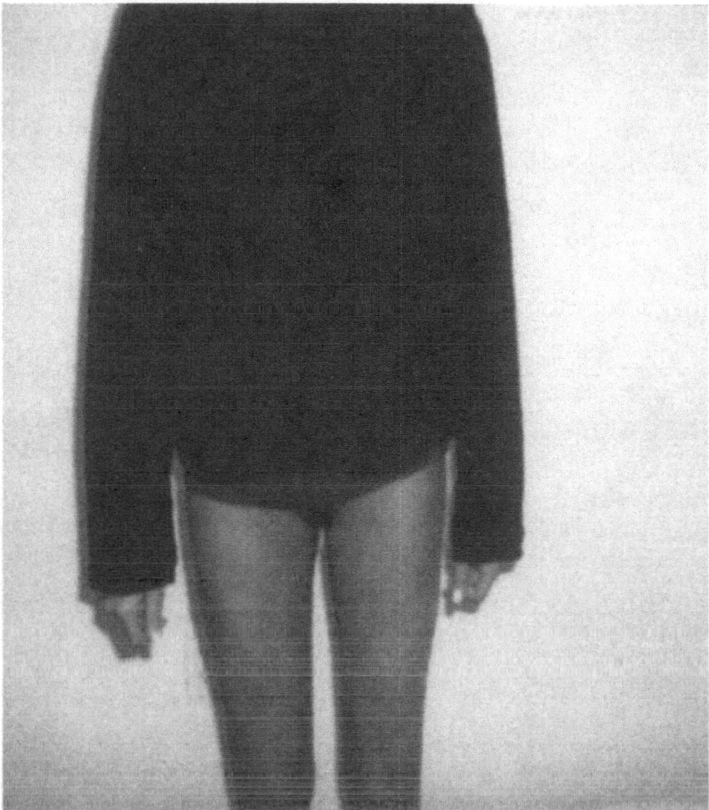

FIGURE 3 Postoperative photo of patient.

The more experienced you become as a liposuction surgeon the more patients will be referred to you for secondary repair. A combination of hand and machine liposuction combined with fat transfer is a useful advanced technique for repair of postliposuction defects along with liposhifting as discussed in Chapter 25.

25

Liposhifting Instead of Lipofilling: Treatment of Postliposuction Irregularities

Ziya Saylan
Saylan Cosmetic Surgery Center, Düsseldorf, Germany

The most common complication after a liposuction is the residual fat (left over) and hollows. Until now we were correcting the postliposuction irregularities with autologous fat injections with no long-term results. Lipofilling alone has proved unsatisfactory in filling the irregularities. Fat transfer as we use and perform it today does not survive and is not a good solution to fill the postliposuction irregularities. After many years of disappointment with fat fillings, I have decided to shift the fat under the skin from the surrounding tissue into the hollow with no suctioning, air contact, or injecting. This author loosens the fatty tissue and shifts it under the skin with no liposuction and does not remove the loosened fat out of the body during this procedure. Afterward a special type of taping and fixation for 5 to 7 days is necessary. The results are so satisfactory that I want to introduce this method to help other plastic and aesthetic surgeons in further development and achievement.

In the European community, about 250,000 liposuctions are performed annually, and this number is increasing rapidly. As the amount of liposuctions performed increases, the number of unsatisfactory results is also increasing. According to a questionnaire from the German Liposuction Society [1], among its members almost 16% of liposuctions needed to be corrected (lipofilled) or reliposuctioned. Gerald Pittmann [2] pointed out that 15% needed "small touch-ups" or lipofillings as "a local treatment in the office," and another 9% needed to undergo a liposuction with lipofilling or reliposuction.

The fat transfer procedure in use today does not achieve optimal and long-lasting results. After few months a large amount of the injected fat disappears and sometimes the patients complain about new hollows on the donor site. My personal experience until now is that lipofilling small post-liposuction irregularities may be helpful but will never offer a long-term result for large irregularities or hollows. This fact forced me to search for a new method. After studying fat transfer and fat damage for years, I came up with the idea of shifting the fat under the skin with no suctioning (damaging) and with no removal from the body (including no pressure and no air contact). Also, reinjection is not necessary because it would apply an extra force on the fat implant. This is in my opinion the best way *not to damage* the fatty tissue and thus let it survive. I would like to share this positive experience of mine with the other plastic and cosmetic surgeons. This new technique that I have developed myself has been applied on 41 patients since August 1996.

TECHNIQUE

This procedure consists of the following stages:

1. Marking the skin while the patient is standing
2. Anesthesia (local) of the skin
3. Tumescent technique
4. Loosening the fat with a Becker cannula
5. Shifting
6. Fixation of the shifted fat (taping and Reston foam fixation)

Marking the Skin

Marking the skin is very important. Marking has to be done while the patient is standing (Fig. 1), which allows the physician to localize the proper places for liposhifting and also gives him or her the possibility of controlling the results. An orthostatic table like Giorgio Fischer's is not always necessary but helpful. In order to achieve better results we allow the patient to stand many times during this procedure (multipositional liposuction). The molds and hollows should be marked with different colors to show the direction of the shifting to give extra help to the surgeon. The surgeon should not forget that as the patient lies on the operating table the fat deposits surrounding the hollow may change position. Also, the amount of fat to be shifted

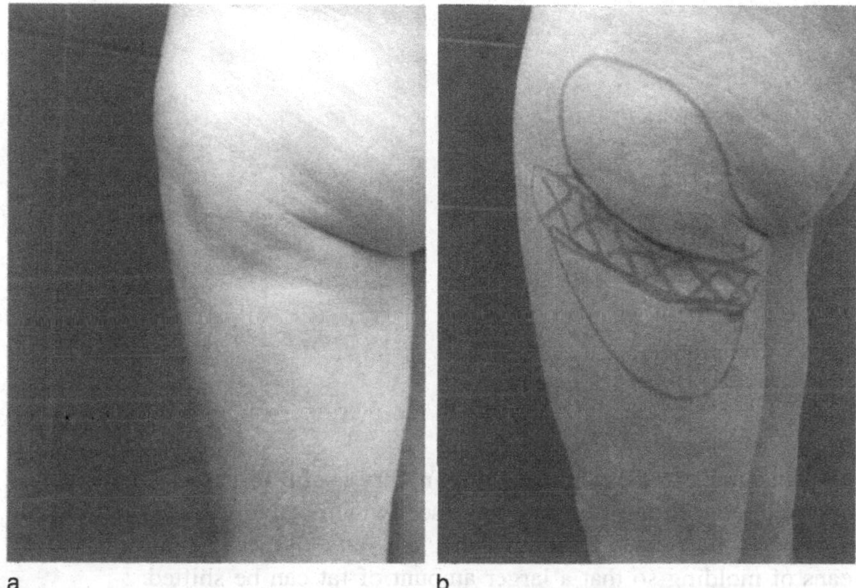

FIGURE 1 (a) Patient standing and (b) marking the skin.

has to be decided before the procedure. The places where large amounts are required should be marked with a third color or should be written on the skin, which makes the whole procedure easier. A documentation by means of photographing is very important for future comparison. We also make a drawing on a piece of paper, which provides further direction.

Anesthesia

General anesthesia is done if the patient wishes to be totally sedated. Normally iv sedation is not necessary. The infiltration of a tumescent solution is all that is required. This allows us to let the patient stand up during the procedure for a better localization of the fat to be shifted. The skin at the sites of the incisions are infiltrated with local anesthesia (we prefer 1% lidocaine with epinephrine; Astra Chemicals).

Tumescent Technique

The tumescent solution is used to loosen the fatty tissue and also to provide anesthesia (Fig. 2). After infiltration of the tumescent solution, time is required to let it take effect and achieve optimal fat loosening and vasoconstriction. A molding of the tissue for 20 min (Giorgio Fischer, personal

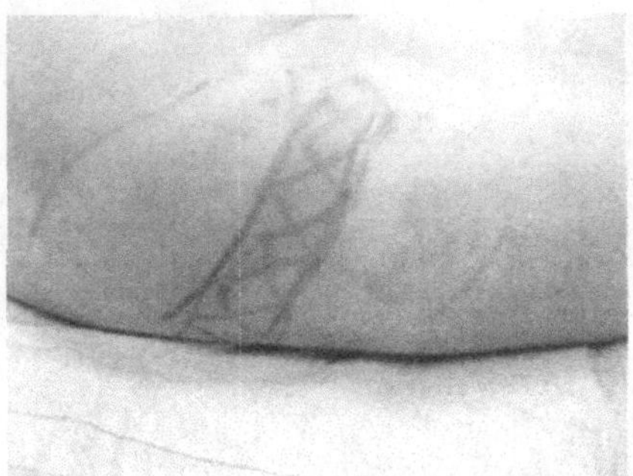

FIGURE 2 Infiltration.

communication, 1997) is in my opinion very useful to obtain a better loosening of the fat. In our study we have seen much better results after molding the place to be treated. I believe that the fatty tissue will be released by means of molding so that a larger amount of fat can be shifted.

Loosening Fat

The tumescent technique has now diluted and loosened the fatty tissue, but now something has to be done in order to free the fatty tissue further from the connective tissue. For this purpose, I use a 26-cm-long, 3-mm-wide Becker cannula (Figs. 3, 4, and 5) from Byron Medical Co. (Tucson, AZ), which is pushed under the skin and moved in a crisscross technique in order to release the fat. Many incisions are required to achieve better results; windshield-wiper movements have to be avoided, otherwise the subcutaneous connective tissue will be damaged and skin will also be loosened, which is not the goal.

Shifting

Pushing or shifting the fat under the skin can now be done (Figs. 6, 7, and 8). An old thick cannula (6–9 mm) which is no longer used can be helpful for this purpose. The cannula is held in both hands and the fatty tissue under the skin is shifted toward the imperfection which has to be filled. The place to be filled has to be observed very closely and when the hollow is filled and has the same level as the surrounding skin, further shifting is required to obtain an overcorrection of 20–30%, which is the amount of tumescent solution that will be absorbed in a few hours.

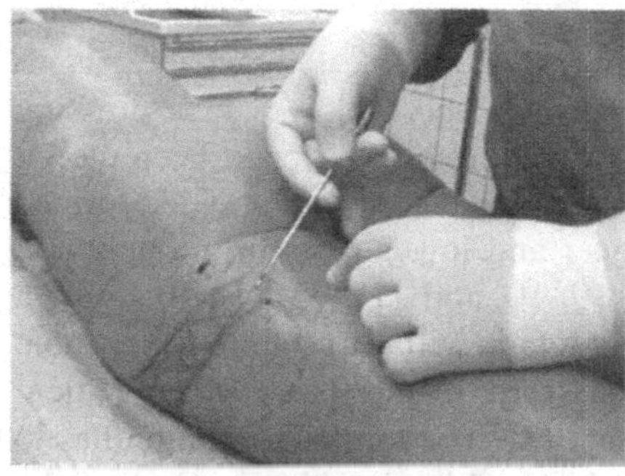

Figure 3 Loosening with a Becker cannula.

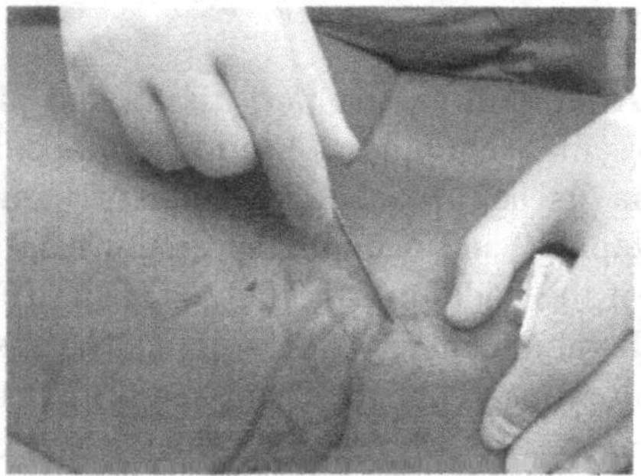

Figure 4 Loosening the fat.

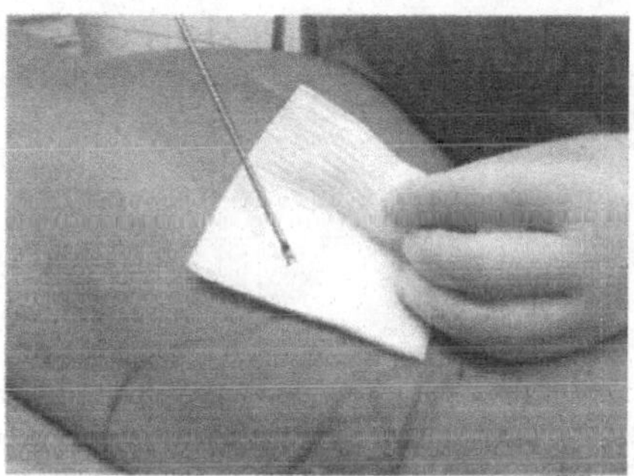

Figure 5 Subcision with a Toledo dissector.

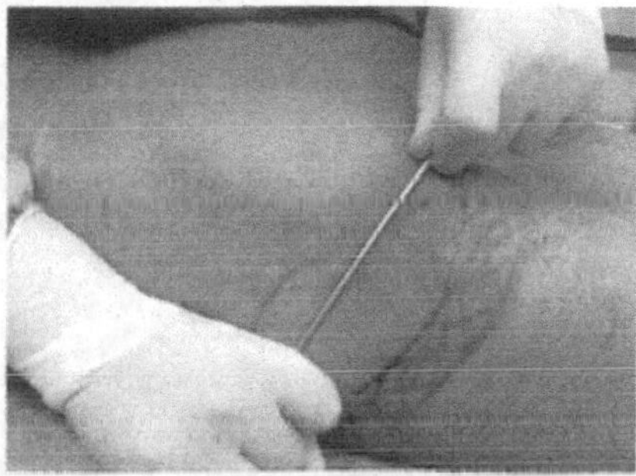

Figure 6 Shifting with the cannula.

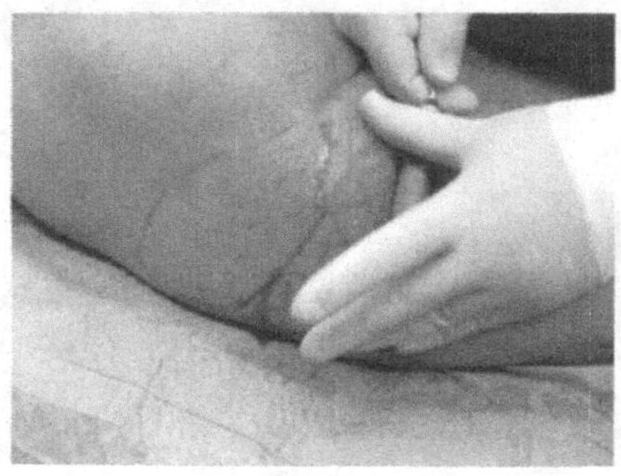

Figure 7 Shifting with the handle.

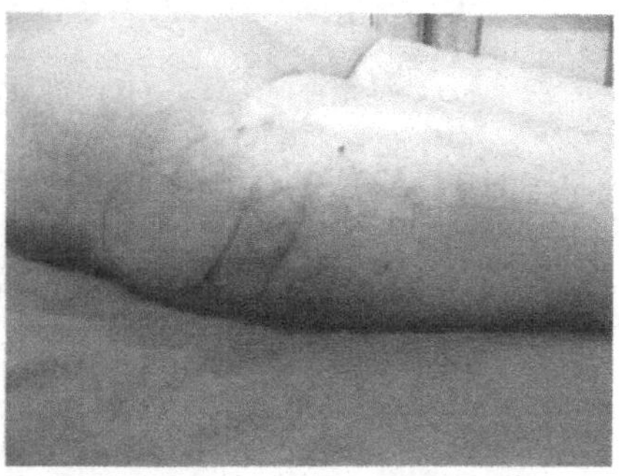

Figure 8 Result of liposhifting.

Fixation

After shifting the fatty tissue and placing it in the hollow a tape dressing (same technique as used in orthopedics) is required in order to keep the fat in its new place. This kind of taping is called "watermelon-slice-formed taping" and it applies pressure from upper and lower parts in the direction of the middle of the tape dressing (Figs. 9, 10, and 11). We usually apply a Reston foam [3] (3M Company) dressing. A tape will also stabilize the whole dressing. This foam applies a kind of massage to the tissue as the patient moves, which reduces bruising and edema [3]. The tape and fixation has to be removed and renewed after 3 or 4 days, which enables control of the area operated on (look for hematoma and infection) and gets rid of the loosened dressing. The fixation is removed after 7 days.

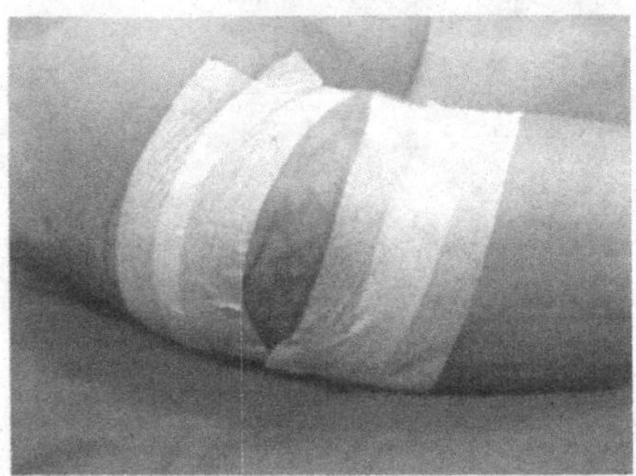

Figure 9 Taping and pushing the fat toward the hollow area.

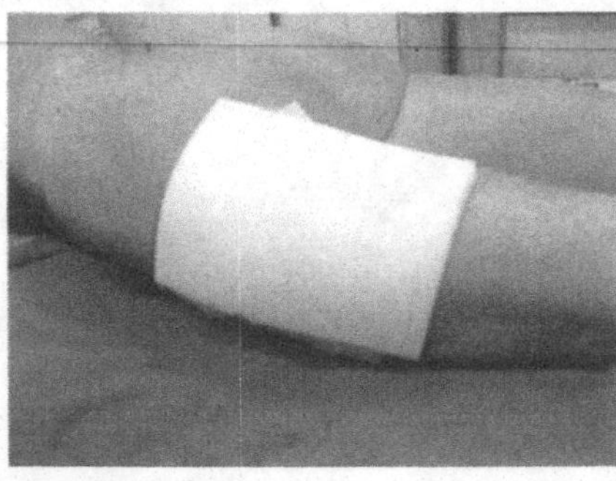

Figure 10 Reston foam fixation.

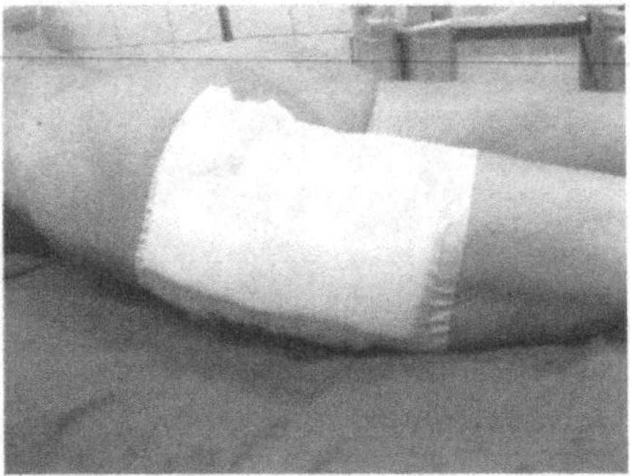

Figure 11 The dressing.

RESULTS

I have applied this technique on 41 patients over a period of 5 years. All patients are female with an average age of 34. The rate of satisfaction is 88% (24 patients). Some cases, with large imperfections, had to be liposhifted more than once (5 cases, 14%). This will be explained to the patient before the surgery to plan a strategy and schedule the surgery. A period of 3–4 months is needed between the two treatments. In 3 cases (11%) the result was not that satisfactory and 2 cases (7%) did not respond to this treatment. The final results were observed only after 3–6 months (Fig. 12).

COMPLICATIONS

The most common complication was hematoma due to fat loosening (5 cases; 12%). This problem was reduced by using the tape and the Reston foam and also by leaving the incisions unsutured. There were no infections. A hyper sensibility of the liposhifted part of the body lasts longer than the liposuctioned parts of the body. Also the hypo sensibility is seen more frequently but disappears after a few weeks. A hemosiderin pigmentation (pigmentation of the skin due to iron in the blood) was seen in two cases who had hematomas which were still there after 6 and 9 months.

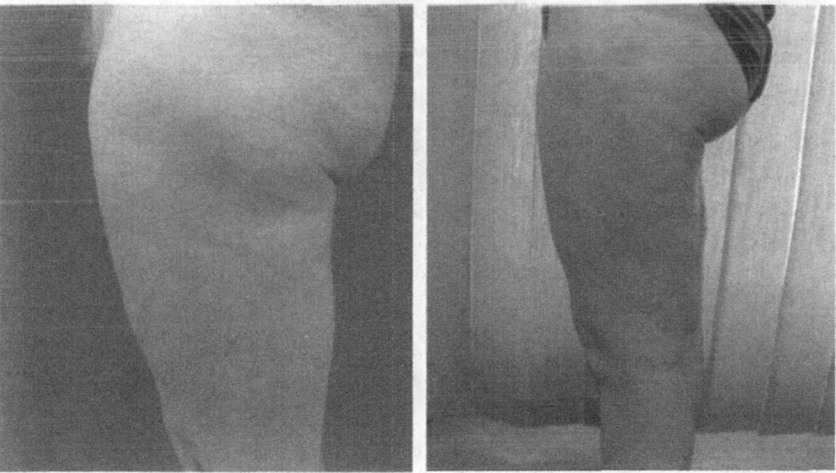

FIGURE 12 Before (left) and after (right) photos of the same female patient 6 months apart.

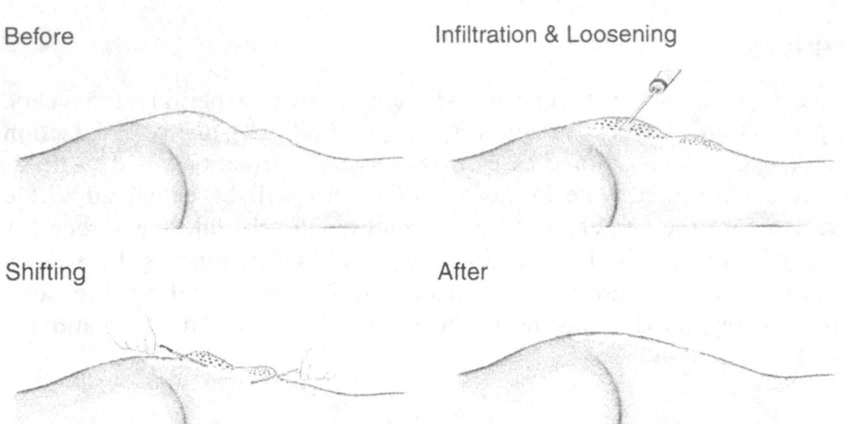

FIGURE 13 The explanation of the liposhifting as shown by drawings.

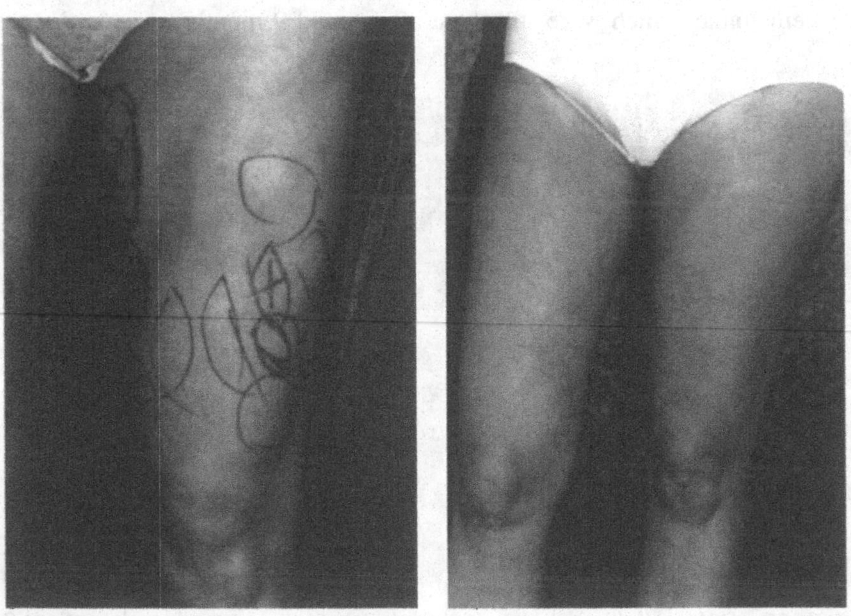

FIGURE 14 Liposhifting before (left) and after (right).

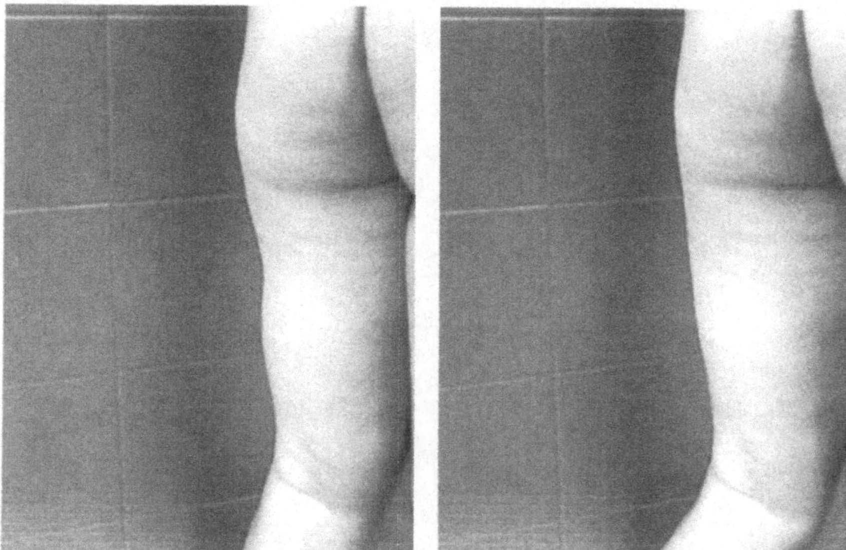

Figure 15 A case of liposhifting after a liposuction deformity.

CONCLUSION

Liposhifting is the only method to eliminate larger irregularities of the skin and the underlying tissue caused by liposuction (Figs. 13–15). It is helpful only in the extremities and in the abdominal wall. It is practical and safe because contamination of the fat transplant via air contact is not possible and the technique requires no training or special instruments. The fixation of the liposhifted part of the body for 1 week is very important to stabilize the shifted fat and make it possible for the fat to survive. More research has to be done to study my technique, which would also make it possible to compare the results with those of other surgeons. The irregularities due to liposuction are still a main problem.

REFERENCES

1. Saylan Z. Liposuction complications. Annual Meeting of the German Liposuction Society, Düsseldorf, Germany, 1996.
2. Pittman G. Liposuction and Aesthetic Medicine. St. Louis, MO: QMP Inc., 1993.
3. Saylan Z. Evaluation of a new kind of dressing after liposuction. Am J Cosmet Surg 1996; 13(2):149–151.

26

Structural Lipoaugmentation

Sydney R. Coleman
Centre for Aesthetic Rejuvenation and Enhancement
New York, New York, U.S.A.

INTRODUCTION

The idea of injecting fillers into the subcutaneous tissues has been entertained since the earliest days of modern aesthetic surgery. In 1911, Fredrick Kolle [1] created a detailed classification of deformities of the forehead, nose, mouth, cheek, chin, neck, and body for the purpose of systematizing subcutaneous injections of paraffin into humans. As injecting paraffin fell out of favor, aesthetic surgeons continued using the injection technique to inject other substances. Charles Conrad Miller described his experiences with infiltration of fat tissue through cannulas in 1926 [2]. Even though Miller reported good results with the injected fat, the technique he described never became popular. With the introduction of liposuction in the 1980s, physicians renewed their interest in the grafting of autologous fat through a cannula [3–6].

In 1987 after successfully grafting fat to correct iatrogenic liposuction deformities, I started infiltrating fat in the face for aesthetic reasons. Even some of my earliest attempts at fat grafting yielded long-term structural changes that have had every indication of permanence [7,8]. From 1987 to 1992, I developed the following approach to fat grafting in order to change facial contours, to revise scars, and to rejuvenate the face. The technique emphasizes respect for handling fat tissue and basic sound surgical technique.

PREPARATION

To obtain predictable results in facial recontouring, planning is essential. The first step is determining the patient's problems. I listen to their desires and complaints and examine them. I ask them to bring photographs of themselves when they were younger or of faces they consider attractive. With the knowledge of a patient's goals and a three-dimensional awareness of the patient's physical appearance, I compare the more idealized versions the patients have of themselves with their current condition.

In the presence of each patient, I study current photographic images in many views and discuss their faces with them to identify their soft tissue deficiencies. Also with the patient present and participating in the decision-making process, I mark my comments on tracings of their faces and create blueprints of the projected plans for augmentation. As I am marking the blueprint, I explain the placement of fat to the patient. On the blueprint, I first note the varying degrees of deficiency of the tissue to be augmented. Then I indicate with colored pens the levels into which the fat is to be layered, the direction of placement, and the projected volumes. Such planning will improve the chances of placing the fat to make a well-thought-out change of the patient's appearance.

However, improvement in the appearance of a patient is not enough for a successful result. Not only does the patient need to be prepared for the changes in their face or body, the patient should understand the details of the planned procedure, the expected postoperative course, their responsibilities during recovery, and any anticipated sequelae and potential complications that can occur. The amount of time I invest in preparation is often equal to or more than the length of the procedure itself. Placement of any amount of structural fat into a patient's face or body should never be done as a spur of the moment inspiration but only after careful planning.

TECHNIQUE

This method of structural fat grafting has been previously described [9–12]. Small intact parcels of fat tissue are harvested and then refined to remove the nonviable components. Gentle positive pressure propels the harvested fat parcels through the lumen of a cannula much smaller than the harvesting cannula to place parcels of fat tissue in a manner that allows nutrition and structural integrity in the host tissues.

Harvesting

Observe sterile technique at all times during the procedure. Prepare the patient with antiseptic soaps and paint the skin with an antiseptic agent such as povodione iodine. Donor sites are selected to improve body contour and avoid deformities.

Employ local anesthesia for harvesting smaller volumes, epidural, or general anesthesia for larger volumes. After depositing 0.5% lidocaine with 1:200,000 of epinephrine at the incision sites with a 27-gauge needle, a no. 11 blade is used for making the incision. Through the incision, infiltrate the appropriate solution using a blunt Lamis infiltrator attached to a 10-cc syringe. When using general anesthesia or epidural anesthesia, infiltrate Ringer's lactate with 1:400,000 of epinephrine infiltrate bluntly into the harvesting sites through a stab incision using a blunt Lamis infiltrator. If only a limited amount of tissue is to be harvested, local anesthesia can be used with infiltration of 0.5% lidocaine with 1:200,000 of epinephrine. The solutions are usually infiltrated in a ratio of 1 cc of solution/cc of fat to be harvested.

A 3-mm two-holed blunt harvesting cannula is connected to a disposable 10-cc Luer-Lok syringe. The entry portal of the cannula is just large enough to allow admittance of fat tissue parcels of a size that will then pass through the lumen of the syringe. Suction created by slowly withdrawing the plunger of this 10-cc syringe combines with the curetting action of the cannula to harvest miniscule intact parcels of fat tissue.

Transfer and Purification

After disconnecting the syringe from the harvesting cannula, the aperture of the syringe is sealed with a cap, and the plunger of the syringe is removed. The capped 10-cc syringe is placed into a sterilized sleeve in a sterilized central rotor of a centrifuge. Spinning the syringes at about 3000 rpm for 3 min separates the harvested material into three layers. The top layer is composed primarily of oil from ruptured parcels of fat; the lowest layer is composed of blood and lidocaine or Ringer's lactate; and the middle layer consists mainly of subcutaneous tissue.

To maintain a vacuum that will hold the fat in place during tilting of the syringe, leave the cap on the Luer-Lok aperture of the syringe while the top oil layer is decanted. Then remove the cap and allow the aqueous, dense lower level to drain. Placing cottonoid surgical strips [13] into the top of the tissue layer wicks off most of the remaining oil. After the oil and aqueous components have been removed, the refined tissue is transferred into 1-cc Luer-Lok syringes.

Placement

One- to two-millimeter incisions are made with a no. 11 blade. If general anesthesia is used, no solutions are infiltrated into the recipient site. Otherwise, anesthesia is provided with a combination of regional nerve blocks and 0.5% lidocaine with 1:100,000 of epinephrine. Infiltration of local anesthesia into the recipient sites with a 25-gauge needle will occasionally induce a hematoma. These hematomas can dramatically impede a surgeon's ability to place an appropriate volume in a smooth fashion. To avoid the formation of hematomas, I now use a blunt fat tissue infiltration cannula for infiltration of local anesthesia.

The cannula used for placement of refined fat is 17-gauge with an ejection aperture close to the distal end. The ejection portal is just large enough to allow passage of small parcels of fat tissue. A cannula connected to a disposable 1-cc Luer-Lok syringe filled with refined fat tissue is inserted through the incision and advanced to the target area. As the cannula is withdrawn, gentle digital pressure on the plunger of the syringe forces fat out through the cannula. Only a minute amount of refined fat is expressed with each pass. At no time is strong positive pressure placed on the plunger. If any resistance is encountered, the cannula is disconnected from the syringe to inspect for the possibility of fibrous tissue or parcels too large to pass through the cannula. With appropriately designed harvesting and infiltration cannulas, this stoppage will rarely happen. The blunt design of the cannulas reduces the chance of damage to underlying structures (nerves, blood vessels, salivary glands, etc). The length, shape, curvature, tip shape, and size of the cannula can vary to facilitate multiple technical considerations.

If multiple-layered placement from the bone outward is planned, advance the cannula tip immediately down to a deeper plane and place the layers closest to the bone first in a fanlike design. Then, infiltrate the middle layers of muscle, subcutaneous tissue, and connective tissues. Finally, infiltrate the subdermal layers. The surgeon should create the desired postoperative shapes during the initial placement. As the tissue is slowly placed, the projected form is created with each pass of the cannula, depositing a miniscule amount of tissue. Each pass must be precise and the correction should be observed immediately after placement of fat tissue.

I believe that the key to consistent results is to place the fat in extremely small amounts with each pass and to use multiple passes. I rarely place more than 1/10th of a cubic centimeter with a single pass, and for most passes I deposit from 1/20th to 1/50th of a cubic centimeter. This maximizes survival, integration, and anchoring of the transplanted fat.

POSTOPERATIVE CARE

Edema is the most consistent postoperative sequelae for this technique. The trauma caused by the multiple passes with a blunt cannula results in remarkable tissue edema. To reduce edema, straps of taut Microfoam tape create a slight compression for 3 or 4 days on the skin of the infiltrated areas. Cold compresses or ice packs are used for 3 days and the patients are instructed to keep their heads elevated above their heart. When they return for facial suture removal three to five days after the procedure the patients are taught to massage selected areas.

Four years ago, I began applying electromagnetic energy postoperatively four or five times a day for 5–7 days postoperatively. This empirically has reduced the recovery time [14]. Even with compression, elevation, cold therapy, massage, and electromagnetic therapy aiding in the recovery process, postoperative edema is still a major impediment.

Patient Examples

Case 1

This 44-year-old male had remarkable pitting and many depressed scars from chronic cystic acne. The deepest scars were lateral to his chin, extending into the submentum (Figs. 1, 2, and 3, left). The patient was most bothered by the lower face scars, but also asked if a minimal amount of correction could be made in his cheeks. Into lateral chin scars at the level of the border of the mandible and slightly above, 8 cc was placed on the left and 11 cc on the right. Into the left lower nasolabial fold, 4 cc was placed on the left

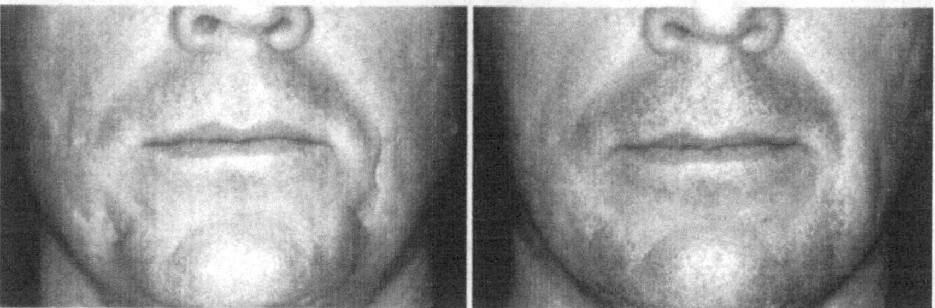

FIGURE 1 Case 1. This 44-year-old patient presented with deep scars around his chin from chronic acne (left). Eight cubic centimeters of fat was grafted into the right submental scar and 4 cc into the left scar along with 5 cc of fat into the right cheek and 3 cc in the left. Four cubic centimeters of fat was also placed in the left nasolabial fold (right).

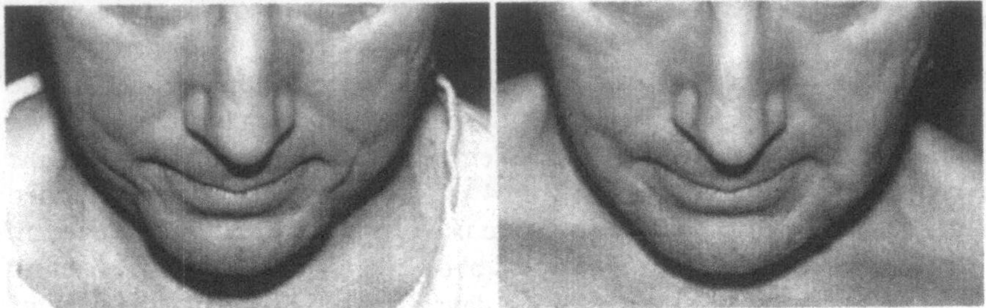

Figure 2 Case 1. Pictures before (left) and after (right) the 1-year follow-up. This tilted downward front view gives a clear idea of the improvement in the appearance of the skin around the submental region, nasolabial folds, and jawline.

only. Into the submental scar, 4 cc of fat was grafted with a nice correction even with the remaining trap door deformity. Finally, 5 cc of fat was feathered over the right cheek and 3 cc over the left. The placement throughout was primarily superficial, against the scarred skin. When the patient returned for follow-up at 1 year he was extremely pleased with the results (Figs. 1, 2, and 3, right).

Case 2

This 43-year-old patient felt she looked "gaunt" and sick even though she was extremely athletic and healthy. She specifically was bothered by the "hollowness" of her cheeks (Fig. 4, left, above and below). Fat was har-

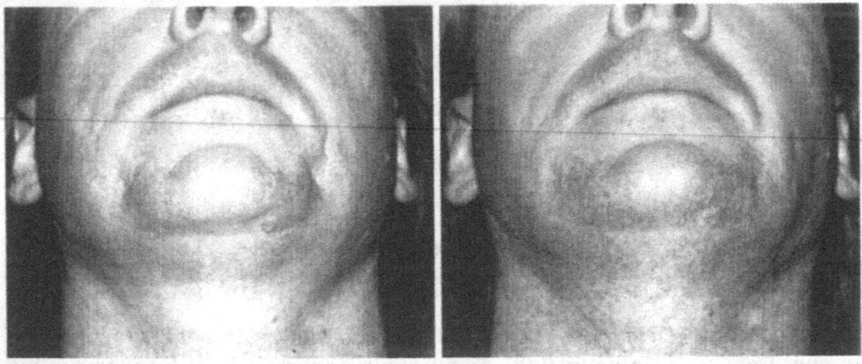

Figure 3 Case 1. Pictures before (left) and after (right) the 1-year follow-up. The upward tilted front view shows a marked improvement in scars around his chin.

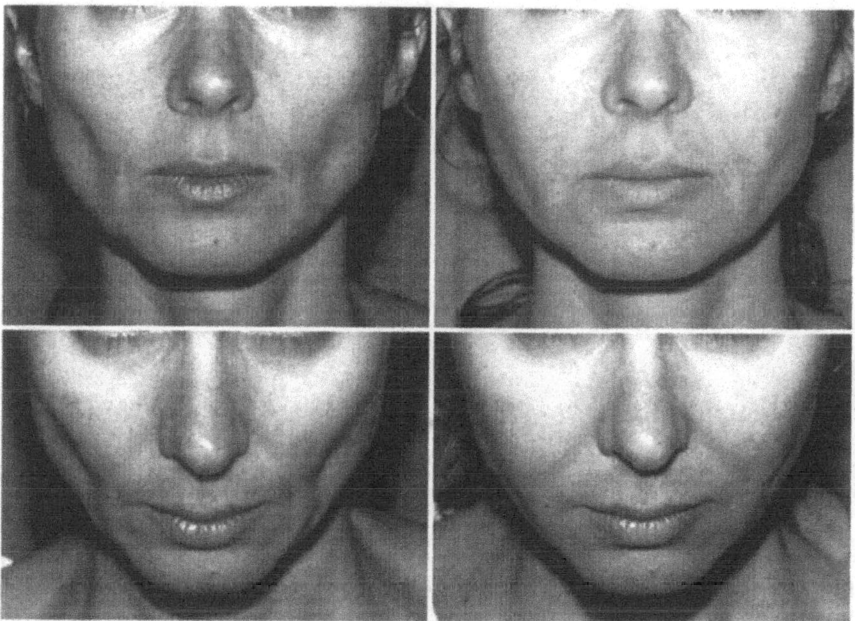

Figure 4 Case 2. This 43-year-old patient presented with "hollows" of her cheeks that gave her the appearance of a sick person (left). After infiltration into her cheeks, nasolabial folds, and marionette regions, she returned at 15 months (right) with a much healthier appearance.

vested from the thighs. Into the right buccal cheek 5 cc was placed and into the left 3.75 cc was placed. Into each nasolabial fold 2 cc was placed and into each marionette region 1 cc was placed. Into the malar cheek 6 cc was placed over the right and 7.5 cc over the left. One cubic centimeter was feathered up into each lower eyelid. She returned 15 months later, feeling that she looked much healthier (Fig. 4, right, above and below).

Case 3

This 52-year-old patient presented with multiple complaints. She reported "holes in my face" referring to the hollowness in her cheeks and upper eyelids. Below the hollows in her cheeks, she felt she had jowls forming emphasized by her marionette frown lines; above her eyelids, her forehead was excessively wrinkled. Overall the patient appeared tired and distressed (Fig. 5, left). Before the first procedure, she was afraid of having bigger lips and did not understand the placement into the glabella or nasion. She asked for me to be extremely conservative in these areas. Fat was grafted in three

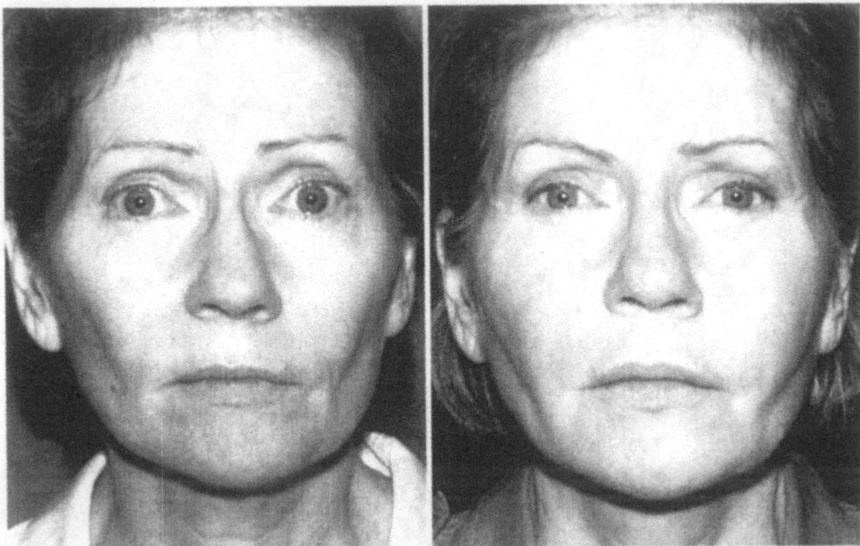

Figure 5 Case 3. This 52-year-old patient was bothered by "holes in my face," referring to the hollowness in her cheeks and upper eyelids (left). Overall, the patient had a very tired and distressed expression on her face. Fifteen months after the last of three fat-grafting procedures, the patient returns with a healthier, rested, emotionally neutral countenance (right).

sessions into various regions of the face to bring about changes that would impart fullness as well as rejuvenate her face. During the first session 22.5 cc of fat was grafted in the forehead, 3 cc in each supraorbital rim, 12.5 cc in each malar cheek, and 1 cc in the glabella and nasion. Four-and-a-half cubic centimeters of fat was added to the right buccal cheek and 4 cc to the left one. In the lip, 1 cc was added to the white roll, 2 cc to the upper lip vermilion, and 1.25 cc to the lower lip. Four cubic centimeters was also added at each angle of the mandible along with 14 cc into the mentum. The patient returned after the procedure excited about how much younger and more attractive she appeared. At that point, she understood my goal with the lips and glabellar placement. She wanted a fuller glabella, as she liked the appearance of the glabella in the immediate postprocedure period. Likewise, she wanted fuller but not big lips. Even though I warned her that it would be difficult to improve the marionette much more, she wanted more added. She also decided to have the left nasolabial fold filled (it had not been done at the last procedure). Finally, we decided to add minor amounts to most areas of her face. Four months after the first procedure, another 5 cc of fat was added to the forehead, 5 cc to the left cheek, 2 cc to the glabella, 2.25 cc in the right supraorbital region, and 4 cc in the left supraorbital region. Into the infraorbital region 0.5 cc was placed in the left side only. Two-and-a-half cubic centimeters was also added to the left nasiolabial fold only, 1.5 cc more was added to the upper lip, and 1.5 cc more to the lower lip. Into the right buccal area, 2.5 cc more was added. Finally, 2 cc more was placed into the left border of the mandible and 2.5 cc to the right border.

She returned 10 months later impressed by the lack of wrinkles in her forehead and the overall improvement in the texture of her skin and young look. However, she wanted more of a change in her lips and she was considering a face-lift to tighten her jawline. I suggested that we could get a little more improvement by adding to the border of the mandible. She was pleased with the appearance of her lower and upper eyelids, but she had noticed some wrinkles left in the crow's feet area where I had not placed fat. She also wanted me to place more into the marionette region even though I told her that it would not improve the area a great deal. And now that she had seen an improvement in the left nasolabial fold, she wanted to add a little more to both sides. Finally, she noted some irregularities in her forehead. Even though she remembers me telling her that irregularities in the forehead are common, and she loved the appearance of the forehead, she wanted me to try and place more fat. A year after the previous procedure, 9.5 cc of fat was added to the forehead, 1.25 cc into each crow's feet area, 4 cc to the left nasolabial fold and 2.5 cc to the right, 2.5 cc to each marionette region, and 5 cc to each border of the mandible. Into the lip, 0.5 cc was added to the white roll. Finally, 1 cc of fat was placed to the upper lip and 5 cc to the lower lip.

Fifteen months after the last procedure, her facial expressions appear softer and calmer. Restoring the fullness to her cheeks, jawline and forehead has created a more youthful, healthy appearance and reduced the wrinkling in these areas (Figs. 6 and 7, right).

DISCUSSION: RATIONALE FOR TECHNIQUE

Harvesting and Refinement

The technique I use for harvesting, refining, and transferring fat was developed to minimize mechanical trauma to the delicate parcels of fat and to limit exposure to air during the harvesting and transfer phases. Successful tissue transplantation of most tissues (skin, cartilage, corneas, and bone) in humans requires that tissue architecture be maintained. Likewise, with fat tissue transplantation, tissue architecture must be respected. To allow placement, the fat should be harvested as an intact parcel already a size that can

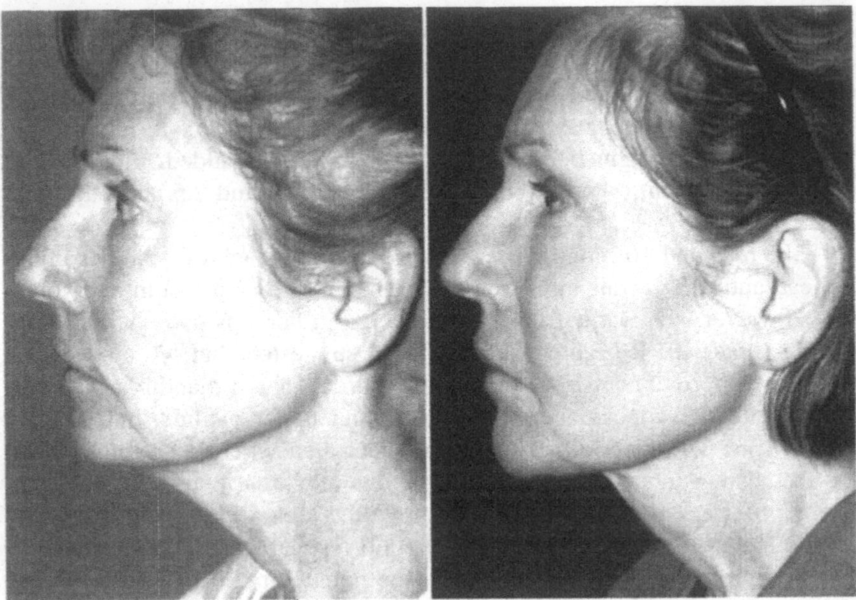

FIGURE 6 Case 3. Picture before (left) and 15 months after (right) the last procedure. The side view of the patient demonstrates a dramatic change in the relationship of the neck with the chin, the size and shape of the lip, as well a subtle change in the shape of the profile of the nose.

easily pass through the lumen of a small cannula. By harvesting fat in this fashion, the operating surgeon does not have to reduce the size of the fat parcel. Reducing the size of larger parcels of fat so that they will move through a smaller needle (straining, chopping, washing, etc.) can disrupt the fragile tissue architecture and other tissue components such as fibrin.

The surgeon must respect that the fragile human fat tissue was never intended to survive unprotected. Without the protection of skin, fat can be easily damaged by mechanical maneuvers and atmospheric changes. For instance, fat tissue is not well equipped to handle the high negative pressures of extraction with a vacuum or the high positive pressures of placement. Exposure to dry air will rapidly cause the fat to desiccate [15]. "Washing" of the harvested tissue, even though advocated by many physicians, can damage fat tissue [16–18]. The mechanical action of "washing" can subject the reticular fibers and connective tissue septae to unnecessary trauma and can disrupt the fragile fat tissue architecture [19]. It is possible that washing the fat will remove fibrin so that it does not anchor to the surrounding tissues as well [20,21]. However, intact parcels of fat tissue harvested in the manner

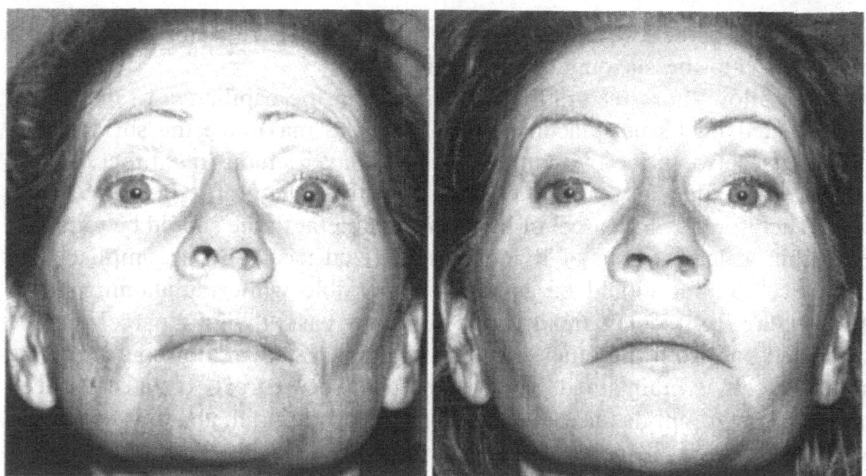

FIGURE 7 Case 3. Picture before (left) and after 15 months (right) of follow-up. This upward tilted front view demonstrates a marked improvement in the forehead wrinkling with no Botox injections and a widening of the nasion and glabella. A significant increase in the buccal cheek volume and chin can also be seen. In addition, the entire lip has been expanded, including the white roll of the upper lip.

described here appear to be able to withstand brief centrifugation to yield long-term results.

Knowing that the infiltrated tissue is relatively pure fat tissue enhances the predictability of fat grafting. Most of the oil, blood, and lidocaine should be gently removed from the harvested tissue by sedimentation or centrifugation. Material harvested by syringe liposuction can contain as little as 10% and as much as 90% of potentially viable fat. Placement of a 10% concentration of fat will obviously give a dramatically different result than will placement of a 90% concentration. To obtain consistent, predictable results, most of the oil, blood, and extracellular aqueous components must be removed without causing significant damage to the fat tissues to be transplanted.

Structural Fat Placement

Harvesting, refinement, and transfer of subcutaneous tissue to provide relatively pure, intact parcels of fat is paramount for successful fat grafting. However, the most challenging exercise of fat grafting is the last phase—the placement of the refined fat into the recipient site. The surgeon should place the fat parcels so that they survive uniformly, are stable, and become integrated into the surrounding recipient tissue.

To allow more respiration diffusion from the capillaries to the newly transplanted fat tissue, placement should try to maximize the surface area of contact between the two entities. Studies have demonstrated that as little as 40% of grafted fat tissue is viable 1 mm from the graft edges at 60 days [22]. Therefore, every parcel of the transplanted fat tissue should be touching or within at least 1 mm of living, vascularized tissue. To accomplish this, the parcels of fat should be as small as possible while maintaining tissue architecture. By placing small parcels in many passes, the fat parcels can be separated one from the other and thereby the surface area of contact of the small parcels is maintained. The distance between parcels of fat does need not to be great, only as large as a capillary. Separating the parcels of fat and keeping them small increases the potential for diffusion, respiration, nutrition, and eventual revascularization.

Integration

This technique emphasizes placement of fat in an integrated fashion. If fat is placed in large clumps, the fat that eventually survives will usually feel and look like lumps of fat. By placing fat into small parcels and separating parcels from each other with the donor site tissues, the transplanted fat is not easily palpable as a discrete entity. Instead, it feels like the tissues into or next to which it is placed. For instance, fat parcels placed into muscle and separated by fibers of muscle will feel not like fat but like a larger and firmer muscle. Fat placed next to skin in a smooth layer will feel like thicker skin, not fat against skin. Fat parcels placed next to cartilage or bone will feel firm like cartilage or bone and will be difficult to distinguish from cartilage or bone by palpation of the area. Finally, this method of placement encourages anchoring of the fat parcels to the host tissue to discourage migration and encourage structural changes.

Levels of Placement

The manner of placement and level of placement will determine the final result of fat grafting. Fat layered deep against bone or cartilage will feel like bone or cartilage and support the overlying tissues. Prime examples are fat placed against the malar and mandibular regions. On the other hand, to soften wrinkles, to decrease the size of pores, or to smooth acne scars, infiltrating the fat immediately under the skin provides dermal support. To fill, plump, or restore fullness, fat tissue is placed from the deepest levels into the intermediate layers and out to the skin. For example, for structured, fuller malar cheeks, first infiltrate a layer against bone, then sequentially place more superficial layers of fat (placing most of the volume in the deepest layers). Placing the fat immediately under skin or mucosa will expand the surface area. For the lips, layering of the transplanted fat against the mucosa can increase the surface area of vermilion show.

Care should be taken to avoid placing fat into unstable planes. For instance, infiltration of the forehead next to the bone is difficult since the areolar plane does not allow for stability of the fat tissue. In such an area, every effort should be made to infiltrate fat tissue into the more superficial facial and muscle layers, as well as under the skin. Accuracy of the initial placement is imperative since placed fat cannot be predictably molded into another shape after placement. If the surgeon accidentally allows a cyst or clump to form, digital manipulation can sometimes flatten such minor irregularities. Check for structural integrity of the placed fat by palpation of the areas after each series of infiltrations. This is not to mold the fat, but to ensure that the newly placed fat has no lumps and feels evenly placed.

Amounts for Placement

Estimating the volume to be placed in each area and situation can be extremely difficult. Because structural fat grafting involves three-dimensional increments that can be as small as 0.5 mm and are rarely more than 3 or 4 mm, there is little room for error. The surgeon must consider numerous elements and must adjust for each one. Some of the fragile fatty tissue will be damaged enough to die no matter how careful the harvesting, refinement, and placement is performed. A minimal compensation should be made for resorption in this situation. Also, the surgeon must bear in mind that the injected material is not entirely composed of fat. Even after refinement, some quantities of blood, xylocaine, and oil will be present in the refined fat tissue.

Swelling of the recipient tissues either during the placement or before can obscure the visual clues that the surgeon can use for determining an endpoint. Infiltrated local anesthesia will distend the tissues prior to placement. A hematoma during local or fat infiltration can sometimes cause dramatic enlargement of the recipient site. Finally, the immediate tissue edema caused by forcing a blunt cannula through living tissue is variable from patient to patient and anatomic area to anatomic area.

The most important single technical point is the use of 1-cc syringes to prevent overzealous augmentation. Initially, it is best to try small volumes of the infiltrate into each area. As the physician becomes familiar with the technique and the results that different volumes create, he or she can increase the amount placed in each area gradually.

COMPLICATIONS

Complications with structural fat grafting have been described previously [9,11,23]. The majority of complications are related to appearance. They are most often associated with the location, manner, and volume in which the fat tissue has been placed into recipient areas. These complications include overcorrection, undercorrection, irregularities, and asymmetries.

Structural fat grafting has other potential complications that it shares with other surgical procedures. Infections are usually associated with intraoral contamination or breaks in technique. Although the cannula is blunt, damage to underlying structures such as nerves, muscles, glands, and blood vessels is possible. Complications associated with incisions and with the harvesting sites are also possible. Fortunately, the complication rate with fat grafting is extremely low compared to that of most open surgical techniques.

CONCLUSION

The predictability and longevity of fat grafting is intrinsically related to the technique used. Harvesting small parcels of intact fat tissue and separating the parcels from each other maximizes the surface area of contact of each parcel of fat tissue with the surrounding host tissues. Increasing the surface area of contact places the transplanted fat cells located at the center of the parcels closer to a blood supply. Since fat is living tissue, this proximity to a nutritional and respiratory source promotes long-term survival. Also, maximizing the surface area of contact encourages integration and anchoring of the newly placed fat tissue. Finally, the anchoring of the fat tissue parcels allows for the potential of dramatic structural changes and the placement of relatively large volumes without migration of the fat from the intended site. In my experience of more than 3000 cases, fat tissue harvested, refined, and placed in the specific manner described here has consistent long-term survival. This provides aesthetic surgeons with a reliable soft tissue filler technique with which to move into this century.

REFERENCES

1. Kolle FS. Hydrocarbon prostheses. In: Plastic and Cosmetic Surgery. New York: D. Appleton & Company, 1911:211–338.
2. Miller CG. Cannula Implants and Review of Implantation Techniques in Esthetic Surgery. Chicago: Oak Press, 1926.
3. Chajchir A, Benzaquen I. Liposuction fat grafts in face wrinkles and hemifacial atrophy. Aesth Plast Surg 1986; 10:115–117.

4. Illouz YG. The fat cell "graft": a new technique to fill depressions. Plast Reconstr Surg 1986; 78:122–123.
5. Teimourian B. Repair of soft tissue contour deficit by means of semi liquid fat graft. Plast Reconstr Surg 1986; 78:123–124.
6. Fournier PM. Who should do syringe liposculpturing? J Derm Surg Oncol 1988; 14:1063–1073.
7. Coleman SR. Early results with fat grafting. American Society of Aeshtetic Plastic Surgery Scientific Session, San Francisco, CA, April, 1988.
8. Coleman SR. Long-term survival of fat transplants: controlled demonstrations. Aesth Plast Surg 1995; 19:421–425.
9. Coleman SR. Facial recontouring with Lipostructure. Clin Plast Surg 1997; 24: 347–360.
10. Coleman SR. My view: Structural fat grafting. Aesth Surg J 1998; 18:386–388.
11. Coleman SR. Structural fat grafts: The ideal filler? Clin Plast Surg 2001; 28: 111–119.
12. Hurwitz DJ, Coleman SR, Katz A. Structural fat grafting of the face: lessons from a teacher and his student. In: Habal MB, Himel HN, Lineaweaver WC, Colon GA, Parsons RW, Woods JE, eds. Key Issues in Plastic and Cosmetic Surgery. Basel: S. Karger, 2001; 17:15–38.
13. Carraway JH, Mello CG. Syringe aspiration and fat concentration: a simple technique for autologous fat injection. Ann Plast Surg 1990; 24:293–296.
14. Kinney BM. The therapeutic use of electromagnetic fields in plastic surgery. Aesth Surg J 1999; 19:86–88.
15. Aboudib JHC, Cardoso de Castro C, Gradel J. Hand rejuvenescence by fat filling. Ann Plast Surg 1992; 28:559–564.
16. Lewis CM. The current status of autologous fat grafting. Aesth Plast Surg 1993; 17:109–112.
17. Toledo LS. Syringe liposculpture: a two-year experience. Aesth Plast Surg 1999; 15:321.
18. Carpaneda C, Ribeiro M. Study of the histologic alterations and viability of the adipose grafts in humans. Aesth Plast Surg 1993; 17:43–47.
19. Horl HW, Feller AM, Biemer E. Technique for liposuction fat reimplantation and long-term volume evaluation by magnetic resonance imaging. Ann Plast Surg 1991; 26:248–258.
20. Niechajev I, Sevcuk O. Long-term results of fat transplantation: clinical and histologic studies. Plast Reconstr Surg 1994; 94:496–506.
21. Chajchir A, Benzaquen I, Wexler E, Arellano AH. Fat injection. Aesth Plast Surg 1990; 14:127–136.
22. Carpaneda CA, Ribeiro MT. Percentage of graft viability versus injected volume in adipose autotransplants. Aesth Plast Surg 1994; 18:17–19.
23. Coleman SR. The technique of periorbital lipoinfiltration. Oper Tech Plast Reconstr Surg 1994; 1:120–126.

27

Syringe Fat Grafting

Pierre F. Fournier
Private Practice
Paris, France

HISTORY OF SYRINGE FAT GRAFTING

Fat grafting is not a new operation. As a filler, as a space-occupying tissue, adipose tissue has always interested the aesthetic surgeon. It started in several different countries. In North America extensive research was done by L. Peer, Gurney, Kanaval, and Stevenson and in Europe by Rossati. Their conclusion was that 50% of the transplanted cells should survive. A cell survival rate of 25–50% seems highly constant.

By serendipity, in September 1985 I "discovered" that adipose tissue could be extracted using a syringe and a needle. The ease of the extraction, done under anaerobic conditions and respecting the integrity and the sterility of the adipose tissue, immediately suggested that I could reinject this extracted fat into other places of the body where needed. Before this "discovery" fat grafting was an open or semiopen procedure with a risk of infection and visible scars when obtaining the adipose tissue. The syringe–needle unit or syringe–canula unit technique was obviously a significant improvement as all the shortcomings of the previous techniques were eliminated.

We shifted from an aerobic technique to an anaerobic technique that is much simpler. It was evident that such an improvement of the conventional technique would be easily accepted by both surgeons and patients. With this new tool, we wanted to prove that syringe fat transfer could achieve the same results as the conventional open or semiopen techniques and could even give better results (Fig. 1). The use of the syringe–needle unit or syringe–canula unit technique gave new life to the old procedure of fat grafting, making it safer and simpler and allowing the surgeon to obtain long-lasting results with repeated injections throughout time. Each injection adds to the partial improvement obtained with the previous injection.

The well-established concept of overcorrection when fat grafting is done in stages, over a period of time, using a simple, easy procedure with repeated injections, is a method that is readily accepted by the patient and the surgeon. We also hoped that the syringe technique could improve the take of adipose tissue and that the cell survival rate of 25–50% could be higher.

ADVANTAGES OF THE SYRINGE TECHNIQUE

The specimen of fat obtained with a 2-mm-diameter needle (14-gauge) and a syringe is made up of cores of adipose tissue, and even though the peripheral part of this sliver of fat is damaged, the central fat is not and contains undamaged fat lobules. It is admitted by all that adipose cells "don't take" only adipose lobule take. Damaged lobules do not take; only those with their vessels and septi intact can do so. This is a closed technique that keeps the removal sterile and whole, and the fat tissue can thus be used

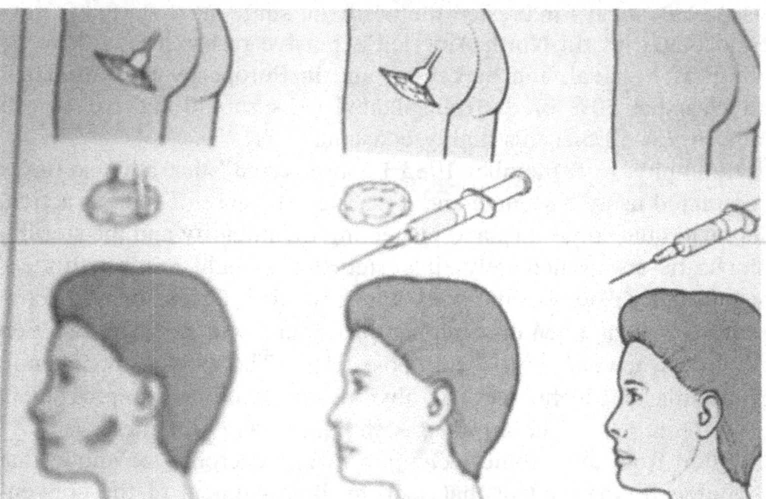

FIGURE 1 Evolution of fat grafting: open procedure, half-open procedure, and closed procedure.

for a transfer. This technique is an innovation in aesthetic plastic surgery, since it permits closed removal and implantation in anaerobic conditions with no scars or overcorrection in volume.

Thus it is possible to perform fat transfers safely since syringe extraction was developed with its ease of transfer and lack of scarring in the extracted and grafted areas. Gentle vacuuming in the syringe may reduce the risk of lysis. The buffering action of the normal saline decreases the impact of the adipose tissue fragments in the syringe, and their transportation is carried out without damage since the whole operation is performed in a fluid medium and not in a vacuum as with the machine. The less nonviable tissue that remains in the sample, the less resorption is expected. The syringe allows the surgeon to aspirate, process, expel, and store adipose tissue using conventional plastic syringes. Overcorrection is still necessary, as it has been since the procedure was first used more than 100 years ago, except today it is no longer necessary to disfigure the patient. It is now possible to do several grafting procedures spread over time. As in any tissue transplant, the smaller the amount, the greater the chance it will take. The result of small and repeated implantations is that the patient can lead a normal social life a few days after the operation and will readily accept this treatment in several stages.

Classical experimentation has been put into practice. The overcorrection necessary to obtain the final result can be accomplished with repeated grafts and is no longer performed in one operation. Patients are thus overcorrected *over time* and *not in space*. Progress has also been made in the instruments used, but this is not due to new scientific data. One of the basic principles of general surgery and general plastic surgery, "respect of the tissues," is accomplished more efficiently with the use of the syringe.

In the history of fat grafting, we must note that the syringe technique has been used in the past, but it was a half-closed technique (or half-open). It was used by Brunnings in 1911 and later by Willy and Sava. Charles Willy, a British aesthetic surgeon, wrote and published a book in 1925 showing photographs of him injecting fat into the face with a syringe for aesthetic reasons. In this procedure the fat was finely chopped with scissors from a block of tissue removed with a scalpel, placed in a syringe, and reinjected. This semiclosed technique was an improvement over the purely open technique. George Sava, another British aesthetic surgeon, used the same procedure to modify the faces of Allied spies sent to the occupied territories during the World War II. Whenever he desired a temporary face change, he used fat taken from another individual. When he desired a permanent result, he took the fat from the same person from another part of the body. The main advance in fat grafting as it is done today is the use of the syringe for extraction of the adipose tissue.

MATERIALS AND METHODS

After we understood the possibilities offered by the syringe–needle unit or syringe–cannula unit we started fat grafting on our own patients. As fat tissue is the most natural tissue to be used on the body whenever it is needed, we gave up completely with all other artifical fillers.

The selection of patients has been done by the aging process. We strongly believe that many of our patients need tissue augmentation, a subcutaneous fill of the face, and not a "pull" or lift of the skin and superficial subcutaneous tissues. Many surgeons do not seem to be aware of tissue involution and tissue proliferation.

Most of our patients have been women, mostly mature, between the ages of 30 and 45. Less than 5% of our patients are men. The exact number cannot be estimated. Our experience is a clinical one. We do not know the exact number of our patients who have had syringe fat grafting. They are several thousands (faces mostly, body defects, breast augmentation, sequelae of reduction liposculpturing, and routine reinjections after reduction liposculpturing) over 15 years and we are positive that syringe fat grafting is efficient.

Indications for Syringe Fat Grafting and Patient Selection

Facial Recontouring

In many cases, one procedure is not enough, and several injections have to be given 3 months apart (building up a chin or in the cheekbone area). In the case of a rejuvenation indication, the older the patient the more injections are needed, since the face's fat reserve decreases considerably with time.

In young or mature people who have "weak points" in the face, fewer procedures are needed. A maximum of four or five injections are necessary to have a permanent result or at least a long-term result. This is why fat grafting should be used as a preventive step in facial recontouring as soon as it is needed and not only as a treatment when the aging process is advanced. We have many long-lasting results (14 years) in young patients who came for repeated injections, and the result is obvious clinically as well as on xerographies. In the face, the results are better in the glabella, forehead, cheekbone area, cheeks, nasolabial furrows, and chin. The least satisfying results are in the lips.

Body Contouring

This has unpredictable results; sometimes only one injection gives long-lasting results, especially where there is scar tissue. In other cases, the injections have to be repeated every 6 months.

Legs

We have had long-lasting results 5 years after one or two procedures were done in cases involving poliomyelitis.

Breasts

We have injected large amounts of fat in the submammary space: 150, 200, and 250 cc. The results have been good for a year or two. Many patients did not come regularly for follow-ups, and we do not know the final results.

We observed an infection (abscess) in one breast and a large oily cyst in another case. We now seldom inject the retroglandular space. Rather, we inject subcutaneously in the four quadrants of the breast, mainly the upper two. The technique is the same as that used in facial recontouring. When injecting the breast retroglandularly or subjectorally or for a body defect, we use a 60-cc syringe and a 4-mm blunt cannula. The fat is washed in most cases, and general anesthesia is used.

Hands

These give the most reliable results, with 12–15 cc being injected subcutaneously in the dorsum of the hand. Long-lasting results are seen after 4 or 5 years. We believe that bones behave as a splint and prevent the retraction of the graft. The technique used for hands is the same as that used for the face.

SYRINGE FACIAL FAT GRAFTING

We now describe in detail the technique of syringe facial fat transfer—syringe lipofilling—which is the most used.

Why Facial Recontouring?

Facial ptosis in the case of tissue involution is due to a loss of volume of the deep structures, particularly of the soft tissues of the lower two-thirds of the face. Therefore what concerns us is to restore the lost volume using the means at our disposal (prostheses made of silicone, bone, cartilage, dermis, or adipose tissue blocks) or by fat grafting when the involution's location allows it.

Until recently, as far as rejuvenation surgery was concerned, the aesthetic surgeon was limited to practicing surface surgery. The concept of volume restoration was never mentioned, whether for a rejuvenation problem or as an embellishment. Surface surgery was supposed to resolve all problems in all cases, the proposed treatment being above all a cutaneous one. According to the importance of the aesthetic anomaly or the age of the patient, different options were available: model lifting, prolonged model lifting, upper lifting, lower lifting, or full lifting. A volume increase of the malar region was done only for the beauty it gave according to the patient's own request and never for rejuvenation purposes (Fig. 2).

It is well known that the full lift had little or no effect on the T-zone of the face, where the structure is bony and ages differently. The loss of volume of the V-zone ("V" in shape as well as a symbol of vulnerability) was never mentioned, even though it was obvious that the support of this zone, representing two-thirds of the medium and inferior laterals of the face, is adipose tissue, both superficial as well as deep. This tissue's involution, its hypotrophy, produces a false ptosis in the lower half of the face (a true ptosis is when there is tissue proliferation). In global aging there is thus an outside and inside aging process; there is a cellular proliferation or involution (Figs. 3 and 4). Professionals such as artists, cartoonists, painters, sculptors, morphologists, aestheticians, and makeup artists clearly distinguish between the full face and the hollow face. Reading their books is infinitely more educational for the aesthetic surgeon than the anatomy textbooks that ignore the aging process.

We thus distinguish between two sorts of wrinkles: tension and pressure wrinkles of the full face on which gravity is acting (ptosis on the

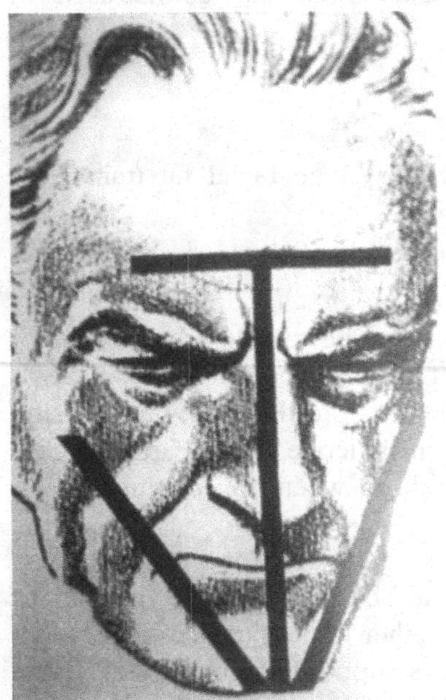

FIGURE 2 The T-zone and the V-zone of the face.

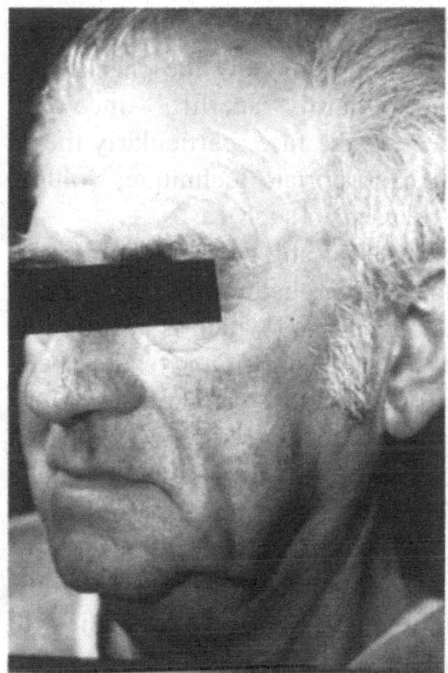

FIGURE 3 Tissue proliferation; tension and pressure wrinkles.

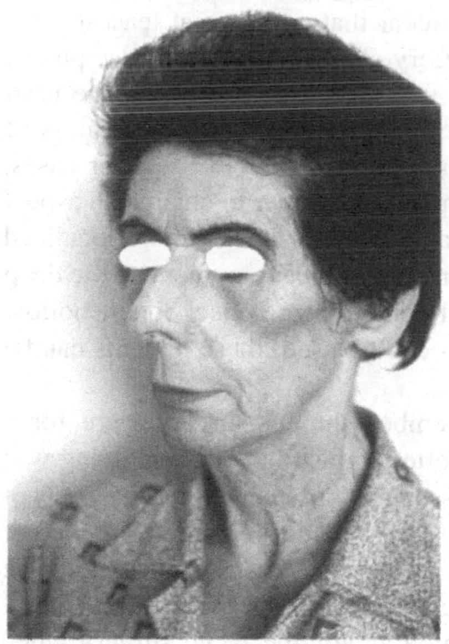

FIGURE 4 Tissue involution; sag and shrinkage wrinkles.

outside) and sag and shrinkage wrinkles of the hollow face on which gravity acts less (ptosis from the inside). A face-lift improves only the cheeks; the term "*meloplasty*" is more appropriate than the term "face-lift," since only the cheeks are helped and not the other areas of the face, particularly the T-zone. Surface surgery for this area is an inappropriate technique; volume surgery is the only technique that should be used in such cases.

Facial analysis is of prime importance before any aesthetic surgery of the face and neck. In cases of tissue involution, there is too much cutaneous covering, which is no longer adapted to its content and which is at the same time its support, structure, and framework. This cutaneous cover has been accused of being the origin of aesthetic anomalies, whereas the true culprit is the hypotrophy of the superficial and deep structures of the V-zone. A face-lift-inappropriate treatment in such cases will have consequences such as unnecessary scars, decrease of the side burns, and a recession and a stepping of the hair line in the postauricular zone.

The essential consequence of aging—tissue involution in the V-zone, which has not been corrected—will continue, and a new false ptosis will occur, more or less rapidly. A volume surgery could avoid or delay this evolution and has the advantage of simplicity. The skin's elasticity will once more be blamed, although it has nothing to do with the deep involution process. Lipofilling is not a panacea, and it is certain that some day we will have other techniques at our disposal. Lipofilling does, however, have the advantage of being the only precise treatment that corrects, at least temporarily, the defect in question. Volume surgery also takes care of false ptosis: Facial skin is only a cover for the deep structures and should not be used as a means of traction or tension to give back the tonicity and firmness of the face when the framework is the source of the problem. In other cases, patients do not come for rejuvenation purposes but rather to change an aspect of their appearance. These patients are candidates for one or more localized volume increases in the face because of insufficient development of the deep structures or a desire to modify a normal contour (e.g., cheekbones, hollow cheeks, and chin). If a silicone prosthesis can be used, these patients can be treated by lipofilling as well.

Aesthetic facial rejuvenation and embellishment surgery were for a long time bidimensional surgery. It was often unjustified because aging was treated in an incomplete manner; the associated tissue involution was not corrected and the previous volume of the face was not restored. The idea of volume surgery must therefore be added to the idea of surface surgery. The latter is in fact incomplete and is justified only in cases of tissue proliferation; it is often performed at the same time as volume facial surgery when there is an associated deep soft tissue proliferation.

The use of adipose tissue or its derivatives is not the only option. Other means (prosthesis or other autologous tissue) leading to a volume increase in the region to be treated can be used. With the volume of the operated regions temporarily or permanently restored by a more logical implantation surgery, the consequence of aging—tissue hypotrophy—can be addressed. Lipofilling easily permits the surgeon to perform trimensional surgery by acting on an element that has previously been ignored: volume.

Preoperative Examination

The preoperative examination is very important. With the help of a mirror and the patient's cooperation, the surgeon should study the weak points of the face, where tissue involution begins, and the other zones of the face for which the patient is seeking to have an aspect modified. If needed, a test can be done to temporarily show the effect obtained by the desired volume. A determined quantity (2, 4, or 6 cc or more) of lidocaine diluted to one-third is injected in the area or areas to be corrected. Thus the surgeon will have an idea of the quantity of adipose tissue needed for the correction.

The procedure for finding the false ptosis needs to be done systematically. The thumb is placed in the cheekbone area and then an up-and-out traction movement is made. If there is a modification in the nasolabial or labiomental furrows or in the jowls, this maneuver shows hypotrophy in the region and the existence of false nasolabial or labiomental furrows and false jowls. The cheekbone region needs to be increased as well as the false nasolabial or labiomental furrows. The cheekbones, together with the chin, are the three pillars of the youth-and-beauty triangle. The cheekbones are the hanger of the face (Figs. 5 and 6).

In the case of wrinkles on the upper lip, the skin should be smoothed out with the help of both index fingers, each being placed on the external part of the white hemilip and performing an outward movement. If the wrinkles totally disappear, they are deep wrinkles caused by the involution of the underlying tissues; lipofilling is therefore indicated. If there is partial or total persistence of wrinkles then these are superficial wrinkles—true wrinkles caused by skin lesions. These lesions will be helped partially by lipofilling, but they will need additional treatment to be completely corrected (mechanical or chemical dermabrasion, laser treatment, or collagen injection). These facts should be carefully explained to the patient. The examination should be done again when the patient has decided to have the operation. The conclusions should be written down, and a diagram of the face should be drawn.

When the operation date is set, generally after a second consultation to give the patient time to think it over, the surgeon will ask for the usual

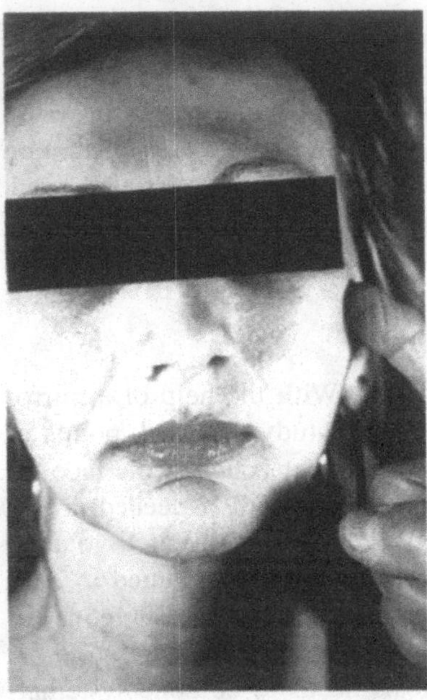

FIGURE 5 The cheekbone-area sign.

preoperative examination for surgery and give routine preoperative treatment (vitamins C and K and phenobarbitone). Photographs should be taken of the face from different angles, and an estimation should be made of the amount of adipose tissue needed to do the filling (usually 30–40 cc in general). Weak points should be isolated. The total amount of local anesthetic to use, the size of the extraction zone, the length of the operation, the postoperative reactions, and the return to normal of the region or regions treated depend heavily on this estimation. These procedures should be explained to the patient, as well as the fact that the treatment affects individuals differently. Written information should also be given to the patient.

FACIAL AND HARVESTING ZONE MARKINGS

A good-quality dermographic pen should be used to mark the patients.

Face

The face is marked first. The marking should be done while the patient is standing and according to the results of the facial analysis. The nasolabial, labiomental, and glabellar furrows are marked with two lines. The cheek-

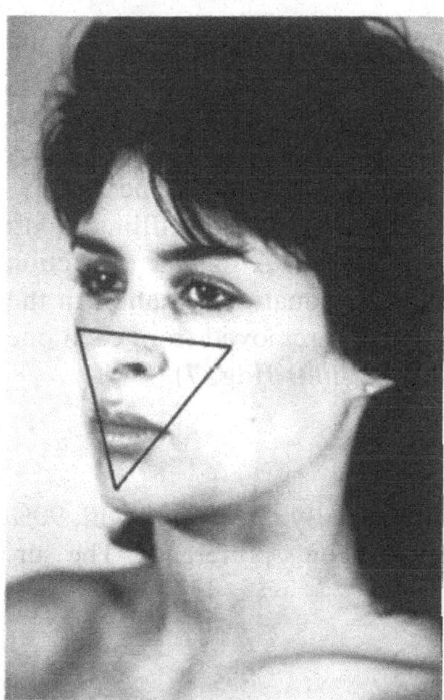

FIGURE 6 The triangle of youth and beauty.

bones and cheeks by a triangle or an oval or a circle. The lips should be marked with a point. These should be symmetrical and identical on each side of the face. Sometimes one side of the face needs more correction than the other side, a very frequent aesthetic anomaly. It may be explained by a prolonged time of pressure on this side during the sleep.

The quantity to inject in each area is evaluated, and the surface of the extraction zone depends on the total volume necessary. In general, 4–6 cc are injected in each malar zone; 2–4 cc in each nasolabial furrow; 1–2 cc in each labiomental furrow; 4–6 cc in each cheek; 2–4 cc in the glabellar region; 8–10 cc in the total frontal area; 6 cc in the temples; 2.5 cc in each upper or lower lip; and 6, 8, 10, or 15 cc in the chin. Once the marking of the face is finished, a photograph is taken and kept in the patient's file.

Harvesting Zones

The extraction zone surface will vary, depending on the quantity of the adipose tissue to be extracted. Obviously this extraction should not leave any surface irregularities. The chosen zone should be marked while the patient is standing if this zone is located in the trochanteric region or the hip. It should be done while the patient is lying down if it is in an exterior buttock or in the abdominal wall, since morphology is modified by the position.

The markings should be either a circle, an oval, a square, or a rectangle. The interior of the marked zone should be subdivided in small rectangles approximately 4 cm long and 3 cm wide. Their number should be approximately equal to the number of syringes necessary to do the filling. With one syringe, 5 cc of adipose tissue can be extracted. A regular extraction can be performed easily and without leaving a residual deformation in the totality of the zone if only 5 cc of adipose tissue is removed from each one of the rectangles, which thus serve as measuring units (Fig. 7).

OPERATIVE ZONE DISINFECTION

Rigorous asepsis is necessary. The tegument is usually disinfected with 90% alcohol or another product, according to the surgeon's preference. The sur-

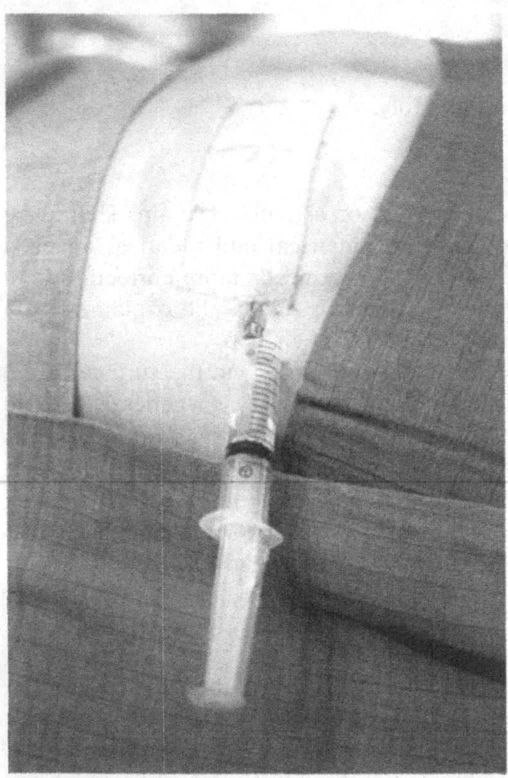

FIGURE 7 The hips and buttocks are excellent harvesting zones.

geon will be gloved and masked. Draping of the operative zone should be done as for any other facial operation, before the anesthesia is given. When using nonsterilized external refrigeration as anesthesia or as a complement to local anesthesia, disinfection should take place and the drape should be placed when this is finished.

OPERATIVE ZONE ANESTHESIA

Anesthesia in the operative zone should be different than the one used for reduction microlipoextraction. Recall that in the case of microlipoextraction for reduction lipoplasty when a reinjection of tissues is not foreseen, "the most important thing is not what one extracts, but what one leaves"; in the case of microlipoextraction to reuse the tissues obtained during the extraction, "the most important thing is not what is left, but what one extracts." In both cases, the tissues must be respected by the surgeon, but the tissues to be respected differ in each case.

The fraction that must live or relive is what matters, not the fraction that will be eliminated. A noninfiltrated extraction is better because the hydraulic traumatism caused by the injection added to the chemical traumatism caused by the injection of adrenaline and lidocane are avoided. Therefore in the case of microlipoextraction and reutilization of the extracted tissue, the utmost care should be taken by the surgeon for the tissue to the reinjected.

Anesthesia of the Harvesting Zone

Anesthesia of the donor zone should be performed first. The following should be done to extract the tissue to be reinjected.

Local Anesthesia

Even if local anaesthesia is not theoretically desirable for the above-mentioned reasons, it is often used. As in the case of a nerve block or regional anesthesia, lidocaine 1% with adrenaline is used. For anesthesia through infiltration, the greater the surface to anesthetize, the weaker the dilution. In general, a dilution to the third is used. The dilution is done using 2°C saline solution. A weaker dilution is perfectly possible (a fourth, a fifth, an eighth, or a tenth).

All the marked regions should be infiltrated at the same time; it will simply take longer for the anesthesia's effect to be felt. The infiltration should be made in all thicknesses of the layer of adipose tissue, but especially in depth. External refrigeration with ice bags should always be used after for 20 min. The purpose is to obtain an extraction with as little bleeding as possible and to reinforce the anesthesia.

Cryoanesthesia

The best method is external cryoanesthesia. However, we shall not describe this here since it deserves an article of its own.

General Anesthesia

Sometimes patients want general anesthesia rather than local. This is inconvenient, since the patient is kept in the clinic longer, but it is the ideal technique for large extractions. Twilight anesthesia can also be used. Two or three zones can be refrigerated simultaneously and the surgeon can perform the extractions satisfactorily. This anesthesia is for ambulatory patients.

Anesthesia of the Facial Zones

Anesthesia of the receiving zone is performed second. Considering the fragility of the adipose tissue, certain precautions should be taken: If the patient is under general or twilight anesthesia, there is no problem.

A nerve block is particularly convenient for the face: a block of the supraorbital nerves for the forehead and the glabella; a block of the infraorbital nerves for the upper lip, the nasolabial furrow, and the cheeks; and a block of the mental nerves for the lower lip and the labiomental furrows. In certain cases, a wheal of lidocaine will be enough. It is the transcutaneous needle penetration that is painful; the subcutaneous injection is not really painful.

We currently use external refrigeration, especially in the glabellar zone. The patient holds a block of ice between two pieces of cotton a few minutes before the injection. The skin should be anesthetized as a priority because the deep tissues are a lot less sensitive. Small plastic bags filled with broken ice cubes are applied on the cheeks for about 10 min. Cryogel can also be useful since it shapes itself to irregular surfaces. It needs special surveillance because it can burn the skin. Giorgio Fischer's technique is recommended: instead of filling the bags with ice and water, he used a mix made of two-thirds tap water and one-third antifreeze, after storing for a while in the freezer. The bags can thus be used several times.

Local anesthesia by infiltration of the zones to be increased is used in most of the cases. There are no special recommendations. In general, a solution to the third is used. All infiltration on the face is preceded by the application of a plastic mask kept in the refrigerator. It is applied from the beginning of the anesthesia of the donor zone. Facial infiltrations are therefore performed with no pain, with the help of an intradermic needle. Once finished, the mask is applied again until the adipose tissue is injected. This preoperatory anesthetic work, both time consuming and demanding a high level of skill, can be carried out by the surgeon or an assistant.

Premedication should be done from the beginning of the operation (0.25 mg of atropine sulfate by subcutaneous injection). An intravenous perfusion of saline solution can be made. If this is not done, a vein should be catheterized from the beginning of the operation. The best premedication is the psychological premedication achieved during the previous consultations.

Observations

External refrigeration of the areas to be operated on should be done before any kind of anesthesia—general, twilight, block, or local—as well as before any kind of extraction or injection of adipose tissue. It should be maintained for about 20 min.

PURE LIPOFILLING TECHNIQUE

Instruments

The equipment necessary for a face fill is minimal as follows: (1) "classical" filling needle (2-mm outside diameter and 4 cm useful length) and disposable ones (14 gauge) (Fig. 8); (2) 30- and 21-gauge needles for local anesthesia; (3) 10-cc disposable plastic syringes; (4) 20-cc saline solution vials at room temperature or at 2°C, which will serve to dilute the local anesthetic, to avoid all dead space in the syringe, to diminish the impact, facilitate the transportation, and to wash the adipose tissue; (5) 2-mm external diameter transfer needle; and (6) wood or metal test tube holder. For the extraction we no longer use 2-cc insulin syringes or 5-cc syringes, which do not permit washing of the extracted adipose tissue. If the face fill is done at the same time as body liposculpturing, the adipose tissue extracted with the help of single-orifice cannulas of 3 or 4 mm outside diameter and 50- or 60-cc syringes can be reused if it is transferred to 5 or 10 cc syringes on which the usual 2 mm outside diameter filling needle has been mounted (14 gauge). Harvesting with a 14-gauge cannula does not give a specimen of fat of the same quality as with the needle and therefore is not recommended.

Extraction Technique

The syringe allows the extraction, preparation, and reinjection of adipose tissue in a closed space, while respecting the integrity and sterility of the

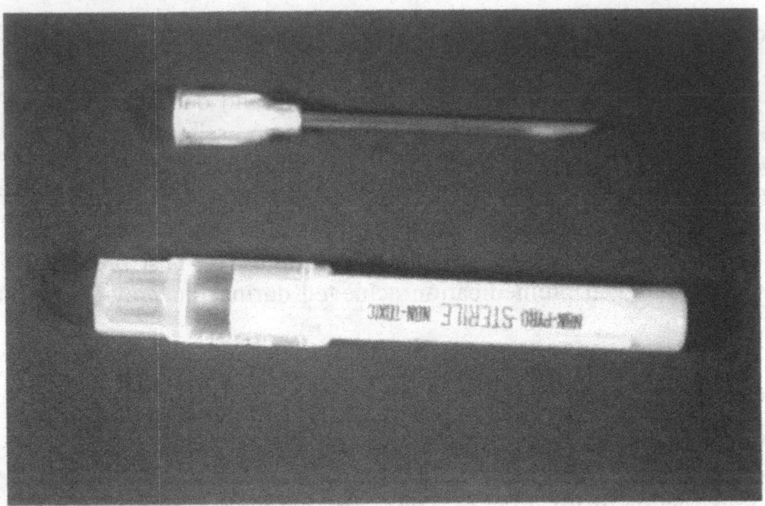

FIGURE 8 The 14-gauge needle.

extraction. It also serves as a reservoir to conserve the extracted tissue in the freezer if necessary.

Extraction of the Adipose Tissue

Using a 2-mm-outside-diameter filling needle mounted on a 10-cc syringe, we first place 2 cc of saline solution at room temperature or at 2°C in the syringe to decrease the impact of the extracted adipose tissue fragments into the syringe. The left hand makes a fold on one of the small rectangles marked on the extraction zone, and the needle is pushed through the skin in the middle of the adipose tissue. The left hand is then placed flat on the extraction zone and will stay that way throughout the operation. The right hand pulls out the syringe plunger completely, and the surgeon begins the extraction. During the whole extraction, the plunger is kept in this same position (Figs. 9 and 10). At different levels back-and-forth movements are made in a fan shape almost the length of the needle. Three to four of these are made in one direction before going to the neighboring region, without taking out the needle, which must remain under the skin. Between 30 and 50 s are needed to obtain 5 cc of adipose tissue. Once the 5 cc have been obtained, the needle is removed and 3 cc of saline solution are drawn into the syringe. The syringe is then placed vertically on a test tube holder, plunger up. The needle that was used for the extraction is mounted on another syringe for use in another rectangle extraction. This takes place while

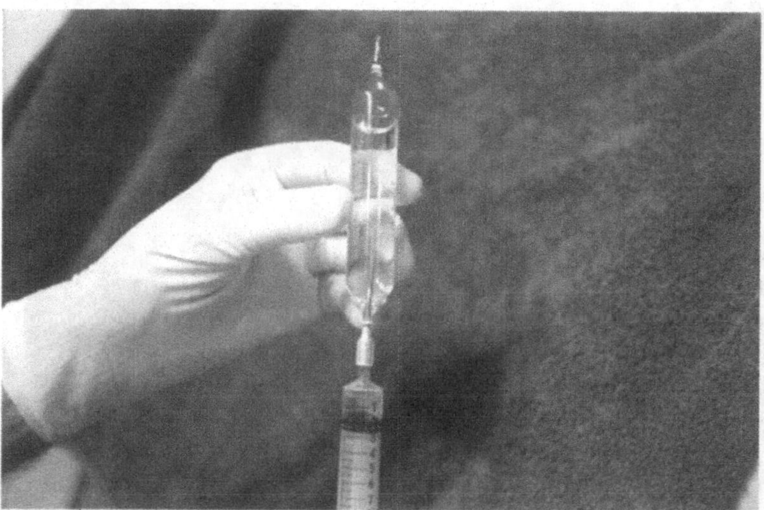

FIGURE 9 Two cubic centimeters of normal saline or 5% glucose solution are aspirated in the syringe before harvesting.

the adipose tissue in the first syringe is going through a period of decantation, the first phase of washing. Once 5 cc of adipose tissue has been extracted with the second syringe in the same way, 3 cc of saline solution should be added and the syringe placed vertically on the test tube holder. The predetermined amount of adipose tissue is removed in each of the rectangles marked on the extraction zone.

Washing

When the extraction is finished the surgeon washes the adipose tissue with the saline solution. Once the 3 cc of saline solution have been drawn into the syringe and it has been placed vertically on the test tube holder, one can see the mixture separate: the adipose tissue on top and the bloody saline solution on the bottom. This separation takes place in a few seconds (Figs. 11 and 12). This hydrohematic fraction is emptied into a cup and 5 cc of saline solution are again drawn into the syringe. The syringe should once again be placed on the test tube holder in order to obtain the separation of the two fractions while performing the same maneuver on the other syringes.

There should be as many washings as necessary to obtain bloodless adipose tissue. In general, two to four washes are necessary, sometimes more if the sample is very bloody or if not enough time is allowed between each wash. A transfer needle allows adipose tissue to pass from one syringe to

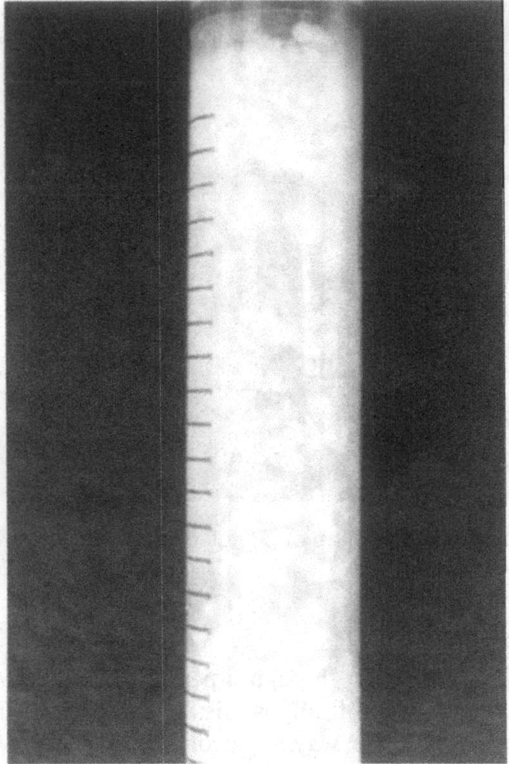

FIGURE 10 Fragmented cylinders obtained.

another in order to get equal amounts for symmetrical regions. The reinjection can be done when all the syringes have been thus prepared. Locally there should be an occlusive, slightly compressing dressing made of a few compresses kept in place by several Elastoplast bands or a layer of Elastoplast. This dressing should be removed after 24–48 hr. It may have to be changed after a faw hours if bleeding persists.

For 10 years now, during the lipoextraction for lipofilling and for washing the fat, we no longer use normal saline (we use it only to dilute the local anesthetic). Instead we use a 5% glucose solution and believe that our results are better than before.

Reinjection

Once the dressing is made, the injections should be done. The needle used for the reinjection should be of the same caliber as that of the extraction,

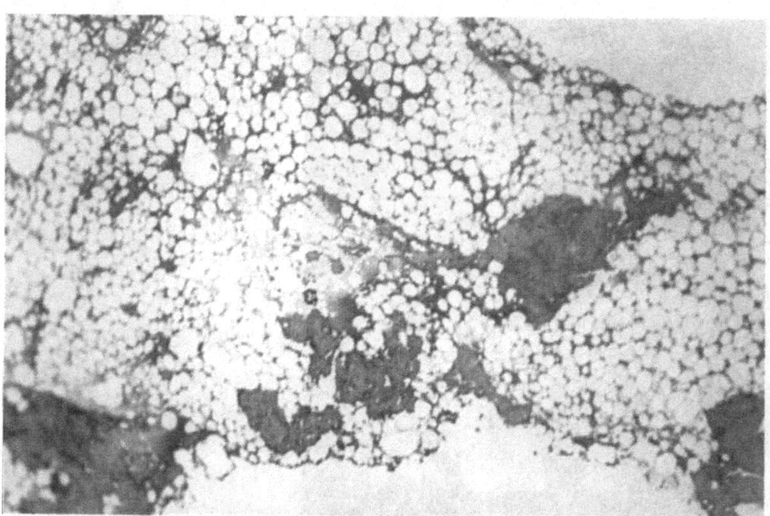

FIGURE 11 Histology of the fat cylinders: normal adipose tissue.

namely 2 mm outside diameter (14 gauge). The needle will penetrate through the skin at the appropriate points of penetration for each region to inject. The vestibular approach is not recommended because of its potential for sepsis. If a 14-gauge cannula is not recommended for harvesting it can be used instead of a 14-gauge needle for the grafting (Fig. 13).

One must inject with caution and make sure not to be in a vessel. This maneuver can be performed if desired with the needle mounted on an empty syringe. Once this is done, the syringe full of adipose tissue is used and the injection begins. This is done in an intermittent fashion, 0.25 or 0.5 cc every centimeter, always in a retrograde direction, while constantly verifying the evacuation of the syringe's contents by its graduated scale. We have to make "pearls and not lakes." This fan-shaped reinjection should be done at different levels to obtain a harmonious result and restore the previous anatomy of the site. The injection's track should be straight or curved, depending on whether the defect is linear or arched (lips or glabellar furrows). In the case of a larger defect (hollow cheeks or cheekbones), several retrograde injections should be made in a fan shape, starting from the subcutaneous penetration orifice. If desired, a regular crossed increase can be performed by using another needle penetration point opposite the first (Fig. 14).

The total content of a syringe should never be injected in the same place. If necessary, the zone to be injected can be prepared with a full instrument (e.g., a tunneller) with a very fine point (e.g., a small awl). The preoperative grid permits a more regular repartition of the ulterior injections

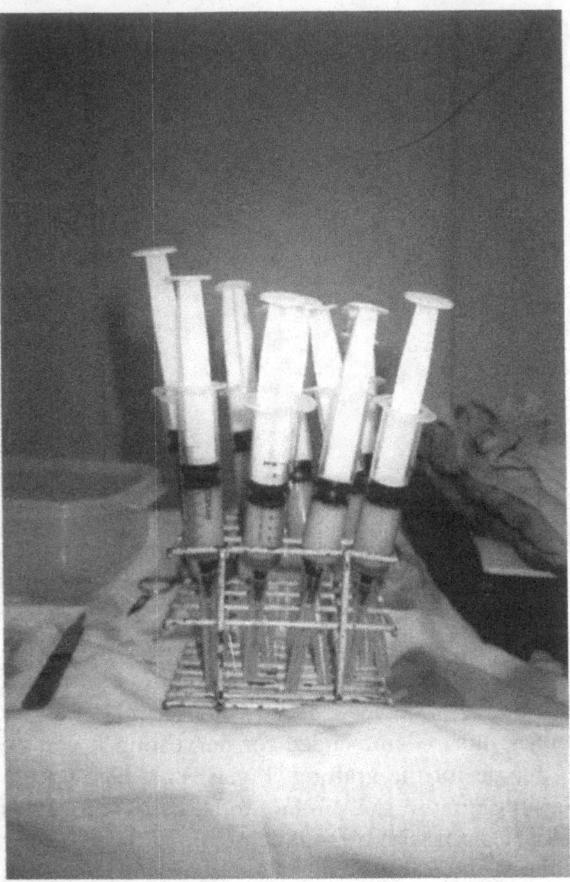

FIGURE 12 The extracted adipose tissue is washed.

and will not overly traumatize the region as would a blunt cannula. Transfering the contents of a 10-cc syringe into 1-cc syringes may be used when desiring more precise work and very small injection amounts.

Remodeling of the Injected Region

After the injection, the operated regions should be remodeled carefully using the thumb and index finger, one of them being in the vestibule in the case of injections in the nasolabial furrows, the cheeks, or the lips. Immobilizing the area with an Elastoplast band is not essential, but it cannot hurt. It is recommended for 2 days. It is necessary after injection in the cheekbone area or chin. This is also true for implantation of prostheses in these areas.

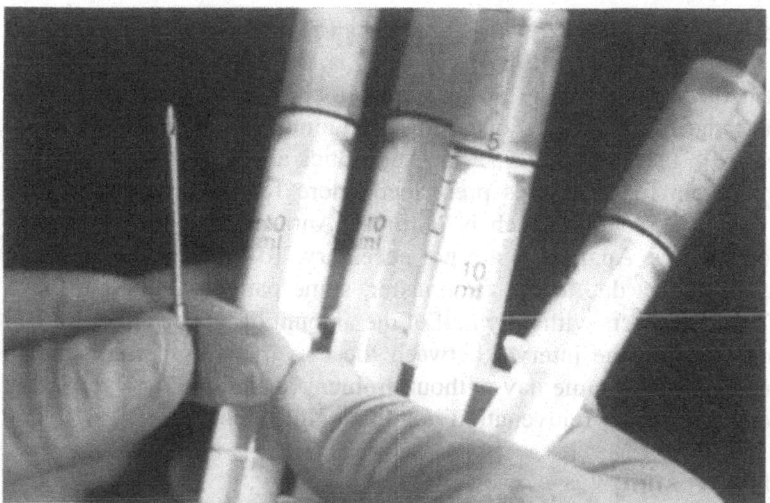

FIGURE 13 A needle of the same diameter (14-gauge) is used for reinjection.

The preoperative course is simple. Edema varies from one patient to another. There are rarely ecchymoses, and patients do not mention any pain or discomfort. The patients have a normal appearance after 3–5 days. The extraction zones take longer to return to normal. They have edema and are indurated for several weeks. Sometimes patients should be warned that they

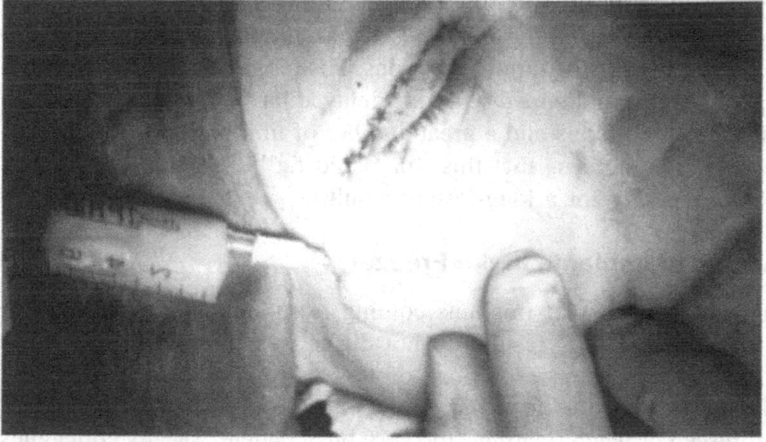

FIGURE 14 "Make pearls and not lakes."

will suffer more from the extraction zones than from the injection zones on the face.

When the filling is done on an ambulatory basis without general or twilight anesthesia, the whole operation, including preparation, operation, and patient rest, takes about 1.5–2 hr. Antibiotics are prescribed systematically; vibramycin for 5 days is prescribed, more for medicolegal reasons than for risk of infection, which is minimal. Anti-inflammatories are prescribed for 15 days. Analgesics are not necessary. To limit the unavoidable postoperative edema due to the fat transfer, some patients request to have two smaller fat transfers with only half of the amount of fat each time instead of the total amount, the interval between the two transfers being 1 week. They can socialize the same day without problem (technique for "very busy people" or "lunch time rejuvenation" or "embellishment").

Delayed Harvesting

A few months after starting syringe fat grafting we thought of preparing the donor area as well as the receiving area to obtain better results and decrease the number of injections necessary for a long-lasting result. The aim is to create an inflammatory condition of the fat tissue and to graft a "healing fat tissue" instead of a normal fat tissue. This possibility is explained to the patient, who will choose between "fresh fat grafting" or "prepared fat grafting." In this latter case, we give a conventional local anesthesia and/or a cryoanesthesia (external), and with a spinal needle or an ordinary 19-gauge needle give repeated strokes for 1 or 2 min in the whole thickness of the fat layer of the harvesting zone. No fat is extracted. A dressing is applied and the patient returns home. The future receiving area may be prepared the same way. After 10 to 12 days, the patient returns and a conventional fat harvesting is performed and the first injection accomplished. The remaining fat is kept in the freezer for future injections. Histologic studies have shown that the specimen of fat obtained with this delayed harvesting has many new vessels, new collagen fibers and a great number of fibroblasts (Fig. 15). Our clinical experience confirms that this "prepared fat" decreases the number of injections necessary for a long-lasting result.

Conservation of Implants in the Freezer

Conservation of all types of implants coming from adipose tissue is easily possible through cold. The results do not differ from those with the fresh implants normally used. The purpose of this conservation is to save the excess implant extracted or to avoid a new extraction when repeated injections are foreseen or when treating "the very busy patient." Many colleagues have followed this path and have confirmed the innocuousness and efficiency

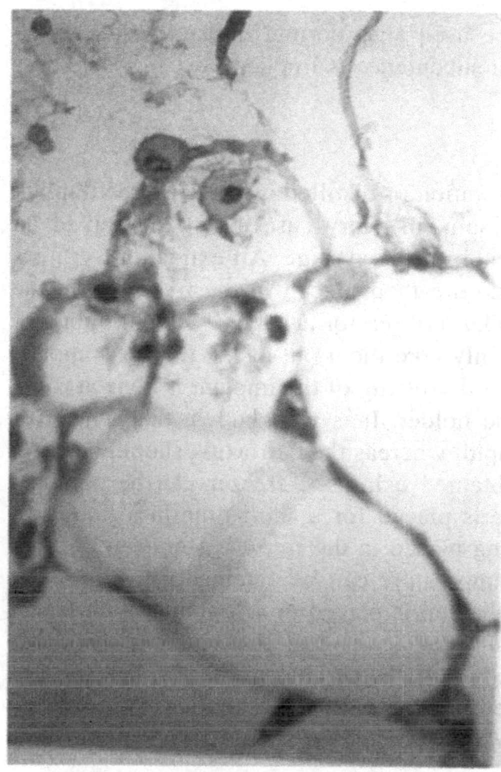

Figure 15 Histology of delayed harvesting.

of this procedure (David Morrow of Palm Springs, California, and Dimitra Dassiou of Volos, Greece, just to cite two).

Tissue conservation by refrigeration is a classic technique, as in the case of other cells (sperm), and the innocuousness and efficiency of the technique are also proven. All types of implants coming from adipose tissue have been kept in the freezer and reused, some after a whole year, for example, (1) adipose tissue cylinder extracted with a 2-mm-diameter needle (washed with saline solution) or glucose 5% solution or Ringer's solution, (2) microimplants extracted with a 12-/10-mm (19-gauge) or an 8-/10-mm (21-gauge) needle (washed with saline solution), (3) implants extracted with 3-/4-mm diameter cannulas and 60-cc syringes that can be used with 5- or 10-cc syringes and the classic 2-mm-diameter fill needle (washed with saline solution or glucose 5% solution), and (4) autologous collagen extracted with a 21-gauge or a 19-gauge needle (washed with distilled water and kept in the freezer). This collagen can be used as a dermal implant (using a 19-gauge needle or dermojet) or as a subcutaneous implant.

TECHNIQUE

After washing with either saline solution or distilled water to rid the implant of all traces of blood or hemoglobin, in every case the sterile cap of an injection needle is placed on the hub of the syringe. All extraction syringes are placed on a test tube rack and are then placed in the freezer with the patient's name on a label (no special refrigerator needed, −30°C is enough). To reuse the implants, one need only take them out of the freezer compartment 1 hr before reutilization. This defrosting of the implant is done at room temperature (22°C) on a test tube holder. It is well known that whenever possible the freezing should be rapid, whereas the defrosting should be slow.

A quicker freezing than obtained using the freezer can be obtained with liquid nitrogen. The syringe is placed for a short time in a liquid nitrogen-filled container before being placed in the freezer. A quicker defrosting than that obtained at room temperature can be obtained in warm water (28° or 30°C). The syringe with the cap is placed in a container with faucet water warmed to this temperature.

Once again, the results obtained with the help of these conserved implants are no different than those obtained with fresh implants (on the face or hands). For some authors anyway preserved fat should give better results.

COMPLICATIONS

Edema is not a complication but rather a part of the operation. It varies from one patient to another: sometimes it is small, and sometimes it deforms the area. The lips react most readily. It is difficult to foresee to which category the patient belongs; that with a small reaction or that with a big one. The importance of this edematous reaction is of course related to the amount of adipose tissue injected (Figs. 16 and 17). Nevertheless, one can tell the patient that in most cases after 3 days the deformation of the treated area will no longer be visible to others—only to the patient. Less often the treated regions can have abnormal edema for about 8 days.

Ecchymoses are rare because the adipose tissue is washed. There can, however, be small ones related to the anesthesia or the adipose tissue injection. Sometimes they are delayed and appear on the second or third day. They can be hidden with makeup. Pain or discomfort are rare complications. This author has never seen liquefaction of the graft and only two cases of infection, one in the cheek and the other in the breast. Often a localized, sensible induration may be noticed in the treated areas, which is more pal-

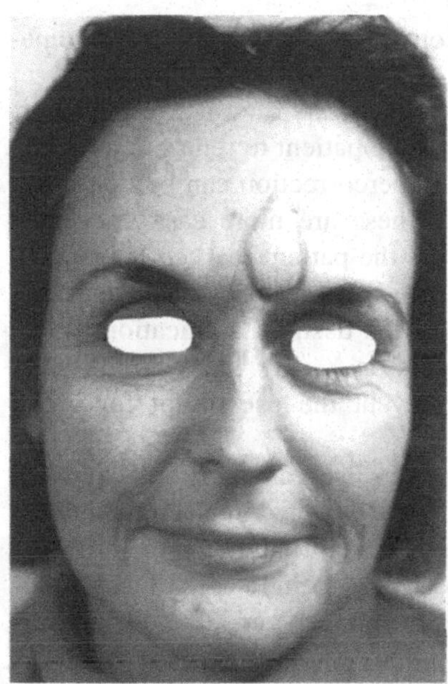

FIGURE 16 Complication: an uneven result in the glabella after 3 years.

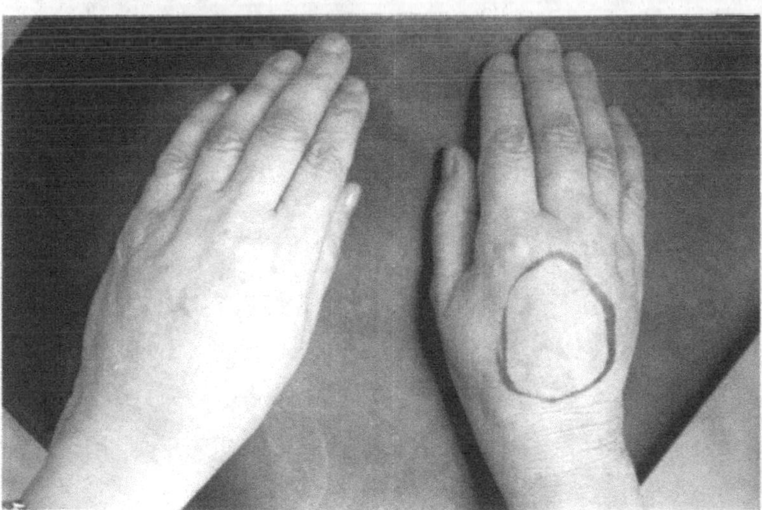

FIGURE 17 Complication: 3 years after lipofilling the removal of fat excesses is requested in one hand.

pable than visible, disappearing spontaneously in a few weeks, and sometimes lasting, several months or years.

In order to avoid significant reactions, it is important not to hypercorrect in volume the region treated. One wants the patient to return to a normal appearance within a few days. Necessary hypercorrection can be done with repeated injections spread out over time. These are more easily accepted than a hypercorrection in volume that leaves the patient marked for a much longer time as a consequence of the operation. Moreover, small quantities take better than larger ones, as with any grafted tissue. Calcifications in the grafted areas may be seen after several years on X rays. They are different of cancer calcifications but such event prevent the use of fat for breast augmentation.

The only unfavorable evolution is the disappearance of the results obtained due to total reabsorption of the graft. This is noted in a certain number of cases. In fact, the reabsorption of the graft is due to the extreme diffusion of the implanted tissue if patients are older and their facial adipose tissue capital has almost disappeared. It is rare for younger patients with individ-

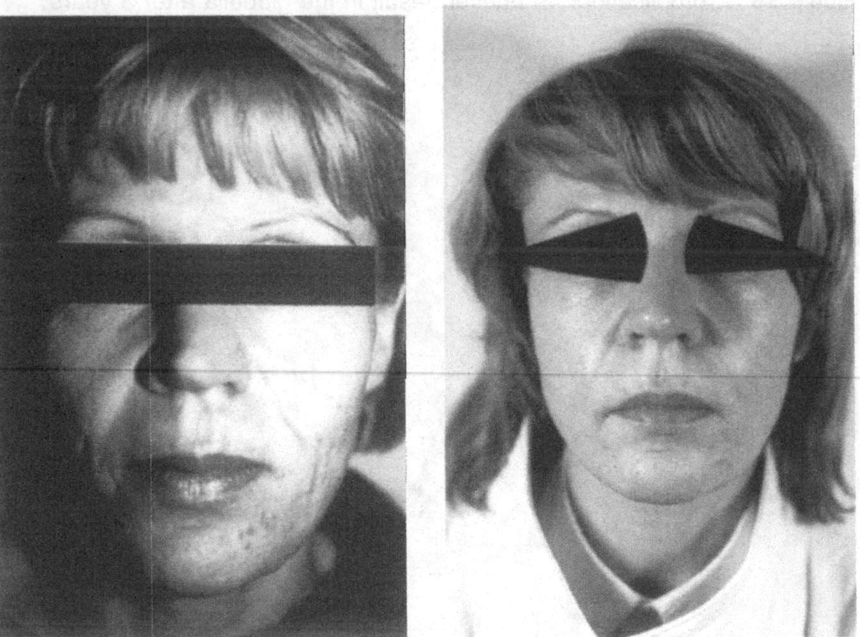

FIGURE 18 Result after 8 years of one injection of 20 cc in the cheeks and cheekbone area.

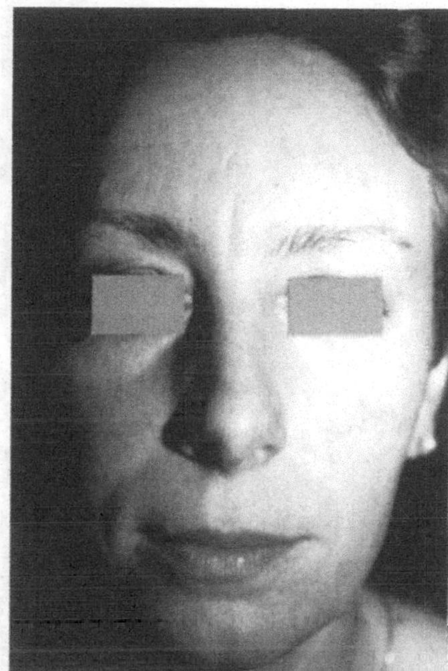

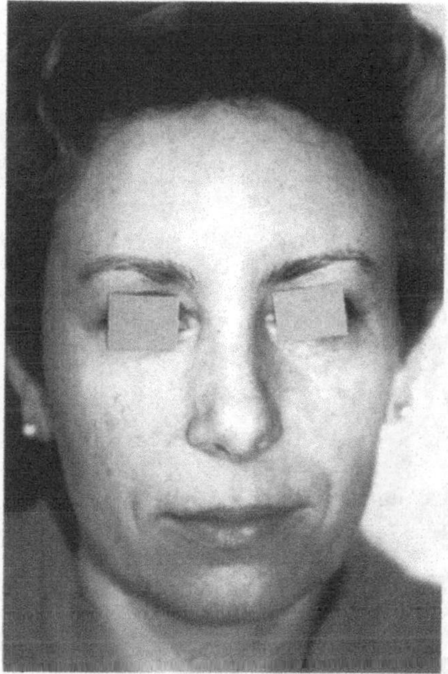

FIGURE 19 Permanent result after 13 years of only one graft of 5 cc in the glabella.

ualized and limited weak points to be dissatisfied with their operations. Of all the facial zones, the most difficult to treat is the lips.

RESULTS AND DISCUSSION

We have only clinical experience. We can state than 80% of our patients are happy with the results if they accept the necessary repeated injections. If the result is objective it is also subjective. In certain cases, the surgeon has moderate enthusiasm about the result and the patient a lot. The reverse is also true when treating the ageing process the moment a new graft is decided by the patient. It may be 1 year, 2 years or 5, 6 or 7 years. When building a chin or cheekbones for aesthetic reasons we always propose four sessions of graft, one every 3 months to obtain a long-lasting result.

The anaerobic technique of fat grafting has confirmed that the accepted figure of 25–50% cell survival rate is mostly constant, but is never sure, as the results of fat grafting are *unpredictable*. It has been confirmed that the take is better with young and thin patients than with mature ones. The tech-

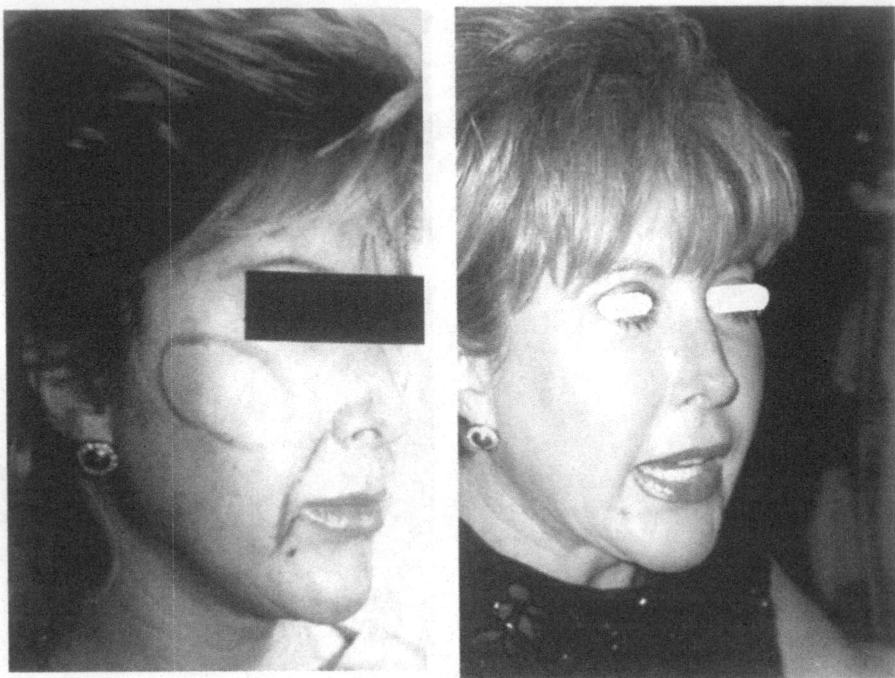

FIGURE 20 Patient grafted three times in over 14 years (1985, 1990, 1995); the last photo on the right was taken 6 years after the last graft.

nique used is also very important. The use of a 14-gauge needle is important; a 14-gauge cannula does not give the same results, as we do not obtain fat slivers of the same quality. The survey of Ed Griffin in 1999 is optimistic: of a sample of 96 physicians in Atlanta in 1999, 85% collected the fat with a syringe, 62% washed the fat, 85% did not centrifuge the fat, 62% did not use a gun injector, and 64% reported survival of 6–10 years.

The washing of the adipose tissue has to be done carefully as well the reinjection. Making "pearls and not lakes" is very important. The donor zone choices we consider the best are the buttock, the hips, and the pubic area. Even if tumescent anesthesia is used for fat grafting we believe that is not the best for fat grafting (hydrolical and chemical trauma). The main improvement in fat grafting up to now has not been a better take than with the conventional semiclosed technique but in a simpler technique, avoiding scars and allowing repeated injections easily accepted by the patients and the surgeon. We must understand that adipose tissue is a filler, a space-occupying tissue. The 25 or 50% of adipose tissue grafted that takes suc-

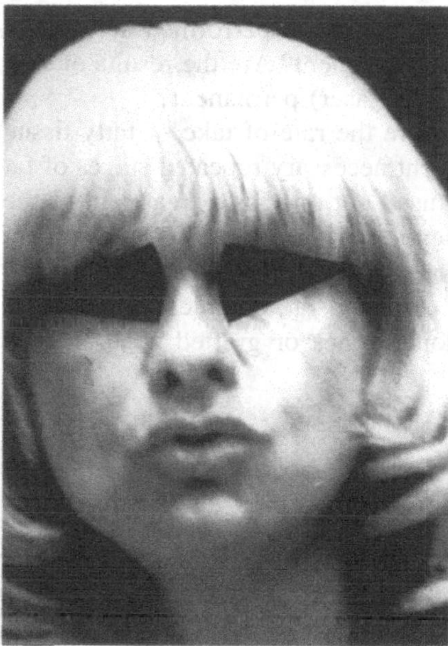

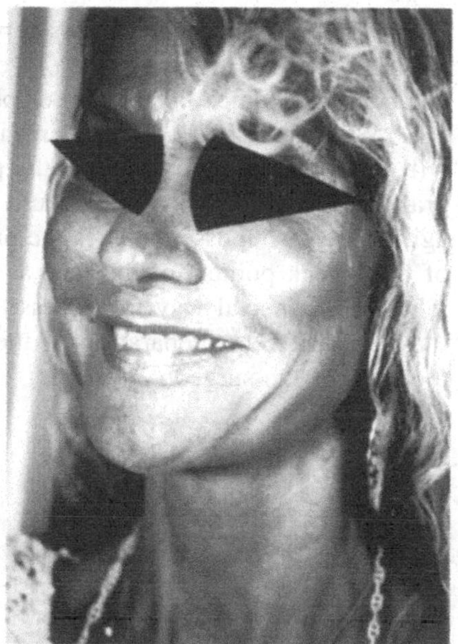

FIGURE 21 This patient had 5 cc of fat injected every 3 months (four injections in 1 year and nothing else), which produced a good result even after 14 years.

cessfully will age just like the neighboring nongrafted adipose tissue and will need to be replaced. Just like face-lifts or chemical peels, collagen, or botox injections the results obtained are not eternal (Figs. 18–21).

CONCLUSION

Our experience of 15 years with syringe fat grafting yields the following: (1) the results of fat grafting are unpredictable, but the accepted rate of take of 20–50% is highly probably in 80% of the patients and this rate has been increased when using the syringe technique for harvesting; (2) repeated grafts are necessary as the grafted fatty tissue *will age as well the neighboring tissue*; (3) the main advance has been the ease of this anaerobic and closed technique of fat harvesting and grafting, which is accepted with enthusiasm by both patients and surgeons; and (4) syringe fat grafting presently cannot be a treatment is one stage except in unpredictables cases as in skin or bone grafting, but it is the best way to decrease, to slow down or decelerate the aging process, and the prevention of this unavoidable process should be the main indication is young and mature people. As it has been said before: We can put back the clock of time but we cannot stop it. The results are not permanent unless repeated grafts are performed at variable intervals. But are the results of a face-lift permanent? Are the results of skin abrasion, mechanical, chemical, or physical (laser) permanent?

We believe and hope that in the future the rate of take of fatty tissue will be increased and will avoid the present necessary repeated stages of fat grafting. Syringe fat grafting should be used not only as a treatment of the aging process but essentially in the prevention of this process. The treatment of the "weak points" of the face as soon as they appear is a must. Maybe it will be a special way to process the extracted fat, chemical or physical; maybe a different preparation of the doner zones or grafted zone. This is the wish of the surgeon.

28

Syringe Techniques Used to Obtain Autolipocollagen

Pierre F. Fournier
Private Practice
Paris, France

We have seen that a removal in the fat tissue made with a 2-mm-external-diameter fill needle (14-gauge) mounted on a syringe is composed of fat tissue cylinders whose center is unharmed and which can be used perfectly for a graft. There are in fact intact lobules surrounded by septi and capillaries. However, if instead of a 2-mm needle (14-gauge), a 12-/10- or 8-/10-mm (19- or 21-gauge) needle is used, one no longer obtains fat columns but microimplants of intact cells or cores of fat tissue, since the needle acts as a veritable circular scalpel by drilling into the fat tissue. These can be seen with the naked eye when the syringe is emptied into a container of normal saline or when the syringe is shaken. When a 5-cc removal is made, approximately one-fifth is liquid fat and four-fifths is a solid portion made up of microimplants (Figs. 1–3).

There are two kinds of microimplants. Some of them, the majority, are rectangular, made up of cellular isles three to five cells thick with or without septum debris adhering to their surface or are made up of pure septum fragments, circular, oval, or elongated because of the action of the needle on the septal walls. The needle acts as a punch, or a circular scalpel, identical to the punch used for hair transplants. These specimen are identical whether or not the removal is accomplished with anesthetic infiltration of the fat

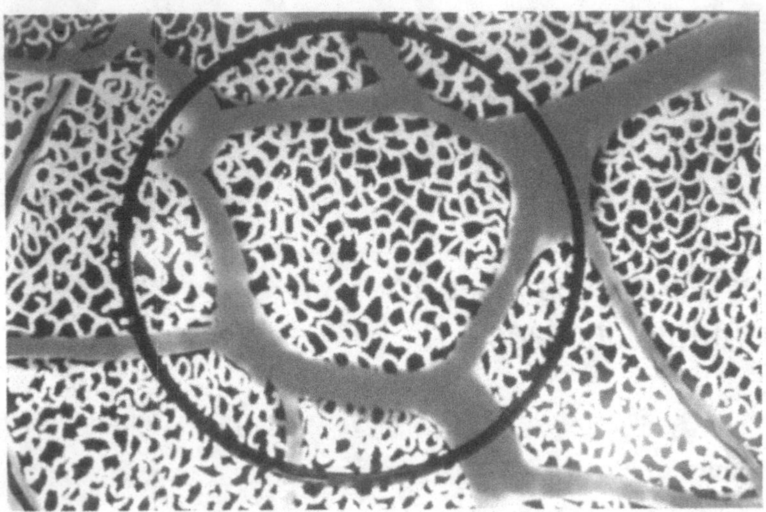

FIGURE 1 The squeleton of adipose tissue is made of collagen.

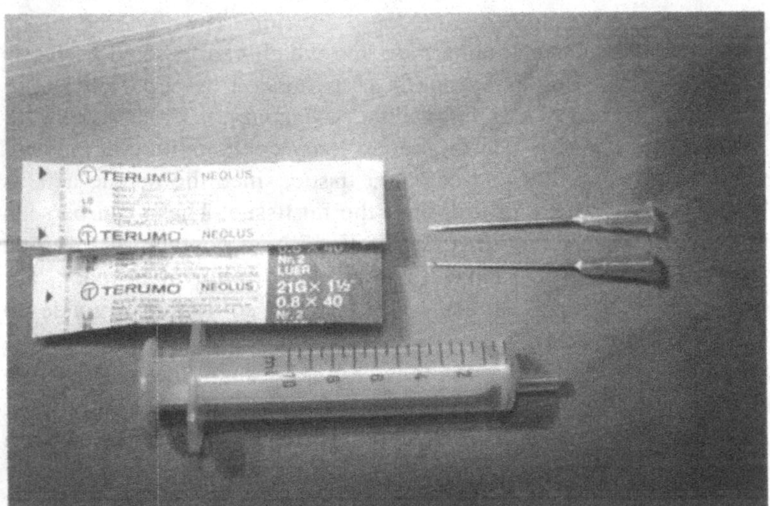

FIGURE 2 Equipment needed to obtain autologous collagen: 10-cc syringe, 19-gauge needle, and 21-gauge needle.

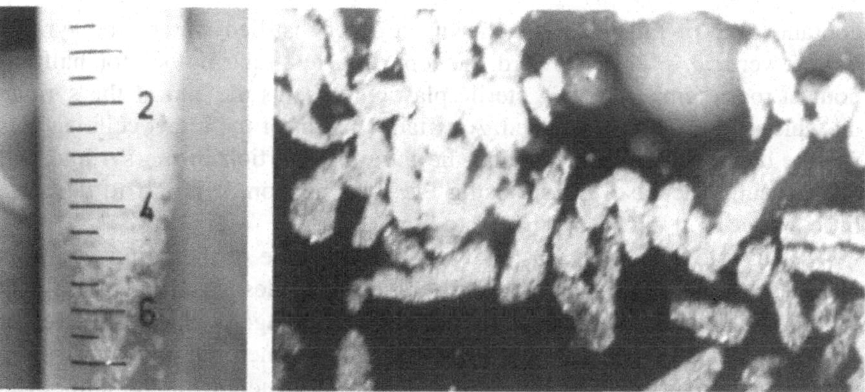

FIGURE 3 Microimplants harvested with a 19 gauge needle.

tissue. It is possible to reuse the microimplants as they are once they have been separated from the liquid portion by decantation or untracentrifugation. A 8-/10-mm needle must be used for the reinjection. Another smaller needle would prevent the implants or septal debris from passing through. During a deep intradermic injection, the pressure on the tissues resulting from the injection under pressure with overcorrecting will splinter the intact cells and their liquid contents will be evacuted through the skin opening created by the needle point. This solid fraction can also be injected with a dermojet. We have accomplished many injections with these methods without any infectious or other complications. Since this solid fraction is not entirely pure, we have tried to obtain a specimen composed solely of collagen, that is to say, only septi cell membranes and cells of the vessels of the adipose tissue.

Different techniques can be used to separate the oily liquid portion contained in the cells from the solid collagenic portion which surrounds it. Thus this collagenic extraction consists of two steps: (1) the removal of the microimplants; and (2) the separation of the solid fraction, in which we are interested, from the liquid fraction by splintering. For this we have used different methods and instruments.

The removal instrument is always a 10-cc syringe mounted with a 8-/10- or 12-/10-mm (21- or 19-gauge) needle. The first modification was suctioning 2-cc of distilled room-temperature water in the syringe before the removal. Five cubic centimeters of fat tissue are extracted and washed in the distilled water as much as necessary to obtain a bloodless removal. Once this is obtained, the syringe is filled completely with distilled water. It then contains 5 cc of fat tissue mixed with 5 cc of distilled water. The syringe is kept vertical, plunger toward the top, on a test-tube holder for half-an-hour at room temperature. A sterile plastic cup seals the end of the syringe on which the needle is mounted. A certain amount of the intact cellular isles will be destroyed by osmosis and the pure oily portion in the syringe will consequently increase. Before using the solid portion, it is left to decant a little longer or it can be centrifugated.

A histological study has shown that only some of the adipocytal isles obtained by the above-mentioned technique were destroyed but not all. In order to completely destroy the intact isles, the syringe is placed in a freezer for 12 hr. A histological study of the thawed specimen (about 1 hr at room temperature for it to thaw) showed complete destruction of the adipocytal isles. The solid portion is then separated from the liquid portion by decanting or, even better, by ultracentrifugation before being reinjected. These results have been verified by different histologists in different countries and they all agree on the above-mentioned method to destroy all of the adipocytal isles. This technique has been widely used before using the "Instant Collagen Technique."

Since their discovery, the properties of ultrasounds have been widely used in biology and medicine. The "cavitation effect" has been used by Michele Zocchi, M.D., in Turin, Italy, to separate the oily portion of the microimplants from the solid collagenic portion. The syringes, filled with microimplants and sealed, are placed in the recipient of an ultrasound surgical instruments cleaner. The recipient is filled with sterile normal saline and the machine activated. After 20 min the microimplants are blasted. These blasted microimplants are then separated by ultracentrifugation. The autolipocollagen obtained in this manner can be used immediately. A special centrifuge machine was created for this purpose by Dr. Zocchi and can hold four syringes.

Later, Katsuya Takasu, M.D., of Tokyo, Japan, also used the ultrasound properties to break up microimplants. This requires using a very powerful machine widely used in the United States which has a sterile stem that can be dipped into a 10-cc test-tube filled with microimplants. Such a machine needs only a few seconds to break the implants which are later centrifuged. The collagen obtained in this manner can be used immediately or stored in a deep freeze. When so desired, we personally use a small ultrasound jewelry cleaner which breaks up the microimplants perfectly in 20 min. The same results could be obtained with a pulsed laser. Though these cell-splintering techniques are perfect, they are time consuming for the patient and the surgeon. It is surely possible to reduce the time in the freezer and obtain satisfactory lysis but a histological study has not yet been done. A dip in liquid nitrogen for a certain amount of time could also cause cellular lysis but here again a histological study has not been done. Though it is preferable to obtain the solid purified portion in as little time as possible, the stakes at hand are large enough to make the 12 hr wait worthwhile. The freezer technique has been used for several years.

Other devices can help speed the lysis of the isles: (1) Using glass syringes which are traumatizing for the fat tissue, two recent publications drew attention to this. (2) Creating a vacuum in the syringe by blocking the plunger which is then pulled as hard as possible. This negative pressure as well as the osmotic action of the distilled water will speed the cellular lysis. Shaking the syringe for a while will also speed the lysis of the contents. (3) Rupturing the implants with gentle pressure once they have been placed on a fine sieve has also been studied. However, this requires handling out in the open and has thus been abandoned. The most widely used technique has been that of placing the implants in a freezer. With the autologous collagen implants, just like with the bovine collagen implants, the patient must visit the doctor's office several times. Though the immediate obtainment of a pure specimen is desirable, using an instrument specially created for this purpose, the "hand-made" techniques are no less valid.

In all cases, whatever technique is used, once the implants have been ruptured and the separation of the lipocollagen from the oily portion obtained, the collagen is used immediately or stored in 1-, 2-, 5-, or 10-cc syringes in the freezer. Each syringe will be sealed with a sterile package containing an intraveinous injection needle or any other kind of sterile obturator. The use of 1 or 2 cc insulin syringes mounted with 8-/10-mm (21-gauge) needles is recommended for these injections. The oily portion is kept in case the surgeon wishes to use it later.

A larger amount of collagen can be obtained after a "delayed harvesting." The donor zone is prepared exactly as for a delayed harvesting of fat cylinders (see Chapter 27). Within 5 days the local fibroblasts will create collagen fibers. This new collagen is of type 3. A peak is reached on the 12th day which is when the delayed harvesting is recommended (Michele Zocchi). Thus, other than the usual quantity of collagen in the intercellular fibrous substances, there is a certain amount of neocollagen fibers created during the delayed harvesting period.

THE INSTANT COLLAGEN TECHNIQUE

The technique that we prefer now is the following one, very simple, allowing the surgeon to obtain a very fine collagen, passing easily through a 30-gauge needle. We call it the Instant Collagen Technique and it has the following requirements:

1. The needles used are the same as with the other technique: 8/10th of a millimeter or 12/10th of a millimeter (19- or 21-gauge). We use the 19-gauge needle most of the time.
2. The anesthesia is carried out in the same way as before, one-third of xylocaine with 1:200,000 epinephrine diluted with two-thirds of chilled saline at 2°C.
3. The harvesting is done in the same places as before.
4. After the extraction zones have been anesthetised (same zones as a lipofilling: buttocks or hips are preferred), the surgeon will wait 10 min to obtain a good anesthesia and a good hemostasis.
5. After 10 min hydroexpansion of the donor zones is obtained with an injection of 200 cc of chilled normal saline using syringes of 60 cc. Tumescent anesthesia may also be used instead of the conventional local anesthesia described.
6. The extraction is performed immediately after (10-cc syringes, 19- or 21-gauge needle). Usually six syringes are needed each containing 5 cc of adipose tissue debris.
7. Washing is performed with normal saline or distilled water if there is any blood, as many times as necessary.
8. Decantation is obtained on a test tube holder. Centrifugation is also possible if desired.
9. The collagen obtained is very fine and pass easily through a 30-gauge needle. In the samples obtained there is no oil visible when a 19-gauge needle is used for extraction. After a conventional local anesthesia the core of tissue in the lumen of the needle has the thickness of four or five adipose cells. After expansion of the donor zone, when the adipose cells have been distended by the injection of 200 cc of saline, the core of tissue in the 19-gauge needle has only the thickness of one adipose cell. When the tissue fragments of cell membranes retinaculum cuti or vessels are in the barrel of the syringe, they shrink and regain the original dimention that they had before the magnification of the adipose tissue (Fig. 4).

Such tissue debris obtained from the skeleton of the adipose tissue are pure collagen and can be injected into the skin or subcutaneously as desired (Fig. 5). This autocollagen can be injected at once or kept in the deep freeze of a refrigerator, as the adipose tissue harvested for a lipofilling with the usual precautions. Thawing take about 1 hr at room temperature.

Autolipocollagen does not give better results than bovine collagen as it is destroyed by collagenase exactly like bovine collagen. This autologous collagen has the same purpose as bovine collagen: to act as a scaffold. The

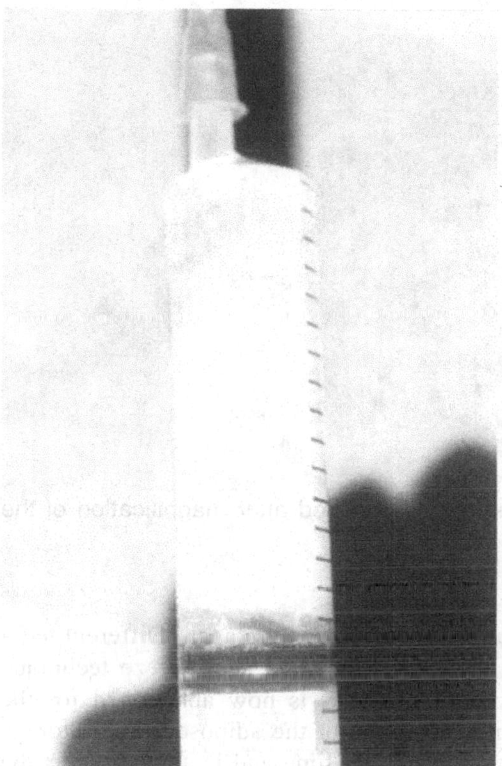

Figure 4 Collagen tissue debris harvested with a 19-gauge needle after magnification of the donor zone.

patient may choose between the two types of collagen: bovine or autologous. No allergy has to be feared. Tests are unnecessary. The amount used is unlimited as it is free.

COMPLICATIONS

We have seen few complications. Some are the same as with bovine collagen: lumps into the skin or redness.

SUMMARY

There is a small amount of human autologous collagen in the fat tissue. Its obtainment by the surgeon, using simple means, is desirable and justified

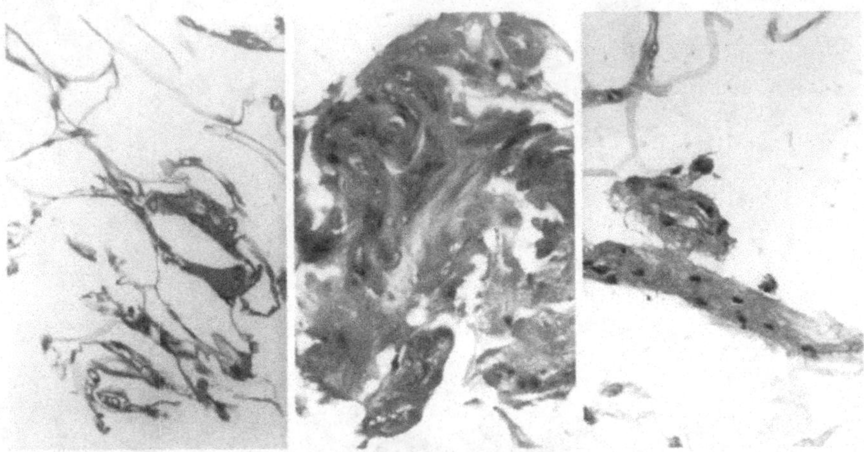

FIGURE 5 Histology of the tissue debris obtained after magnification of the donor zone.

by the cost and possible harmful effects of bovine collagen. Different technical means are described and commented on. The deep freeze technique recommended for its simplicity and reliability is now abandoned for the Instant Collagen Technique by magnification of the adipose tissue. Storage by deep freezing can be used for a very long time and is as reliable as the storage of fat cylinders used for a lipofilling.

29

Periorbital Lipoaugmentation

Lisa M. Donofrio
Yale University School of Medicine
New Haven, Connecticut, U.S.A.

INTRODUCTION

Periorbital augmentation with autologous fat is an excellent way to restore youthful fullness to the upper face. The normal aging changes of the periorbital area render it hollow, baggy, and sharply demarcated from the neighboring cheek mass. The smooth taught rounded surfaces of youth are lost. Compounding the problem are "rejuvenation" procedures such as blepharoplasty and laser resurfacing, which often further hollow, sculpt, and contract the periorbital tissues. The time has come to take pause and reevaluate the changes in the periobital area that occur with aging.

ANATOMY

Deep to the skin in the suborbital area is a thin layer of subcutaneous fat. Inferiorly at the margin of the lower orbital rim the subcutaneous fat lies superficial to the superior border of the malar fat pad. Deep to the fat lies the orbicularis oculi muscle whch at its lower border is continuous with the superficial musculoaponeurotic system. At the level of the orbital rim deep to the orbicularis muscle is the fibrous orbital septum which originates at the arcus marginalus and courses superiorly to insert in the inferior tarsal muscle. The arcus forms a "sling" containing the medial, middle, and lateral orbital fat pads. The anatomy of the upper lid is identical with the exception that the orbital septum inserts into the levator aponeurosis and there are only two orbital fat pads, medial and lateral (Fig. 1) [1,2].

MORPHOLOGY

The morphology of the periorbital tissues in youth is represented by the presence of anteriorly projected arcs and broad convexities. The arc of the upper lid/brow complex is contiguous with the convexity of the forehead and the temple. The lower lid forms a sweeping continuous arc from the tarsus to the anterior jaw. With aging, however, the architecture of these arcs is lost and the tissues flatten resulting in a relative excess of skin (Fig. 2). Additionally with the loss of subcutaneous fat comes demarcation of the inferior orbital rim. The skin becomes adherent in this area due to the rigidity and anchoring provided by the arcus marginalus. There are two distinctive patterns of suborbital aging the atropic and hypertrophic variants (Fig. 3). The atrophic variant is characterized by hollowing of the suborbital area. This is even more apparent in heavy individuals with a full cheek mass. The globe appears sunken, and patients with this type of aging change commonly complain of undereye circles due to the concavity of the area (Fig. 4). The second, hypertrophic variant is equally disfiguring, with the accentuation of suborbital fat in pockets or festoons. Due again to the immobility of the arcus marginalus, this fat is sequestered and separated from the cheek mass

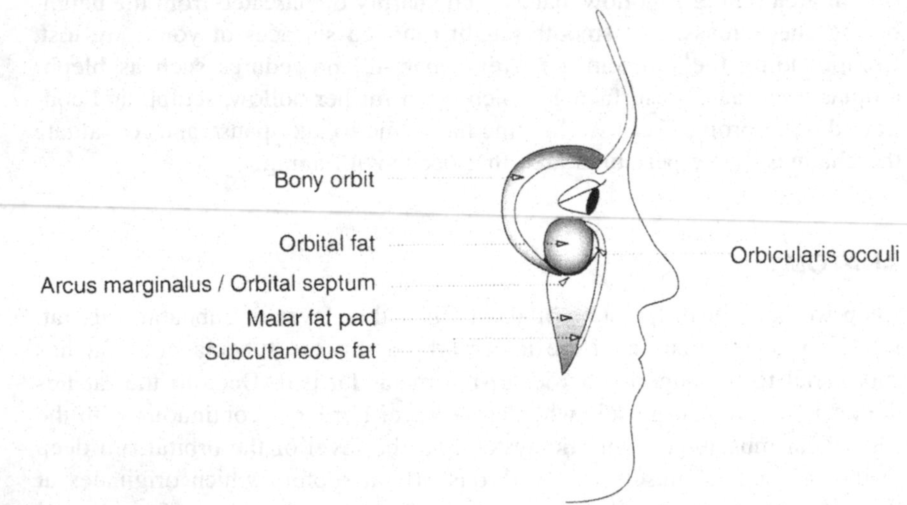

FIGURE 1 Orbital anatomy.

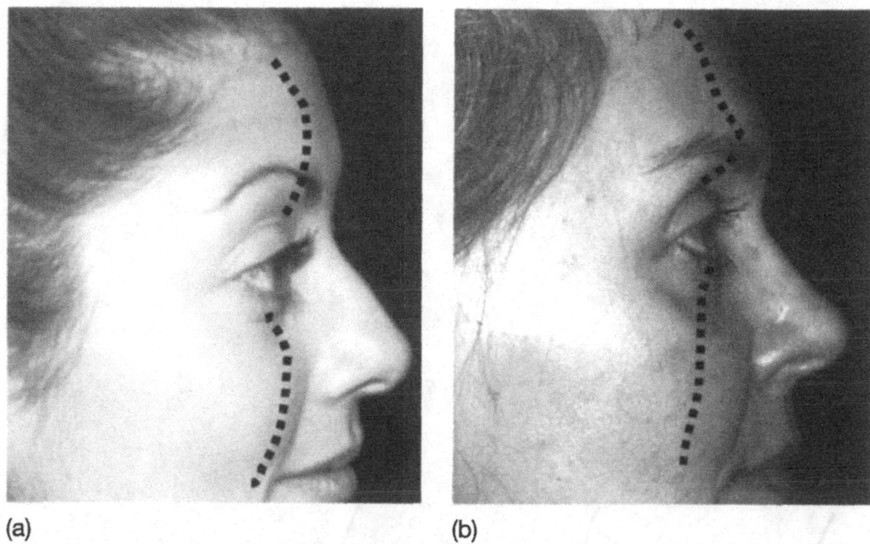

(a) (b)

FIGURE 2 (a) Morphology of the young face; (b) morphology of the aged face.

by a line of demarcation (Fig. 5). Some patients in this category probably represent a true hypertrophy of suborbital fat such as that seen in adolescents with an atopic diathesis. However, in the majority of cases the suborbital fat displays a relative hypertrophy which is a visual phenomenon related to atrophy of the upper central cheek mass. In both the atrophic and hypertrophic variants of periorbital aging, fat augmentation is an invaluable tool for restoring the normal contour of the eye/cheek complex.

The upper lid and brow display a relative excess of skin due not only to the shrinkage of subcutaneous tissue in the area but also to that occurring in the neighboring forehead and scalp. This causes a downward descent of the brow and lid. Loss of the superior most extension of the buccal fat pad in the temple causes a lateral descending of the brow. Blepharoplasty of the upper lid causes a scooped-out, hollow eyelid/brow complex with more lid show. By filling up the brow, temple, and forehead with fat and restoring the youthful convexities one can reposition the brow and tent out the loose skin (Figs. 6 and 7).

UNDEREYE CIRCLES

One of the most common complaints of all ages is undereye circles. There are three causes for suborbital circles and a patient may display one or all of these. The first as described above is due to a pooling of shadow just

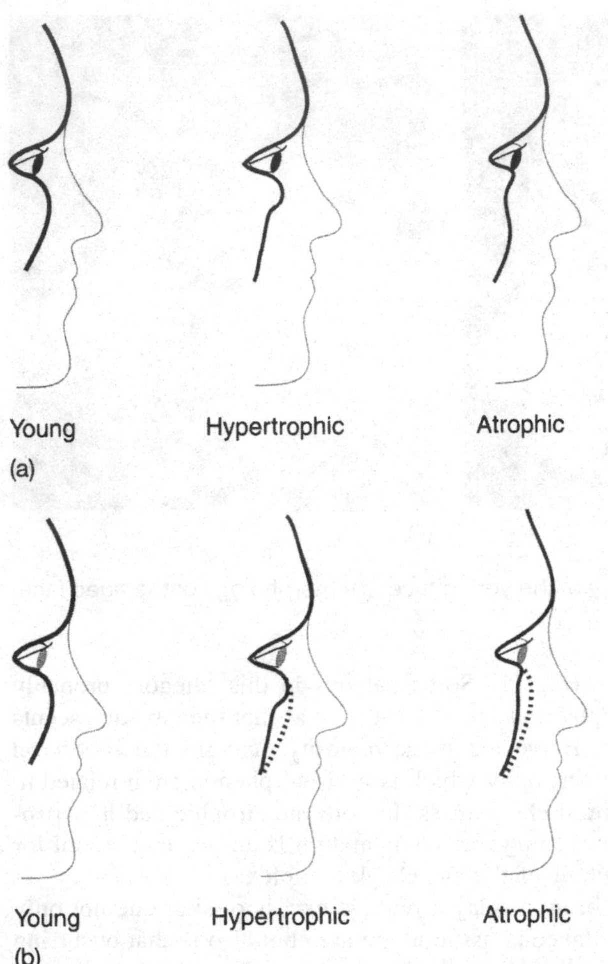

FIGURE 3 (a) Suborbital aging patterns; (b) correction with augmentation.

above the orbital rim. This is most often seen in the concavity that results from atropic suborbital aging, but can also be seen in the sulcus caused by the tethering of the arcus marginalus in the hypertrophic variant. It is also commonly called the tear trough deformity. By changing the concavity of the tear trough to a convexity the shadow can be altered to a point of highlight and the circle eliminated (Fig. 8). The second cause is from true hyperpigmentation of the skin in the suborbital area. This is seen most commonly in Mediterranean skin tones and is easy to spot due to the accentu-

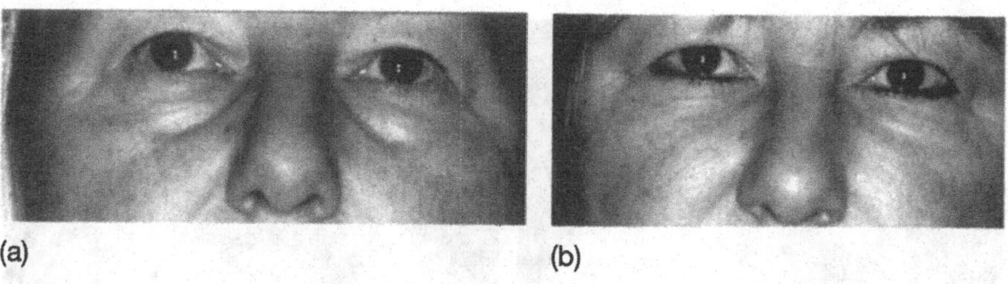

(a) (b)

FIGURE 4 Atrophic suborbital aging (a) before and (b) after periorbital lipoaugmentation.

ation of the pigment with a Wood's lamp [3]. Less commonly the skin in this area can display a false hyperpigmentation due to acanthotic epidermal changes. Both these conditions are epidermal problems and attenuated with topicals that suppress melanin production or smooth out the skin surface [4]. The third cause is from increased vascularity in the suborbital tissues. This may be seen as early as childhood secondary to allergies, but is also seen in the aging adult as a result of subcutaneous fat atrophy and a "demasking" of the suborbital vasculature. In this case, when fat is placed diffusely high in the subcutaneous plane it can add opacity to these tissues and camouflage the ectatic vessels (Fig. 9).

IATROGENIC PERIORBITAL AGING

Ironically, most procedures designed to correct periorbital aging changes often make them worse. Blepharoplasties performed for "excess skin" as seen in atrophic periorbital aging and for "excess fat" in hypertrophic periorbital aging are rife with problems. Skin and fat tailoring most often produce canthal rounding and a skeletonization of the occular area with increased lid show, overaccentuation of the inner upper and lower orbital sulcus, demarcation of the orbital rim, and scarring (Fig. 10) [5]. Transconjunctival techniques, while avoiding the tarsal disruption and canthal rounding, are rarely done conservatively and can lead to demarcation of the orbital rim and a flattening or hollowing of the midface that worsens over time. These procedures, while eliminating an undereye bulge, ignore the important arc of the midface seen in youth and establish a new straighter plane. It is common practice to follow a transconjunctival blepharoplasty with CO_2 laser resurfacing of the periorbital area to cause contraction of the "excess skin" [6]. This only accentuates the bony underlying architecture further and in the case of aggressive resurfacing leads to a shiny atrophic skin texture. Newer blepharoplasty techniques which release the arcus marginalus and

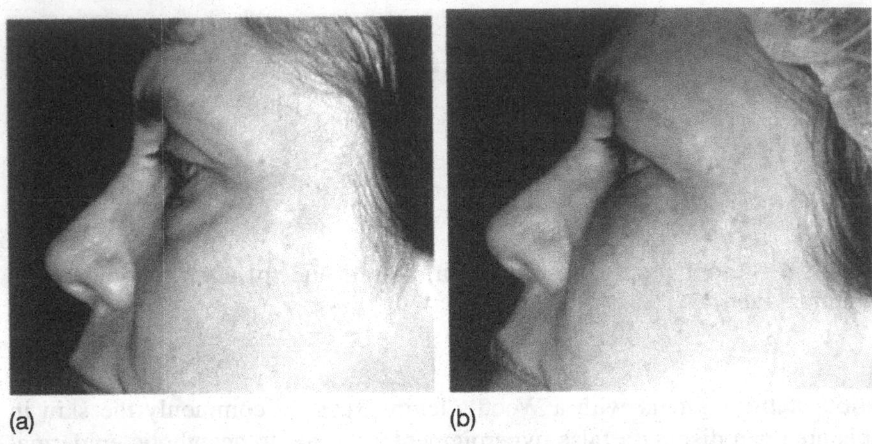

(a) (b)

Figure 5 Hypertrophic suborbital aging (a) before and (b) after periorbital lipoaumentation.

reposition rather than excise the orbital fat look promising, but are difficult and rarely done [7]. One of the primary indications for periorbital autologous fat augmentation is in the correction of postblepharoplasty and postlaser deformities.

CANDIDATE SELECTION

Patients with both the atropic and hypertrophic variants of periorbital aging are good candidates for autologous augmentation as are those with tear trough deformity, postblepharoplasty dysmorphism, postlaser cutaneous atrophy, and hypervascularity. The rationale behind using autologous fat in each one of these cases is different as is the technique employed. Practitioners attempting to place fat in the periorbital area should be well versed and comfortable with structural augmentation in other parts of the face. The periorbital area is highly unforgiving of unscrupulously placed fat and fat retention rates are surprisingly high in this area. The best approach therefore is the conservative one and patients need to be made aware of the subtle change that each transfer will accomplish and the need for multiple sessions to achieve a satisfactory final result. Lifestyle demands need to be considered since the periorbital tissues are prone to prolonged ecchymosis and edema. Patient education is an invaluable tool. In the initial consultation the causes of periorbital aging should be discussed as they relate to the patient. An early photograph is highly instructive to refresh their memory of what they used to look like. Patients are often mislead to believe that the post surgical

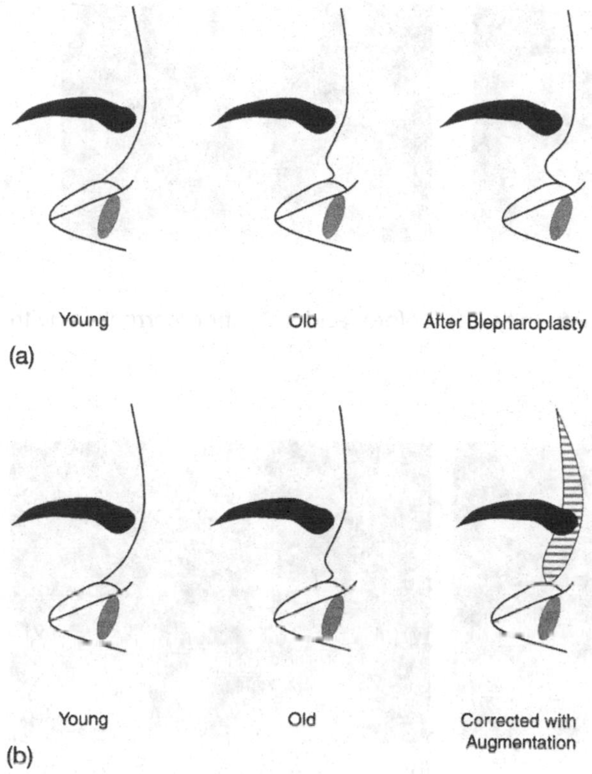

FIGURE 6 Two options for fixing the aging lid: (a) blepharoplasty and (b) lipoaugmentation.

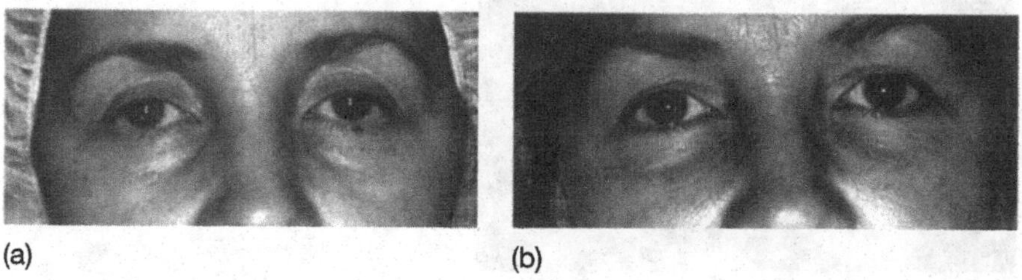

FIGURE 7 A 42-year-old woman with aging lids (a) before and (b) after lipoaugmentation.

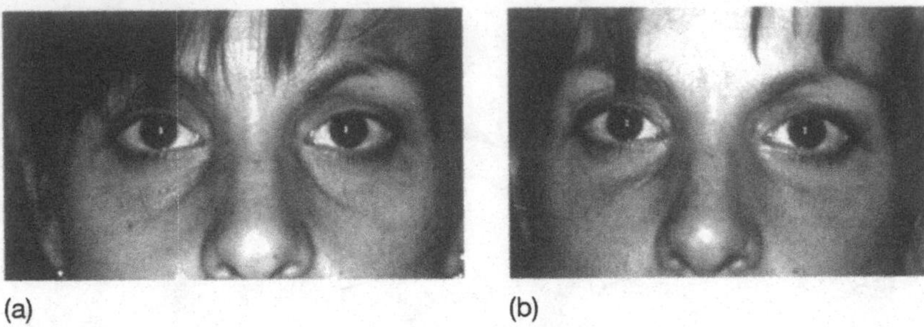

(a) (b)

FIGURE 8 Tear trough deformity (a) before and (b) after correction with lipoaugmentation.

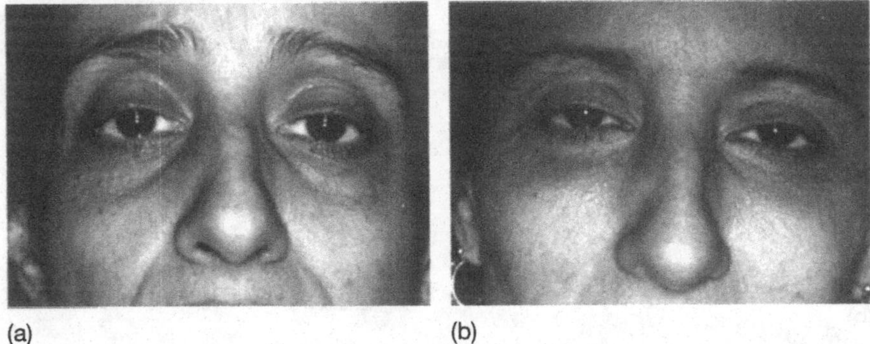

(a) (b)

FIGURE 9 Undereye circles (a) before and (b) after correction with lipoaugmentation.

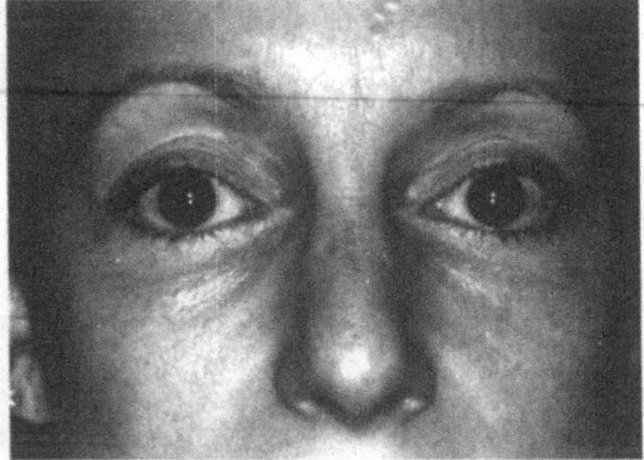

FIGURE 10 A 39-year-old female with typical hollowing and contracture after blepharoplasty.

"sculpted eye" is what they should be seeking, when in truth a deeper set fuller eye is what was seen in youth (Fig. 11). Dealing with expectations before the procedure can save unnecessary disappointment later on. Surprisingly the majority of patients are highly receptive to concept of "filling them out" and welcome a more natural alternative to traditional lifting procedures. Patients on anticoagulant therapy or those with serious heart problems are not candidates for this procedure. Relative contraindications include cancer, history of deep vein thrombosis or pulmonary embolus, heavy smoking, or history of poor retention from a prior fat transfer. Relative contraindications require a physician to use his or her clinical judgment on an individual basis.

PATIENT PREPARATION

After the initial consultation is completed a map or blueprint of the patient's face is drawn on paper and then transferred to their face on the day of the procedure with a marking pen (Fig. 12). Preoperatively cephalexin at a dose of 500 mg twice a day is started the day before the procedure and continued for 6 days afterward. To decrease bruising tendency patients are warned to stay off all vitamin E-containing products as well as nonsteroidal anti-inflammatory agents, ginko biloba, St John's wort, ginseng, ginger, and alcohol for 1 week prior to the procedure. Diazepam (5–10 mg) or alprazolam (1–2 mg) may be given orally to ease anxiety. Patients with a history of tacchycardia from dental visits may benefit from 25 mg of atenolol administered 2 hr before the procedure. Patients are instructed to wear loose, dark

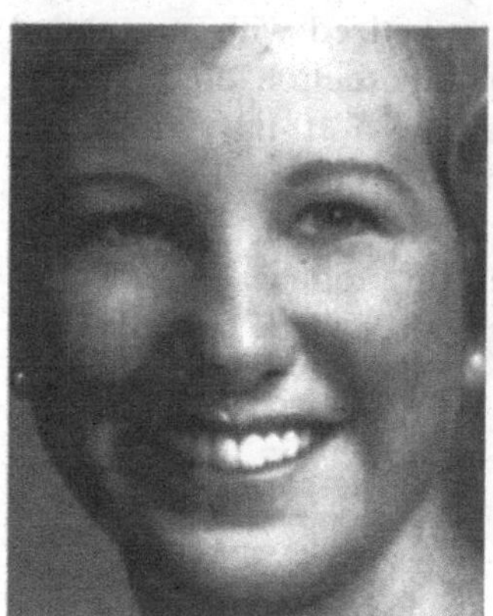

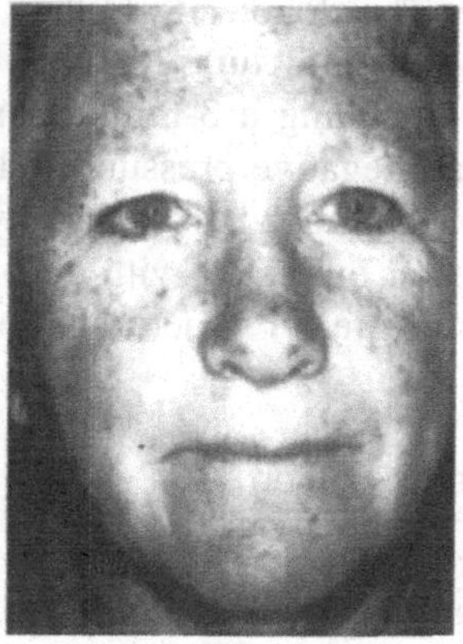

FIGURE 11 (a) Age 20; (b) age 55. Notice how fullness, not more lid show, was seen in her youth.

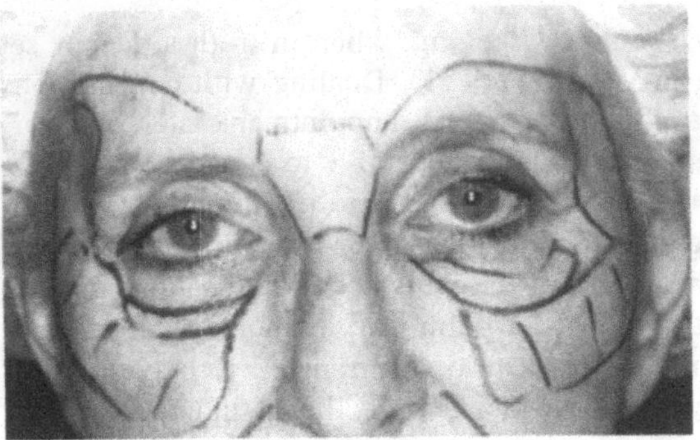

FIGURE 12 Preoperative markings.

clothing and bring a girdle or tight biking shorts for postoperative donor site compression.

THE PROCEDURE

The donor site is selected from an area that will aesthetically benefit the patient; however, every attempt should be made to harvest fat from sites with high lipogenic activity such as the outer thigh, buttocks and abdomen [8]. The author has found that dense outer thigh fat is preferable to fibrous abdominal fat both in the ease of harvesting and in the smoothness of transplant. Too much fibrous tissue in the adipose tissue will clog the transplant cannulas and lead to uneven injection of fat in the periorbital tissue. The donor site is circled with a marking pen and the patient placed on a draped procedure room table. The donor site is then anesthetized with a modified Klein tumescent solution until turgid (Table 1). Liposuction of the donor site is carried out by attaching a 3-mm cannula onto a 10-ml syringe and generating only manual negative pressure of 1 ml at all times (Fig. 13). An open-tipped cannula such as the Coleman extractor (Byron, Tucson, AZ) should be used, since fat extracted with an open tip produces cylinders of fatty tissue which posses greater structural integrity than single fat cells (Fig.

TABLE 1 Modified Klein Solution

1 liter lactated Ringer's solution
12.5 meq sodium bicarbonate
500 mg lidocaine
1 mg epinephrine

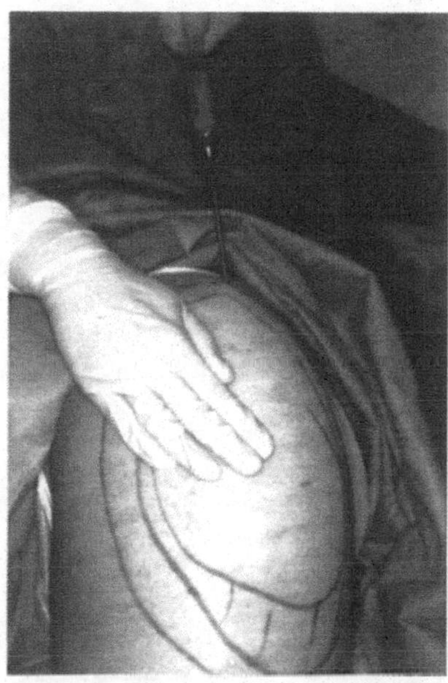

Figure 13 Extraction of fat is done by hand with less than 1 ml of negative pressure generated in a 10-ml syringe.

14). The basic science literature supports this by noting greater survival of cylindrical fat transplants as opposed to adipocyte suspensions [9]. The amount of fat extracted depends on whether frozen fat storage is to occur. Typically the author will extract 20–60 ml when the periorbital area exclusively is to be addressed and 60–120 ml when pan-facial augmentation is desired. The periorbital area alone will use no more than 10 ml of fat per visit and the unused fat extracted on the initial visit can be frozen in 10-ml syringes for later use. Frozen fat viability is controversial but the author routinely uses it with good lasting results. The collected fat is then centrifuged for 20 s at 3400 rpm to separate off the tumescent fluid from the fat and triglyceride layer, both which are discarded. The compacted fat is transferred to 1-ml syringes with a female–female large lumen transfer device in preparation for transplant. Only 1-ml syringes are used in this procedure since they allow greater control over the placement of very small aliquots of fat.

FACIAL ANESTHESIA

By blocking the infraorbital nerve as it exits the infraorbital foramen, good anesthesia of the midface and lower lid can be easily achieved. This can be

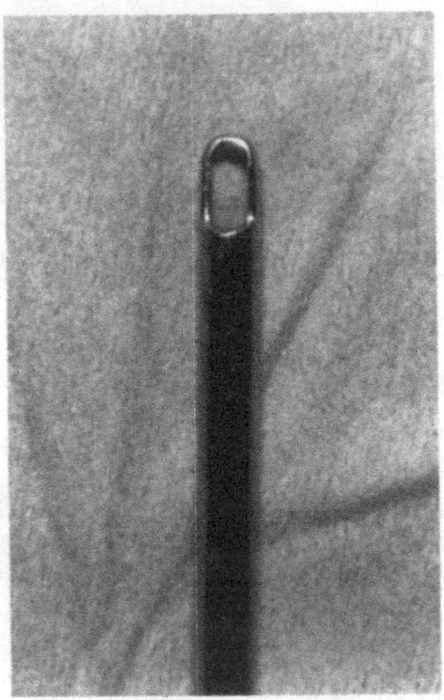

FIGURE 14 Open-tipped extractor (Byron, Tucson, AZ).

accomplished by either the intraoral or transcutaneous route using a $1\frac{1}{2}$ in. 30-gauge needle. One percent lidocaine with epinephrine is commonly used; however, in certain patients this can lead to tachycardia and a solution without epinephrine is substituted. The lateral eye, temple, and upper lid are infiltrated with additional 1% lidocaine with epinephrine steering clear of superficial visible vessels. While waiting the 10 min required for maximum vasoconstriction, the patient can pre-ice the periorbital area with moldable ice packs; this further inhibits ecchymosis and provides additional anesthesia.

PERIORBITAL AUGMENTATION TECHNIQUE

Periorbital fat augmentation is carried out with only blunt 18-gauge instruments like the Coleman I and Coleman II infiltrators (Byron, Tucson, AZ) or a modified microcannula (Fig. 15). Blunt instruments allow the fat to be placed in multiple deep planes without the risk of perforation of the orbital septum that sharp instruments would incur. The internal 18-gauge diameter insures that the fatty parcels pass through unharmed. Entry sites on the face are made with an 18-gauge NoKor™ needle at points of entry that allow easy access (Fig. 16). When treating both the hypertropic and atrophic variants of periorbital aging it is necessary to strengthen the structural integrity

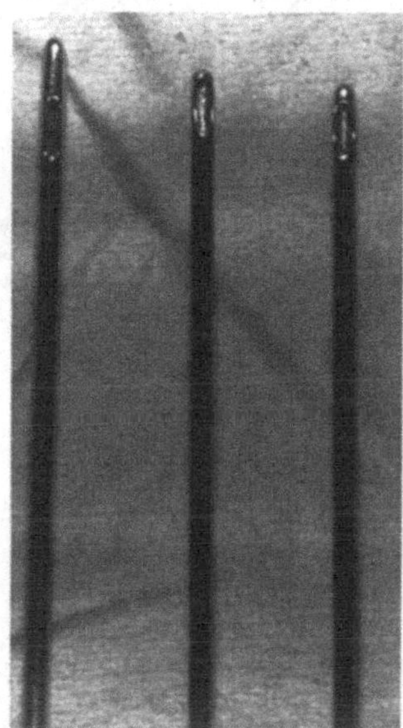

FIGURE 15 Blunt-tipped infiltrators.

of the inferior orbital rim by augmenting this area. From an entry site either in the midcheek of nasolabial fold, tiny pearls of fat are placed in a plane very close to the bone moving medial to lateral (Fig. 17). These pearls of fat are less than 0.1 ml in volume and evenly distributed along this deep plane. In patients with hypertrophic suborbital fat and atrophy of the upper

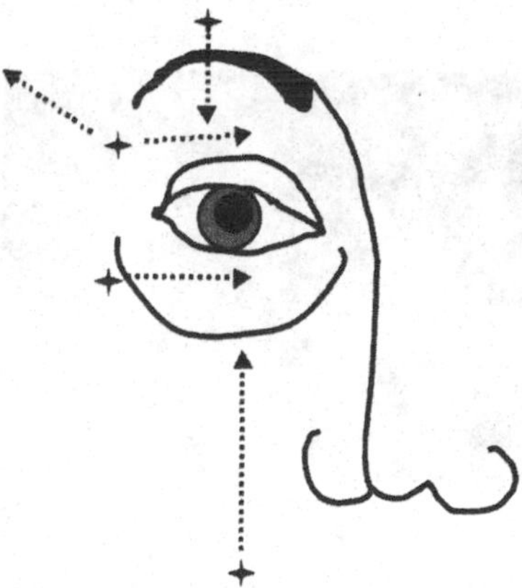

FIGURE 16 Example of entry sites and direction of infiltration.

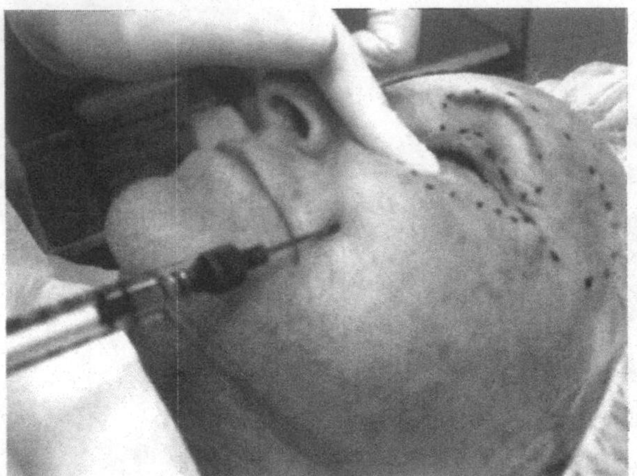

FIGURE 17 Technique of orbital ridge infiltration.

cheek mass, the end point is a projection of the cheek mass to the level of the suborbital bulge (Fig. 18). This typically takes 1–3 ml of fat. If the trough at the level of the arcus marginalus is still evident, careful placement of a strand of 0.1–0.3 ml of fat can be placed in the subcutaneous plane using a lateral approach. When treating the atrophic variant of suborbital aging, the above method is employed along the orbital rim, extending the droplets of fat more superiorly to the level of the base of the globe. Then a lateral approach is employed, staying deep to the orbicularis oculi muscle and placing linear fat deposits perpendicular to the initial fat placement (Fig. 19). A maximum of 2 ml of fat is placed from this lateral approach. Expe-

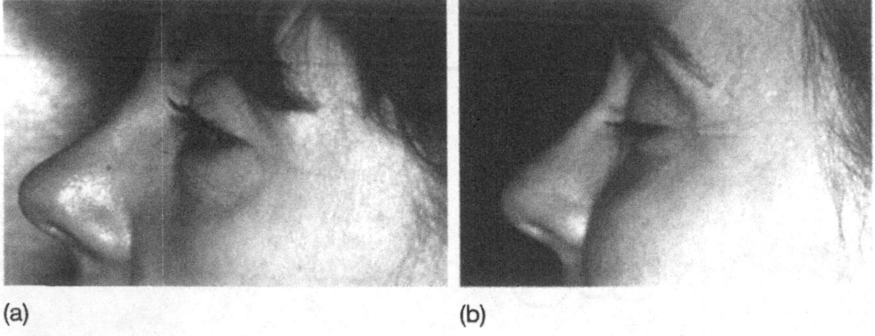

(a) (b)

FIGURE 18 Hypertrophic suborbital aging (a) before and (b) after lipoaugmentation.

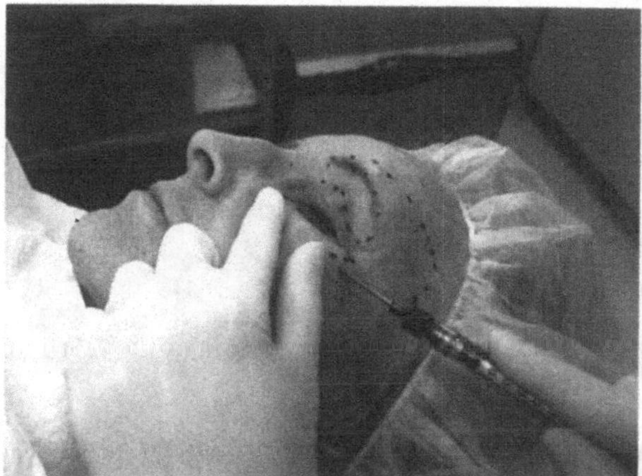

FIGURE 19 Technique of infraorbital infiltration.

rienced fat transfer surgeons can then place 0.5–1 ml of fat in the immediate subcutaneous plane, taking 20–50 passes to empty a 1-ml syringe. This is the most unforgiving part of this technique and multiple passes of fine fat filaments are more likely to insure an acceptable result. Fat when placed in this superficial plane lends a textural improvement to the overlying cutis and fills in the atrophic suborbital hollow (Fig. 20). The temple can also be filled from this lateral incision. Augmentation in the temple takes place in the subcutaneous plane above the temporalis fascia. It is placed in thin strands over multiple passes in a fanlike distribution from medial to lateral. For even, smooth distribution an additional entry site at the lateral margin of the temple in the hairline may be utilized to afford crosshatching of the fat (Fig. 21). One milliliter of fat is usually adequate to fill this area since any more leads to lumpy postoperative edema. The brow and upper lid is approached through either a lateral or superior incision. Since horizontal ridging is common in this area when a lateral approach alone is used, an additional superior entry site is desirable. Fat is placed in smaller than 0.1-ml droplets very close to the superior orbital ridge moving from medial to lateral (Fig. 22). Fat may then be placed higher in the subcutis in fine filaments, weaving in a crosshatched manner from both entry sites. A maximum of 2 ml can be placed in the brow in this manner. The goal of brow augmentation is to drop the orbital ridge and "tent" the lid/brow in an anterior direction. Any hollow just superior to the brow in the forehead can also be filled with 1–2 ml of fat, staying superior to the alveolar plane in the forehead to elevate the brow (Fig. 23). In the unique situation of periorbital fibrosis of the skin secondary to aggressive blepharoplasty 0.1–0.3 ml of fat can be carefully placed with

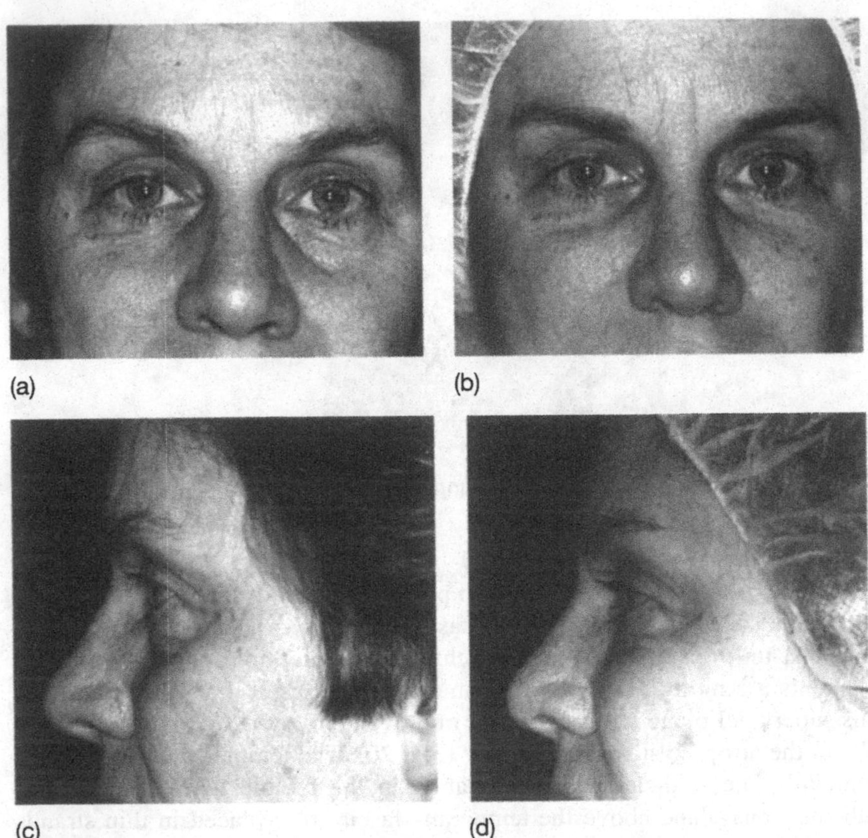

FIGURE 20 Atrophic suborbital aging front view (a) before and (b) after lipoaugmentation. Side view (c) before and (d) after lipoaugmentation.

a sharp 18- to 20-gauge needle subcising the scar tissue and releasing the adhesions. This is very difficult and should be tried only when the fat transfer surgeon is highly accomplished in this technique.

POSTOPERATIVE

Ice is immediately applied to the transplanted area and for 10 min every hour for the rest of the day. One concern with over icing is the compromise of blood supply to the newly transplanted fatty tissue. However, with correctly placed fat in thin strands it should not be a problem and markedly decreases the postoperative bruising. Since cooling tissue further decreases the need for an immediate oxygen supply, the prudent application of post-

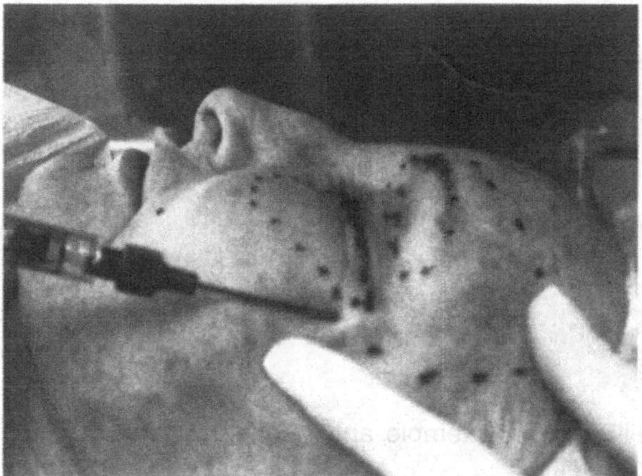

FIGURE 21 Technique of temple infiltration.

operative ice should not be harmful [10]. Six milligrams of betamethasone acetonide is given intramuscularly in the gluteus or deltoid to decrease swelling. The donor site is dressed with an absorbent dressing and compressed with a girdle or tight biking shorts. Acetaminophen is satisfactory for postoperative pain management. Edema occurring after the first postoperative day responds to warm compresses, and any ecchymosis may be camouflaged with opaque makeup.

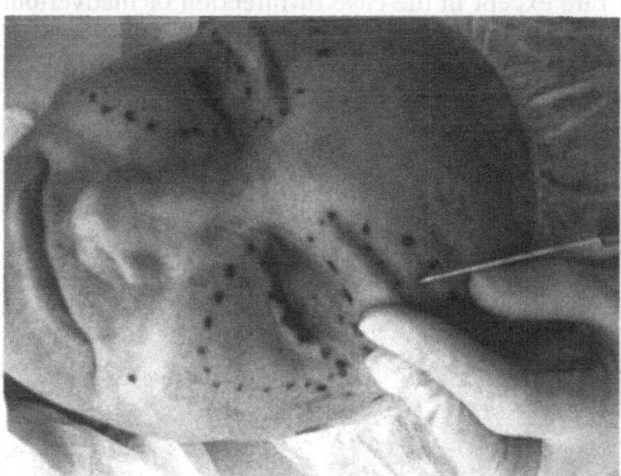

FIGURE 22 Technique of brow infiltration.

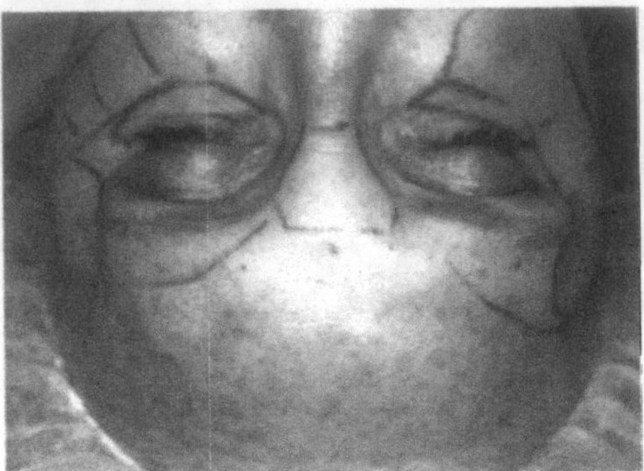

Figure 23 Patient after filling of right temple and forehead. Note elevation on right side as compared to left.

COMPLICATIONS

The most common postoperative complications are ecchymosis and edema. These are most often seen in the initial transfer and not in the touch-up procedures. Fat lumps and cysts are usually due to incorrectly placed fat or excessive amounts and can be avoided with conservative meticulous technique. Persistent fat lumps of greater than 3 months' duration can be treated with 2–4 mg/ml of dilute triamcinolone acetonide injected repeatedly at 2-week intervals or additional fat may be placed in the surrounding area to "blend in" the lump. If these fail, an attempt to remove them via microliposuction or direct excision can be tried (Fig. 24). Persistently visible entry sites are possible but very rare except in the case of infection or inadvertent tattooing of the marking ink. Overaggressive fat placement or the use of

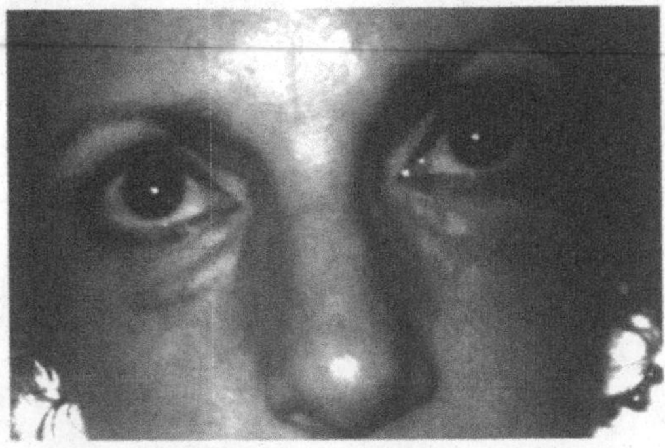

Figure 24 Periorbital fat lumps seen with overcorrection and poor technique.

sharp instruments increases the risk of perforation of the orbital septum. Fat retention is usually very good in the periorbital area, but like all living grafts may occasionally die and be absorbed. Other rare side effects include infection of the donor and recipient sites, hematoma formation, and temporary paresthesias. There are no documented cases of blindness following blunt infiltration of fat in the periorbital area.

TOUCH-UP PROCEDURES

Using the conservative approach lessens the risks of lumping and overcorrection, but falls short of complete augmentation. Additional touch-up transfers using the same or smaller amounts are often required. For the correction of periorbital aging changes in the middle-aged patient a total of four to eight transfers are usually adequate. Younger patients with early aging changes of in need of correction from aggressive blepharoplasty procedures may achieve complete correction in the initial procedure. Touch-ups present an excellent indication for the use of frozen stored fat. This lessens the time required to perform the procedure as well as the recovery for the patient. Fat intended for later use should be labeled with name, date, and social security number on the day of the extraction and placed in a freezer at −30°C with continuous temperature monitoring and a minimum temperature alarm. It may be kept in this manner for up to 2 years with retained viability. Frozen fat is transferred exactly the same as fresh fat using 1-ml syringes, blunt instruments, and the above-mentioned microtransfer technique.

CONCLUSION

Periorbital augmentation is a necessary part of the surgical antiaging armamentarium. It allows for the gradual restoration of the normal youthful contours of the face. It is an excellent complement to botox injection of the periorbital area and a wonderful way to correct the hollow pinched look that results from blepharoplasty and face-lifting procedures. The textural improvement seen with diffusely placed fat in the periorbital skin is a more natural-looking improvement than that seen with resurfacing procedures. The difficulty of learning the technique of periorbital augmentation is attenuated by a slow conservative approach with multiple touch-up procedures.

REFERENCES

1. Shorr N, Enzer Y. Considerations on aesthetic eyelid surgery. J Dermatol Surg Oncol 1992; 18:1081–1095.

2. Dailey RA, Wobig JI. Eyelid anatomy. J Dermatol Surg and Oncol 1992; 18: 1023–1027.
3. Gilchrest BA, Fitzpatrick TB, Anderson RR, Parrish JA. Localization of malanin pigmentation in the skin with Wood's lamp. Br J Dermatol 1977; 96(3): 245–248.
4. Bhawan J. Short- and long-term histologic effects of topical tretinoin on photodamaged skin. Int J Dermatol 1998; 37(4):286–292.
5. Campbell JP, Lisman R. Complications of blepharoplasty. Facial Plast Surg 2000; 8(3):303–327.
6. Seckel BR, Kovanda CJ, Cetrulo CL, Passmore AK, Meneses PG, White T. Laser blepharoplasty with transconjunctival orbicularis muscle/septum tightening and periocular skin resurfacing: a safe and advantageous technique. Plast Reconstr Surg 2000; 106(5):1127–1141.
7. Baker SR. Orbital fat preservation in lower lid blepharoplasty. Arch Facial Plast Surg 1999; 1:33–39.
8. Arner P, Engfeldt P, Lithell H. Site differences in the basal metabolism of subcutaneous fat in obese women. J Clin Endocrinol Metab 1981; 53(5):948–952.
9. Fagrell D, Enestrom S, Berggren A, Kniola B. Fat cylinder transplantation: an experimental comparative study of three different kinds of fat transplants. Plast Reconstr Surg 1996; 98(1):90–98.
10. Nedelcu J, Klein MA, Aguzzi A, Martin E. Resuscitative hyperthermia protects the neonatal rat brain from hypoxic-ischemic injury. Brain Pathol 2000; 10(1): 61–71.

30

Reduction Syringe Liposculpting

Pierre F. Fournier
Private Practice
Paris, France

HISTORY OF SYRINGE LIPOSCULPTURING

It was in September 1985, 7 years after Giorgio Fischer's first demonstration of machine liposuction in Paris, that I discovered by accident that adipose tissue could be extracted using a syringe. One of my patients wanted to have liposculpturing of the knees, but she was frightened (for unknown reasons) about the use of anesthesia, either local or general, as well as about drugs for premedication or sedation. As she was highly motivated, I performed the operation with the only anesthetic possibility left: cryanesthesia.

She was admitted to my clinic as an outpatient. In the operating room, ice packs were applied to the knees for 20 min; normal saline with epinephrine (1 mg/liter) chilled at 2°C was injected subcutaneously (roughly 200 ml in each knee); and external cryoanesthesia was carried out again for another 30 min. The operation was then performed with absolutely no pain, according to the patient, and with the use of the suction machine. I removed, without difficulty, 100 cc of fat on one side and 120 cc on the other.

As I was a bit doubtful about the absence of pain experienced by the patient (maybe she was a masochist), I wanted to determine, on myself, if such anesthesia was really so effective. That evening, at home, I injected subcutaneously 40 cc of chilled (at 2°C) normal saline (without epinephrine) into my left iliac fossa. After 5 min I took a 5-cc syringe on which was mounted a 19-gauge needle and used multiple strokes on the fatty layer, in a fan-shaped area, after I had punctured the skin.

My left hand stabilized the skin and my right hand held the syringe during the few minutes needed for the procedure. I felt no pain whatsoever, except when inadvertently I reached the inner aspect of the skin. However, I suffered no pain while the needle was moved to and fro in the adipose tissue.

After I was convinced of the anesthetic power of the chilled, normal saline, I removed the needle and, to my great surprise, saw that the syringe was half-filled with adipose tissue. In order to have a firmer grip on the syringe, as it was a small one (5 cc), I was simultaneously holding the barrel and the fully extended plunger, which I had unintentionally pulled to the end. This simply demonstrated that by giving strokes, fat slivers are mechanically placed in the needle and that the negative pressure created in the syringe by the pull of the plunger transports the fat slivers into the barrel of the syringe. This specimen of extracted fat was later given to my pathologist, who reported the fatty tissue to be undamaged.

The ease of this extraction—done under anaerobic conditions and respecting the integrity and the sterility of the adipose tissue—immediately suggested that I could reinject this extracted fat into other places of the body where needed. Obviously, this procedure would require larger needles and cannulas mounted on larger syringes if I wished to extract larger amounts of fat and to sculpt the body.

The day after my "discovery" two patients were scheduled to have their nasolabial folds decreased, which I usually performed with small cannulas and the suction machine. I used, as the day before, a 5-cc syringe and a 19-gauge needle. The procedure went as smoothly as the day before. I removed 2 cc of fat from each side and at the moment realized that one of the advantages of syringe liposculpturing was the ability to measure exactly the amount of fat extracted from each area (Figs. 1–6).

I began to use larger (14-gauge) needles and manufactured small cannulas (14-gauge) with one, two, or three openings that I mounted on 10-cc syringes for working on double chins and other small areas. The bleeding was lighter than when using needles, and for a while I worked on small adiposities with such equipment. One day, as large cannulas were not available for mounting on 60-cc syringes, I cut the handle of a common Karman abortion cannula, used for liposculpturing, and passed it through the dilated hub of the syringe. To avoid the deadspace that exists in such equipment, I primed the syringe with normal saline before I started. After this maneuver it was easier to pull the plunger (the lock was not yet created), and I was surprised to see that the extracted fat contained less blood than with the machine. After 2 years of working with such equipment (60-cc syringes and

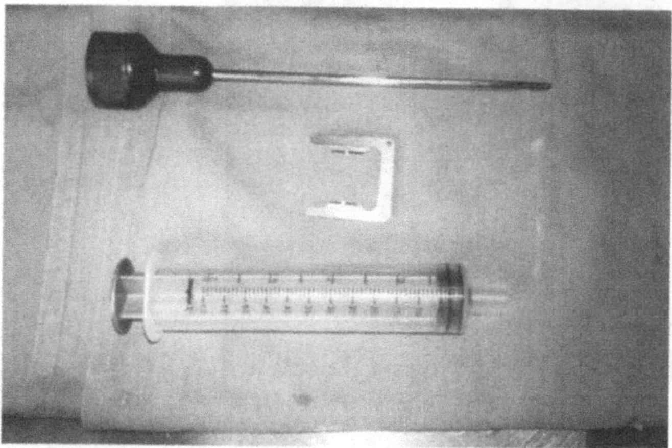

FIGURE 1 All the equipment needed: a Toomey syringe, a Tulip cannula, and a lock.

Karman abortion cannulas with cut handles), the manufacturers came to understand the advantages of these instruments and they then perfected cannulas, either passed through the hub (French model) or mounted externally on the syringe (Tulip model created by John Johnson) (Fig. 7).

Little by little the advantages of the syringe over the machine became obvious, and I thus elaborated the theory of the "buffering phenomenon." In the November 1983 issue of the *Journal of Plastic and Reconstructive*

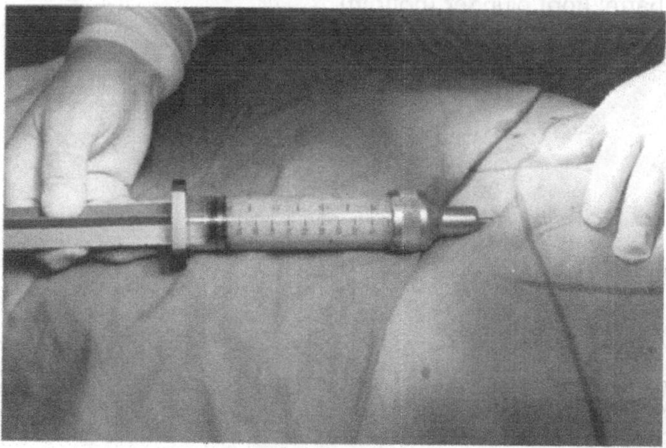

FIGURE 2 It takes 12 s to fill a 60-cc syringe after infiltration.

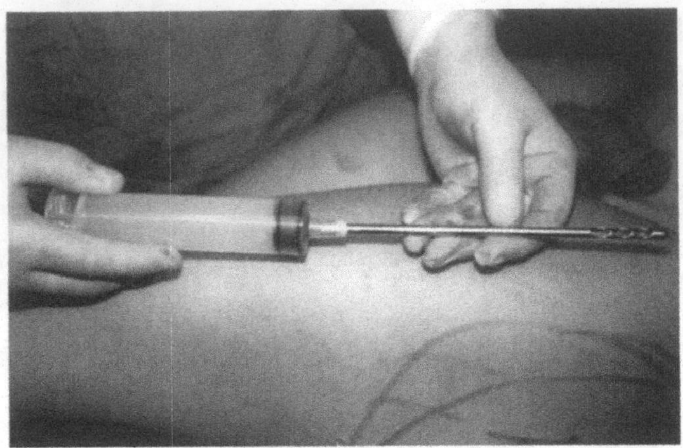

FIGURE 3 Makeshift equipment.

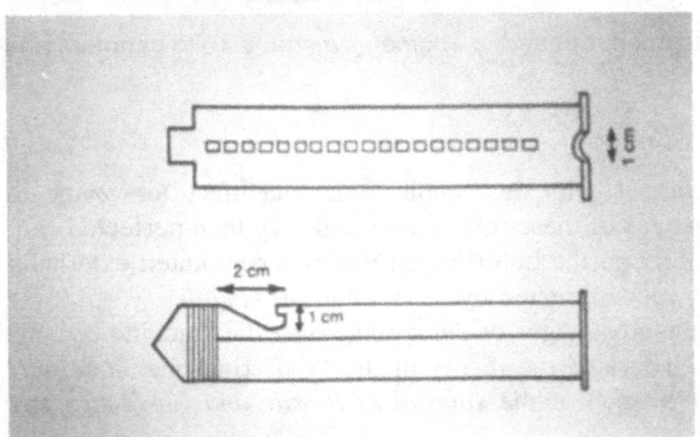

FIGURE 4 Syringe barrel (top) plunger (bottom).

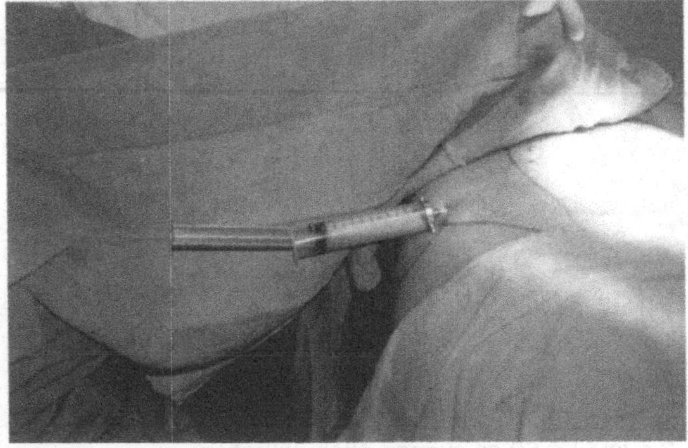

FIGURES 4 AND 5 The makeshift lock.

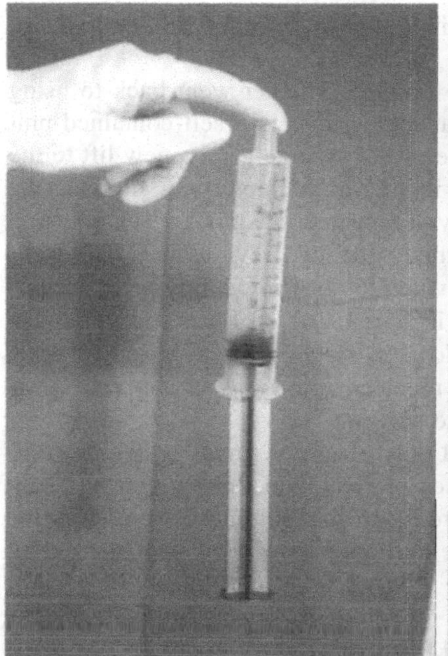

FIGURE 6 Testing the lock.

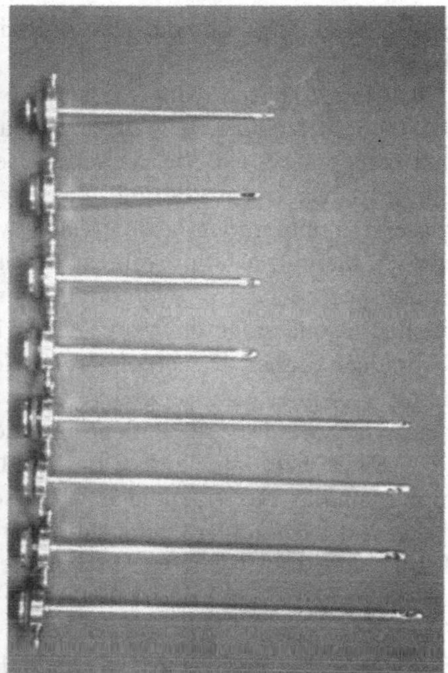

FIGURE 7 The French cannula (passes through the syringe). They may be used with all kinds of 50- or 60-cc syringes and not only with Toomey syringes.

Surgery, devoted to liposuction, an excellent article appeared written by Frederick Grazer with the help of Guenter Grams that explained, wonderfully well, that, whereas air can be compressed as many times as desired, a vacuum (or the absence of air) can be obtained only once. Thus syringe liposculpturing is as powerful as machine liposculpturing but with the advantage that there is a buffering system with the syringe method; this system cannot exist when the suction machine is used.

With the syringe the operation is performed in a fluid medium, whereas with the machine it is performed in a vacuum. The advantages of syringe liposculpturing can be explained by the fact that this buffering system (or shock-absorbing system, the syringe being primed with normal saline before liposculpturing) is placed between the adipose tissue and the negative pressure created by the syringe. The advantages derived from such a system are also valid for pure lipoextraction as well as when the adipose tissue is to be recycled. The advantages of syringe liposculpturing are outlined in Table 1.

Once I started using the syringe in 1985, I never went back to using the suction machine. It is obvious that the syringe is a self-contained unit that is far superior to the machine. Use of the syringe gave a new lift to the old procedure of fat grafting, making it safer and simpler and allowing the surgeon to obtain long-lasting results with repeated injections. Each injection adds to the partial improvement obtained with the previous one. The well-established concept of overcorrection when fat grafting is no longer accomplished in one stage anymore, nor is it done using an open and unreliable technique. Rather, the procedure is done in stages over a period of time, using a simple, easy procedure with repeated injections, a method that is readily accepted by the patient and the surgeon.

Since 1985, this author has used only plastic syringes on which common cannulas are mounted in all cases of reduction liposculpturing. Cannulas and syringes are selected according to the volume of the adiposity. Table 1 illustrates why the use of the syringe is preferred over the use of the machine.

SYRINGE REDUCTION LIPOSCULPTURING

Equipment

Lipodissectors (Cannulas)

Cannulas are classfied according to their outside diameter. They are made of metal. Those of very small external diameter (microcannulas) measure 2 or 2.5 mm. Useful lengths are 7, 12, and 24 cm. They have a blunt opening and a blunt tip, which is round or bullet-shaped. Those of average external diameter (minicannulas) measure 3, 3.5, and 4 mm. Useful lengths are 14 and 24 cm, and they also have a round or bullet-shaped tip and one blunt opening. Others have a diameter equal to 5 mm (macrocannulas). They have a useful length of 15–24 cm. The cannulas are mounted on the syringe either externally (Tulip) or pass through the syringe (French model). Special annuals can be easily mounted on 50- to 60-cc syringes with a long hub, as used by urologists.

When cannulas are reused, metal cleaners should be used before sterilization. Future cannulas will be made of hard plastic. They will be sterile, disposable, of all lengths, and of all diameters. It would be ideal to have a sterile, disposable cannula and syringe made in one piece.

Syringes

Syringes of average size (10 or 20 cc) are made of plastic and are sterile and disposable. They are used with microcannulas or minicannulas. Small

TABLE 1 Comparison between Syringe and Machine Liposculpturing

	Machine	Syringe
Cost of the material	High	Not high
Disposable	No	Yes. Future technique: syringes and cannulae in one piece, sterile and disposable.
Transport	Constraints	No constraints
Encumbering/Maintenance	High	Not a factor
Machine Breakdown	Always possible	No effect on the technique
Easy use	Heavy equipment more difficult to use	Light equipment easy to use
Surgical Control	More difficult	Easy due to lightness of equipment
Surgical Precision	Less precision—no exact measure of resected quantities	Very precise since there is a measuring unit of resected volumes: the syringe.
Lipoextraction power	One atmosphere	One atmosphere—a vacuum can only be obtained once
Lipoextraction speed	Same as syringe	Same as machine
Dead space	Yes. Large amount	No. Thanks to saline solution drawn into syringe before adipose tissue is added.
Buffering effect	No. Impossible	Yes. Thanks to saline solution drawn into syringe before adipose tissue is added.
Surgeon's fatigue	More tiring than the syringe	Less tiring than the machine. Both require same back and forth movements but the syringe is much lighter to work with.
Quality of results	Good but uncertain. Possible mistakes	Excellent. Technique more reliable. Few errors possible.

TABLE 1 Continued

	Machine	Syringe
Symmetry of results in large pair adiposities.	Approximative. More difficult to estimate in large containers.	Very precise. Syringe is a measuring unit in volume surgery.
Symmetry of results in small pair adiposities.	Very approximative estimate.	Extreme precision verified in syringe's graduated scale.
Noise during operation.	More or less strong depending on machine. Problem for patients under local or twilight anesthesia.	Total silence. Good environment for patient and surgeon, who can then do more creative work.
Liposanguine aerosols.	Yes if filter is inapproprite (AIDS, herpes, hepatitis).	No risks.
Adipose tissue and nerve trauma.	Some. Negative pressure transmitted to inside of dissected areas. Operation takes place in a vacuum.	Very little. Buffer liquid between negative pressure and dissected areas. Operation takes place in a liquid environment.
Shock possibility.	Higher because of adipose tissue nerve trauma.	A lot less because of buffering effect of the syringe.
Peroperatory bleeding.	Higher because of direct negative pressure on capillaries.	A lot less again because of buffering effect of syringe.
Transfusion possibility.	Always possible.	Less probable.
Amount of adipose tissue resected in same area.	Less. Limited by precocious bleeding.	More. Bleeding occurs much later.
Amount of adipose tissue resected without risking shock, large hemorrhage, or transfusion.	About two liters.	Four or more liters.

Work for two trained operators.	Risky due to possible asymmetry of results. Equipment problems.	No problem since precise estimate of resected volume by each operator on pair adiposities. Desirable to treat large, medium, multiple or pair adiposities.
Advantages of operation done by two trained operators.		Operatory and anesthesia time decreased. Hospitalization and convalescence time shorter. Less fatigue for operators.
In case of reutilization of resected adipose tissue.	Vaporisation and trauma of tissues. Transport in a vacuum with brutal impact.	No tissue vaporisation. Transport in liquid environment. Buffering of impact. Syringe allows extraction, treatment (washing) and reinjection of adipose tissue by a closed technique, respecting integrity and sterility of extraction. If needed, can be kept refrigerated.
Why there are not more practitioners using the syringe.	Machine seems to give more importance. Patients think machine does operation, not surgeon, thereby believing all practitioners can obtain equal results. Also, lack of information or surgeon's resistance to change techniques.	Using an old instrument like a syringe simplifies operation too much, demystifying the suction machine, once considered to be indispensable, possessing magical powers.
Democratization of operation among surgeons and potential patients.	Difficult.	Easy.

syringes do not need a lock. The plunger is locked with a plastic needle cap.

Large-volume syringes are used with macrocannulas (50 and 60 cc). These are used by urologists and by gynecologists (for abortions). These syringes are plastic, sterile, and disposable. They should have a large outside-diameter opening of 5 mm or more. The implantation of a cone on the syringe has an 8- to 10-mm external diameter (Toomey Tip). A lock (snapper) is necessary to immobilize the plunger. It is best to fill the syringe with a few cubic centimeters of normal saline before the extraction to avoid any dead space.

The Lock

A lock is necessary when using 60-cc syringes. Different models exist. We recommend the "Johnny lock" (John Johnson). We use only the makeshift one, which is excellent. The lightness of our equipment decreases possible bleeding.

The Awl or Ice Pick

To avoid incision scars, punctures are made through the skin with an awl. This opening can be dilated with a hemostat to allow entry of the cannula. The puncture of the skin made by the awl heals better than an incision with a scalpel and is almost invisible. This puncture needs to be dilated with an artery forceps to avoid friction with the skin, which may give a pigmented spot at the place of the puncture.

Cautions

The larger the diameter and capacity of a syringe, the less its suitability for transportation of the fat. This is why it is much better to use a syringe adapted to the volume of the adiposity and to the volume of fat to be extracted. The outside diameter of the syringe should be as small as possible. This is why a 2-cc syringe for insulin injections is superior to the standard 2-cc syringe, which is much shorter.

The cannulas should also be chosen according to the volume of the adiposity. If specially made cannulas are not available for mounting on plastic syringes, it is a simple task to use the standard machine Karman cannulas. The machine mounting is first sawed off, and then the cannula is passed through the barrel of the plastic syringe and pushed with long scissors in a screw-type motion through the plastic cone after the opening has been appropriately cut. It may be necessary to use an ice pick or hemostat to dilate the plastic cone still further. The cannulas have to be adapted perfectly to the cone and syringe.

This equipment is as useful as any specially manufactured lipodissector for syringe-assisted liposculpturing. The equipment is tight, waterproof, and airproof. Surgeons who choose to make their own equipment can obtain the syringes in medical, dental, or veterinary supply stores. Cannulas of 2, 2.5, and 3 mm can be mounted externally, as their inside diameter corresponds to the inside diameter of the small syringes.

In all systems described, suction is as fast as with the machine, is less shocking, provokes less bleeding, and is less tiring.

Reduction Syringe Liposculpturing Technique

The goal of the procedure is to perform a partial lipectomy in the localized adiposity. Four steps are required: (1) removal of the excess adipose tissue in a crisscross dissection/extraction (lesional lipectomy or mesh lipoextraction); (2) remodeling of the remaining crisscrossed adipose tissue; (3) redistribution of the skin after a wide peripheral mesh undermining of the neighboring normal adipose tissue has been done with a cannula (perilesional mesh lipoplasty; no removal of adipose tissue during the peripheral undermining has to be done); and (4) adequate immobilization of the treated area until shrinkage and healing proceed satisfactorily. In some cases, after performing reduction liposculpturing on one or several adipose regions, it is worth using part of the harvested fat (60 cc usually) to fill in the neighboring depressions. The final result will be improved.

The surgeon must keep in mind that closed liposculpturing is an artistic, three-dimensional, architectural technique of body contouring. It is essentially a tactile operation with the surgeon working almost blindly. We are dealing with a volume of space-covering tissue, the skin. Fat is highly vascularized; consequently, a lipectomy has to be performed using a blunt cannula to create crisscrossed dissection/extraction channels. It is imperative to avoid excessive bleeding through the use of vasconstrictors. It is also crucial to reposition the skin and underlying fat using the shrinking properties of the skin and the technique of peripheral mesh undermining. Finally, adequate immobilization is vital to liposculpturing.

Basic Principles

The following are some of the basic principles in reduction syringe liposculpturing:

1. A crisscrossed lipectomy (tunnels, columns of fat, lattice, and mesh lipectomy) has to be performed. Several approaches have to be made.

2. A peripheral mesh undermining technique is usually part of the operation (without fat extraction). This is mostly important when the skin is of average quality such as with mature patients.
3. Dissecting hydrotomy with vasconstrictors (chilled normal saline at 2°C and 1 mg/liter of adrenalin) is necessary.
4. The required instruments include a small blunt-tipped cannula with one blunt opening, an ice pick, and syringes.
5. The shrinking properties of the skin should be utilized after repositioning and immobilizing the tissues.

Preestimation of the Quantity to be Resected

The amount of adipose tissue to be resected during liposculpturing must be calculated during the patient's various preoperative examinations. This is a matter of experience and judgment and can be acquired only with time after assisting the operations performed by other surgeons. Only then can an accurate estimate be made. During the operation, this estimate can be more or less modified, but overall the surgeon has a relatively good idea of the amount of tissue to be resected. It is not a "suck as you go procedure."

Preestimation required the same kind of judgment that is necessary for other aesthetic operations. The eye will examine the state of the skin (thick, with or without stretch marks); the fingers will test the tonicity of the areas to be treated by using the pinch test in a standing position, lying down, while the underlying muscles are contracted, and while walking. The preestimation of a region such as the saddlebag area can be done only after a careful study of the neighboring adipose areas that can play a role in the origin of the saddlebags: hips, buttocks, and the lower buttocks fold. One must therefore differentiate between true saddlebags, false saddlebags, and mixed cases. Squeezing of the buttocks is requested to differentiate false saddlebags from true ones and mixed cases.

Xerographies, echographies, scanners, or other complementary examinations can be useful but are never demanded because the preestimation is above all clinical. The preestimation is noted on the patient's card, on special diagrams, or on the Polaroid photos made during the course of the first visit. Computer study may also be used.

Notes

We once more insist that the surgeon needs to know the approximate amount of adipose tissue to be resected before the operation. The following items depend on the quantity to be resected: (1) whether the operation can be done all at once or over several procedures; (2) whether conventional, tumescent, local, general, or epidural anesthesia is to be utilized (the dose of local anesthesia also needs to be estimated); (3) the amount of fluids and electrolytes needed; (4) the length of hospitalization (whether the patient is ambulatory); (5) whether a blood transfusion needs to be considered even if this is not frequent nowadays; and (6) the approximate length of the operation and of the convalescence.

"Good judgment comes with experience, and experience with bad judgment."

Marking the Patient

Marking the patient is done in the standing position, just before the operation (Fig. 8). We use a green Pentel pen; the skin marker must be of good quality to resist the preparations. We mark (1) the adiposity by encircling it, (2) 1–1.5 cm around the previous circle (Fig. 9) (the tip of the cannula will be pushed until the second marking, so there will be no stair-step deformity), and (3) beyond the adiposity between 2 and 8 cm from the second marking. This corresponds to the extent of the peripheral mesh undermining. Finally, the openings (or incisions) will be marked by a circle to avoid any permanent or transient tattooing from the ink of the marking pen. All the adipose regions are marked before the operation, as is the site of the intended inci-

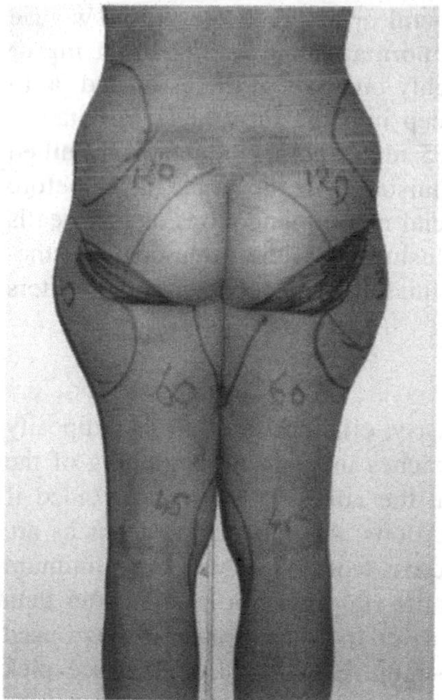

FIGURE 8 Marking the patient.

sions or openings. The appropriate amount of resection will be marked in the middle of the adiposity.

Anesthesia

Reduction liposculpturing can be done according to the type of anesthesia that the patient desires—general, twilight, epidural, local, or cryoanesthesia. Local anesthesia is the preferred method. We have used the Klein tumescent technique for many years; chilled saline at 2°C is used instead of saline at room temperature. We consider chilling very important with tumescent anesthesia. The colder temperature increases the anesthesia, decreases the bleeding, and prevents shock. A thorough study of tumescent anesthesia is a must before practicing liposculpturing.

External cryoanesthesia can be used in addition to local anesthesia. Ice packs will improve the anesthesia and decrease the bleeding. If refrigerated bags are used, one should watch the patient carefully because the bags can cause skin burns or pigmentation. This does not occur with ice cubes.

Preparation of the Area

In all cases of reduction liposculpturing, the area should be injected to decrease bleeding as well as to enhance the procedure. A syringe or a pump are used for this preparation. During general or epidural anesthesia, we use the following solution: 1 liter of chilled normal saline at 2°C and 1 mg of epinephrine. The amount injected is roughly one-half of the estimated fat to be removed. This solution is injected deep into the fatty layer to obtain a spasm of the vessels at this level. After 5 min, another injection of chilled saline at 2°C, with epinephrine, is administered in the upper layer before starting the procedure. There are no special recommendations as the area is prepared with the local anesthesia when using the Klein tumescent anesthesia. The tumescent solution is always chilled at 2°C. Between 1 and 4 liters are injected in the average cases.

Approaches in Liposculpturing

The planned approach has to allow for easy, efficient work in the adiposity to obtain the best possible result. Approaches used at the beginning of the procedure which are concealed far from the adiposity must be avoided if they interfere with proper working conditions. As many approaches as are necessary will be performed for the crisscross work; there will be a minimum of two (Fig. 13). Puncturing the skin in the right tension line is better than incising it. In all of the approaches used for the past years, we have used an awl or an ice pick to make the opening. Should the awl or ice pick puncture be too small to allow the passage of the cannula, the hole can be dilated by passing first one branch and then the second branch of a hemostat,

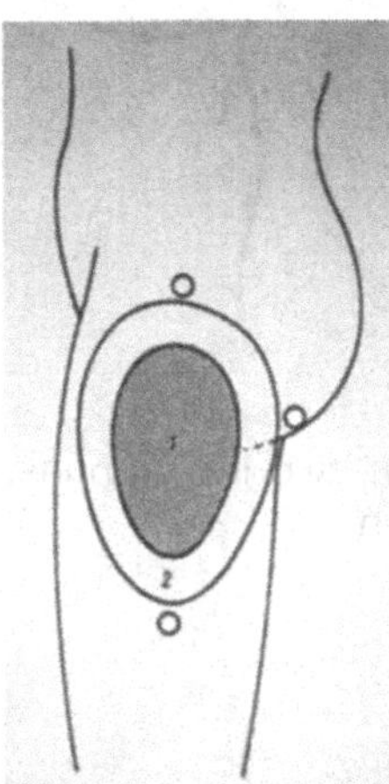

FIGURE 9 Three approaches are used in saddlebag liposculpture. The central crisscrossed lipoextraction zone. Peripheral mesh undermining.

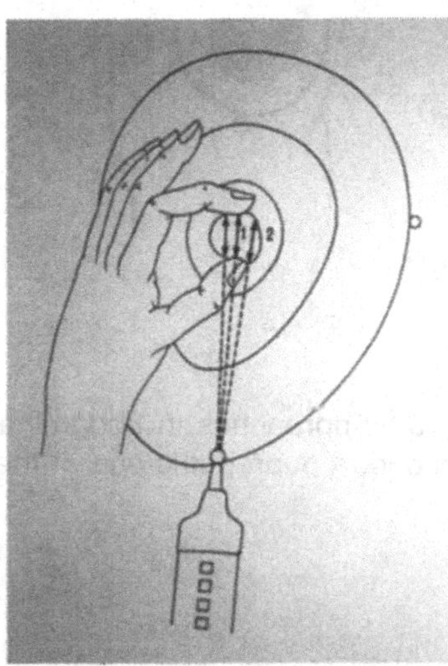

FIGURE 10 Saddlebags liposculpture. Small strokes are used in the center to "decapitate" the adiposity.

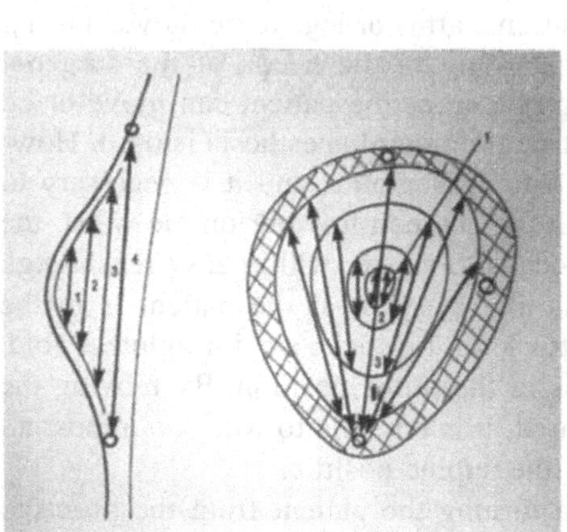

FIGURE 11 Diagram of the short and long strokes to level the adiposity.

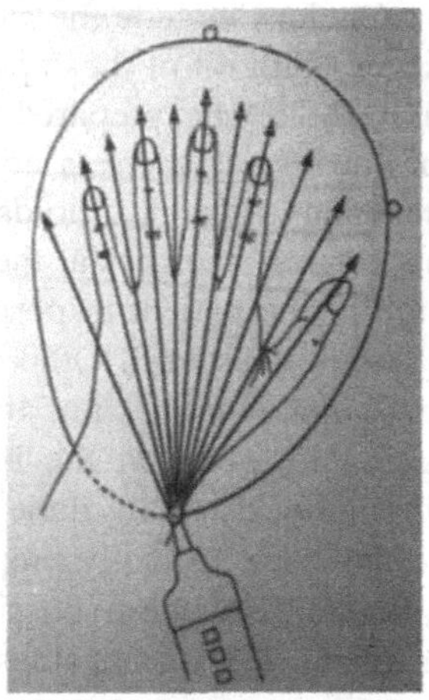

FIGURE 12 The hand is a guide—no more than three strokes are used in the same direction.

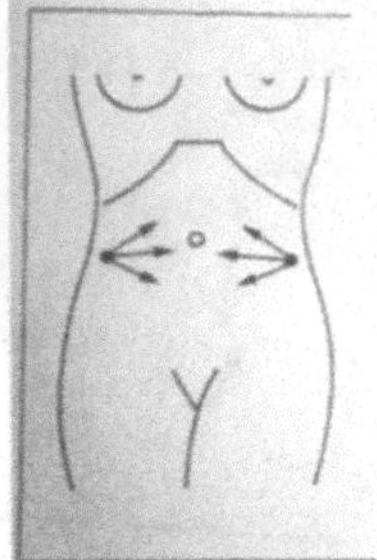
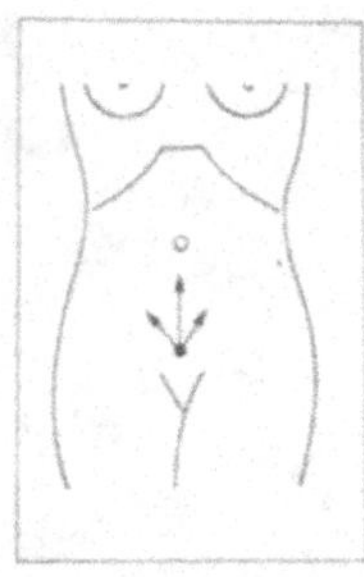
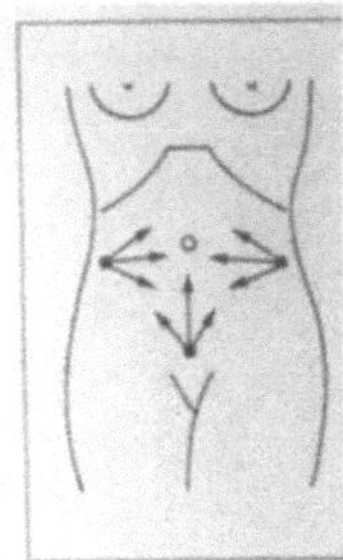

FIGURE 13 Approaches in abdominal liopsculpturing: first, two lateral ones, and, second, a suprapubic one at the end of the operation.

which are separated very gently. As there is no incision of the skin, the healing of the wound is far superior to a standard incision and is almost invisible. The wound needs to be closed in most of the cases by a fine nylon 5-0 suture or by an inverted stitch of resorbable material.

Positioning the Patient

The position of the patient should be the most adequate and convenient for the surgeon. Choices include the supine position, the prone position, and the lateral position. With all of these positions, arms or legs to be moved during the operation should be prepared according to the needs of the surgeon. Under local anesthesia, there is no problem, as the patient can move or be moved if necessary. This also holds true if epidural anesthesia is used. However, during general anesthesia, the patient is supine, and it is necessary to elevate a side of the patient to permit the surgeon to work on the waist, the hip, or the lateral chest roll. Other localizations are within easy reach, e.g., thighs, knees, and double chin. It is also possible if the patient is in the supine position to work on the buttock or to create an infragluteal fold, although this is not as easily done as in the prone position. By moving the patient who has been specially prepared, it is possible to work on almost all localized adiposities of the pelvis in the supine position.

When using general anesthesia turning the patient from the prone to the supine position or vice versa during a liposculpturing procedure should be avoided whenever possible. Nevertheless, it is sometimes necessary to do this, and special precautions should be observed by the surgeon and the anesthesiologist. For safety reasons, it is much better to do the requested procedures in two stages instead of taking risks with the patient when a change of position is needed.

A word of caution: positioning the patient is important, as the surgeon should not be working in unfavorable conditions. The surgeon should always have easy access to the different approaches needed during the procedure in order to do the best work possible. Tumescent anesthesia allows the surgeon to work in the best conditions as the position of the patient is easily modified.

Surgical Technique

In describing surgical technique, the work on a hip with a 3- or 4-mm cannula and a 60-cc syringe will be used as an example. At the previously marked sites, incisions or openings are made (we prefer the puncture) and are dilated with a hemostat. Pretunneling is not absolutely necessary but is recommended if the fat is hard. The cannula is directed in the area before liposculpturing is begun. Before it starts, one should fill the syringe with 5 cc of chilled saline; this will then act as a buffer. The cannula is then passed through the opening while the left hand folds temporarily the skin.

The plunger is withdrawn and kept withdrawn by the surgeon's right hand. The maneuver is not difficult and can be made easier by the use of a stop. The cannula is moved in a fanshaped motion, approximately three times in the same direction (we do not recommend that it stay in the same tunnel). The strength of the surgeon is exerted when pushing the cannula into the adipose tissue, not when pulling it. The opening of the cannula will face down during this maneuver. After 60 cc of fat is collected in the barrel, the syringe will be emptied into a basin on the operating table. The same procedure will follow using another approach and so on to perform an even crisscrossed work.

When the adiposity is conical (saddle bags or abdomen) the surgeon (1) has to work in the middle of the adiposity, below the conical portion, giving small strokes to "decapitate" this adiposity; and (2) also has to use long strokes to "level" the adiposity, using different approaches to obtain a crisscrossed work. Three approaches are used when treating saddle bags in a clockwise direction. Three approaches are also used for an abdomen. An even crisscrossed work is achieved when using a different approach to fill a syringe. The left hand still guides and follows the work of the right hand. Liposculpturing is a tactile operation. The work of the hands is summarized in Table 2. The division of labor between the two hands is opposite to standard surgery, in which the right hand is the one that dominates. With liposculpturing the left hand is the "brain hand," and the right one is a mere piston. One may in some circumstances use a smaller cannula (no. 2) to do the crisscrossing at a different level. At intervals, the left hand will pinch the skin (pinch test) between the index and the thumb to evaluate the thickness of the fold. The surgeon will usually monitor the modification of the

TABLE 2 Duties of Each Hand during Liposculpture

Left hand	Right hand
Stabilize	Pushes
Lift	Pulls
Grasp	Dissects
Harden	Fills the syringe
Guide	Empties the syringe
Localize	Pulls on the plunger
Palpates	Measures the amount of the fat extracted
Monitors	
Carries out the pinch tests	

contour of the area treated to avoid an overcorrection and will also check the volume of fat removed against the preestimate. A 1-cm uniform thickness of fat covering the area should be left, and this result is controlled by a pinch test made with the left hand. Should the fat in the syringe show too much blood, the surgeon must stop suctioning the area and work on another part of the adiposity. Should the patient complain under local anesthesia, the surgeon should inject more of the anesthetic solution. It should be noted that the skin has to be grasped in order to place the cannula in the right place. The left hand should be flat during the whole operation to stabilize the tissues and should exert some pressure on the tissues.

When the lipectomy has been completed and the expected amount of fat removed the surgeon performs a peripheral mesh undermining using the same openings and the same instruments. No suction is done during this procedure. The cannula is pushed in a fan-shaped motion until it reaches the marked line of the mesh undermining. This mesh is also done in a crisscross fashion through the area already lipectomized. The peripheral mesh undermining allows the excess skin that is covering the crisscross lipectomized adiposity to fit better in its new bed; less resistance will be encountered in the neighboring tissues because many retinacula cutis will have been severed. The peripheral mesh undermining must be proportional to the amount of fat removed and also to the quality of the skin. When a small amount of fat is removed in a young patient it is unnecessary.

When one area is completely treated, the surgeon will work on the opposite paired adiposity unless another well-trained lipoplastic surgeon has already done the second side. When a neighboring depressed area has to be grafted, part of the fat that has been harvested will be washed with normal saline and reinjected in a crisscross manner. This area will be remodeled with the surgeon's left hand and immobilized together with the other treated areas. Remodeling of the adipose area is done with the surgeon's left hand. We never drain.

When some patients have heavy legs we use the Cherif Zahar technique under general anesthesia, and a tourniquet is applied on the thigh (Fig. 14) after emptying the leg of its blood using an elastic bandage (Figs. 15 and 16). No infiltration is necessary. There is no bleeding during the operation and the results are excellent.

Dressing

Unless a special garment is used, the surgeon dresses the area using Elastoplast. Several layers have to be used because the dressing acts as an external splint.

Fluid and Electrolyte Balance

When using general or epidural anesthesia the anesthesiologist will take care of the problem of fluid and electrolyte balance. Roughly double the

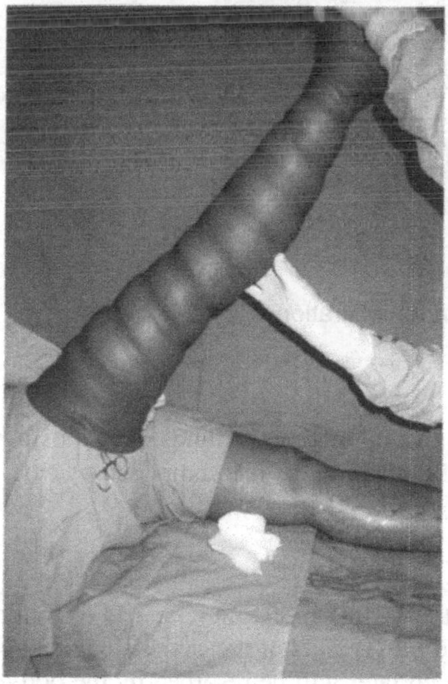

Figure 14 Applying the tourniquet during the Cherif Zahar technique.

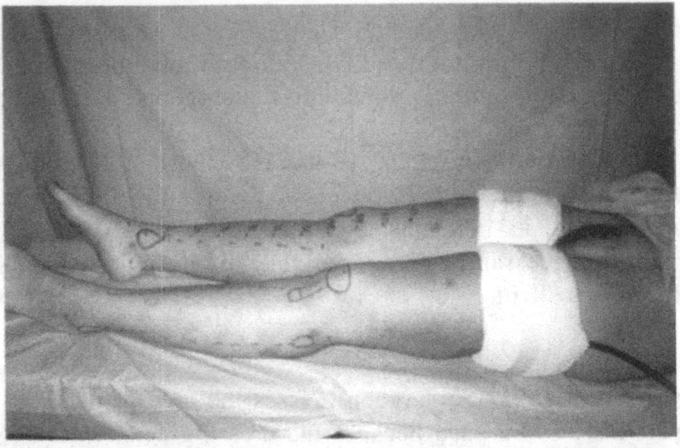

FIGURE 15 Tourniquet in place.

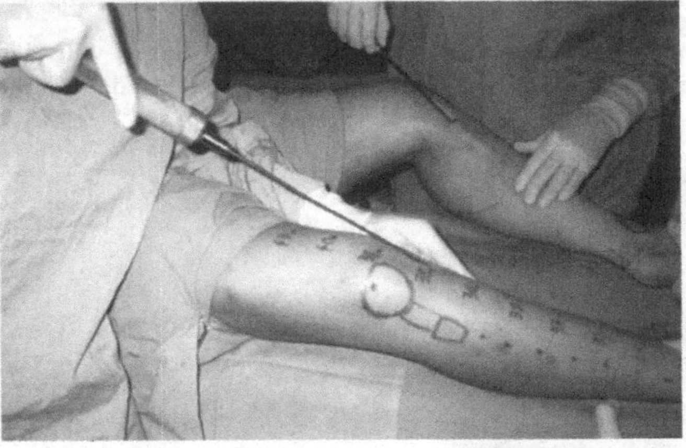

FIGURE 16 Cherif Zahar technique without infiltration.

amount of fat removed has to be given to the patient in fluids. When using tumescent anesthesia no fluid should be given iv, as recommended by Jeffrey Klein.

Technical Considerations

The quantity of fat to be removed is the visible resection. One has to think that during the procedure the to-and-fro movements of the cannula devitalize a certain amount of adipose tissue, which later will be resorbed by the body. This is the invisible or biologic resection. During the procedure, there is

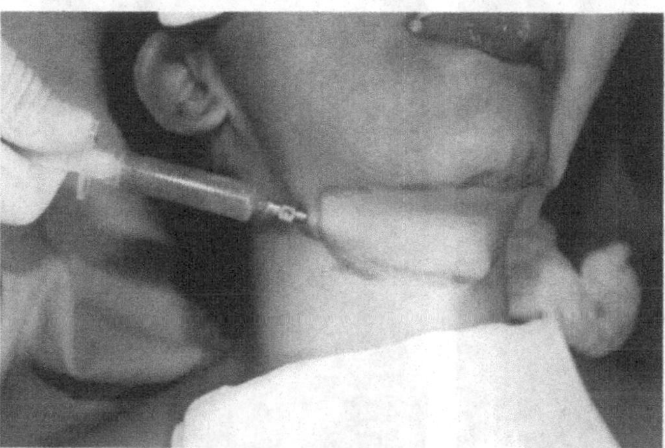

FIGURE 17 Neck liposculpturing with a 10-cc syringe and a 12-cm cannula (14-gauge diameter).

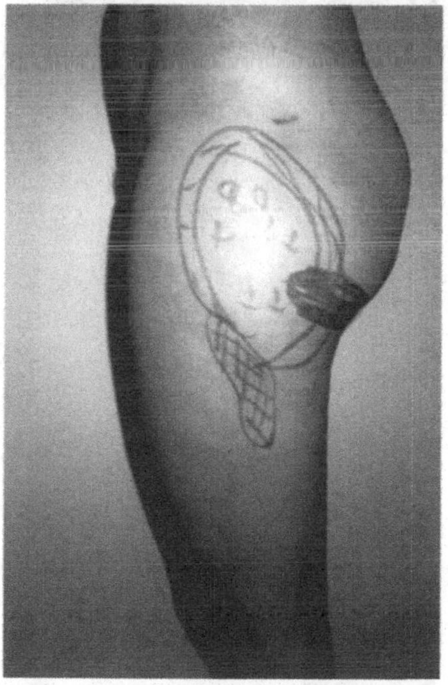

FIGURE 18 Syringe fat grafting is used to treat an uneven surface.

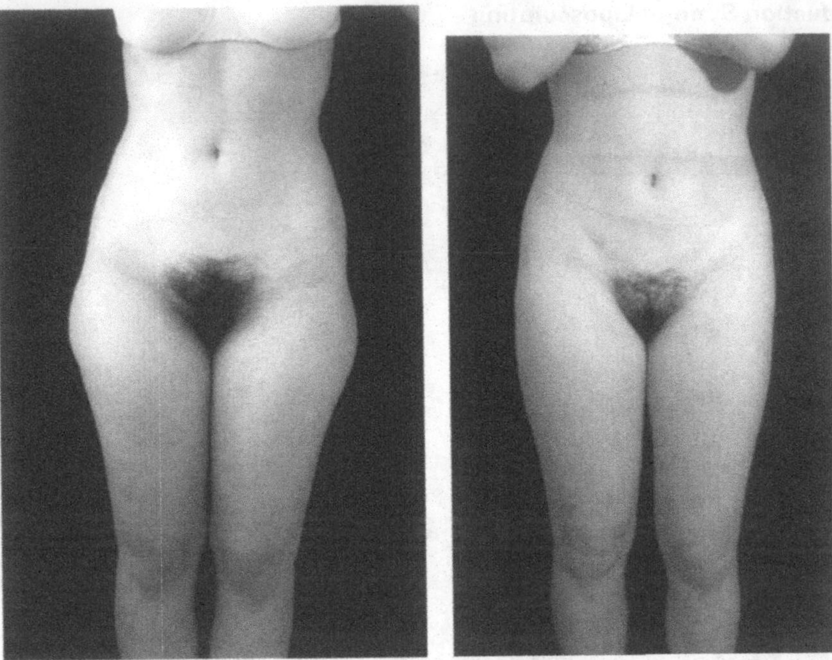

FIGURE 19 Before (left) and after (right) hip and saddlebags liposculpture on a young patient.

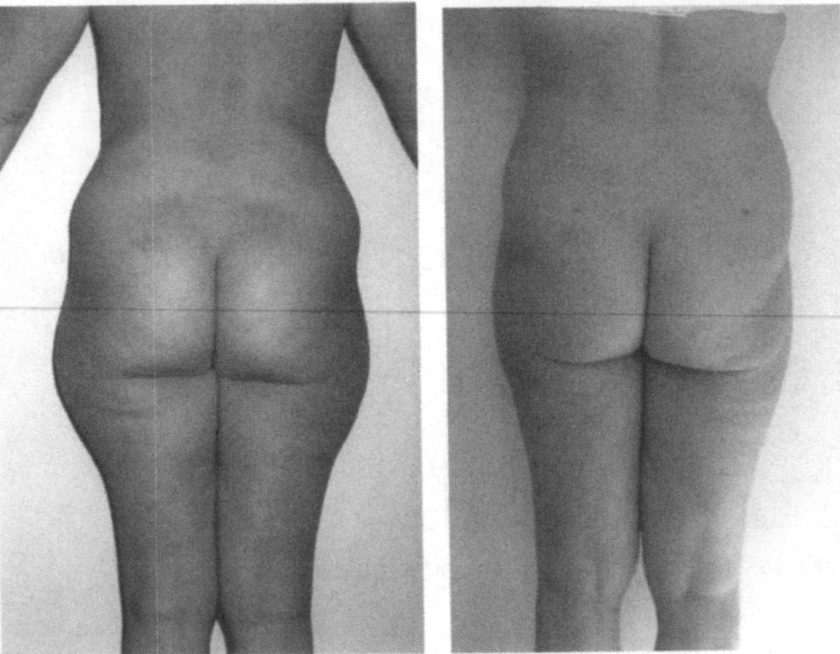

FIGURE 20 Before (left) and after (right) hip and saddlebags, infra gluteal sulcus, and inner-thighs liposculpture on a mature patient.

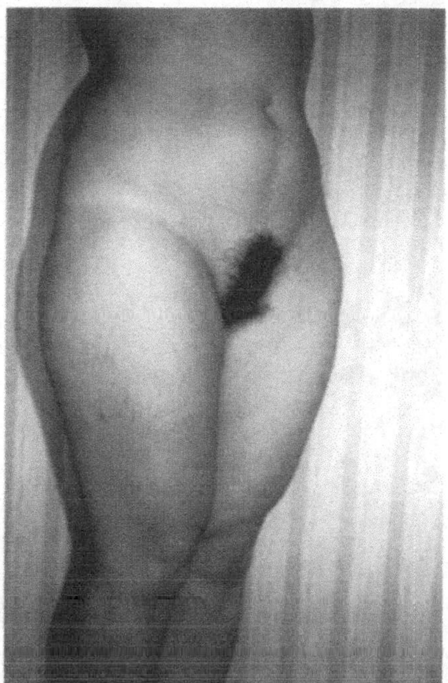
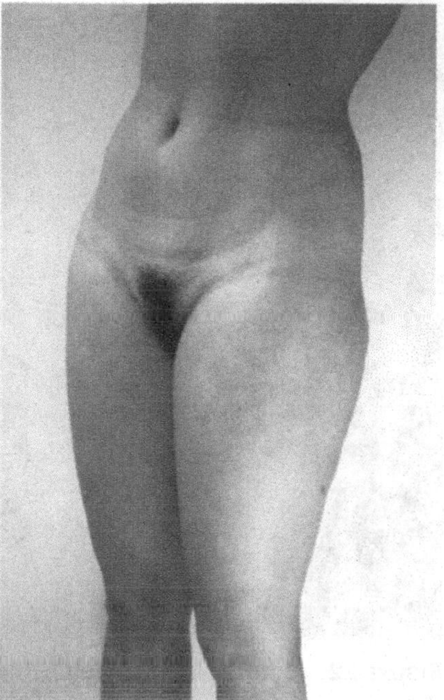

FIGURE 21 Before (left) and after (right) circumferential thigh and hip liposculpture.

destruction of adipose tissue. The volume of fat reduction is obtained in two different ways: mechanical disruption and suction friction scraping.

The visible resection is the one obtained by the scraping motion of the cannula, which also removes a part of the fat that has been mechanically disrupted. The invisible resection is made up of most of the devitalized fat obtained by the friction of the cannula and of some of the mechanically disrupted fat. After a certain period of time, the procedure will create scar tissue, which will be followed by contractions, as is true for any operation on or below the skin. This consideration enhances the prognosis for a thorough and even lipectomy. The peripheral mesh undermining in the whole area treated is to obtain a homogeneous contraction of the scar tissue.

The skin will be affected by the primary contraction of the muscular fibers (immediate, active process). The adipose tissue will be modified by the contraction of the fibrous tissue (passive contraction, delayed). After a liposculpturing procedure, there is an immediate improvement in contour due to the biologic resection. The skin will also be modified immediately

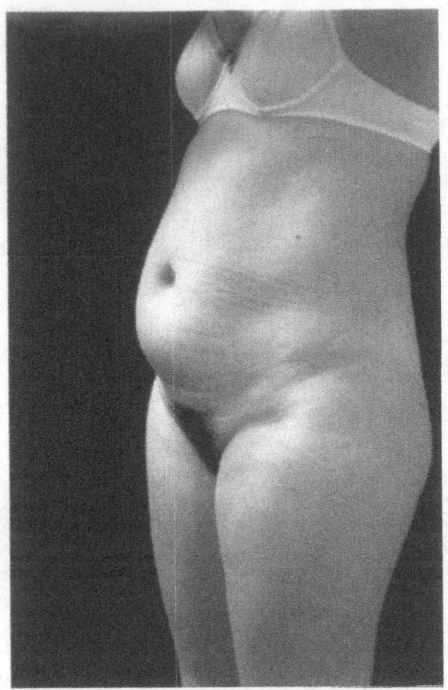
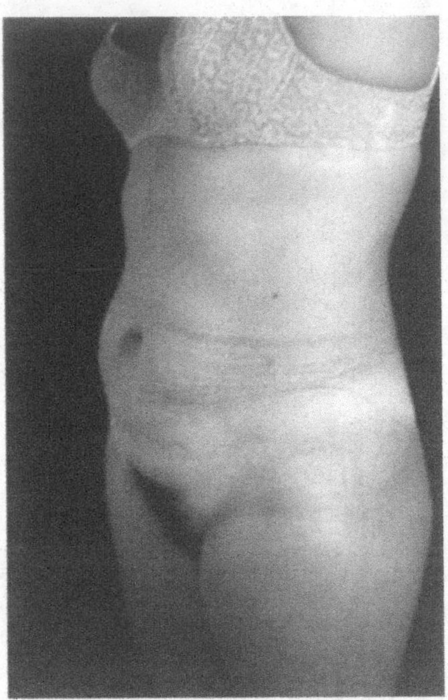

FIGURE 22 Before (left) and after (right) liposculpture of the abdomen.

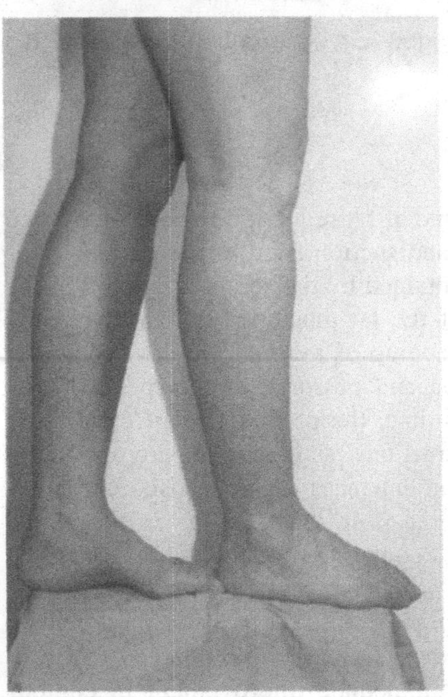
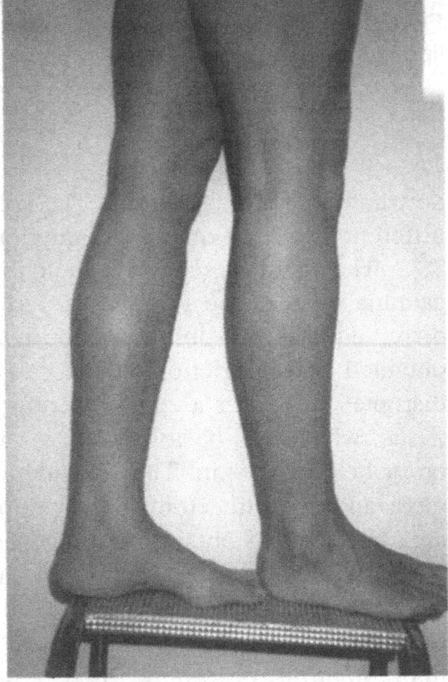

FIGURE 23 Before (left) and after (right) (1 year later) liposculpture of ankles and calves.

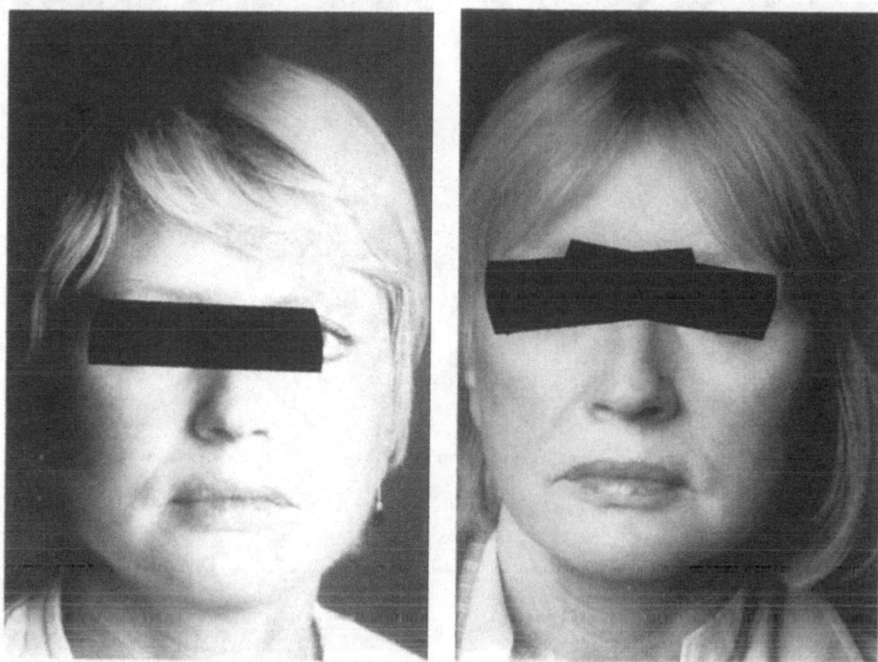

FIGURE 24 Before (left) and after (right) facial liposculpturing.

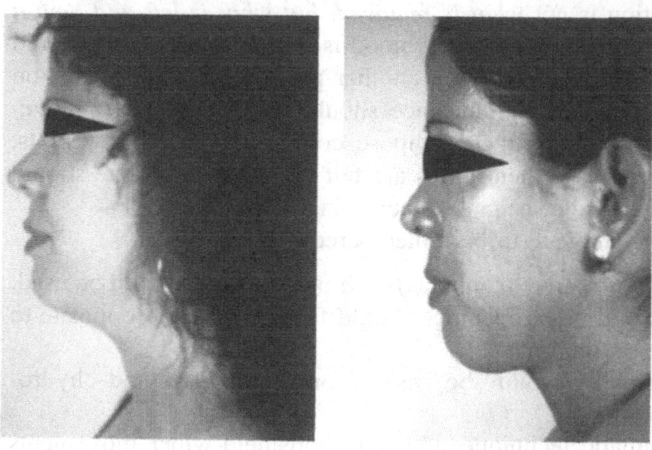

FIGURE 25 Before and after neck liposculpturing.

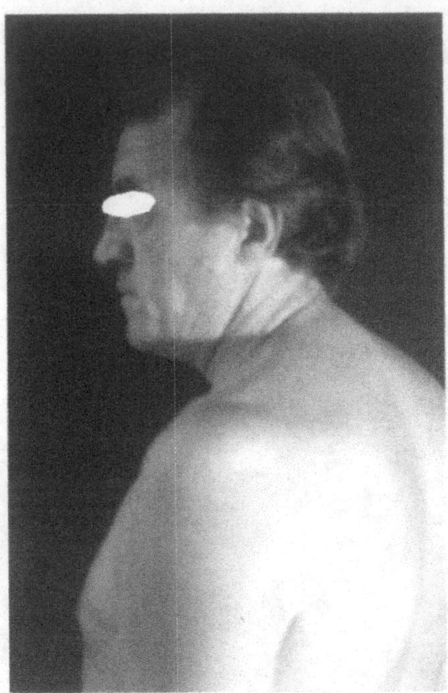
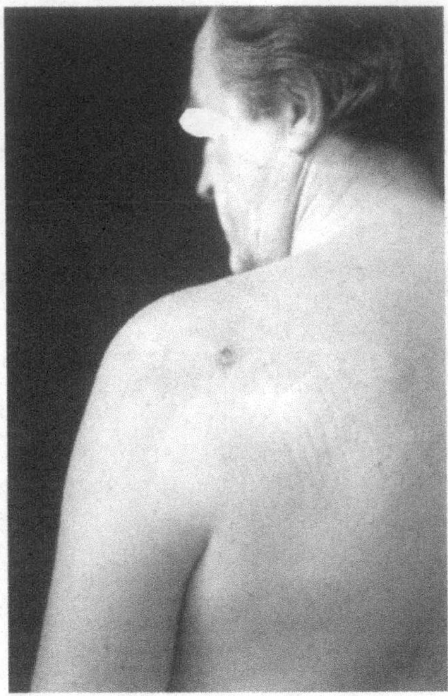

FIGURE 26 Before (left) and after (right) removal of lipoma.

by the primary contraction of elastic fibers and later by the contraction of the underlying fibrous scar tissue.

Surgeons performing liposculpturing should remember that the most important consideration is not *what is removed, but what is left and how it is left* (as in a rhinoplasty). If too much blood is in the aspirate, one should stop working in the area and work on another part of the adiposity or on another adiposity. Under no circumstance should windshield-wiper movements be done, as they will cut the adipose columns that harbor vessels, nerves, and lymph vessels. When lumps are felt under the skin, one should work on them with a smaller cannula (decreasing work).

The following points are to be remembered:

1. Small lipodissectors (cannulas) with one opening should be used.
2. Blunt tip and blunt openings should face downward (opposite to the scale on the syringe).
3. The syringe should be used for extraction and hydrocryodissection.
4. An atraumatic technique with no windshield-wiper movements should always be used.

5. Tunnels should be fan-shaped, starting from the puncture wound.
6. Dissection should be blunt and deep, using the direct approach and puncturing with an ice pick.
7. Crisscrossing (tunnels and fat columns, lattice work) should be done. Two or more approaches can be used.
8. The left hand should direct the operation.
9. Peripheral mesh undermining should be performed when necessary.
10. Remodeling and immobilizing should be done.
11. Grafting the neighboring depressed areas has to be considered sometimes.

Cautions in Liposculpturing

The following cautions should be kept in mind: (1) never use sharp cannulas; (2) the opening should always look down opposite to the scale of the syringe; (3) never do windshield-wiper movements; and (4) decreasing work may be useful in certain circumstances; i.e., the use of a smaller cannula after a larger one has been used. Asepsy is very important. The incision is minor but the wound is major.

Pushing the cannula below the skin and waiting, without moving it, does not remove fat; when using a suction machine or syringe, it is necessary to move the syringe in the fat to see the fat flow in the syringe or in the tube. This is why liposuction is not a good term for the procedure. Lipoextraction is a more accurate word. Lipoextraction carried out artistically is liposculpturing. Liposuction makes one think of a passive act without possible complications, whereas liposculpturing makes one think of an active act with possible complications.

Larger diameter cannulas produce more damage to the fat. A large contour defect can be created very rapidly and is difficult to treat. Smaller cannulas (3 or 4 mm in external diameter) are advised. Because 1 cm of fat has to be left below the skin, all contour defects, such as cottage cheese deformity, can be treated later in a separate procedure (e.g., cutting the subcutaneous connections with a 14-gauge needle and grafting a few cubic centimeters of autologous fat) or superficial liposculpturing. Superficial liposculpturing with a small cannula (2 mm) can be performed during the main procedure if necessary.

Complications

It has been said that there are complications but many errors in liposculpture. When using the syringe cannula technique many complications are complications of "beginners." All "unpleasant events" of anesthesia (general, epidural, or local) can be seen but are rare. It is the same with surgical complications (hemorrhage, infection, etc.) in trained hands. There is less bleeding, edema, and shock with the syringe during major cases. The complications that we have encountered with the syringe are mostly aesthetic complications (insufficient resection, a resection that is too large or irregular, cutaneous waves due to a bad skin tonicity, and postlipoplasty irregularities). A good selection of candidates and a rigorous technique following a lengthy practical and theoretic training will help avoid most complications.

When treating postlipoplasty irregularities the syringe fat-grafting or the liposhifting technique as described by Ziya Saylan can be used (loosening the fat subcutaneously, shifting the fat externally, and fixating of the fat). As Giorgio Fischer says, "Lipoextraction is easy, liposculpture is difficult."

Results

As the results obtained with the syringe cannula are as good as with other instruments (machine, ultrasonic, powered) and the technique is safer and simpler, we recommend the syringe cannula technique. We should remember that what matters is not what is in our hand, but what is in our head. It is not the instrument which is doing the operation, it is the liposuction surgeon. No instrument can replace talent and experience.

SUMMARY

The use of the syringe is an advance in reduction and incremental liposculpturing. A real democratization in the medicosurgical group has been possible due to the simplification of the equipment. The shock-absorbing action of the syringe makes the operation safer. Excellent results are obtained because one does a perfectly symmetrical work. The syringe is a unit of measurement as this surgery is concerned with volume.

31

Facial Volume Restoration with the Fat Autograft Muscle Injection Technique: Preliminary Experience with a New Technique

Kimberly J. Butterwick
Dermatology Associates
La Jolla, California, U.S.A.

Edward B. Lack
The Center for Liposculpture and Cosmetic Laser Surgery
Chicago, Illinois, U.S.A.

A relatively new concept in rejuvenation of the aging face is replacement of soft tissue volume, not simply under specific rhytids and furrows, but full face volume restoration [1]. As one ages, volume diminishes around the eyes, the perioral regions, the cheeks, and the mandibular areas with flattening of the natural arcs of fullness about the face [2] (Fig. 1). This loss of soft tissue volume cannot be corrected with rhytidectomy or laser resurfacing. Fat augmentation has been recommended to restore youthful fullness with good results [3,4]. However, longevity and symmetry of fat augmentation have been problematic [5]. In addition, prolonged edema for months has limited patient acceptance when large volumes are replaced. In order to minimize downtime for patients, multiple sessions with small volumes of frozen fat have been recommended [6,7]. A new method for facial volume restoration with adipose tissue that potentially circumvents these problems

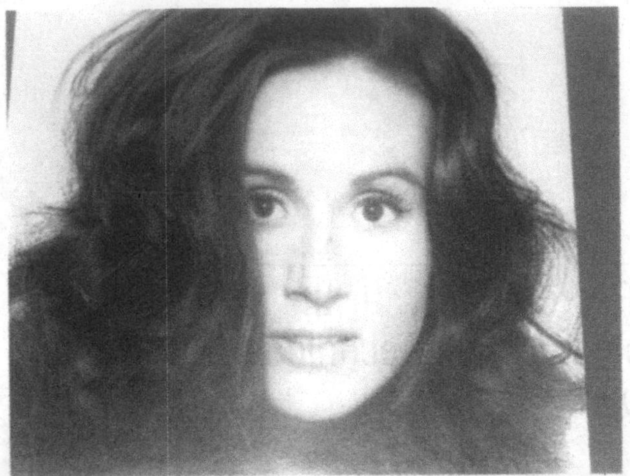

(a)

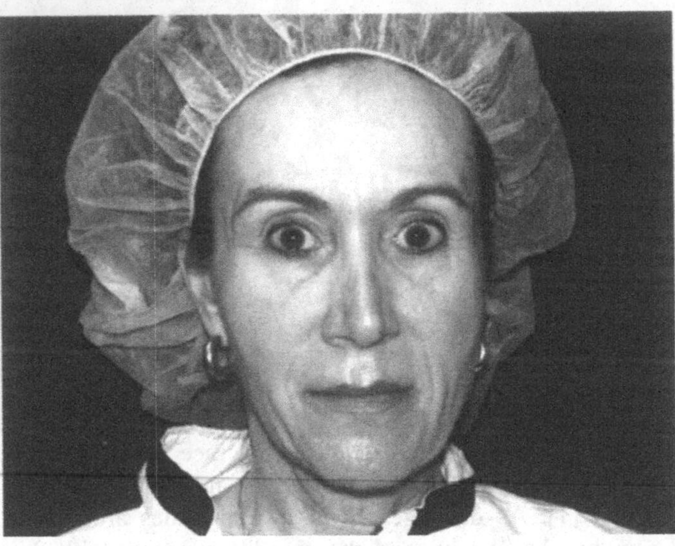

(b)

FIGURE 1 (a) Patient as she appeared 30 years prior to her evaluation. (b) A 63-year-old patient. Note loss of volume in the perioribital and perioral regions. The temples, cheeks, and mandibular regions also demonstrate volume loss.

is known as fat autograft muscle injection (FAMI). With this technique, adipose tissue is injected within or adjacent to the facial expression muscles to restore facial fullness and optimize longevity of the grafted tissue. Downtime for patients has been reduced to 5–7 days.

EVOLUTION OF THE FAMI TECHNIQUE

The FAMI technique was developed by French plastic surgeon and anatomist Roger E. Amar [8]. The French have long been pioneers not only in liposuction, but in fat augmentation as well. Illouz revived interest in fat augmentation in the early 1980s with new instrumentation and techniques [9]. Fournier introduced liposuction and lipoaugmentation by the syringe technique [10]. Amar was further influenced by Coleman's work in the early 1990s on Lipostructure [11]. Coleman is credited with the concept of three-dimensional full-face volume replacement with small "parcels" of fat injected in multiple planes in the subcutaneous fat. He reasoned that small parcels of fat had the best chance of developing a blood supply and surviving, in contrast to the technique of overcorrecting 30 to 50% as was then popular. In 1996 a pivotal study was published by GuerroSantos, who demonstrated 5-year survival of fat in rat muscle [12]. Amar's background in anatomy and cervical muscle lifting [13] combined with this new knowledge of long-term survival of fat within the muscle inspired him to attempt fat injections within the facial expression muscles. He reported 3-year survival of fat in 1999 and has now reported 5-year survival of fat within the facial expression muscles [14]. The FAMI technique was introduced in the United States in February 2001.

THEORY

The FAMI technique is based on two premises. First, that the volume lost during aging involves atrophy of not only fat but muscle and bone as well. The second premise is that transplanted fat survives best next to muscle.

Atrophy of fat, muscle, and bone is a well-documented aspect of the aging process. Even as early as 1893, Neuber, the first to describe fat augmentation in the face, noted loss of both fat and muscle in his dissections of the face [15]. Gonzales Ulloa described atrophic changes of the senile face, primarily in the subcutaneous plane [16]. Berman noted three types of subcutaneous fat in the face, all of which atrophy over time, superficial and deep subcutaneous fat and a distinct type of perimuscular fat [17]. Sarcopenia, the involuntary atrophy of all skeletal muscles with aging, has been well described in the literature [18–20]. It is a natural process that exists in essentially all older individuals [18]. Loss of bone and dental structures has also been documented as part of the aging process [21–26] and recognized in the plastic surgery literature [27].

There is ample evidence that fat survives optimally near muscle. Nguyen demonstrated in 1990 that muscle was the ideal recipient site when autologous fat was injected into rats [28]. At 9 months, fat injected into the subcutaneous plane was completely absorbed and the only site in which autologous fat remained was that injected in the muscle. GuerroSantos's study in 1996 demonstrated 5-year survival in rat muscle as described. He further found that the muscle thickness continued to increase for 6 months following fat grafting within the muscle. This may explain why fat injection into muscles has been helpful in other fields of medicine. In 1994 Zaretsky used fat to augment vocal cord muscle, noting improved muscle function after fat injections [29]. This work in otolaryngology has been collaborated by others [30,31]. Fat injection into muscle has also been used in urology to augment the sphincter tone of the bladder neck muscle [32]. The rationale of transplanting small quantities of fat in contact with well-vascularized tissue has been confirmed by many histologic studies [33–35]. A survey of 37 experienced cosmetic surgeons further found that 52% reported the best survival when fat was injected next to muscle versus other locations [36]. Fulton recommends fat augmentation into muscle "wherever muscle is available" [37]. Ultimately, in the FAMI technique, fat implantation hypertrophies the vectors of the muscles of facial expression. This duplicates the contour and support of these muscles in youth, restoring normal volume to the cosmetic units of the face.

INDICATIONS

The FAMI procedure involves injection of autologous fat in or near the muscles of facial expression. Because it parallels the blood supply, trauma is minimized and, as described, survival of the fat is optimized. The goals of this technique are seen in Table 1.

Ideal candidates are those with SMAS integrity but pan-facial volume loss. These patients are usually ages 30–50. The FAMI procedure is also ideal for postrhytidectomy patients, who are generally ages 45–70. These

Table 1 Goals of the FAMI Technique

- Restore youthful projections of the aging face
- Restore continuity of cosmetic units and jawline
- Support free margins of the face
- Restore aesthetic proportions

patients in particular want to avoid a pulled or stretched appearance with second or third lifting procedures. Localized volume loss in areas such as the lips, tear trough deformity, nasolabial folds, and chin and perioral areas is also an indication for FAMI. This technique is not used to directly fill holes or valleys, but rather to restore the volume surrounding these defects. In restoring the natural projections of the face, the FAMI procedure transforms these defects to the smooth attractive contours of youth.

Poor candidates for the FAMI procedure are those with excess SMAS laxity, those with exaggerated nasolabial folds, and those with a ptotic cheek merging with a ptotic neck. These patients would be better served with rhytidectomy. In addition, patients with significant superficial rhytids (Glogau's types III–IV) are likely to be better candidates for facial resurfacing.

PREOPERATIVE EVALUATION

At the initial consultation, patients are advised to bring photographs of themselves 10 to 20 years prior. A digital photograph is then taken at the consultation of the patient which can be compared to the earlier photographs. The loss of volume in particular areas, as well as the expected results, can be demonstrated and discussed with the patient. The fact that this is a new technique is discussed with the patient and therefore long-term results cannot be guaranteed. Some patients may wish to store frozen fat for later touch-ups as needed. Most patients prefer this option of freezing additional fat in the event they want larger lips or subtle changes. They find it comforting that adjustments and fine tuning are readily available, despite being informed that the longevity of frozen fat is under debate [38].

The preoperative evaluation also includes a second pre-op visit during which a history and physical are performed, instructions reviewed, and consents signed. The patient is further instructed to avoid aspirin, nonsteroidal anti-inflammatory agents, and other anticoagulants (herbal formulas, vitamin E, etc.) for 10 days to 2 weeks prior to the procedure. A preoperative antibiotic is prescribed to start the day before surgery.

PROCEDURE

Harvesting

The preferred donor site is generally the medial knee. This site is relatively resistant to changes in weight, either weight loss or gain. The outer thigh is similarly suitable for harvesting. The fibro-fatty tissue in the abdomen is less suitable for grafting in most individuals but could be used in those with central adiposity. The donor site is prepped and draped in a sterile fashion.

The standard Klein tumescent solution is then infiltrated into the donor site. Dr. Amar prefers to infiltrate around the perimeter of the donor tissue, leaving the donor cells relatively untouched by lidocaine, which has been shown to affect fat cell viability [39]. Harvesting is performed in a sterile fashion with a harvesting cannula attached to a 10-cc syringe with hand-held low-vacuum pressure. Six- to 12-cc syringes are filled, capped, and set upright to allow fluid separation. The infranatant fluid is then discarded and the fat is centrifuged sterilely at 3600 rpm for 3 min (Fig. 2). The infranatant and supranatant fractions are removed and the fat is transferred aseptically to 1-cc syringes.

Anesthesia

Most FAMI procedures are performed with regional nerve blocks and supplemented with oral or intramuscular (IM) analgesia. For full-face procedures, some patients have low needle tolerance and prefer the option of intravenous (IV) sedation administered by an anesthesiologist. We typically use lorazepam 1 mg po and low-dose demerol and phenergan im, similarly to our liposuction protocol.

Injection

Specific injection cannulae have been developed for specific muscle groups (Fig. 3). The fat is injected in a retrograde fashion along the length of the

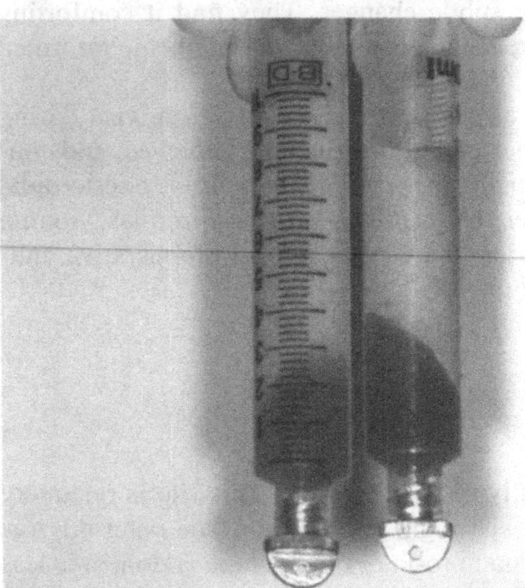

FIGURE 2 Ten-cubic-centimeter syringes after centrifugation. The infranatant fluid will be discarded and the supranatant oil fraction will be decanted.

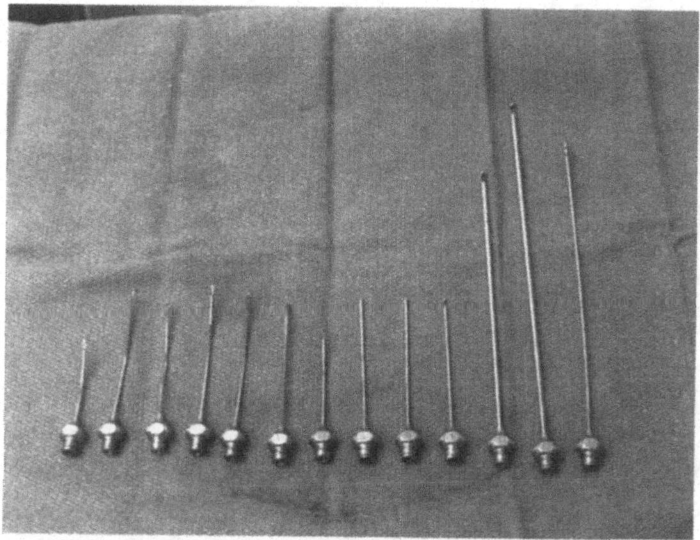

Figure 3 A set of Amar injection and harvesting cannulas.

muscle, usually from the origin to the insertion of that muscle. The muscle bundle is filled with one to three passes of the syringe and generally 1 to 3 ccs per muscle. Each cannula is designed to fit the contour of the skeleton and the curve of the muscle bundle (Figs. 4 and 5). Total volumes range from 3 cc in a small case to 65 cc in larger cases. There are more than 30 facial expression muscles, which occur in three planes, superficial, middle, and deep. Precise placement within the muscle requires detailed knowledge of the origin and insertion of each muscle in the face as well as familiarity with the depth of the muscle planes and the contours of the skull (Fig. 6 and Table 2) [40,41].

POSTOPERATIVE COURSE

Patients experience edema with minimal bruising for 5–7 days. The edema may be significant and patients need to expect this during the first postoperative week. There is essentially no postoperative pain and minimal soreness. There have been no serious complications such as infection or hematoma. There may be temporary palpable lumpiness particularly in the perioral region, which is palpable but not generally visible (Fig. 7). Swelling and subsidence of swelling occurs in a surprisingly symmetric fashion. After the period of initial edema there is gradual symmetric loss of edema, stabilizing at 2–3 months.

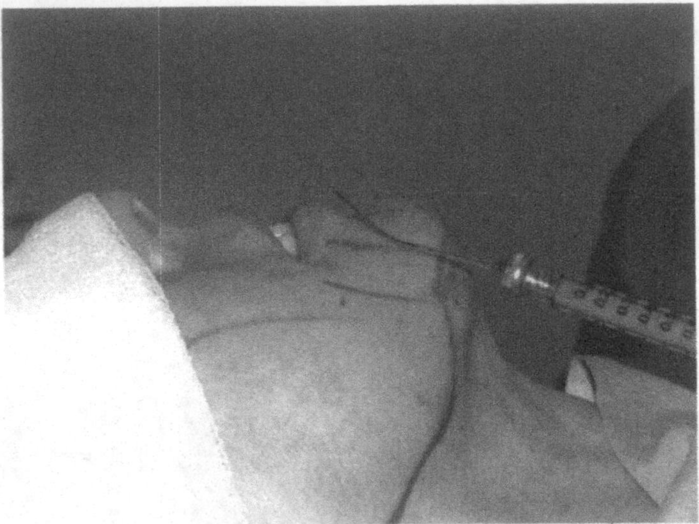

FIGURE 4 Injection cannula no. 7, designed to fit the contour of the depressor labii inferioris muscle as it blends with the fibers of the orbicularis oris muscle.

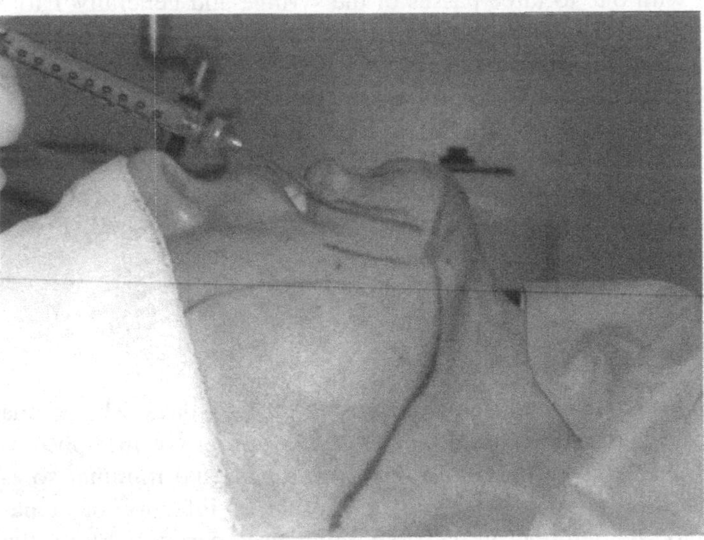

FIGURE 5 Injection cannula no. 3 is for injecting the platysma muscle as a portion of the muscle crosses the mandible and passes to the angle of the mouth.

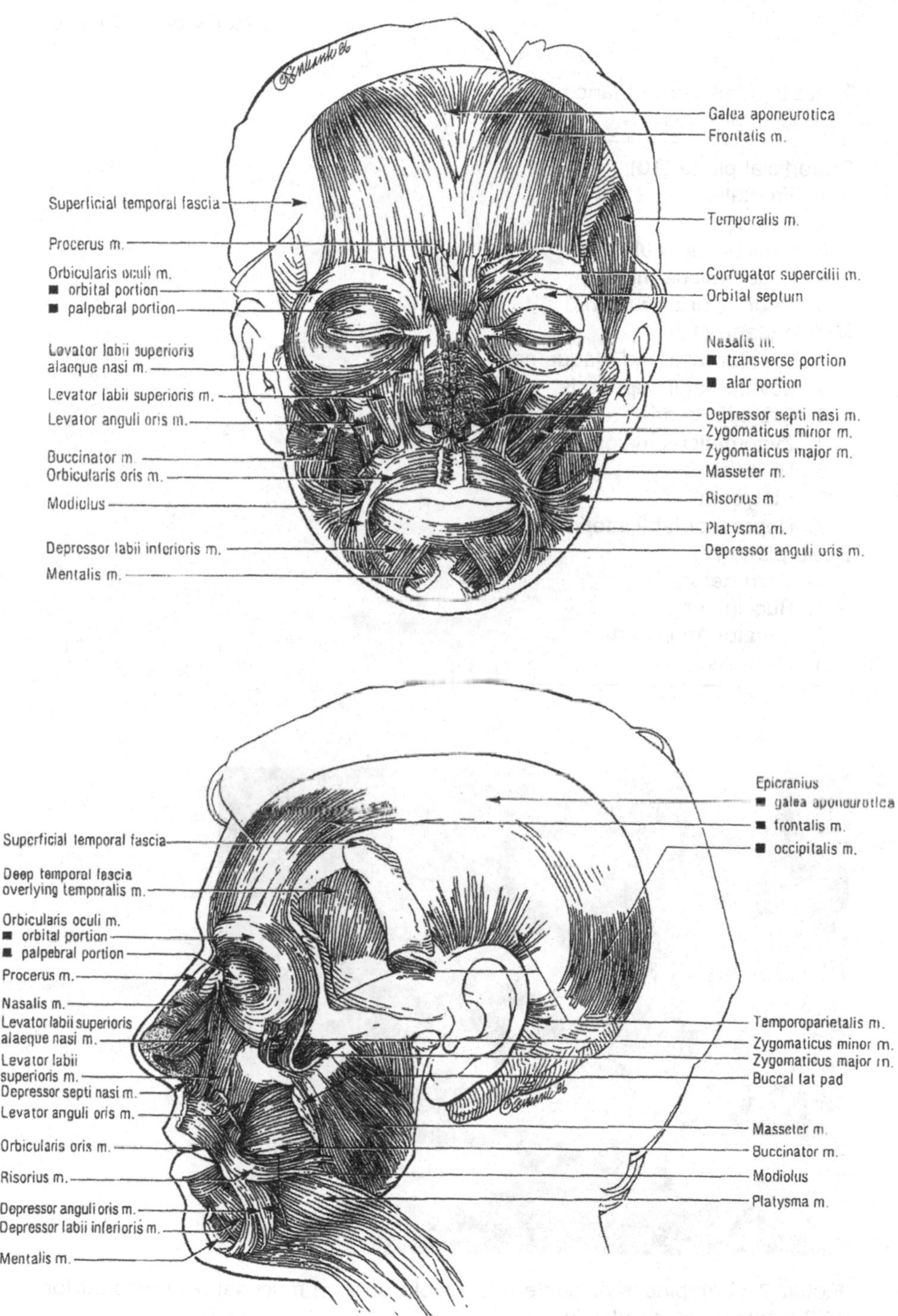

FIGURE 6 Anatomy of the facial musculature. (From Ref. 40 with permission.)

TABLE 2 The Three Planes of the 30 Facial Muscles

Superficial plane (10)
1. Frontalis
2. Procerus
3. Orbicularis oculii
4. Zygomaticus minor
5. Depressor anguli oris
Middle plane (13)
1. Levator labii and alaque nasi
2. Levator labii superioris
3. Orbicularis oris
4. Zygomaticus major
5. Risorius
6. Platysma
7. Depressor labii inferioris
Deep plane (7)
1. Corrugator
2. Buccinator
3. Levator anguli oris
4. Mentalis

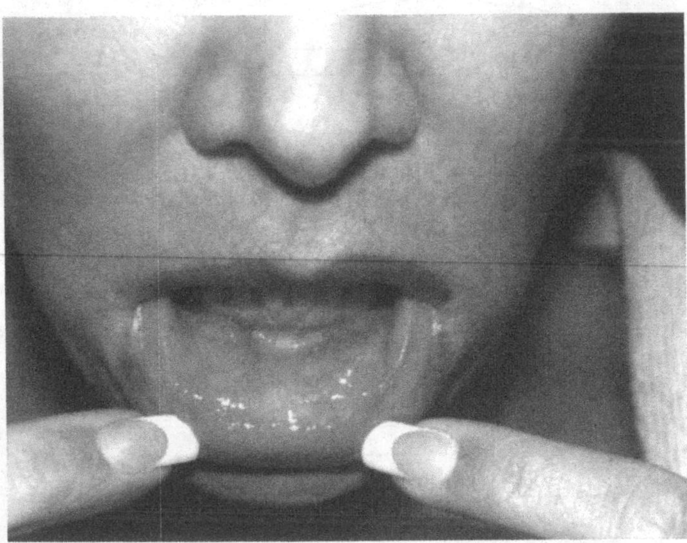

FIGURE 7 Lumpiness palpable and visible only on mucosal side present for 1–2 weeks postoperatively.

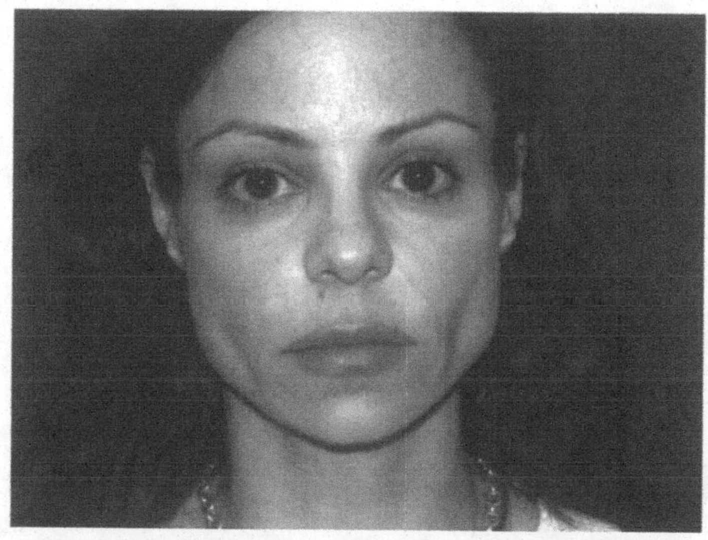

(a)

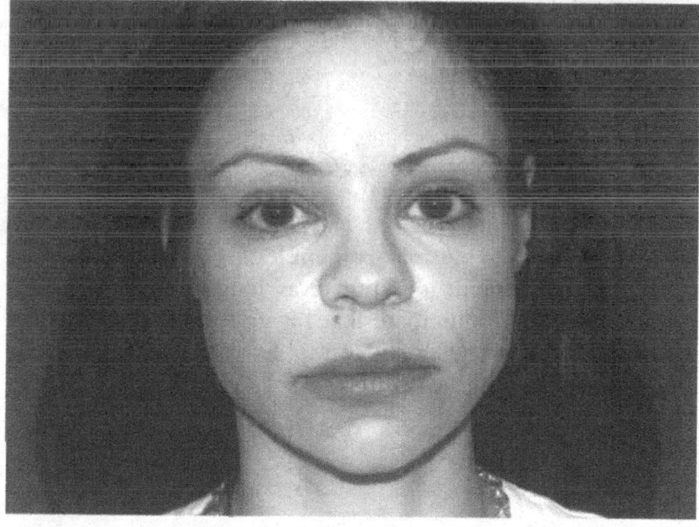

(b)

Figure 8 (a) Pre- and (b) postoperative photograph of patient in her mid-30s. Lower facial musculature injected with 24.7 cc.

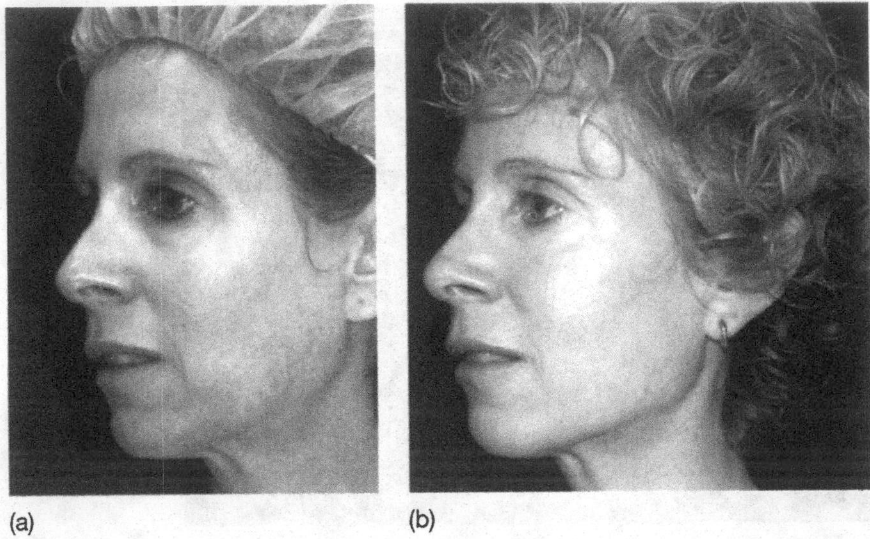

(a) (b)

FIGURE 9 (a) Pre- and (b) postoperative photographs of patient in her mid-40s. The perioral and mentalis muscles were treated with 19.5 ccs to achieve a more aesthetic profile and reduce early jowling.

RESULTS

In our experience performing over 100 FAMI procedures, patients have been uniformly satisfied with the results (Figs. 8 and 9). They are pleased that FAMI does not alter their features but makes them look younger and softer. Longevity of the fat graft is difficult to estimate as long-term data are not available at this time. One could anticipate that fat grafting that persists at 6 months will endure [42]. Amar's data suggest 3- to 5-year long-term survival. We will report our experience with longevity in our patient group in the future.

CONCLUSIONS

Fat autograph muscle injection offers the potential for long-term volume replacement of the aging face. It is a rejuvenating procedure with results that cannot be achieved with current modalities such as facial resurfacing or face-lifting. However, it does not replace the need for these other procedures and all three can be utilized sequentially in a patient's lifetime, depending on his or her needs. Fat autograph muscle injection appears to be a symmetric predictable procedure with high patient satisfaction. It is a precise systematic technique that can be learned and incorporated into a dermatological surgical practice.

REFERENCES

1. Coleman S. Long-term survival of fat transplants: controlled demonstration. Adv Plast Surg 1995; 19:421–425.
2. Donofrio LM. Fat distribution: a morphologic study of the aging face. Dermatol Surg 2000; 26:1107–1112.
3. Eremia S, Newman N. Long-term follow-up after autologous fat grafting: analysis of results from 116 patients followed at least 12 months after receiving the last of a minimum of two treatments. Dermatol Surg 2000; 26:1148–1158.
4. Pinski K. Fat transplantation and autlologous collagen: a decade of experience. Am J Cosmet Surg 1999; 16(3):217–224.
5. Markey A, Glogau R. Autologous fat grafting: comparision of techniques. Dermatol Surg 2000; 26:1135–1139.
6. Donofrio LM. Structural autologous lipoaugmentation: a pan-facial technique. Dermatol Surg 2000; 26:1129–1134.
7. Fulton JE, Suarez M. Silverton K, Barnes T. Small volume fat transfer Dermatol Surg 1998; 24:857–865.
8. Amar RE. Microinfiltration adipocytaire (MIA) au niveau de la face, ou restructuration tissulaire par greffe de tissu adipeux. Ann Chir Plast Esthét 1999; 44(6):593–608.
9. Illouz YG. The fat cell "graft," a new technique to fill depressions. Plast Reconstr Surg 1986; 78:122–123.
10. Fournier PF. Facial recontouring with fat grafting. Dermatol Clin 1990; 8(3): 523–537.
11. Coleman SR. Facial recontouring with lipostructure. Clin Plast Surg 1997; 24(2):347–367.
12. GuerreroSantos J, Gonzalez-Mendoza A, Masmela Y, Gonzalez MA, Deos M, Diaz P. Long-term survival of free fat grafts in muscle: an experimental study in rats. Aesthet Plast Surg 1996; 20:403–408.
13. Amar RE. Lifting tri-muscular de la face et du cou. Lifting de l'Orbiculaire, du Platysma et eu (complexe zygomatique). Ann de chir past Fev 1996; 41: 25–36.
14. Amar RE. Fat autograft muscle injection. AACS Annual Meeting, 2002.
15. Neuber F. Fat transplantation. Chir Kongr Verhandl Dsch Gesellch Chir 1893; 20:66.
16. Gonzalez-Ulloa M, Flores F. Senility of the face—basic study to understand its causes and effects. Plast Reconstr Surg 1965; 36:239–246.
17. Berman M. The aging face: a different perspective on pathology and treatment. Am J Cosmet Surg 1998; 15(2):167–172.
18. Roubenoff R, Castaneda C. Sarcopenia—understanding the dynamics of aging muscle. J Am Med Assoc 2001; 286(10):1228–1231.

19. Volpi E, Sheffield-Moore M, Rasmussen BB, Wolfe RR. Basal muscle amino acid kinetics and protein synthesis in healthy young and older men. J Am Med Assoc 2001; 286(10):1206–1212.
20. Lexell J. Human aging, muscle mass, and fiber type composition. J Gerontol 1995; 50:11–16.
21. Whitmore E, Levine MA. Risk factors for reduced skin thickness and bone density: possible clues regarding pathophysiology, prevention, and treatment. J Am Acad Dermatol 1998; 38:248–255.
22. Chappard D, Alexandre Ch, Robert J-M, Riffat G. Relationships between bone and skin atrophies during aging. Acta Anat 1991; 141:239–244.
23. Boyde A, Kingsmill VJ. Age changes in bone. Gerontol 1998; 15(1):25–34.
24. Knapp KM, Blake GM, Spector TD, Fogelman I. Multisite quantitative ultrasound: precision, age- and menopause-related changes, fracture discrimination, and T-score equivalence with dual-energy ray absortiometry. Osteoporos Int 2001; 12(6):456–464.
25. Payne JB, Reinhardt RA, Nummikoski PV, Patil KD. Longitudinal alveolar bone loss in postmenopausal osteoporotic/osteopenic women. Osteoporos Int 1999; 10(1):34–40.
26. Morse DR. Age-related changes of the dental pulp complex and their relationship to systemic aging. Oral Surg Oral Med Oral Pathol 1991; 72(6):721–745.
27. Mittleman H. The anatomy of the aging mandible and its importance to facelift surgery. Facial Plast Surg Clin N Am 1994; 2(3):301–309.
28. Nguyen A, Pasyk KA, Bouvier TN, Hassett CA, Argenta LC. Comparative study of survival of autologous adipose tissue taken and transplanted by different techniques. Plas Reconstr Surg 1990; 378–386.
29. Zaretsky LS, Shindo ML, deTar M, Rice DH. Autologous fat injection for vocal fold paralysis: long-term histologic evaluation. Ann Otol Rhinol Laryngol 1995; 104(1):1–4.
30. Mikaelian DO, Lowry LD, Sataloff RT. Lipoinjection for unilateral vocal cord paralysis. Laryngoscope 1991; 101:465–468.
31. Bauer CA, Valentino J, Hoffman HT. Long term result of vocal cord augmentation with autogenous fat. Ann Otol Rhinol Laryngol 1995; 104:871–874.
32. Gonzalez de Garibay AS, Castillo Jimeno JM, Villaneuva Perex I et al. Treatment of urinary stress incontinence using paraurethral injection of autologous fat. Arch Esp Urol 1991; 44:595–600.
33. Niechajev I, Sevuk O. Long term results of fat transplantation: clinical and histologic studies. Plast Reconstr Surg 1994; 94:496–506.
34. Peer LA. Transplantation of Tissues. Baltimore: Williams & Wilkins.
35. Carpaneda CA, Ribeiro MT. Study of the histological alterations and viability of the adipose graft in humans. Aesth Plast Surg 1993; 17:43.
36. Griffin EI. Autologous fat grafting: survey results and analysis. American Academy of Dermatology Annual Meeting, Mar 21, 1999.
37. Fulton JE. Fat transfer: historical perspectives. Am J Cosmet Surg 1999; 16(3): 193–194.
38. Kaminer MS, Omura NE. Autologous fat transplantation. Arch Dermatol 2001; 137(6):812–814.

39. Moore JH Jr, Kolaczynski JW, Morales LM, Considine RV, Pietrzkowski Z, Noto PF, Caro JF. Viability of fat obtained by syringe suction lipectomy: effects of local anesthesia with lidocaine. Aesth Plast Surg 1995; 19:335–339.
40. Salasche SJ, Bernstein G, Senkarik M. Muscles of facial expression. In: Surgical Anatomy of the Skin. Appleton & Lance, 1988:69–87.
41. Gray H. The facial muscles. In: Gross CM, ed. Anatomy of the Human Body. 107th ed. Phildelphia: Lea & Febiger, 1969:382–390.
42. Pinski KS, Roenigk HH. Autlogous fat transplantation: a long term follow-up. J Dermatol Surg Oncol 1992; 18:179–184.

32

Fat Viability Studies

Neil S. Sadick
Weil Medical College of Cornell University
New York, New York, U.S.A.

INTRODUCTION

Long-term adipocyte survival is an achievable goal following lipotransfer. The importance of harvesting and injection techniques as well as adipose tissue characteristics are discussed in the present chapter.

Transplanted autologous adipose tissue is an increasingly popular material for soft tissue augmentation in aesthetic and reconstructive surgery [1–3]. Advances in the technique of liposuction surgery, the relative case of adipose tissue harvesting, and the advance of the antigenic and inflammatory responses from allergenic or alloplastic materials are factors which have increased interest in adipose tissue as a successful filler [4,5]. Although most commonly employed for correcting facial rhytides, fat transplants have also been used for augmentation of congenital defects; scarring diseases such as linear amorphea, lupus erythematosis, and atrophoderma of Pasini and Pierini; and the posttraumatic scars and augmentation of aging hands and breasts [5–12]. Despite the expanding use of transplanted adipose tissue the literature is devoid of objective studies which document the persistence of the grafted material and the time course of resorption.

A review of the literature on human fat transfer with multiple techniques for both harvesting and transplantation reveals a wide range of graft survival from 0 to 8% [14,15]. In animal models prolonged survival of fat transplants has been demonstrated with and without the addition of nutrients such as vitamin E and fetal bovine serum [16–18]. Past studies of assessing adipose viability have been based on histologic studies of evaluation by photography and other imaging techniques [13,18–22]. Major questions asked in studies involving lipotransfer are listed in Table 1.

REGIONAL VARIATIONS OF ADIPOCYTE CONTENT

The fatty acid composition of adipose tissue depends primarily on the type of dietary fat consumed over the previous 2 to 3 years [23]. There are small site-specific differences in fatty acid composition which are useful in a "fingerprint" that may be utilized as a marker of the persistence of transplanted fat—subcutaneous fat from the face, breast, and abdomen has higher concentrations of saturated fatty acids and lower concentrations of monosaturated fatty acids than fat from the gluteal region and lower extremities [24–26]. The cause for these differences is unknown, but has been attributed to temperature-induced modulation of the fluidity (unsaturation) of stored fat or innate-specific differences in the adipocytes (e.g., in selective fatty acid uptake, release or synthesis, or in Δ9 desaturase activity).

TABLE 1 Practical and Theoretical Questions Related to Adipocyte Viability in Lipotransfer

Is low vascularity of the donor site optimal?
Is high vascularity of the recipient site optimal?
Does low-pressure fat aspiration increase adipocyte viability?
Does filtering and washing of harvested adipocytes diminish viability?
Does use of a ≥2-mm cannula for injection minimize adipocyte injury?
Is a multilayered approach to deposition of fat in the recipient site desirable?
Is overcorrection of the recipient site desirable?
Can improved viability of adipocyte be accomplished using dyes?
Does the tumescent technique enhance adipocyte viability?
Does the syringe technique enhance viability as compared to mechanical liposuction?
What is the optimal cannula size for harvesting?
Is there a viability difference between donor sites?
Can adipose tissue be stored for use at a later time and still maintain adipocyte viability?
What is the optimal method of storage?

THEORIES OF PERSISTENCE OF LIPOTRANSFER

There are two theories which have been postulated to explain clinical success after fat transplantation [27–36]. The host replacement theory claims that histiocytes scavenge lipid material and lead to a fibrotic response which may replace adipose tissue [36]. The survival theory postulates that the fat graft tissue survives after the host reaction subsides [37]. The surgically transplanted fat becomes ischemic following transfer into the recipient site. Some cells die, some survive as adipocytes, and others differentiate from preadipocyte cells. After recovery from the transfer process, the preadipocyte cells become functional adipocytes and accumulate fat once the fat graft regains it blood supply from the periphery.

PREVIOUSLY REPORTED STUDIES

The literature is laden with subjective reports of long-term augmentation following fat implantation [27–35]. However, few reports document the scientific basis of this assumption. In a landmark study the author documented the use of site-specific fatty acid patterns of adipose tissue to document the persistence at 2 years of transplanted fat as documented by gas chromatographic analysis after adipose tissue was extracted and examined by the Folch technique utilizing a flame ionization detector and a forced silica column. Although evident in only one of six patients, this study supports the long-term potential of this natural autologous filler (Fig. 1) [38].

Published histologic studies from humans have demonstrated both healthy and fibrous fatty tissue after fat transplant [39–41]. The relative importance of fibrosis versus fat engraftment for the long-term clinical filler effect of autologous transplanted fat remains unknown to date. An in vitro study evaluating the long-term viability of human adipocytes and preadipocytes harvested by a closed-syringe tumescent liposuction technique, such as used in this study, showed that a significant percentage of cells can survive the harvest and thrive in cell culture [42]. A more recent report documented that human adipocytes maintained their viability in culture for up to two months after the closed syringe liposuction harvest [43].

Published histologic studies from humans have demonstrated both healthy and fibrous fatty tissue after fat transplant [39–41]. The relative importance of fibrosis versus fat engraftment for the long-term clinical filler effect of autologous transplanted fat remains unknown to date. An in vitro study evaluating the long-term viability of human adipocytes and preadipocytes harvested by a closed-syringe tumescent liposuction technique showed that a significant percentage of cells can survive the harvest and thrive in cell culture [42]. A more recent report documented that human

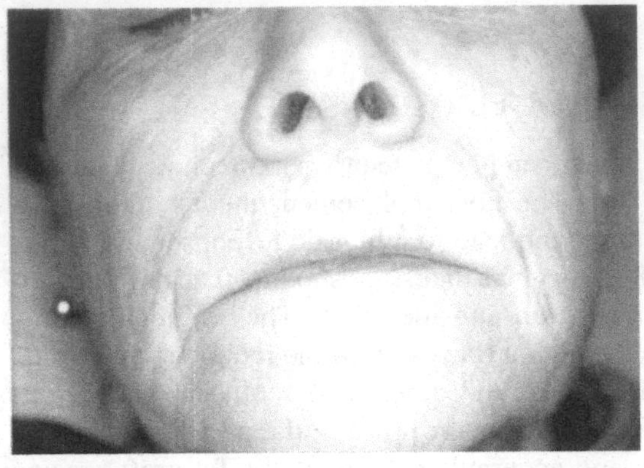

(a)

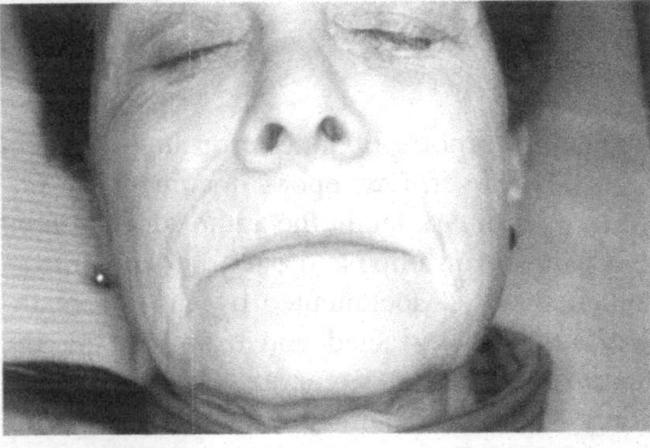

(b)

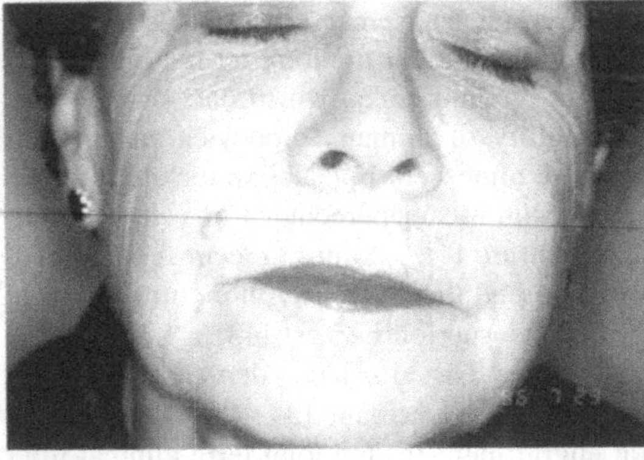

(c)

FIGURE 1 Long-term lipotransfer study. Patient at (a) prelipotransfer, (b) 6 months postlipotransfer, and (c) 12 months postlipotransfer. The patient, of thin genetic constitution, was one of six in the present study who manifested long-term adipocyte survival.

adipocytes maintained their viability in culture for up to 2 months after closed-syringe liposuction harvest [43].

Schuller-Petrovic found living fat cells; some collapsed at 2 weeks after injection [44]. Carapenda studied collagen alterations in adipose tissue autografts to the abdominal subcutaneous fat in patients prior to abdominoplasty. He found a Type I collagen capsule circumscribing the graft in addition to several alterations in the synthesis degradation and remodeling of Type I and Type II collagen within the transplanted tissue. An increased and decreased inflammatory response in a time sequence was shown as well as a shift in the inflammatory process from the peripheral viable region to the central inviable region where small pseudocytes and nonnucleated adipocytes were present [45,46].

Coleman transplanted mechanically disrupted adipocytes and found rounded vacuoles 1 week after the transplantation at the injection site and the intact adipocytes. At 1 month, previous cellular spaces widened and contained sparse lymphocytic infiltrates. A new zone of connective tissue between the reticular dermis and the subcutaneous fat developed [47].

Guerrosantos et al. found that in Wistar rats fat transplanted into subcutaneous tissue was impossible to identify or separate from the already existing fat. Only part of the fat implanted into subcutaneous tissue seemed to survive while fat strips implanted intramuscularly not only survived, but also showed augmentation in size in relation to the initial size of the graft [48].

Other studies have attempted to document the persistence of transplanted fat with imaging techniques. Horb et al. examined the patients for 1 year with magnetic resonance imaging. He noticed a 55% loss at 6 months with regular negligible decreases in volume between 9 and 12 months as documented by the quantitative imaging technology [21]. Goldman et al. used ultrasound to document the retention up to 1 year of transplanted fat in patients with focal depression syndrome (i.e., Romberg's syndrome, Lupus) [22]. Long-term correction of lipodystrophy and coup'de Sabre deformities have also been reported by Glogau utilizing an ultrasound imaging technique.

Harvesting and injection methods may influence the longevity of lipotransfer. Important variables may include syringe and cannula size, anesthesia, degree of overcorrection, frequency of treatments, donor site depth, technique of placement, sample washing, and sterility. McCurdy analyzed fat cell survival clinically and concluded that the following technical characteristics prolonged graft survival: (1) low vascularity of the donor site, (2) high vascularity of the recipient site, (3) low-pressure technique of aspirate of fat, (4) filtered and washed harvested adipocytes, (5) use of ≥2-mm cannula for injection to minimize adipocyte injury, (6) multilayered deposit

Table 2 Studies on Graft Survival and Longevity in Autologous Syringe Fat Transfer

Year	Human/ animal/ *in vitro* study	Anesthesia	Harvesting technique	Fat processing	Reinjection technique	Site of injection
2001	Human (*N* = 6)	0.1% lidocaine with epinephrine	Syringe, 14-gauge	Extraction cannula	16- to 18-gauge needle; overcorrection 30–50%	Subcutaneous
1997	Human (*N* = 176)	Tumescent local anesthesia 0.1% lidocaine with epinephrine	Syringe, 1.5- to 2-mm cannula, or 14-gauge needle	Washing with saline; gravity separation; freezing −20°C	16- to 18-gauge needle; overcorrection 30–50%	Subcutaneous (sc)
1992	Human (*N* = 4)	Local anesthesia 0.5%; lidocaine with epinephrine	Syringe, 3-mm cannula, or 14-gauge needle	Washing with ringer; gravity separation	18-gauge needle; overcorrection	Subcutaneous (sc)
1996	Rats (*N* = 120)	im general	Sharp excision and cutting of graft	None	14-gauge needle, no local anesthesia	Subcutaneous and intramuscularly
1996	Human (*N* = 140)	Peridural block; saline and epinephrine locally	Cannula, 3- to 5 mm	Washing with saline; gravity separation	Cannulas, 3-mm	Subcutaneous deep plane of legs
1990	Human (*N* = 50)	Tumescent local anesthesia, 0.25% lidocaine with epinephrine	Syringe, 14-gauge extraction cannula	No washing because of tumescent fluid	18-gauge needle	Subcutaneous (sc)

Evaluation	Histology	Longevity	Conclusion of authors	Comments
Gas chromatography RAI of fatty acids	None	2 years	Best results in thin individuals	Long-term potential of transplanted fat at 2 years
Clinical, histology	2 weeks after injection; living fat cells, some collapsed	Up to 8 years clinically	Best results in facial hemiatrophy, scars and posttraumatic atrophy; living fat cells even after defrosting, demonstrated by trypan blue staining; method of choice	Important study with high number of documented patients with different indications; good description of technique; long documented follow-up; important: high number of viable cells even after defrosting
Clinical	None	"Significant augmentation persists" after 3 years; multiple reinjections; persistence of 30–50% each session	Method of choice	Clinical observation with good description of technique
Histology	im injection: survival of all of the injected adipocytes. sc injection: survival of part of the graft; very difficult to identify or separate from preexisting fat, lymphocyte migration and strong fibrotic process	im injection: very good survival after 3, 6, 9, and 12 months. sc: failure of most adipocytes to survive transplantation	Good survival in muscle because of higher vascularity than in subcutaneous tissue	Large animal study with sufficiency high numbers; animal studies may not be fully comparable with human skin, though
Clinical observation	None	"About 80%" persistence of fat as observed over 5 years	Low absorption rate because leg is not highly vascularized	Good description of technique; other studies have shown that low absorption rates are due to intramuscular injection, not high vascularization
Clinical observation	None	6 months: substantial degree of correction. 3 years: at least 50% augmentation remaining	Treatment of choice for augmentation of facial lines	Good description of technique

Table 2 Continued

Year	Human/ animal/ *in vitro* study	Anesthesia	Harvesting technique	Fat processing	Reinjection technique	Site of injection
1990	Human ($N = 50$)	Tumescent local anesthesia 0.25% lidocaine with epinephrine	Syringe, 14-gauge extraction cannula	No washing because of tumescent fluid	18-gauge needle	Subcutaneous (sc)
1990	Human ($N = 25$)	Tumescent local anesthesia 0.07% lidocaine with epinephrine	Syringe, 14-gauge blunt minicannula	No washing; gravity separation	With trocar, diameter not stated	Deep subcutaneous
1993	Human ($N = 4$)	Tumescent local anesthesia 0.05% lidocaine with epinephrine	Syringe, 14-gauge needle	Centrifuge at 1000 rpm for 1 min; mechanical disruption of cell walls	25-gauge needle	Intradermal
1996	Human (N = not stated)	General anesthesia	Suction machine and syringe, cannulas 5–8 mm	Not stated	Not stated	Subcutaneous (sc)
1990	Human ($N = 43$)	Dermis: local anesthesia; subcutis: chilling with saline	Syringe, 14-gauge needle	Washing with saline	14-gauge needle; side-by-side comparison of reinjected fat vs. Zyplast	Subcutaneous (sc)

Evaluation	Histology	Longevity	Conclusion of authors	Comments
Clinical observation	None	6 months: substantial degree of correction; 3 years: at least 50% augmentation remaining	Treatment of choice for augmentation of facial lines	Good description of technique
Clinical observation	None	Not exactly determined	"Gratifying"	Good description of technique
Hydroxyprolene to determine collagen content in graft; Western blot for collagen differentiation; histology after removal	At 1 week: no intact injected adipocytes; vacuoles (microcysts). At 1 month: new zone of fibrous tissue at junction reticular dermis, sc; at 3 months: condensed fibrotic scar, mild dermal fibrosis, dermal expansion	"Longevity of results rivals Zyplast"; longevity of cells is short; these are replaced by fibrosis	Cells do not survive intended with this technique. Augmentation effect through dermal fibrosis. Safe, effective, reproducible. Animal models may not be comparable to the human skin	Thorough histologic examinations; very good demonstration of technique; cell walls in this technique are purposely destroyed after harvest
Clinical observation	None	Not stated exactly; variable	Variable and unpredictable longevity; improvement of overlying skin; fat graft has place in contour correction	No important data concerning patients or technique are given; largest extraction cannulas used
Clinical observation and photographically using 3-dimensional optical profilometry of replica surface from 18 subjects	None	Longevity determined after 3, 5, and 12 months; ~75% of correction lost after 6 months; 22% of collagen-treated subjects maintained at least 30% of correction after 1 year; 44% of fat augmented subjects maintained at least 30% correction after 1 year		

TABLE 2 Continued

Year	Human/ animal/ *in vitro* study	Anesthesia	Harvesting technique	Fat processing	Reinjection technique	Site of injection
1992	Human (*N* = 43)	Local anesthesia	Suction machine with filter trap; 3-mm blunt cannula	No washing; gravitational pooling	15-gauge and 18-gauge needles	Subcutaneous (sc)
1996	Human (*N* = 45)	Not stated; probably general anesthesia	Suction machine and syringe; 3- to 5-mm one- to three-hole cannulas	Washing with saline; anticoagulant agent; centrifugation 1000 rpm, 5 min	Not applicable	Not applicable
1998	Human (*N* = 40)	General anesthesia	Suction machine and syringe, vacuum between 500 and 500 mmHg; liposuction cannula 4 mm	Addition of saline solution and collagenase; centrifuge 600 rpm, 1 min	Not applicable	Not applicable
1991	Human (*N* = 53)	Local anesthesia with hyaluronidase	Suction machine	Washing with Ringer's solution	Large lumen cannula	Subcutaneous (sc); injection in facial defects

Evaluation	Histology	Longevity	Conclusion of authors	Comments
Clinical observation and patient assessment questionnaire	None	Longevity determined after 3, 6, 9, and 12 months; depending on underlying condition, remaining augmentation was between 30 and 50% at 12 months with linear morphea having the least amount of fat resorption	Thigh is ideal donor site; autologous fat transplantation is safe and effective; longevity as clinically and patient assessed, is satisfactory	Long follow-up, some cases 48 months; results are discussed as "graft viability," a term that may only be used after histologic assessment
Not applicable	H&E staining; demonstration of all cellular, humoral and structural components of fat; tissue damage suggested by free fat, hemoglobin, and clots	Not applicable	Tissue damage after both machine and syringe harvesting leads to release of inflammation mediators. Washing eliminates free fat and blood, thus decreasing inflammatory response to graft	Thorough report of technique and negative pressures used; tumescent anesthesia would help to decrease tissue trauma and blood in aspirate in the first place
Not applicable	Sudan black staining, red blood cell counter	Not applicable	Live fat cells from syringe harvest on average: 15700/mm^3; live fat cell from cannula harvest: 14000/mm^3; more blood means less living adipocytes	Novaes developed a technique that quantifies the number of fat cells in 1 ml of injection; Sudan stains nonruptured fat cells; the high numbers per milliliter prove the theories of complete damage of suctioned fat wrong
Magnetic resonance imaging at 1 day preoperatively, 5, 12 days, and 3, 6, 9, and 12 months	Aspirated cells: 40% had defective cell membranes, without hyaluronidase 50%	Volume loss at 3 months 49%, at 6 months 55%, at 9 months 55%, at 12 months (10 patients) 55%	Autogenous fat transplantation after liposuction only suitable for repair of small soft tissue defects. Individual deposits should not exceed 1 ml	MRI provides objective evaluation of volume loss with an error of 5%

TABLE 2 Continued

Year	Human/ animal/ *in vitro* study	Anesthesia	Harvesting technique	Fat processing	Reinjection technique	Site of injection
1993	Animal; New Zealand white rabbit ($N = 16$)	No local anesthesia	14-gauge needle	No washing	14-gauge needle	To subcutaneous pockets in the ear
1994	Human ($N = 15$)	Local anesthesia, lidocaine	20-ml syringe and liposuction 3-mm cannula	Not applicable	Not applicable	Not applicable
1995	Human ($N = 2$)	0.5% lidocaine with 1:200,000 epinephrine	Syringe, three-holed blunt-tipped cannula	No washing; gravity separation	16-gauge needle	Subcutaneous (sc)

of fat, and (7) overcorrection of the recipient site [43]. Schiffman found that the size of the cannulae used to remove fat did not significantly affect fat cell integrity [49]. Brandon et al. found that the type of anesthesia, needle shape, and suctioning technique did not influence fat survival [50]. Takasu et al. found that freezing of fat for variable periods of time did not improve survival [51,52]. No prospective studies have been performed to establish a clear preferred donor site, although it is likely that the choice of donor site location is important [53–55].

Differing dilutions of tumescent anesthesia have been used with or without epinephrine vasoconstriction versus increased adipocyte metabo-

Evaluation	Histology	Longevity	Conclusion of authors	Comments
Histology	Fibrous connective tissue was more prevalent in suctioned fat grafts compared to surgically removed fat grafts	At 9 months: 42.2% of surgically excised fat shows maintenance of volume compared to 31.6% of suction-assisted fat grafts	Both suctioned and surgically removed fat grafts undergo significant volume reduction	Depending on point of view, a volume maintenance of 31.6% after 9 months in transplantation into a sc pocket may be regarded as fairly high. Animal models may not be comparable to human skin
Chemical assay	None	Not applicable	Isolated adipocytes remained highly viable, as evidenced by glucose transport under both basal and maximal insulin-stimulated conditions	Liposuction minicannula yields highly viable adipocytes
Clinical (photography)	None	More than 6 years clinically	Very good longevity of fat grafts when placing small amounts of fatty tissue in multiple tunnels; emphasis on proper injection technique and good primary correction	Description of the Fournier technique with photodocumentation of very good longevity in two cases

lism. The role of bicarbonate in this setting is unclear. An approximate ratio of 5:1 of anesthetic infiltrate to the desired volume of harvested fat is used. Waiting for 15–20 min to allow for skin blanching to occur (where epinephrine has been used) to limit the amount of blood contaminant is of import. A small nick with a No-Kor needle or microblade over an anesthetized wheal of the donor area will allow for relatively atraumatic entry of the harvesting needle [56].

In terms of fat separation, if the surgeon chooses to wash the fat, Ringer's lactate rather than saline is the preferred lavage solution as previous studies have shown less stimulation of the glucose metabolism pathway utilizing the former. If centrifugation is performed, it has been shown that this must be formed with care in order to minimize the changes of torsional damage to the adipocytes [57,58].

No correlation can be found between survival of fat harvested with syringe or machine aspiration. A syringe produces a relative vacuum of about −0.6 atm. Only if maximum negative pressure of −0.95 atm in machine aspiration is applied may partial breakage and vaporization of fatty tissue occurs. The diameter of the fat cells is mechanically distended and is larger than in lipocytes extracted at −0.5 atm [59].

No correlation can be found between survival of fat harvested with a liposuction cannula versus 14-gauge needle. Isolated adipocytes remain highly visible after harvesting with a 3-mm liposuction cannula, as evidenced by glucose transport assays, and may even be used for metabolic studies in obese patients [60].

Sudan black stain may be used to demonstrate viable fat cells. An average of 14.00 and 15.28 live fat cells at 1 mm for cannula and syringe harvesting have been shown in a respective study conducted by Novas et al. [61]. Continuous suction leads to a constantly reduced maximum suction pressure if the maximum suction pressure of the mechanical aspirator never exceeds −8 bar. Reduced flux during aspiration leads to reduced adipocyte tissue trauma and increased viability [62]. Most studies state that blood in transplanted fat accelerates degradation of transplanted fat [63–65].

Slow freezing of the tissue to −20°C shortly after harvesting has no harmful effect on the adipocytes. Studies have shown that there are a high number of viable adipocytes, whereas flash freezing may be used to destroy adipocytes as in lipocytic dermal augmentation [66]. A storing period of up to 6 months has been recommended. Skin freezing to −20°C is preferable if one wants to transplant viable adipocytes, whereas flash freezing may be used to destroy adipocytes as in lipocytic dermal augmentation [66]. Most surgeons use 14- to 25-gauge needles for reinjection depending on harvesting and processing techniques. Studies have shown no correlation between the diameter of the needle and longevity of correction. Short time intervals of recycling for 4 to 12 weeks and many repeat treatments have been shown to lead to perpetuation of the inflammatory reaction at the site of injection [62]. Finally Brandon has stated that body fatness and physical fitness may influence the survival rate of transplanted fat. He theorized that smaller fat cells with higher quantities of collagen surrounding the globules decrease the trauma during fat transfer and thus improve the quality of the graft once it reaches the recipient site [50]. This is in concert with the study of Sadick et al. where the patient with the longest retention of fat at 2 years had the thinnest genetic constitution [38]. A summation of many of the above-mentioned studies is presented in Table 2.

CONCLUSIONS

The present chapter substantiates the fact that long-term success of fat transplantation has not been fully elucidated but is certainly potentially achievable. Further studies elucidating the role of harvesting and implantation variables and adipose tissue characteristics are in progress. These studies will likely provide greater insight into the mechanism of adipocyte retention observed by the practicing cosmetic surgeon.

REFERENCES

1. Gurney CE. Studies on the fate of free transplants of fat. Proc Staff Meet Mayo Clin 1937; 12:317.
2. Smith V. Morphological studies of human subcutaneous adipose tissue in vitro. Anat Rec 1971; 169:97.
3. Pinski KS. Fat transplantation autologous collagen: a decade of experience. Am J Cosmet Surg 1999; 16:217–223.
4. Peer LA. Loss of weight and volume in human fat grafts. Plast Reconstr Surg 1950; 5:217.
5. Ersek RA. Transplantation of purified autologous fat: a 3-year follow-up is disappointing. Plast Reconstr Surg 1991; 87:219.
6. Klein JA. The tumescent technique for liposuction surgery. Am J Cosmet Surg 1987; 4:263–267.
7. Moskowicz L. Treatment of facial hemiatrophy by transplantation of fat tissues. Med Clin 1930; 26:1172.
8. Pinski KS, Roenigk HH. Autologous fat transplantation: long term follow-up. J Dermatol Surg Oncol 1992; 18:179–184.
9. Charjchir A. Liposuction fat grafts and face wrinkles. Adv Plast Surg 1986; 10:115–121.
10. Coleman SR. Facial recontouring with lipoculture. Clinics Plast Surg 1997; 24: 347–367.
11. Vita VT. Lipoinjection and aging hands. Am J Cosmet Surg 1989; 6:27–32.
12. Hin LC. Syringe liposuction with immediate lipotransplantation. Am J Cosmet Surg 1985; 5:243–248.
13. Glogau R. Microlipoinjection: autologous fat grafting. Arch Dermatol 1988; 124:1343–1350.
14. Gurney CE. Experimental study of the behavior of free fat transplants. Surg 1938; 3:680.
15. Gurney CE. Studies on the fate of free transplants of fat. Proc Staff Meet Mayo Clinic 1937; 12:317.
16. Ullmann Y, Hyams M, Ramon Y et al. Enhancing the survival of aspirated human fat injected in nude mice. Plast Reconstr Surg 1998; 101:1940–1944.
17. Moscana R, Shoshanzolichtig H et al. Viability of adipose tissue injected and treated by different methods: an experimental study in the fats. Ann Plast Surg 1994; 33:500–506.

18. Niechajev J, Secuk O. Long-term results of fat transplantation: clinical and histologic studies. Plastic Reconstr Surg 1994; 94:490–506.
19. Carpareta C. Percentage of graft viability versus injection of volume in adipose autotransplant. Adv Plast Surg 1994; 18:16–19.
20. Coleman SR. Long-term survival of fat transplants controlled demonstrations. Aesth Plast Surg 1995; 19:421–423.
21. Horb HW, Feller AM, Biener E. Technique for liposuction fat re-implantation and long-term volume evaluation by magnetic resonance imaging. Ann Plast Surg 1991; 26:248–257.
22. Goldman R, Carmargo CP, Goldman B. Fat transplantation and facial contour. Ann J Cosmet Surg 1998; 15:41–44.
23. Ito Y, Hudgins LC, Hirsch J, Shike M. Adipose tissue fatty acid composition in recipients of long-term total parenteral nutrition (TPN). Am J Clin Nutr 1991; 53:1487–1492.
24. Hudgins LC, Hirsch J. Changes in abdominal and gluteal adipose tissue fatty acid compositions in obese subjects after weight gain and weight loss. Am J Clin Nutr 1991; 53:1372–1377.
25. Petreck JA, Hudgins LC, Levine B, Ho M, Hirsch J. Breast cancer risk and fatty acids in the breast and abdominal adipose tissues. J Nat Cancer Inst 1994; 86:53–56.
26. Malcolm GT, Bhattacharya AK, Velez-Duran M, Guzman MA, Galmann MC, Strong JP. Fatty acid composition of adipose tissue in humans: differences between subcutaneous sites. Am J Clin Nutr 1989; 50:288–291.
27. Folch J, Lees M, Sloane-Stanley G. A simple method for the isolation and purification of total lipids from animal tissue. J Biol Chem 1957; 226:497–509.
28. Takasu K, Takasu S. Long-term frozen fat for tissue augmentation. J Aesth Derm Cosmet Surg 1999; 1:173–178.
29. Jackson RF. Eight years of fat transplantation experience. Am J Cosmet Surg 1999; 16:287–290.
30. Hernandez-Perez E, Lozana-Guarn C. Fat grafting: techniques and uses on different anatomic areas. Am J Cosmet Surg 1999; 16:197–204.
31. Coleman WP. Fat transplantation. Dermatol Clin 1999; 17:891–898.
32. Bircoll M. A nine-year experience with autologous fat transplantation. Am J Cosmet Surg 1992; 9:55–59.
33. Hernandez-Perez E. Bi-level lipoinjection for facial wrinkles. Am J Cosmet Surg 1992; 9:73–75.
34. Scarborough DA, Schuen W, Bisaccia E. Fat transfer for aging skin. Technique in rhytides. J Dermatol Surg Oncol 1990; 16:651–655.
35. Gurney CE. Studies on the fate of free fat transplants. Proc Staff Meet Mao Clinic 1937; 12:34.
36. Van RLR, Roncar DAK. Isolation of fat cell precursors from adult rat adipose tissue. Cell Tissue Res 1977; 181:197.
37. Asken S. Microliposuction and autologous fat transplantation for aesthetic enhancement of the aging face. J Dermatol Surg Oncol 1991; 5:968–972.

38. Sadick NS. Fatty acid analysis of transplanted adipose tissue. Arch Dermatol 2001; 137:723–729.
39. Chajchr A, Benzaquen I. Fat-grafting injection for soft tissue augmentation. Plast Reconstr Surg 1989; 85:921–934.
40. Vasquez BA, Ontiveror S, Gonzalez G. Histologic study of aspirated fat. Am J Cosmet Surg 1985; 2:15–17.
41. Van RL, Bayliss CE, Roncari DA. Autologic and enzymological characterization of adult human adipocyte precursors in culture. J Clin Invest 1976; 58: 699.
42. Jones JU, Lyles ME. The viability of human adipocytes after closed syringe liposuction harvest. Am J Cosmet Surg 1997; 14:275–280.
43. McCurdy JA Jr. Five years of experience using fat for leg contouring (commentary). Am J Cosmet Surg 1995; 12:228.
44. Schuller-Petrovics. Improving the aesthetic aspect of soft tissue defects on the face using autologous fat transplantation. Facial Plast Surg 1997; 13:119–124.
45. Carapenda CA. Collagen alteration in adipose autografts. Aesthet Plast Surg 1994; 18:5–11.
46. Sommer B, Sattler G. Current concepts of fat graft survival: histology of aspirated adipose tissue and review of the literature. Dermatol Surg 2000; 28: 1159–1166.
47. Coleman WP III, Lawrence N, Sherman RN, Reed RJ, Pinsky KS. Autologous collagen? Lipocytic dermal augmentation: a histopathologic study. J Dermatol Surg Oncol 1993; 19:1032–1040.
48. Guerrosantos J, Gonzales-Mendoza A, Masmela A, Gonzalez MA, Deop M, Diaz P. Long-term survival of free fat grafts in muscle: an experimental study in rats. Aesthetic Plast Surg 1996; 20:403–408.
49. Shiffman MA. Effect of various networks of fat harvesting and re-injection. J Aesthet Dermatol Cosmet Surg 2000; 1:231–235.
50. Brandon IL, Newman J. Facial multilayered micro lipo augmentation. Int J Aesthet Restorat Surg 1996; 4:95–110.
51. Takasu K, Takasu S. Long-term frozen fat for tissue augmentation. Aesthet Dermatol Cosmet Surg 1999; 1:173–178.
52. Takasu K, Takasu S. Long-term frozen fat for tissue augmentation. Am J Cosmet Surg 1999; 16:231–235.
53. Markey AC, Glogau RG. Autologous fat grafting: comparison of techniques. Dermatol Surg 2000; 26:1135–1139.
54. Fourner PF. Fat grafting: my technique. Dermatol Surg 2000; 26:1111–1128.
55. Hernandez-Perez E, Lozano-Guarin C. Fat grafting techniques and uses in different anatomical areas. Am J Cosmet Surg 1999; 16:197–204.
56. Skoyge JW. The biochemistry and development of adipose tissue and the pathophysiology of obesity as it relates to liposuction surgery. Dermatol Clin 1990; 8:385–393.
57. DePedroza LV. Fat transplantation to the buttocks and legs for aesthetic enhancement or correction of deformities: long term results of large volumes for transplant. Dermatol Surg 2000; 26:1105–1149.

58. Donofrio LM. A structure autologous lipo augmentation: a pan-facial technique. Dermatol Surg 2000; 26:1129–1134.
59. Niechajev I. Sevcuk O. Long-term results of fat transplantation: clinical and histologic studies. Plast Reconstr Surg 1994; 94:496–506.
60. Bastart JP, Cuenes J, Cohen S, Jardar C, Hsinque B. Percutaneous adipose tissue biopsy by mini-liposuction for metabolic studies. J Parenteral Nutr 1994; 18:466–468.
61. Novas F, dos Reis, N, Baroudi R. Contouring method of live fat cells used in liposuction procedures. Aesthet Plast Surg 1998:12:225.
62. Sattler G, Sommer B. Liporecycling: a technique for facial rejuvenation and body contouring. Dermatol Surg 2000; 26:1140–1144.
63. Pinski KS. Fat transplantation and autologous collagen: a decade of experience. Am J Cosmet Surg 1996; 16:217–224.
64. Guerreosantis J. Long-term outcome of autologous fat transplantation in aesthetic facial recontouring. Clin Plast Surg 2000; 27:515–543.
65. Ellenbogen R. Fat transfer: current use in practice. Clin Plast Surg 2000; 4: 545–556.
66. Drake LA, Dinehart SM, Former, ER et al. Guidelines of care for soft tissue augmentation: fat transplantation. J Am Acad Dermatol 1996; 34:690–694.

33

Anticellulite Creams, Endermology, and Other Nonsurgical Methods for Treating Excess Adipose Tissue

Zoe Diana Draelos
Wake Forest University School of Medicine
Winston-Salem, North Carolina, U.S.A.

Excess adipose tissue, more commonly known as cellulite, is a common condition about which relatively little is known. In the medical literature, cellulite is known as adisposis edematosa, dermopanniculosis deformans, status protrusus cutis, and so on [1]. What exactly is cellulite and how does it arise? These are currently unanswerable questions, yet this chapter examines purported theories regarding its etiology to better understand the treatments that are currently in the marketplace. This chapter is more to provoke thought and survey the options rather than to present scientific fact, which is yet lacking in this area.

APPEARANCE

Cellulite is perceived as uneven bumpy skin texture seen especially with side lighting of the affected area. It has been described as a "orange peel" or "cottage cheese" skin appearance. This appearance is due to projections of subcutaneous fat into the reticular and papillary dermis. These herniations can be documented via ultrasound as low-density regions among the denser dermal tissue [2]. Scientifically, the severity of cellulite or the effectiveness of various cellulite therapies is documented through the number and degree of these subcutaneous fat projections.

LOCATION

Cellulite can be located anywhere on the body that contains subcutaneous fat. Certain areas are more likely than others, however. Cellulite is most commonly seen on the upper outer thighs, the posterior thighs (banana roll), and buttocks, but can also be seen on the breasts and upper arms. It seems to be found in areas where excess adipose tissue is deposited, although obesity is not necessary for the presence of cellulite. The pattern of adipose deposit that leads to cellulite may be genetically determined [3].

AFFECTED POPULATION

The appearance of cellulite is not observed until after puberty in females. It is uncommonly seen in men, perhaps because cellulite is hormone mediated and female subcutaneous fat is sequestered into discrete pockets by the presence of septa. Cellulite may be considered a normal body change associated with puberty and cannot be considered a disease, since it is estimated that 85% of females are afflicted with the condition [4].

There are some interesting racial differences in the presence of cellulite, however. Cellulite is more commonly seen in Caucasian females than in Asian females. It is true that it is easier to visualize skin texture irregularities in fair skin, yet Asian females still seem to demonstrate less cellulite. Many theories have been advanced to try and explain this difference. Some feel that the reduced consumption of cow's milk in Asia is the reason, since much of the milk consumed in the United States contains estrogens that enter the milk from the food fed to the cows. Anther possible explanation is reduced endogenous estrogen production in Asian females who consume large amounts of fermented soy in the form of tofu or soy nuts. Fermented soy is high in phytoestrogens, which may suppress adrenal and ovarian estrogen production, which is not the case with the estrogens ingested in cow's milk.

ETIOLOGY

The exact etiology of cellulite is unknown, but several theories deserve mention. The theories fall under several categories: vascular, structural, and inflammatory.

Vascular Theory

Some investigators have postulated that cellulite is a degradation process initiated by deterioration of the dermal vasculature, particularly loss of the capillary networks [5]. As a result, excess fluid is retained with the dermal and subcutaneous tissues [6]. This loss of the capillary network is thought to be due to engorged fat cells clumping together and inhibiting venous return [7].

After the capillary networks have been damaged, vascular changes begin to occur within the dermis, resulting in decreased protein synthesis and an inability to repair tissue damage. Clumps of protein are deposited around the fatty deposits beneath the skin causing an "orange peel" appearance to the skin as it is pinched between the thumb and forefinger. At this stage, however, there is no visual evidence of cellulite. The characteristic appearance of cellulite is only seen after hard nodules composed of fat surrounded by hard reticular protein form within the dermis. Ultrasound imaging of skin affected by cellulite at this stage reveals thinning of the dermis with subcutaneous fat pushing upward, which translates into the rumpled skin known as cellulite.

Thus, this theory holds that hormonally mediated fat deposition, fat lobule compression of capillary vasculature, decreased venous return, formation of clumped fat lobules, and deposition of protein substances around clumped fat lobules leads to the appearance of cellulite. Cellulite treatments employing vascular manipulations are based on this theory.

Structural Theory

Some investigators have observed that cellulite is more common in overweight and obese women. This felt to be due to the presence of copious fat lobules within the subcutaneous tissue encased in fibrous septae with dermal attachments. These fibrous attachments surrounding abundant fat lead to the rumpled appearance of the skin characteristic of cellulite. Thus, weight loss, which reduces the size of the fat lobules, improves the appearance of cellulite. Improvement can also be achieved with exercise, since improved muscle tone creates a better foundation to support the overlying fat. This structural theory of cellulite is the least commonly accepted at the time of this writing.

Inflammatory Theory

Other researchers feel that cellulite is an inflammatory process that results in breakdown of the collagen in the dermis, providing for the subcutaneous fat herniations seen on ultrasound (personal conversation, Peter Pugliese, MD).

The onset of cellulite with puberty and menstruation has caused some researchers to evaluate the hormonal changes necessary for sloughing of the endometrium [8]. It appears that menstruation requires the secretion of metalloproteases (MMP) such as collagenase (collagenase-1, MMP-1) and gelatinase (gelatinase A, MMP-2) [9]. The endometrial glandular and stromal cells secrete these enzymes to allow menstrual bleeding to occur. Collagenases cleave the triple helical domain of fibrillar collagens at a neutral pH and are secreted just prior to menstruation. However, the collagenase may not only break down the fibrillar collagens present in the endometrium, but also in the dermis. Furthermore, gelatinase B is produced by stromal cells or mast cells during the late proliferative endometrial phase and just after ovulation. Gelatinase B is associated with an influx of polymorphonuclear leukocytes, macrophages, and eosinophils, which also contribute to inflammation [10]. A marker for this inflammation is the synthesis of dermal glycosaminoglycans, which enhance water binding further worsening the appearance of the cellulite through swelling. The presence of these glycosaminoglycans has been observed on ultrasound as low-density echoes at the lower dermal/subcutaneous junction [11].

The secretion of endometrial collagenase to initiate menstruation also provides for collagen breakdown in the dermis [12]. With repeated cyclical collagenase production, more and more dermal collagen is destroyed accounting for the worsening of cellulite seen with age. Eventually enough collagen is destroyed to weaken the reticular and papillary dermis and allow subcutaneous fat to herniate between the structural fibrous septa found in female fat. Obviously, if more subcutaneous fat is present, more pronounced herniation can occur. At present, this theory of cellulite formation to support ongoing inflammation in the dermis has the most scientific data in the obstetrics literature.

EVALUATION OF TREATMENT EFFICACY

Treatments abound for cellulite; however, scientifically demonstrating their efficacy is a challenge. Traditional biopsy techniques used in dermatology for diagnostic purposes are not useful in cellulite, since it is a condition involving broad areas, not just one point on the skin. Biopsies may be helpful to determine the amount of inflammatory cells (PMNs, mast cells, eosinophils, etc.); however, the inflammation in cellulite is cyclical and low grade, making sampling error a problem. Noninvasive cellulite assessment methods include photography, thigh diameter measurements, weight measurements, trained observer clinical assessment, skin firmness evaluation, ultrasound skin imaging, and laser.

Doppler Blood Flow Assessment

Photography is the most common assessment method used to determine cellulite treatment efficacy. Camera mounts have been developed to perform standardized posterior thigh and buttock photos with optimal lighting (Canfield Scientific). The key to accurate photos is standardized cross lighting of the subject. It is possible to maximize or minimize the appearance of cellulite through slight changes in the lighting angle of the subject. It should also be recognized that darkening of the skin, either through sun exposure or use of a self-tanning cream, also minimizes the appearance of cellulite.

Methods of evaluating cellulite treatment efficacy that do not involved sophisticated equipment are simply measuring the diameter of the thigh with a flexible tape measure correlated with total body weight before and after a specified treatment period with the topical product under study. This is the most common technique used and is certainly prone to error depending on the tightness with which the tape is pulled, the distance between the feet during thigh measurement, the flexed or relaxed state of the thigh muscles, and the time of day the measurements are obtained. Trained observer evaluations are usually performed on an arbitrary numerical scale assessing visual improvement in the appearance of the cellulite.

Skin firmness assessment, on the other hand, requires a piece of equipment known as a ballistometer. The ballistometer measures skin rebound, which is directly related to skin firmness. More exact images of skin thickness can be obtained with a 20-MHz transducer and M mode ultrasound. Here the intrusion of the subcutaneous fat on a thinned dermal can be measured and evaluated for improvement. Skin thickness can be compared between body areas affected by cellulite and unaffected sites. Last, laser Doppler blood flow assessment can measure the amount of venous congestion present and note any improvement following treatment.

Treatments

The treatments for cellulite have been formulated on the theories previously discussed. Treatments designed to improve cellulite through the enhancement of venous and lymphatic flow include herbals, skin kneading, and massage. Treatments designed to enhance the structure of the overlying skin include retinoids and alpha hydroxy acids. Other treatments, attempting to decrease the presence of the subcutaneous fat, include xanthines and exercise. Unfortunately, liposuction does not necessarily improve the appearance of cellulite, even though the amount of subcutaneous fat has been reduced [13].

Herbals

Herbal treatments for cellulite abound, usually containing a complex mixture of numerous botanical extracts. The exact mechanism of action of some of the extracts is unknown, nevertheless examples of extracts used topically for slimming purposes is listed in Table 1. Some of the extracts contain xanthine derivatives, which have been thought to act as tissue decongestants by increasing "veinotonic activity." In other words, substances such as sweet clover, ivy, and barley improve the peripheral microcirculation, which facilitates lymphatic drainage and enhances edema removal [14].

A study by Bascaglia et al. examined the effect of an herbal cream containing caffeine and horsechestnut, ivy, algae, bladderwrack, thermal plankton, butcherbroom, and soy protein when applied to the thigh for 30 days [15]. They used ultrasound to demonstrate a 2.8-mm mean decrease in subcutaneous fat thickness. The subcutaneous fat thickness began to return to normal once the cream application ceased. They theorized that the cream broke bonds between the adipocytes, allowing the fat to become more compact, but could not explain how reaccumulation could occur so rapidly following discontinuation of treatment. It is also unclear as to whether the effect on the adipocytes could be maintained.

Exothermic Herbal Packs

Many spas employ a combination of herbal packs and heat to purportedly reduce cellulite. Warm herb pastes composed of botanical extracts listed in Table 1 are applied to the upper thighs and buttocks combined with lym-

TABLE 1 Herbal Extracts Incorporated into Topical Cellulite Treatments

Botanical name	Common name
Aloysia triphylla	Verbena
Camellia japonica	Japanese green tea
Citrus limon	Lemon
Cola acuminata	Kola nut
Foeniculum officinale	Fennel
Fucus vesiculosus	Algae
Hedera helix	Ivy
Hordeum	Barley
Mitchella repens	Strawberry
Origanum vulgare	Marjoram
Trifolium subterraneum	Sweet clover

phatic drainage massage. Sometimes externally applied heating pads or warm towels are placed over the herbal pastes to allowed prolonged retention of heat.

For individuals with decreased venous return, the diameter of the thigh can be reduced following vigorous lymphatic massage designed to encourage venous drainage. Change in thigh diameter can be demonstrated in venous insufficiency patients with a decrease immediately upon arising from bed and an increased following prolonged periods of standing. Furthermore, thigh diameter increases in some women prior to and during menstruation due to increased interstitial fluids. This is not surprising since the body is a dynamic organ always in a state of flux. Problems arise, however, when small changes in thigh measurements are used to substantiate cellulite treatment efficacy claims.

Xanthines

Methylxanthines have been touted for their effects on lipolysis. Naturally occurring xanthines include caffeine, while aminophylline and theophylline represent substances traditionally available by prescription. All of these substances inhibit phosphodiesterase and provide β-adrenergic stimulation. β-Adrenergic receptors stimulate the hydrolysis of fat stored as triglycerides. Thus, xanthines promote lipolysis by inhibiting phosphodiesterase, which transforms cAMP into AMP, leading to the conversion of triglycerides into free fatty acids and glycerol. This would ultimately reduce the amount of fat herniating into the overlying dermis. Any change in thigh diameter due to the use of xanthines would occur slowly, over months, rather than days or weeks. Of course, continued application of the xanthines would be necessary to maintain any effect [16]. Current technologies are focusing on the introduction of methylxanthines into clothing worn on the legs, such as panty hose, that would deliver a steady supply to the legs with the friction of walking. It is also possible to design the panty hose such that lymphatic and venous return could be improved through the use of graduated compression.

Retinoids

Retinoids have been evaluated for their effectiveness in the treatment of cellulite. It is thought that cellulite is partly due to decreased firmness and elasticity of the skin. Retinoids, such as prescription tretinoin, improve the denseness of the epidermis, induce the formation of dermal collagen, and stimulate angiogenesis, which would be beneficial in cellulite treatment. Collagen regeneration may decrease the herniations of the subcutaneous fat into the dermis. No large-scale studies demonstrating a positive effect have been published, however. Many topical cellulite treatments are now employing retinol, an over-the-counter vitamin retinoid, which is converted by the skin in small quantites to tretinoin.

Lactic Acid

Lactic acid has also been studied in the treatment of cellulite. It was thought that perhaps by improving the condition of the stratum corneum, the appearance of the cellulite might be lessened. There are no published reports demonstrating the effectiveness of lactic acid or other alpha hydroxy acids in the treatment of cellulite.

Massage and Manipulation

Massage and manipulation are used as cellulite treatments to reduce the amount of interstitial fluid based on the theory that cellulite is caused by poor lymphatic and venous return. Vigorous lymphatic massage, also known as Swedish massage, in the direction of blood flow can reduce the amount of extravascular fluid, reduce thigh diameter, and decrease the appearance of cellulite. Fat is not removed with this technique; however, the dimpled appearance may be improved as tissue edema is reduced. Enhanced tissue edema during menses and after prolonged periods of standing may account for normal fluctuations seen in the appearance of cellulite.

Skin Kneading

Skin kneading, also known as endermologie (LPG, Fort Lauderdale, FL), is a purported cellulite treatment based on the use of a patented machine. The machine, developed about a 15 years ago in France, involves rubbing the skin with an electrically powered hand-held box containing two rollers connected to vacuum suction. The skin is sucked between the two rollers by the vacuum and kneaded. A technician moves the machine over the hips, stomach, legs, and buttocks, which are covered with a nylon stocking to reduce friction. The treatments last between 35 and 45 min. Fifteen treatments are required to see an effect followed by monthly treatments required to maintain the effect.

No articles regarding this technology are published in the English medical literature. But, the French medical literature claims that the skin kneading improves the appearance of cellulite through enhanced circulation, reduced tissue congestion, and the removal of waste products [17]. Company literature is careful to state that the endermologie technique only reduces the appearance of cellulite. It does not remove cellulite. A proprietary study demonstrated a 1.186-mm decrease in perpendicular skin thickness following 12 treatments [18].

Exercise and Weight Control

Last, cellulite can be managed through a reduction in the size of the lipocytes from weight loss. Any decrease in the lipocytes would result in less subcutaneous fat herniation and a physiologic reduction in cellulite. Similarly, an increase in muscle mass would provide better support for the subcutaneous fat and also improve the appearance of cellulite.

SUMMARY

This chapter has reviewed the purported etiologies for cellulite, which provide insight into the treatments that are currently available. Unfortunately, liposuction cannot be guaranteed to reduce the appearance of cellulite. This may be due to the fact that destruction of the dermis is more important than the presence of subcutaneous fat. Alternatively, the poor lymphatic and venous return may not be improved, but rather inhibited by aggressive liposuction. Cellulite is a common condition that currently remains a treatment enigma.

REFERENCES

1. Dahl PR, Salla MJ, Winkelmann RK. Localized involutional lipoatrophy: a clinicopathologic study of 16 patients. J Am Acad Dermatol 1996; 35:523–528.
2. Salter DC, Hanley M, Tynan A, McCook JP. In-vivo high definition ultrasound studies of subdermal fat lobules associated with cellulite. J Invest Dermatol 1990; 29:272–274.
3. Scherwitz C, Braun-Falco O. So-called cellulite. J Dermatol Surg Oncol 1978; 4:230–234.
4. Nurnberger F, Muller G. So-called cellulite: an invented disease. J Dermatol Surg Oncol 1978; 4:221–229.
5. Smith WF. Cellulite treatments: snake oil or skin science. Cosmet Toilet 1995; 110:61–70.
6. Curri SB. Cellulite and fatty tissue microcirculation. Cosmet Toilet 1993; 108: 51–58.
7. Curri SB, Bombardelli E. Local lipodystrophy and districtual microcirculation. Cosmet Toilet 1994; 109:51–65.
8. Marbaix E, Kokorine I, Henriet P, Donnez J, Courtoy PJ, Eeckhout Y. The expresssion of interstitial collagenase in human endometrium is controlled by progesterone and by oestadiol and is related to menstruation. Biochem J 1995; 305:1027–1030.
9. Singer CF, Marbaix E, Lemoine P, Courtoy PJ, Eeckhout Y. Local cytokines induce differrential expression of matrix metalloproteinases but not their tissue inhibitors in human endometrial fibroblasts. Eur J Biochem 1999; 259(1–2): 40–45.

10. Jeziorska M, Nagasae H, Salamonsen LA, Woolley DE. Immunolocalization of the matrix metalloproteinases gelatinase B and stromelysin 1 in juman endometrium throughout the menstrual cycle. J Reprod Fertil 1996; 107(1):43–51.
11. Lotti T, Ghersetich MD, Grappone C, Dini G. Proteoglycans in so-called cellulite. Int J Dermatol 1990; 29:272–274.
12. Marbaix E, Kokorine I, Donnez J, Eeckhout Y, Courtoy PJ. Regulation and restricted expression of interstitial collagenase suggest a pivotal role in the initiation of menstruation. Hum Reprod 1996; 11(suppl 2):134–143.
13. Coleman WP, Hanke CW, Alt TH, Asken S. Liposuction. In: Cosmetic Surgery of the Skin: Principles and Practice. Philadelphia: Decker Inc., 1991:213–238.
14. Di Salvo RM. Controlling the appearance of cellulite. Cosmet Toilet 1995; 110:50–59.
15. Bascaglia DA, Conte ET, McCain W, Frideman S. The treatment of cellulite with methylxanthine and herbal extract based cream: an ultrasonographic analysis. Cosmet Dermatol 1996; 9:30–40.
16. Jackson EM. Substantiating the efficacy of thigh creams. Cosmet Dermatol 1995; 8:31–41.
17. Vergereau R. Use of mechanical skin fold rolling in cosmetic medicine. J Cosmet Med Dermatol Surg (French) 1995; 39:49–53.
18. Marchand JP, Privat Y. A new instrumental method for the treatment of cellulite. Medecine au Feminin (French) 1991; 39:25–34.

34

Nutrition and the Liposuction Patient

W. Patrick Coleman IV
Tulane University School of Medicine
New Orleans, Louisiana, U.S.A.

Timothy Corcoran Flynn
University of North Carolina
Chapel Hill, North Carolina, U.S.A.

Tumescent liposuction, used to remove localized areas of adiposity, has now been performed worldwide for almost 2 decades. Experience has shown that liposuction is a safe and effective treatment for these shape-altering fat deposits, which often are resistant to improvement with diet or exercise. This is because many aspects of weight and body shape have a strong genetic component. Caloric restriction or increased energy expenditure can change overall body weight, but stubborn areas of subcutaneous fat often remain. Liposuction is needed to improve the shape of these areas of excess fat.

Obesity in the United States has been increasing over the past 20 years [1]. Of all people having a body mass index of over 27, almost two-thirds of women and half of men have tried to lose weight [2]. Statistics show that many adults who initially succeed in losing weight regain most or all of the weight within 5 years [3]. Research has been done to explain this failure of weight loss programs with inconclusive results. New weight control programs, new diets, and behavior modification routines are flourishing in an attempt to control the increasing weight of the population. Patients' motivations to lose this increased weight vary [4]. Some may wish to be healthier, others have a desire to change their appearance, while others hope to have greater social interaction or have more enjoyment out of life.

In a survey of body image, Garner found that as many as 52% of men and 66% of women report dissatisfaction or inadequacy regarding body weight [5]. This phenomenon has been labeled "body image distress," and psychologists have recognized this as an addressable problem. While body image distress seems to be on the rise among men [6], it still is predominantly a problem among women. Studies suggest that the prevalence of pathological weight loss behavior is increasing as a result of increasing body image dissatisfaction [7]. Thirty-five percent of dieters in the United States may engage in pathologic attempts to lose weight such as anorexic or bulimic behaviors, and one-quarter of pathologic dieters may go on to develop subthreshold or full-syndrome eating disorders [8]. The liposuction surgeon may want to counsel and advise his or her patients on nutrition and healthy eating to ensure that they have a healthy correct approach to eating.

Although liposuction is not a weight-loss procedure, many patients secretly hope that liposuction will allow them to eat as they please and still not gain weight. If they continue to eat as they please and put on weight, they may develop increased fat in areas with which they did not previously have problems. People who eat excessively after liposuction will often gain weight following the procedure and erroneously conclude, "the liposuction didn't work." Visceral fat stores can also increase after liposuction if the patient gains weight.

Counseling the liposuction patient about good nutrition is advisable for several reasons. Regular exercise and maintaining good eating habits can lead to greater satisfaction with their liposuction procedure and their overall sense of well-being. Some patients use their procedure as a "jump-start" to help them lose some extra weight. Liposuction surgeons who counsel their patients postoperatively about fitness and nutrition often get the best results. Patients who are satisfied with one area that has been improved with liposuction often return to have their silhouette improved by undergoing another procedure on a different area.

A variety of professionals can be utilized to counsel the liposuction patient about diet and exercise. Registered dietitians graduate with a 4-year college degree in food and nutritional sciences. Clinical dietitians study nutrition as well as pathophysiology and are qualified to counsel patients. Patients may need lifestyle modification to make changes in diet and physical activity patterns. Research has shown that encouragement and reinforcement is valuable helping patients to maintain proper eating habits. Eating properly is a habit that must constantly be reinforced in order to achieve a long-term pattern of healthy nutrition.

Exercise counselors can also assist the patient. Joining a health club or gymnasium can help develop and reinforce the benefits of regular exercise. Exercise also must be developed into a habit. Each individual should find a type of exercise they enjoy doing in order to maximize success. Psychologists can teach stress reduction techniques to patients who may need them. Liposuction surgeons should familiarize themselves with available personnel and resources in their community. Assembling a team of professionals to assist the liposuction patient to learn about proper nutrition and exercise is rewarding to the patient.

There is much misinformation regarding what constitutes good nutrition. The media are often discussing nutrition in contradictory ways and patients can be confused about what good eating habits are. For example, many patients tell us that they believe the key to not gaining weight is to eat a low-fat diet. We find it useful to remind the patient that if they ate nothing but granulated sugar they would be on a low-fat diet. Patients must be taught how to eat in a nutritious fashion and eat smaller portion meals more often. They must be instructed how to count calories and how to ascertain the total grams of fat, protein, and carbohydrates in meals. Efforts directed toward proper nutrition will pay off with more satisfied patients.

A nutrition plan must be customized for the individual patient. Each person has individual needs, work schedules, food tastes, and cultural aspects of eating. A proper nutrition plan must take many variables into account. Information which is needed to create a diet and exercise plan is readily available from a variety of reliable sources.

Inquiring about the patient's current eating habits is a good starting point when discussing nutrition. Asking the patient what, when, and where they are eating along with their responsibilities during what they would describe as a "normal day" is very useful. This invaluable discussion will take little time and should begin with the patient basically listing some of the foods and times that they eat throughout the day. This often reveals aspects of nutrition about which they might be confused or have questions. This initial discussion is invaluable in that it gives the physician a chance to assess their patients' nutritional knowledge and forces the patient to actively focus on the types and quantities of food that they are actually eating during the day.

The next step in counseling the patient is instructing the patient that each item of food contains a number of calories further broken down into constituent grams of carbohydrates, protein, and fat. Most patients may focus only on low fat or low-carbohydrate foods without considering their total caloric value. They must be taught to rapidly calculate the total calories and the percentage of carbohydrates, protein, and fat for any food that they consume. By subscribing to this method of eating, one is able to individualize each meal. Within specific calorie and consumption guidelines set forth for each meal, limitless combinations of food are possible. One is forced to evaluate each type of food as to its composition and selectively choose a combination that will provide him or her with a balanced meal.

It is important to understand each patient's potential for a prolonged commitment to healthy nutrition. The most vital concept, inherent to nutritional success, is the realization that this is not a short-term "diet," but a plan for a lifetime of balanced eating. Implied in the word "*diet*" is the notion of transiently restricting one's eating in order to achieve a relatively immediate endpoint (e.g., to lose 15 pounds). For example, a patient may have an immediate goal to fit into a pair of pants, to feel more comfortable in a bathing suit, or to look good for a wedding or a holiday party. This viewpoint leads to a conscious struggle of desires with each meal: the desire to lose weight and that of eating what is enjoyable yet forbidden. Many individuals become frustrated by the difficulty in reaching what is viewed as an unobtainable goal. If, however, that goal is realized, the changes in diet that brought it about are very often discarded for previous more pleasurable habits. The concept of proper nutrition must instead be viewed simply as an aspect of lifestyle that will lead to persistent body weight and composition changes.

Another problem with the traditional concept of a diet is the idea that to lose weight there must be a significant cutback in calories, often to the point of starvation. This method promotes the so called "yo-yo" effect where individuals basically starve themselves to achieve a short-term weight goal and then go back to eating in their usual manner. This becomes an endless cycle of gaining and losing and is an ineffective way to lose body weight. There is scientific evidence to support that crash dieting makes subsequent weight loss more difficult [10]. Crash dieting can please people who rate success by concrete numbers on the scale. But with the individual's decrease in total body weight, a decrease in lean body mass occurs due to under consumption of the basic number of calories required to maintain body function. This promotes an undesirable change in body composition with an increase in body fat and decrease in lean body mass over time. This occurs because of an eventual decrease in lean body mass to such a low level that this individual can no longer lose any further weight in this manner.

The liposuction surgeon should realize that this may be the first time that his or her patient has thought about eating correctly to change body composition. Since liposuction patients have widely different levels of diet and exercise, individualized approaches are in order. Patients with a high attention to fitness may be easiest to work with. They often simply need fine-tuning as they may already be obtaining the majority of their calories from lower glycemic sources. For these patients, working out a calorie plan balanced in carbohydrates, protein, and fat divided into smaller meals throughout the day makes more sense than the traditional breakfast, lunch, and dinner. Patients who have a high percentage of body fat often are not cognizant of basic nutritional principles. These patients often do not realize how many calories a day they consume or the calorie contents of their preferred foods. Patients with high body fat require basic nutritional education such as teaching them to read the package of food products which delineates amount of calories in the food as well as the number of grams of protein, fat, and carbohydrate.

One of the most important issues in helping patients to lose weight or change body composition is to determine the patient's specific daily caloric need. This is defined as the number of calories required to perform activities and tasks encountered during the day in addition to those exhausted by basal metabolic rate. Calories required for maintenance vary with each individual based on age, sex, weight, and level of activity. The physician must individually assess each patient to determine the number of calories needed to maintain, increase, or decrease weight and body composition.

Next, we recommend instructing the patient on different components of different foods. Again, it is important to be able to rate the patient's knowledge on diet to determine at what level to begin when discussing these issues. At the most basic level, foods can be broken up into three components: carbohydrates, proteins, and fats. Examples of food containing primarily carbohydrates are pasta, fruit, breads, cereals, and sugars. In general each gram of carbohydrates contains 4 calories/g. However, not all carbohydrates are so simply comparable. The glycemic index stratifies foods by the length of time it takes the body to digest the various forms of carbohydrates. Lower glycemic index ratings correspond to more complex carbohydrates which are digested over a longer period of time as compared to the simple sugars at the higher end of the index that are metabolized more rapidly. A common goal should be to limit carbohydrates categorized as high glycemic foods in favor of those that rank lower on the scale. Some feel that by consuming foods that are metabolized at a slower rate, the body is less apt to store those calories as fat. Instead, the slower digestion provides a more constant and necessary source of energy that is more likely to be "burned" than the high glycemic simple sugars.

Like carbohydrates, protein also contains 4 calories/g. Foods containing primarily protein are beef, pork, fish, and poultry. Eggs, nuts, and dairy products also contain protein. For many patients, it is the protein component that is most difficult to tailor into the diet. There are many reasons for this phenomenon. Protein products are often more time consuming to prepare. For example, it is much easier for a busy person to grab a bagel in the morning than it is to scramble some eggs. This food group also requires some more expertise in the kitchen. Preparing a tasty, properly cooked fillet of fresh fish is significantly more difficult than simply boiling water and throwing in pasta. Furthermore, there may be cultural, religious, or personal convictions that may prevent patients from eating pork or certain meat products. It is extremely important to determine whether protein is underrepresented in the liposuction patient's diet. Many suggestions and alternatives may be implemented. For example, vegetarians can increase protein using whey or soy proteins, and busy people can be taught to grab a protein bar instead of the bagel. A problem that patients may encounter when beginning a diet that is higher in protein than they are used to is finding enjoyable protein sources. Variety is another problem. High-protein, low-fat foods are limited compared to the ubiquitous high-carbohydrate foods. There is also increased time involved to prepare many good protein sources.

Patients should be aware of the importance of having a ready source of preprepared proteins, which can be very helpful in promoting the intake of a higher protein diet. Commercial protein supplements (Fig. 1) are a luxury that allow a patient to continue a diet when there is not the time available to prepare a protein source such as chicken, beef, pork, or eggs. These

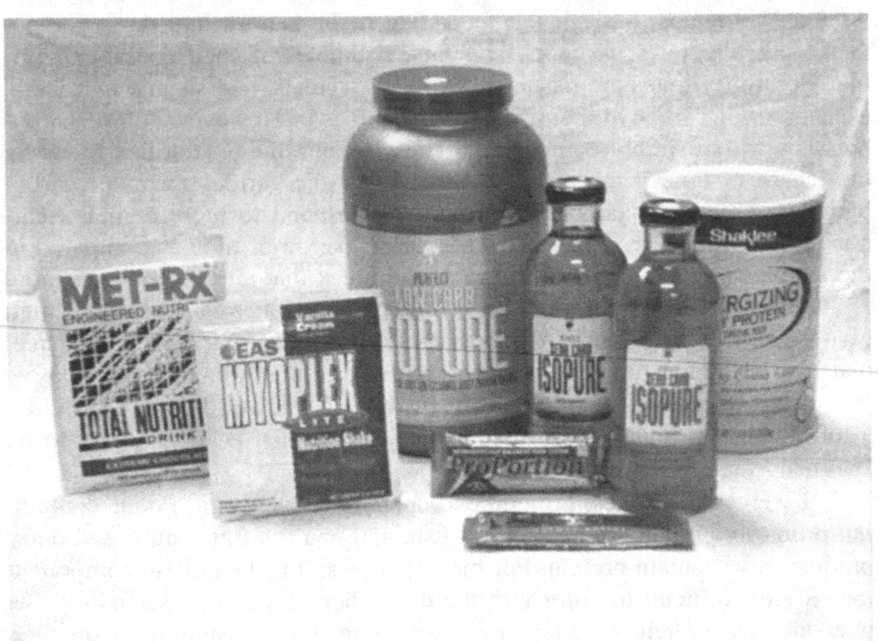

FIGURE 1 Examples of meal replacement and protein supplements.

supplements are available in various powder and solid sources, including bars and even cookies and chips. They are readily available at nutrition stores, through the Internet, and in the "nutrition aisle" in most major grocery stores. However, patients should be counseled not to rely exclusively on these prepackaged foods, but instead to use them as a supplement to natural sources of protein. Patients may also consider having readily available sources of protein with them at work. Cartons of low-fat cottage cheese or cans of tuna fish (in water) are hardy sources of high-grade protein.

Fat contains over twice as many calories per gram than carbohydrates or proteins: 9 as compared to 4. Some examples of fat sources include butter, oils, and margarine. It is fat that gives food "palatability" and what professional chefs call a wonderful "mouth feel." It must be stressed to most patients that the widely held concept that eating foods containing fat correlates with increased stored body fat is absolutely untrue. In fact, a diet that has a moderate amount of carbohydrates and fat has been shown to be superior in respect to loss of weight while retaining or improving body composition of lean body mass to body fat when compared to a diet of high carbohydrates and low fat. Low-fat diets have been shown to alter intramuscular substrates and reduce lipolysis and fat oxidation during exercise [9].

An ideal diet, both to establish good health and to lose or maintain weight, is a simple balanced diet consisting of 40% carbohydrates, 30% proteins, and 30% fats by calorie, not gram. For the average American, this would mean decreasing carbohydrate intake and increasing protein, with or without a restriction of fat depending on the individual's eating habits. For the more motivated patient, a diet should be based on calories needed for their estimated energy expenditure on a given day. To calculate the number of calories required for an individual to maintain their current weight, simply multiply their body weight in pounds by 12 if a person is "inactive" or 15 if a person is "active." Rating a patient as "active" or "inactive" is done through assessing the energy the patient expends throughout the day to carry out their activities. This is just a general way to give a good starting point for maintenance calories that can be tweaked over the initial month that the patient begins this way of eating. The patient may tailor his or her food intake to the recommended numbers and have a large number of options. At a more basic level, other patients may benefit from sample diets in which foods are already broken down by the numbers of carbohydrates, proteins, and fats. Entire meals may be planned around the number of recommended calories.

Here are some diets of selected number of calories broken down into carbohydrates, proteins, and fats for 1500- and 2000-calorie diets distributed among four separate meals (Table 1).

Table 1 1500- and 2000-Calorie Diets

1500-Calorie diet

Meal 1 (400 calories)
40 g carbohydrates; 30 g protein; 13 g fat
Meal 2 (350 calories)
35 g carbohydrates; 26 g protein; 12 g fat
Meal 3 (350 calories)
35 g carbohydrates; 26 g protein; 12 g fat
Meal 4 (400 calories)
40 g carbohydrates; 30 g protein; 13 g fat

Meal 1
Choose A, B, C, or D
A. 1 whole wheat or grain bagel
1 scoop protein powder in 1 cup 1% milk
B. 1 protein bar and 1 cup 1% milk
C. A whole bagel with low-fat mozzarella cheese and 2 boiled eggs (whites only)
D. 3-egg omelet (only use 2 of the yolks) with ham and some low-fat cheese with 2 pieces of wheat toast

Meals 2 and 3 (these meals have the same calories; choose 1 selection for each meal)
Choose one from A–G
A. 4 oz. of lean chicken (cooked in pan with 1 tablespoon of olive oil) or 3–4 ounces of turkey and 2 pieces of wheat or whole-grain bread
B. Salad with 2 tablespoons of full-fat dressing or $2\frac{1}{2}$ teaspoons of oil and as much vinegar as you like and 1 chicken breast or 1 fish filet grilled or 1 can albacore
1 piece of wheat toast
C. 1 protein bar and 1 cup 1% milk
D. 6-inch Subway (turkey, chicken, roast beef, or ham); ask for double meat and 2 slices Swiss cheese, no mayonnaise
E. Burger King: 1 BK broiler, no mayonnaise
F. 1 high-protein smoothie from Smoothie King (flavors: chocolate, banana, lemon, or pineapple)
G. 1 large Wendy's chili

Meal 4
Choose one from A–F
A. 1 and $\frac{1}{2}$ PR Ironman Bars
B. 1 serving of pasta tossed in 2 teaspoons of olive oil
1 chicken breast or tuna steak grilled with no added oils

TABLE 1 Continued

C. Salad with 2 teaspoons of oil and as much vinegar as you like, a piece of lean chicken or fish grilled, and 2 pieces of wheat bread or 1 medium sweet potato
D. A filet of lean meat (4 oz.) grilled or 4 oz. lean ground beef or other beef with less than 7% fat; 1 medium sweet potato with low-fat sour cream
E. Domino's thin-crust cheese pizza with any vegetables that you like. Serving size $\frac{1}{4}$ of the pizza
F. 1 cup whole-grain cereal or $\frac{1}{2}$ cup of oatmeal or $\frac{1}{4}$ cup of grits
   1 cup 1% milk
   1 scoop protein powder in 1 cup water

2000 Calories (5 meals a day)

Meal 1 (475 calories)
  47 g carbohydrates, 36 g protein, 16 g fat
Meal 2 (375 calories)
  37 g carbohydrates, 28 g protein, 12 g fat
Meal 3 (375 calories)
  37 g carbohydrates, 28 g protein, 12 g fat
Meal 4 (475 calories)
  47 g carbohydrates, 36 g protein; 16 g fat
Meal 5 (300 calories)
  30 g carbohydrates, 22 g protein; 10 g fat

Meal 1 (475 calories)
A. $1\frac{1}{2}$ cups of cereal
   1 cup 2% milk
   $1\frac{1}{2}$ scoops Designer Protein
B. 1 half bagel or 1 slice toast
   MetRx Protein Plus bar
   1 cup 2% milk
C. 3 egg omelet (only use 2 of the yolks) with ham and some low fat cheese with 2 pieces of wheat toast
D. A whole bagel with low-fat mozzarella cheese and 2 boiled eggs (whites only)

Meals 2 and 3 (these meals have same calories; choose one selection for each meal) (375 calories)
A. 1 Healthy Choice microwave pizza
   1 scoop Designer Protein mixed in water
B. 3–4 oz. cold cut (turkey, chicken, ham, low-fat roast beef)
   2 pieces of 7- or 12 grain bread with low-fat mayonnaise

TABLE 1 Continued

C. 1 can tuna fish mixed with low-fat mayonnaise
2 pieces 7-grain or 12-grain bread
D. 1 bag microwave popcorn (get the "light" not the "low fat")
1 scoop Designer Protein
E. 1 salad; add chicken with any light, not low-fat, dressing
1 piece of 7- or 12-grain bread
F. 1 high-protein smoothie (chocolate, pineapple, or almond mocha); ask for no turbinado but to add 2 packets of Equal
G. 1 large Wendy's chili

Meal 4 (475 calories)
A. 1 BK Broiler, no mayonnaise
B. 1 bag microwave popcorn (get the light not the low fat)
1 scoop Designer Protein
C. $\frac{3}{4}$ cup rice with gravy
1 chicken breast
D. $\frac{1}{4}$ of Domino's thin-crust cheese pizza
1 scoop Protein or $\frac{1}{2}$ chicken breast
E. 1 cup wheat pasta (I use spirals because it is possible to measure them by the cup this way)
1 chicken breast
Toss in 2 teaspoons of olive oil and spice with an all purpose seasoning
F. 6-inch Subway (turkey, chicken, roast beef, or ham)
Ask for double meat and 2 slices Swiss cheese, no mayonnaise

Meal 5 (300 calories)
For this meal try to eat a protein bar of your choice or another serving of protein such as a chicken breast, or 3–4 oz. of deli meat. Especially if you are eating this meal within 3 hours of when you go to sleep try to make the meal consist of all protein.

Try to eat meals about 3 to 4 hours apart. Try to make a double-size meal for meals 2 and 3 so that if you are on the go, you can eat half and then 3 hours later the other. When you are trying to "eye" food, the best thing for you to do is to try to eat more protein and cut down on the carbohydrates. Worry about excess carbohydrates and keep fat intake moderate. You can add infinite variety to your meals by using the calories per meal provided and adding the numbers on the back of packages and labels of the foods that you are eating into the calories broken down into carbohydrates, proteins, and fats.

We explain to patients that losing weight while preserving lean body mass really comes down to fooling the body into doing something that it does not want to do. The innate objective of the body is to store energy in the form of fat in preparation for a time when food is not readily available. While this may have been an effective system for human evolution and advancement, it is in direct opposition to the individual whose goal is to lose body fat stores. Just dropping calorie intake to a significant amount below what is required for initial weight loss will initially lead to rapid weight loss, but the body will quickly adjust, changing into a "pseudohibernation state" where it favors storing of energy as fat and conversion of lean body mass into fat [11]. To facilitate weight loss, a 10–15% drop below maintenance calories will result in significant weight loss that can be seen in the short term and continue in the long term for the patient to realize his or her goals.

Any increase in energy expenditure without an increase in calorie intake will lead to weight loss. An exercise program that suits the patient's schedule and intensity should be suggested to complement any nutrition program. The benefits of increased physical activity are well established, and we know exercise can reduce morbidity and mortality [12–14]. Exercise can maintain a lower body weight by multiple mechanisms [15], including increased lean body mass, elevated resting metabolic rate, increased concentrations of metabolic hormones, decreased preference for high-fat foods, and increased psychologic well-being.

The type of exercise that the patient participates in is not as important as the frequency in which the patient participates in the exercise. It has been shown that 30–40 min of aerobic exercise that maintains the heart rate at 65–75% of its maximum (which depends on age and other factors) is beneficial. Larger, more overweight patients should be consulted to participate in exercises that are low impact (such as bike riding as opposed to jogging) to put less stress on their joints. A weight-lifting routine (resistance training) should also be encouraged as being part of any complete exercise program. It increases muscular strength, preserves fat-free mass, and increases daily caloric expenditure [16]. Increasing lifestyle activity can have healthy benefits similar to that of aerobic exercise. For example, patients can be encouraged to park farther away from the office and walk a bit more or take the stairs rather than the elevator.

Many resources are available to help the liposuction patient with nutrition. Obtaining cookbooks that have the food calories broken down into carbohydrates, proteins, and fats for servings of food is helpful. Another very helpful option to promote a variety of choices for patients is a calorie counter book. After rating the patient and placing him or her on a specific number of calories, a calorie book encourages variety by allowing the patient to choose foods that they enjoy and put them together into meals that add to the number of calories that they are currently using to lose weight.

Liposuction patients can also benefit from behavior modification techniques designed to improve nutrition. Many people find clubs or programs that rigidly control their intake of food helpful. Low-calorie diets (1200–1500 cal/day) combined with careful controlled food selections are the basis of many commercial programs such as Jenny Craig, Weight Watchers, Nutri/System, and Diet Center. Goal setting (usually 1–2 lbs/week) and reinforcement techniques are used in order to help achieve weight loss and weight maintenance.

Other behavioral techniques can be used to assist with weight control. Self-monitoring (diaries of food intake and physical activity) helps identify problem patterns. Stimulus control techniques can also be used. Stimulus control (cuing) suggests that a behavior is automatic in response to specific stimuli. For example, preparing a gym bag full of exercise clothes the night before planned physical activity can help stimulate the desired response of exercise. Contracting techniques can be used to assist the patient in adhering to desired behaviors. To be effective, contracts should involve the patient in making the contract, be written clearly outlining what behaviors are expected, and provide incentives to change. Stress management techniques are important for overeaters because stress is one of the causes of problems with weight control or overeating [17]. Social support, financial incentives, and relapse prevention are helpful.

In summary, many liposuction patients can benefit from nutritional education. Proper eating habits and nutritious foods can assist the patient in maintaining lean body mass while achieving a normal weight/height ratio. Exercise has numerous health benefits and also helps maintain proper weight and body shape. Establishing a team of individuals who are available to assist the liposuction patient can be rewarding to the liposuction surgeon as well as the patient.

REFERENCES

1. Center for Disease Control and Prevention Update. Prevalence of overweight among children, adolescents, and adults, United States 1988–1994. Morb Mortal Wkly Rep 1997; 46(RR-9):199–202.
2. Green KL, Cameron R, Polivy J et al. Weight dissatisfaction and weight loss attempts among Canadian adults: Canadian Heart Health Surveys Research Group. Can Med Assoc J 1997; 57(suppl 1):S17–SA25.
3. Wilson GT. Behavioral treatment of obesity: thirty years and counting. Adv Behav Res Ther 1994; 16:31–75.
4. Cheslun LJ, Donze LF. Appearance vs. health as motivators for weight loss. J Am Med Assoc 2001; 286:2160.

5. Garner DM. Body image survey. Psychol Today 1997; 30:30–84.
6. Pope HG Jr, Phillips KA, Olivandia R. The Adonis Complex: The Secret Crisis of Male Body Obsession. New York: The Free Press, 2000.
7. Devlin MJ, Zhu AJ. Body image in the balance. J Am Med Assoc 2001; 286: 2159.
8. Shisslak CM, Crago M, Estes LS. The spectrum of eating disturbances. Int J Eat Disord 1995; 18:209–219.
9. Coyle EF, Jeukendrup AE, Oseto MC, Hodgkinson JB, Zderic TW. Low-fat diet alters intramuscular substrates and reduces lipolysis and fat oxidation during exercise. Am J Physiol Endocrinol Metab 2001; 280:E391–E398.
10. Brownell KD, Greenwood MR, Stellar E, Shrager EE. The effects of repeated cycles of weight loss and regain in rats. Physiol Behav 1986; 38:459–464.
11. Karbowska J, Kochan Z, Swierczynski J. Increase of lipogenic enzyme mRNA levels in rat white adipose tissue after multiple cycles of starvation-refeeding. Metabolism 2001; 50(6):734–738.
12. Wannamethee SG, Shaper AG, Walker M. Changes in physical activity, motivation, and incidence of coronary heart disease in older men. Lancet 1998; 351:1603–1609.
13. Wei M, Kamper JB, Barlow CE, Nichaman MZ, Gibbons LW, Paffenbarger RS, Blain SN. Relationship between low cardiorespiratory fitness and mortality in normal-weight, overweight, and obese men. J Am Med Assoc 1999; 282: 1547–1553.
14. Blair SN, Kohl HW, Barlow CE, Paffenbarger RS, Gibbons LW, Macera CA. Changes in physical fitness and all-cause mortality. A prospective study of healthy and unhealthy men. J Am Med Assoc 1995; 273:1093–1098.
15. Poston WSC, Hyden M, O'Byrne KK, Forey JP. Where do diets, exercise, and behavior modification fit in the treatment of obesity? Endocrine 2000; 13:187–192.
16. Ballor DL, Poehlmam EP, Toth MJ. In: Bray GA, Bouchard C, James WPT, eds. Hardbook of Obesity. New York: Marcel Dekker, 1998.
17. Foreyt JP, Poston WSC. What is the role of cognative-behavior therapy in patient management? Obesity Res 1998; 6:18S–22S.

Index

About the Editor

RHODA S. NARINS is Director of the Dermatology Surgery and Laser Center, New York and White Plains, New York, and Clinical Professor of Dermatology and Chief of the Liposuction Surgery Unit, New York University Medical Center, New York. The author of numerous books including *Cosmetic Surgery* (Marcel Dekker, Inc.), book chapters, and journal articles, she is a Fellow of the American Academy of Dermatology, a Fellow and President-elect of the American Society for Dermatologic Surgery, where she has been on the Board of Directors, and a member of the American Society of Liposuction Surgery, the American Society for Laser Medicine and Surgery, the American Academy of Cosmetic Surgery, and the International Society for Dermatologic Surgery, where she also served on the Board of Directors. Dr. Narins has been selected by her peers as one of only 12 dermatologists in the United States listed in "Best Doctors in America" under Aesthetic Surgery and named several times by New York Magazine as one of the "Best Doctors in New York." She received an M.D. degree (1965) from the New York University School of Medicine, New York, and is board certified by the American Board of Dermatology. Dr. Narins is on the liposuction council of both the American Academy of Dermatology and the American Academy of Dermatologic Surgery.

Printed in the United States
by Baker & Taylor Publisher Services